ATLAS OF NERVE CONDUCTION STUDIES

AND ELECTROMYOGRAPHY

ATLAS OF NERVE CONDUCTION STUDIES AND ELECTROMYOGRAPHY

A. Arturo Leis, MD

CLINICAL PROFESSOR OF NEUROLOGY
UNIVERSITY OF MISSISSIPPI MEDICAL CENTER
ELECTRODIAGNOSTIC CONSULTANT
MISSISSIPPI METHODIST
REHABILITATION CENTER
JACKSON, MISSISSIPPI

Michael P. Schenk, MS, CMI, FAMI

DIRECTOR, DEPARTMENT OF
BIOMEDICAL ILLUSTRATION SERVICES
UNIVERSITY OF MISSISSIPPI MEDICAL CENTER
JACKSON, MISSISSIPPI

OXFORD
UNIVERSITY PRESS

OXFORD
UNIVERSITY PRESS

Oxford University Press is a department of the University of Oxford. It furthers the University's objective of excellence in research, scholarship, and education by publishing worldwide.

Oxford New York
Auckland Cape Town Dar es Salaam Hong Kong Karachi
Kuala Lumpur Madrid Melbourne Mexico City Nairobi
New Delhi Shanghai Taipei Toronto

With offices in
Argentina Austria Brazil Chile Czech Republic France Greece
Guatemala Hungary Italy Japan Poland Portugal Singapore
South Korea Switzerland Thailand Turkey Ukraine Vietnam

Published in the United States of America by
Oxford University Press
198 Madison Avenue, New York, NY 10016

Library of Congress Cataloging-in-Publication Data
Leis, A. Arturo.
Atlas of nerve conduction studies and electromyography / A. Arturo Leis, Michael P. Schenk.
p. ; cm.
Includes bibliographical references.
ISBN 978–0–19–975463–2 (hardcover)
1. Neural conduction—Atlases. 2. Electromyography—Atlases. I. Schenk, Michael P. II. Title.
[DNLM: 1. Neural Conduction—physiology—Atlases. 2. Electromyography—Atlases. WL 17]
QP363.L445 2012
616.7′407547—dc23 2011018570

ISBN 978–0–19–975463–2

To my wife Donna,
for her love and support,
and to my parents,
Drs. José and Bertha Leis,
who taught me the value of an education.
—A.A.L.

To my wife Laura,
for her love,
and my parents,
Dr. C. Perry and †Lola Margaret Gleason Schenk,
for exposing me to the world of art and science.
—M.P.S.

CONTENTS

FOREWORD

It is with pleasure that I prepare this foreword to a work from a colleague whose professional accomplishments I have continued to follow closely for the past twenty years. As one of his mentors during his fellowship years at the University of Iowa, I have witnessed firsthand Dr. Leis's proficiency in clinical neurophysiology and his insatiable desire to learn and to teach, which early on culminated in the Golseth Award from the American Association of Neuromuscular and Electrodiagnostic Medicine (AANEM).

Dr. Leis's scientific achievements in the areas of motor control and clinical neurophysiology subsequently propelled him to the rank of professor of neurology at the University of Mississippi Medical Center, but his academic accomplishments have not overshadowed his desire to educate a new generation of clinical neurophysiologists. Although he has since left the institution in pursuit of clinical practice, he continues to teach the neurology residents and fellows. He has received numerous Teacher of the Year awards, attesting both to his scholarship and his ability to explain complex problems with utmost clarity. I believe this *Atlas of Electromyography and Nerve Conduction Studies* amply reflects Dr. Leis's passion for teaching and his expert skills in presentation.

The readers, regardless of their prior experience in this field, will enjoy the visually alluring anatomical illustrations of nerves and muscles, and the corresponding human photographs that serve as a simple guide to muscle localization. Clinical comments pertinent to the nerve or muscle of interest will help to ease the beginner's anxiety about performing nerve conduction studies and the needle examination. The more experienced electromyographer will appreciate the well organized, practical outlines of clinical conditions and entrapment syndromes that include lists of etiologies, clinical features, and electrodiagnostic strategies. Both novice and expert will benefit from the numerous aids to the examination of the peripheral nervous system.

I take great pride in knowing that Dr. Leis's second atlas represents the work of one of our former students. This book meets the practical needs of physicians who perform the art of nerve conduction studies and electromyography, and provides a commonsense approach to problem solving for frequently encountered neuromuscular lesions. I have no doubt that the atlas will be used widely by residents, fellows, and practitioners. I anticipate that, like his first book, this atlas will also gain an excellent reputation and become a standard guide in electrodiagnostic medicine. I hope that its use will not only enhance the electrodiagnostic evaluation, but also encourage research and teaching in the field of clinical neurophysiology.

Jun Kimura, MD
Professor Emeritus
Kyoto University
Kyoto, Japan, and
Professor
Department of Neurology
University of Iowa Hospitals and Clinics
Iowa City, Iowa

PREFACE

The seed for this book was planted by Vicente ("Enzo") Trapani in 1998, who, as a resident in neurology, desired a handbook in electromyography (EMG) that emphasized both muscle localization and clinical pearls. Trapani envisioned a text that would provide high-quality illustrations of skeletal muscles that included nerve, plexus, and root supply; photographs of each muscle in a healthy subject to identify optimum site of EMG needle insertion; clinical features of the major conditions affecting peripheral nerves; and electrodiagnostic strategies for confirming suspected lesions of the peripheral nervous system. Trapani's vision culminated in the very successful *Atlas of Electromyography*, published by Oxford University Press in 2000, which he coauthored with me. Although Trapani is no longer pursuing book writing, this new atlas would not exist without his original contribution.

The current book was also nurtured by my personal experience as an educator, and the many residents and colleagues who offered encouragement and constructive criticism. This added further incentive to expand the content to include nerve conduction studies and to make it more useful for trainees in neurology and physical medicine and rehabilitation programs. This book should be of value to these trainees and to practicing electromyographers, regardless of their clinical disciplines. The book also provides numerous aids to the examination of the peripheral nervous system, which should prove useful to members of other specialties, including critical care medicine, neurological surgery, and family practice. The general practitioner may also choose to use this book as an anatomical guide.

Many of the anatomical and clinical descriptions contained in this book are derived from reviews of several editions of *Gray's Anatomy*, as well as Sunderland's writings on peripheral nerves and nerve injuries. Major books in clinical neurophysiology, such as the ones written by Kimura and by Preston and Shapiro, served as a foundation for this book. Additionally, publications by the American Association of Neuromuscular and Electrodiagnostic Medicine proved invaluable. Therefore, this book should ideally be used in conjunction with these other sources.

The book is divided into sections based on the major peripheral nerves. Each nerve is illustrated, and its anatomy is reviewed in the text. This is followed by a detailed outline of the clinical conditions and entrapment syndromes that affect the nerve, including a list of the etiologies, clinical features, and electrodiagnostic strategies used for each syndrome. General comments about the syndrome are also provided. Routine and special motor and sensory nerve conduction studies are shown in an anatomical illustration. Finally, each muscle supplied by the peripheral nerve is illustrated and accompanied by a corresponding human photograph. The illustration shows the root, plexus, and peripheral nerve supply to the muscle. Written text provides information about the nerve conduction studies, muscle origin, tendon insertion, voluntary activation maneuver, and site of optimum needle insertion. The latter is identified by a black dot (or sometimes a needle electrode) in both the anatomical illustration and the corresponding human photograph. This ensures that pertinent bony, muscular, and soft tissue landmarks can be used to guide the electromyographer to a specific point on the skin for needle insertion. Potential pitfalls associated with nerve conduction studies, as well as the needle insertion, are pointed out. Clinical correlates pertinent to the nerve conduction studies and the muscle being examined are also added.

I hope that use of this book will help to raise the quality of practitioners of electrodiagnostic medicine, and will promote interest and research in peripheral neuroanatomy and clinical neurophysiology.

A.A.L.
Methodist Rehabilitation Center
Jackson, Mississippi

ACKNOWLEDGMENTS

We are grateful to Kyle Cunningham, MS, Department of Biomedical Illustration Services, University of Mississippi Medical Center, for his technical and administrative assistance in preparing this book; and Robert Waldo Gray and Charles P. Runyan, Medical Photography Department, University of Mississippi Medical Center. We thank Mary Mann Austin, Alfredo Gomez, and Melissa Grimes for serving as models for some of the photographs.

I (A. Leis) am indebted to Jun Kimura, MD, for teaching me the principles and practice of clinical neurophysiology, and to Mark A. Ross, MD, and his colleagues at the "three" Mayo Clinics for guiding me through their writings and friendship. Special thanks also go to Dobrivoje S. Stokic, MD, and the Wilson Research Foundation for fostering a climate conducive to clinical research at the Methodist Rehabilitation Center, Jackson, MS.

I (M. Schenk) wish to thank past, present, and future colleagues for sharing their ideas, techniques, and support throughout my professional career.

ATLAS OF NERVE CONDUCTION STUDIES AND ELECTROMYOGRAPHY

OVERVIEW OF NERVE CONDUCTION STUDIES

1

HOW THE PERIPHERAL NERVOUS SYSTEM CONVEYS INFORMATION

THE PERIPHERAL NERVOUS SYSTEM conveys information through sensory and motor impulses (action potentials) that propagate along nerve fibers. In myelinated nerve fibers, action potentials occur only at the nodes of Ranvier, where the axons are exposed and action potentials produce local currents that jump from one node to the next. This type of saltatory conduction propagates rapidly compared with the continuous slow propagation in unmyelinated nerve fibers. In nature, impulses propagate only in the physiologic or *orthodromic* direction. For example, conduction of impulses in motor fibers occurs only toward the muscle (orthodromic motor impulses), while impulses in sensory fibers propagate toward the spinal cord (orthodromic sensory impulses). However, in the electrodiagnostic laboratory, axons within a mixed peripheral nerve that are directly activated by an electrical stimulus carry bidirectional volleys of impulses—those that ascend to the spinal cord, and those that descend toward the muscle or cutaneous distribution of the nerve (Figure 1-1). Thus, sensory and motor impulses can conduct in an *antidromic* direction, opposite to normal physiologic conduction; i.e., conduction of impulses in motor fibers proceeds toward the spinal cord (antidromic motor impulses), while impulses in sensory fibers propagate in the direction of the cutaneous distribution of the nerve (antidromic sensory impulses).

Orthodromic impulses in motor fibers give rise to a motor response known as the *compound muscle action potential* (CMAP) or *M-wave*, which is routinely recorded with surface electrodes placed over a muscle supplied by the nerve. Antidromic motor impulses elicit late responses called *F-waves*, due to antidromic activation of spinal motor neurons, which are also recorded with surface electrodes placed over the same muscle. F-waves provide information about the physiology of proximal motor nerve segments and the excitability of the motor neuron pool (Fisher, 1992). In the case of sensory conduction, antidromic sensory impulses generate a *sensory nerve action potential* (SNAP) that is routinely recorded with surface electrodes placed over the cutaneous distribution of the nerve, although orthodromic sensory impulses can also be recorded with surface electrodes placed over the nerve. In addition, orthodromic sensory impulses traveling in Ia afferent fibers elicit the spinal monosynaptic *H-reflex* (Kimura, 1989). The ascending sensory volley also elicits other spinal reflexes, and continues to ascend in the dorsal columns of the spinal cord and medial lemniscus of the brainstem to reach the thalamus and primary sensory cortex of the brain. Recording orthodromic sensory volleys from the central nervous system is the basis of somatosensory evoked potential (SSEP) studies. After an electrical stimulus to a nerve, the recorded response also depends on the fiber types activated by the stimulus. For example, a low-intensity stimulus will preferentially generate responses mediated by lower-threshold, larger-diameter myelinated fibers, whereas a high-intensity stimulus to the same nerve will generate responses that are also mediated by higher-threshold, smaller-diameter fibers. In addition, there is a direct relationship between fiber size and conduction velocity in myelinated fibers (Levin and Luders, 2000). The proper analysis of the various waveforms produced by electrical stimulation of a nerve plays a crucial role in the assessment of nerve and muscle function.

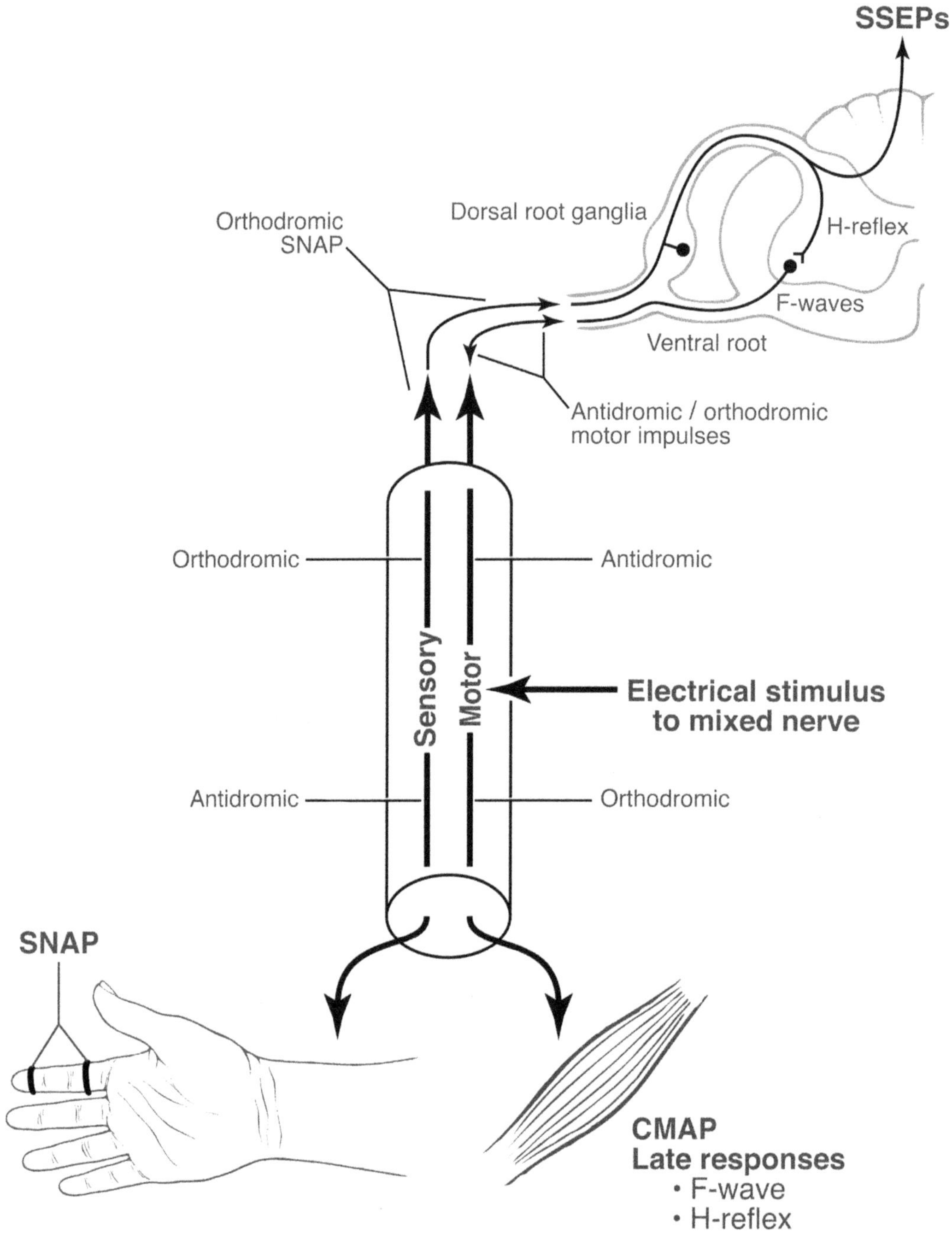

FIGURE 1-1 Electrical stimulation of a mixed peripheral nerve (i.e., a nerve that contains both sensory and motor axons) evokes bidirectional action potential volleys that travel in opposite directions away from the site of nerve depolarization. Knowing how to optimally record the various sensory and motor responses produced by the different volleys is one of the fundamentals of electrodiagnostic medicine. SNAP, sensory nerve action potential; CMAP, compound muscle action potential; SSEP, somatosensory evoked potentials.

STIMULATING AND RECORDING ELECTRODES

For routine nerve conduction studies, the stimulating electrodes consist of a cathode (negative pole) and anode (positive pole), usually spaced about 3 cm apart. Nerve depolarization occurs under the cathode, so accurate calculation of distal latency and conduction velocity depend on proper distance measurements between cathode and recording electrode, and between consecutive cathodal stimulation points along a nerve. Hence, surface measurements are based on the position of the cathode. One must avoid inadvertent surface measurements from the cathode at one stimulus site to the anode at a second site, which results in an error in distance measurement and leads to an erroneous conduction velocity. Similarly, confusing the cathode and anode will lead to an erroneous measurement of distal latency. In theory, nerve hyperpolarization can occur under the anode, producing an anodal conduction block. In routine clinical practice, this is not observed (Wee et al., 2000).

Most commercially available stimulators provide an electrical square wave of variable duration, usually ranging from 0.05 ms to 1.0 ms. Surface stimulation of 0.1 ms duration and a current of 10 mA to 50 mA or voltage of 100 V to 300 V are usually sufficient to activate a healthy nerve. Usually, stimulation is initiated with low current intensity (~10 mA) and gradually increased until the desired response reaches maximal amplitude. The use of a 10 % supramaximal stimulus guarantees the activation of all the axons necessary to generate the maximal SNAP or CMAP. The intensity required to maximally activate a nerve varies greatly between individuals, and from one nerve to another in the same subject. In particular, obese or muscular subjects will require a higher stimulus intensity to depolarize a nerve, especially during the assessment of proximal nerves in the lower limbs. Sometimes, even maximal stimulus intensity may be insufficient to fully depolarize a nerve (e.g., tibial nerve in the popliteal fossa or femoral nerve in the thigh). Similarly, diseased nerves may require higher stimulus intensities. In contrast, one of the most common sources of technical error arises when inappropriately high stimulus intensities are used (Dumitru, 2002). Over-stimulation increases stimulus artifact that can obscure the desired responses. This is particularly problematic when there are short distances between the stimulating and recording electrodes. Over-stimulation also causes the stimulating current to spread to adjacent nerves that are not being tested, which further confounds interpretation of latencies and wave morphology.

For optimal stimulation, the skin should be cleansed with alcohol, and electrolyte gel should be applied under the cathode and anode. This minimizes impedance and improves electrical conductivity. However, too much gel can form a bridge between the cathode and anode, essentially forming a short circuit between these electrodes. Excessive perspiration can also act in this manner, so the skin should be dried. The patient should also be instructed to avoid body lotion prior to the procedure.

The recording electrodes for CMAPs or SNAPs are usually square or round metal plates with average dimension of 1 cm by 1 cm. The electrodes are commercially available as "bar" electrodes with metal plates permanently fixed about 3 cm apart, or "loose" electrodes in which the inter-electrode distance can be varied. When recording CMAPs, these electrodes are taped on the surface of the skin ("surface electrodes") with the active electrode placed over the belly of the muscle and the indifferent or reference electrode placed on the tendon (belly-tendon recording). For recording of antidromic SNAPs, the surface electrodes are positioned so that the active electrode is over the desired cutaneous distribution, with the reference electrode placed 3 cm to 4 cm distally. Metal "ring" electrodes are commonly used for digital SNAP recordings. To record orthodromic SNAPs, surface electrodes are placed proximally over the corresponding nerve, with the active electrode closest to the stimulating electrode and the reference electrode 3 cm to 4 cm proximally along the nerve. For best recordings, the skin should be cleansed with alcohol and electrolyte gel should be applied under each electrode.

By clinical neurophysiologic convention, when the propagating action potential reaches the active electrode it becomes negative relative to the reference electrode, resulting in an upward deflection of the tracing. Conversely, when the propagating action potential moves farther away from the active electrode and toward the reference electrode, the active electrode becomes positive relative to the reference electrode (or the reference electrode becomes negative relative to the active electrode), resulting in a downward deflection of the tracing. If the active electrode is improperly positioned away from the nerve propagating action potential, or inadvertently placed off the motor point in a CMAP recording, an initial downward (positive) deflection will be seen. This results in the characteristic *volume-conducted response*. In some situations, the propagating depolarization never passes directly under the active electrode, and a downward deflection is predominantly or exclusively recorded. This may occur when stimulating one nerve and recording from a nearby muscle innervated by another nerve (e.g., stimulating median nerve and recording from first dorsal interosseous), or when the muscle is absent or markedly atrophic (e.g., recording from thenar muscles in end-stage carpal tunnel syndrome). However, in most cases, a volume-conducted response implies improper placement of the active electrode.

ELECTRODE AMPLIFIERS AND GROUND ELECTRODE

The potentials assessed during routine nerve conduction studies range in amplitude from microvolts (μV) to millivolts (mV). In general, SNAPs are measured in microvolts, with most upper limb sensory responses ≥ 20 μV and lower limb sensory responses typically ≥ 10 μV. In contrast, CMAPs are a factor of one thousand times larger and measured in millivolts, with most upper and lower limb motor responses typically ≥ 5 mV. Hence, stimulus artifact, electrical interference, electromagnetic "noise," and technical difficulties affect the smaller SNAPs much more than the larger CMAPs. Fortunately, the amplifiers used in most commercially available equipment are "differential amplifiers" that amplify only the voltage difference between the two input terminals connected to the recording electrodes and reject "common mode" voltages that appear between the two input terminals and the common ground electrode (Figure 1-2). In routine nerve conduction studies, the ground

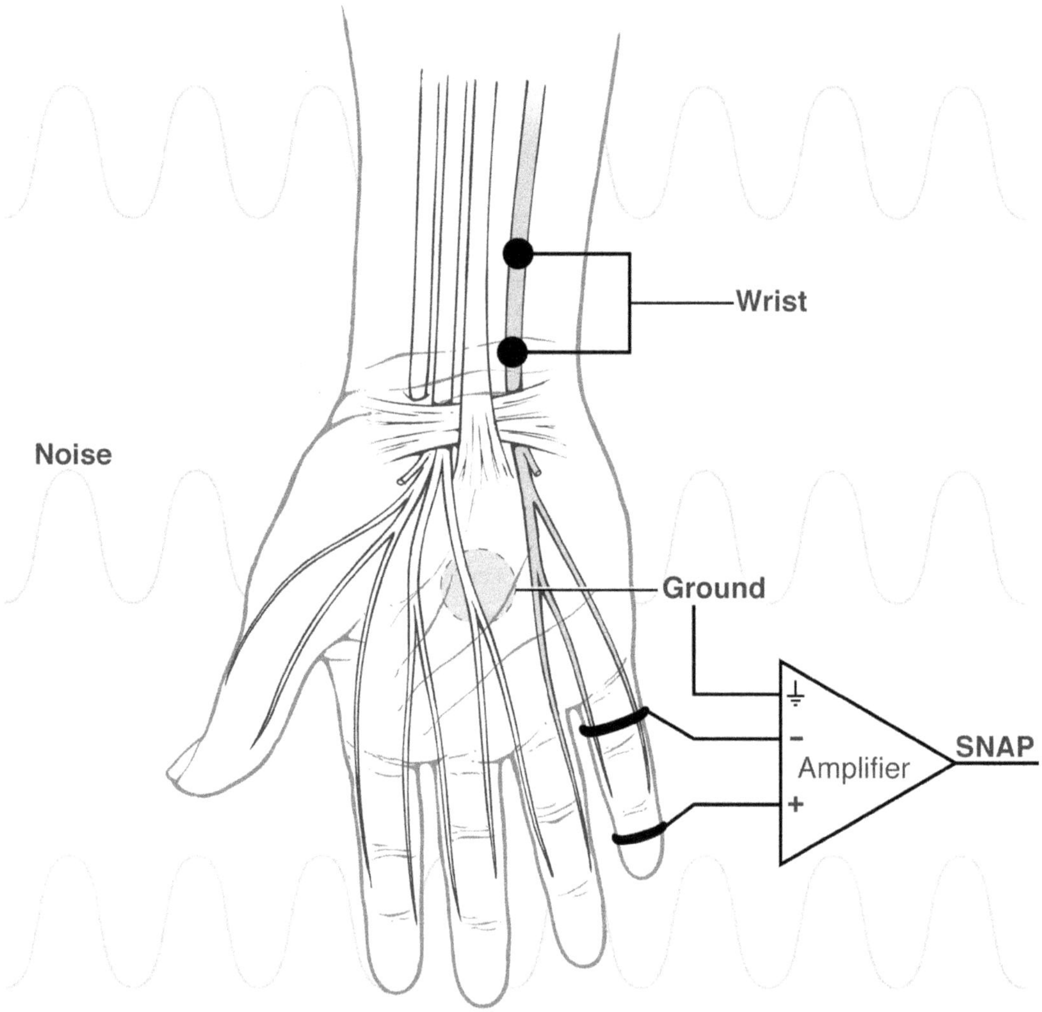

FIGURE 1-2 Differential amplifier. The amplifier eliminates random voltages caused by electrical noise by subtracting the signal from the ground electrode from the signals received from the recording electrodes, magnifying only the desired response (in this case, an antidromic sensory nerve action potential, SNAP).

electrode is usually placed between the stimulating electrodes and the recording electrodes. Without the ground electrode, it would be technically impossible to record SNAPs.

REDUCING ARTIFACTS AND INTERFERENCE

Other precautions may be taken to minimize electromagnetic noise. Major interference arises from poorly shielded power cords running to other appliances in the vicinity of the recording instrument. This is what makes recordings in the intensive care unit so technically difficult. Whenever possible, unplug unnecessary equipment. In addition, inspect the room for loose electrical outlets with loose wiring, and have the outlets repaired. Almost all commercially available equipment comes with variable high and low frequency filters that are automatically adjusted to reduce unwanted frequencies, including interfering high-frequency noise and low-frequency drift. The result of the filters is to emphasize the fundamental frequency of the desired response.

ELECTRICAL SAFETY

The manufacturers of commercially available equipment ensure that their instruments meet electrical safety requirements. However, the operator of the equipment is responsible for ensuring periodic electrical safety checks by biomedical engineers or other qualified personnel familiar with electrical instruments and current leakage (Dumitru, 2002). Relatively simple safety measures can be implemented to maximize patient safety, including routine inspections of equipment and electrical outlets, avoiding extension cords that may increase leakage current, plugging all electrical devices attached to the patient into the same outlet to share a common ground, and attaching only one ground to the patient during the examination. Awareness of these safety measures will permit the safe acquisition of data with minimal risk to the patient.

TEMPERATURE EFFECT

Temperature has a profound effect on nerve conduction studies (Kimura, 1989; Denys 1991). The conduction velocity decreases almost linearly by 2.4 m/s as the temperature measured near the nerve decreases from 38° C to 29° C. Similarly, distal latencies increase

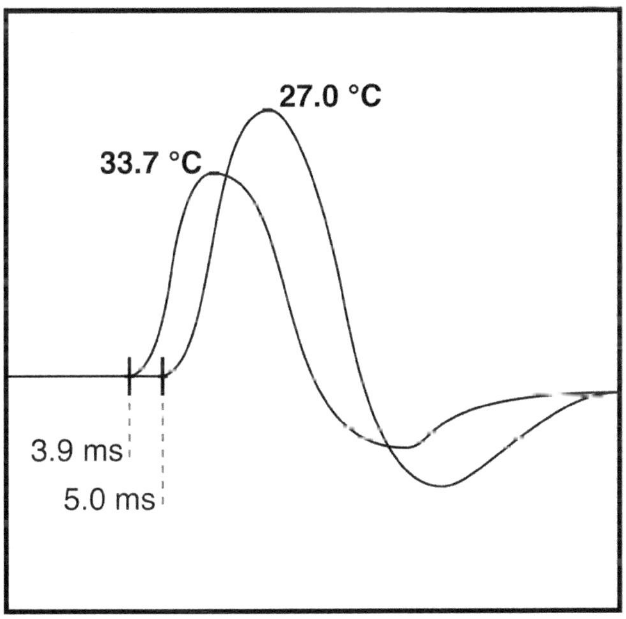

FIGURE 1-3 Temperature effect on the median compound muscle action potential (CMAP) recording from thenar eminence. Cooling the subject's hand from 33.7° C to 27.0° C resulted in a 1.1 ms delay and a 30% increase in CMAP amplitude. To avoid erroneous diagnoses, skin temperature must be controlled.

by about 0.2 ms per degree for both median and ulnar nerves upon cooling the hand (Figure 1-3). Lower temperatures also increase the amplitude of the sensory and motor responses, and can mask a defect in neuromuscular transmission. For routine nerve conduction studies, a skin temperature of 34° C or above corresponds to a muscle temperature close to 37° C. However, repeated stimulation of the hand causes reflex sweating and cooling of the hand, which prolongs latencies, slows conduction velocity, and increases amplitudes. Accordingly, limb temperature should be controlled throughout the nerve conduction studies. This can usually be accomplished easily with portable heaters.

EFFECT OF AGING

In full term infants, normal nerve conduction velocity is about 20 m/s to 30 m/s but by 3 to 5 years of age it increases rapidly as myelination advances to the adult range of 50 m/s to 70 m/s in upper limbs and 40 m/s to 60 m/s in lower limbs (Kimura, 1989). Conduction velocity begins to gradually decline after about age 40, although even in elderly subjects between 60 and 80 years of age the overall slowing of conduction velocity is only about 10 m/s. Aging also causes a decrease in SNAP and CMAP amplitudes and an increase in F-wave and H-reflex latencies (Levin and Luders, 2000). Although the changes with aging are relatively small per decade, they may be enough to make recording of small sensory or mixed nerve responses technically difficult (e.g., sural or plantar nerve responses, respectively).

MOTOR NERVE CONDUCTION

For most motor nerve conduction studies, the desired nerve is stimulated at two or more points along its course, with the cathode distal to the anode (Kimura, 1989). The recorded CMAP is analyzed for *distal latency, amplitude, nerve conduction velocity,* and *waveform configuration* (Figure 1-4). The distal latency includes nerve conduction from the point of stimulation to the axon terminal and time of neuromuscular transmission, including time required to generate the muscle action potential. The distal latency and conduction velocity reflect the speed of conduction in the fastest motor fibers. In contrast, the amplitude and waveform morphology reflect the number of fibers conducting. In most electrodiagnostic laboratories, the CMAP amplitude is measured from baseline to negative peak, although peak to peak amplitude can also be used.

To calculate the conduction velocity in a motor nerve, the time associated with neuromuscular transmission must be eliminated, since this time may be variable. Hence, conduction velocity is determined for the nerve segment between consecutive cathodal stimulation points along the motor nerve, excluding the distal component common to both stimuli. The formula for calculating conduction velocity is: $CV=\Delta D/\Delta T$, where CV is conduction velocity in meters per second, ΔD is total distance between cathodal stimulation points in millimeters, and ΔT is total time in milliseconds for the nerve impulse to travel between cathodal points. A reliable value of conduction velocity depends on accurately measuring the length of the nerve segment between cathodal stimulation points. In most normal subjects, conduction velocity is 50 m/s to 70 m/s in upper limbs and 40 m/s to 60 m/s in lower limbs. Stimulation at multiple points along the motor nerve allows calculation of segmental conduction velocities. In some cases, incremental stimulation across shorter segments can detect an abrupt change in CMAP latency or waveform at the site of nerve compression. This short segment or "inching technique" aids in the precise localization of a nerve lesion (Kimura, 1989).

SENSORY NERVE CONDUCTION

Following stimulation to a sensory nerve, the antidromic volley usually gives rise to a potential that is greater in amplitude than the orthodromic response. For this reason, in routine clinical practice, the antidromic sensory volley is usually preferred to generate the sensory nerve action potential (SNAP). In addition, stimulation to a mixed nerve will usually produce a well-defined antidromic SNAP that can usually be distinguished from

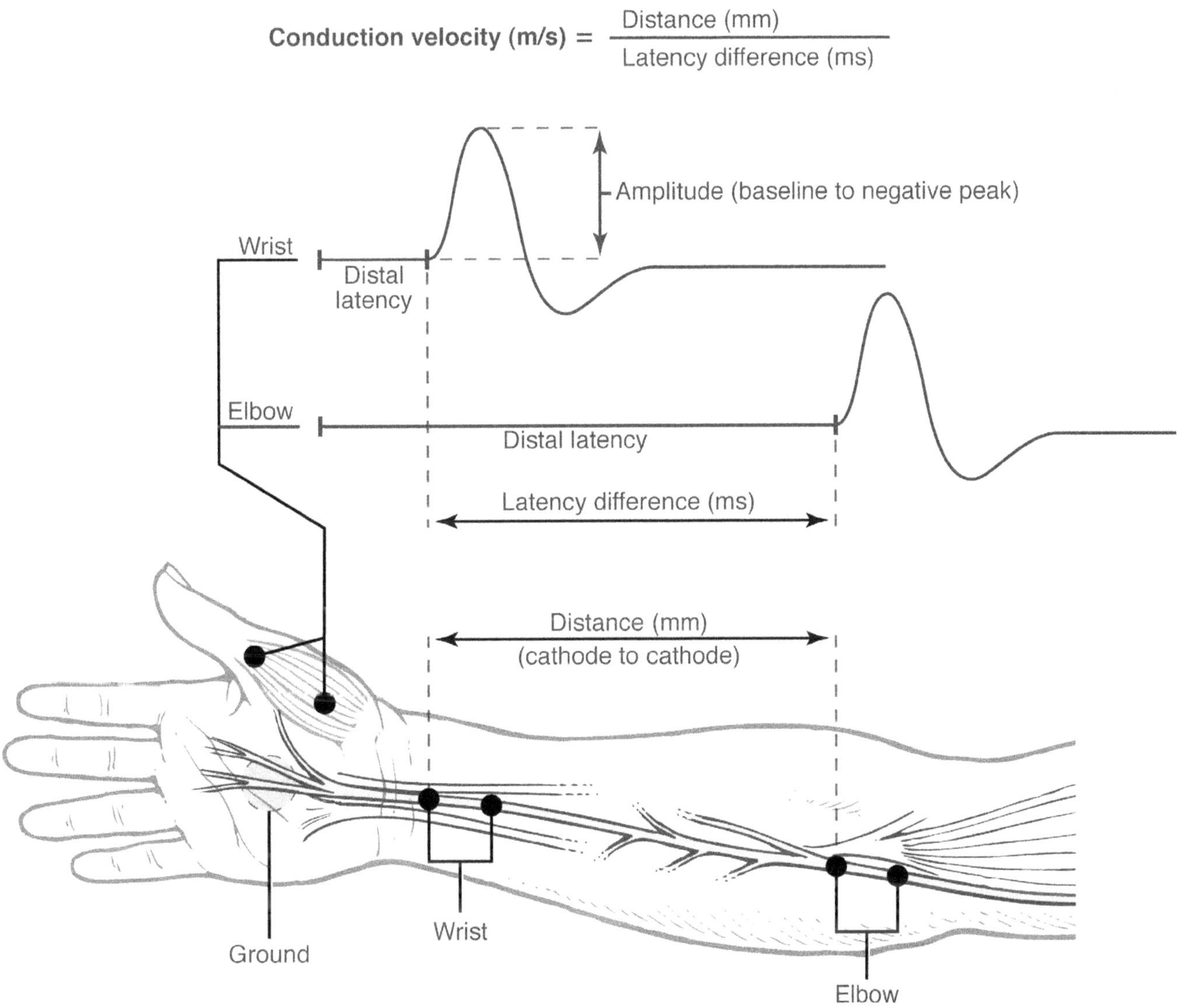

FIGURE 1-4 Measurements of the compound muscle action potential (CMAP).

the motor response, because cutaneous and motor distributions of the nerve may not overlap (e.g., median nerve distributions in the hand) and because sensory fibers have lower thresholds and conduct faster than motor fibers by about 10% (Dawson, 1956). Thus, mixed nerve potentials typically allow sufficient determination of the antidromic SNAP from the orthodromic CMAP.

The recorded SNAP is analyzed for latency, amplitude, and nerve conduction velocity (Figure 1-5). The latency and conduction velocity reflect the speed of conduction in the fastest sensory fibers, whereas the amplitude reflects the number of conducting sensory fibers. Sensory conduction velocity can be calculated in the distal nerve segment because, unlike the CMAP, there is no neuromuscular junction and no time apportioned to neuromuscular transmission. The latency is the nerve conduction time from the point of stimulation to generation of the SNAP. In many electrodiagnostic laboratories, the latency is measured at the onset of the negative peak (Kimura, 1989), although other laboratories use peak latency measurements (e.g., Mayo Clinic). The distance is the length measurement of the nerve segment between stimulation point and recording electrode. The SNAP amplitude is commonly measured from baseline to negative peak, although peak to peak amplitude can also be used. The SNAP elicited by proximal stimulation

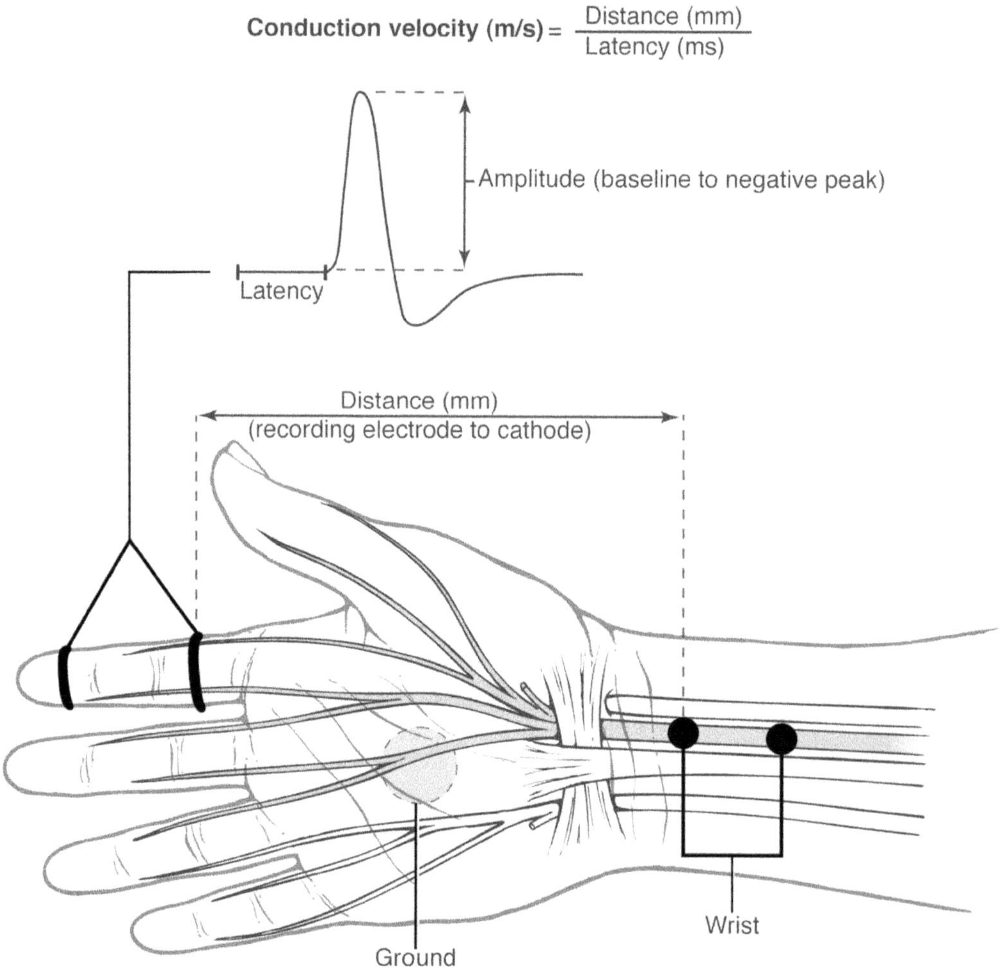

FIGURE 1-5 Measurements of the sensory nerve action potential (SNAP).

(e.g., median nerve stimulation at the elbow) is lower in amplitude and increased in duration compared with the response produced by distal stimulation (e.g., wrist stimulation). Factors that contribute to this effect include dispersion of the waveform that occurs due to the differences in individual fiber conduction velocities magnified by the greater distance of travel, resulting in phase cancellation of arriving nerve fiber action potentials (Levin and Luders, 2000). The disparity between the responses elicited by proximal versus distal stimulation is much more pronounced in sensory than in motor responses because of the relative amplitudes and durations of the responses: SNAPs are a factor of one thousand times smaller than CMAPs and have much shorter durations (usually about 2 ms) compared with CMAPs (usually about 10 ms). Accordingly, a small decrease in synchrony will have a much greater impact on a smaller, shorter response. For these reasons, many experienced electromyographers are cautious of SNAP data elicited by proximal stimulation.

ROLE OF DORSAL ROOT GANGLIA (DRG) IN LOCALIZING LESIONS

The cell bodies for sensory nerve fibers are located in the dorsal root ganglia (DRG), which are commonly situated at the level of the intervertebral foramina and are, therefore, not intraspinal. The SNAP reflects the integrity of DRG cells and their peripheral axons. Hence, SNAPs help to localize nerve disorders (Figure 1-6). An absent or reduced SNAP indicates abnormality at or distal to the DRG (i.e., a *postganglionic lesion*). Entrapment

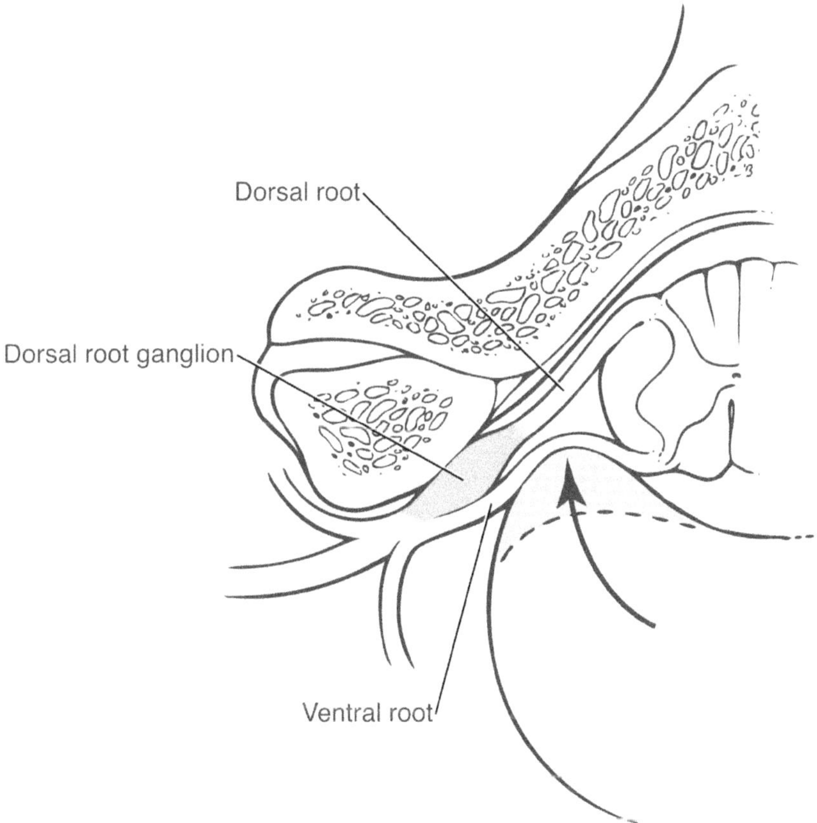

FIGURE 1-6 The role of the dorsal root ganglia (DRG) in localizing lesions. In the majority of cases of disc herniation or spondylosis (arrow), the DRG is spared because it lies outside the spinal canal. Hence, a preserved sensory nerve action potential (SNAP) is seen with disorders causing sensory loss proximal to the DRG (a preganglionic lesion). In contrast, a reduced or absent SNAP indicates a peripheral nerve disorder at or distal to the DRG (a postganglionic lesion).

neuropathies, plexopathies, peripheral nerve injuries, diffuse polyneuropathy, and sensory neuronopathies such as dorsal root ganglionitis are examples of postganglionic lesions. In contrast, a *preganglionic lesion* affects the central sensory fibers between the DRG and the spinal cord, sparing the DRG. Radiculopathy caused by a herniated disc, cervical spondylosis, root avulsion, and other disorders causing sensory loss proximal to the DRG are examples of preganglionic lesions. In preganglionic lesions, the SNAP is normal. Thus, preserved SNAPs serve to differentiate preganglionic from postganglionic disorders. In pathologic processes that infiltrate or extend from the intraspinal space into the dorsal root ganglion, such as malignancy, infection, or meningiomas, the DRG can be injured, resulting in loss of the SNAP. Uncommonly, due to anatomical variation, the DRG in the lumbar and sacral region may be situated proximal to the intervertebral foramina (i.e., intraspinal), making them vulnerable to compression by lateral disc herniations or spondylosis (Levin and Luders, 2000).

LATE RESPONSES: F-WAVE AND H-REFLEX

Routine nerve conduction studies typically assess conduction in distal nerve segments where the nerves are more anatomically accessible. In contrast, F-wave and H-reflex responses also assess conduction in proximal nerve segments. Accordingly, a distinct advantage of performing these late responses is that they detect conduction abnormalities over nerve segments not tested by routine studies. Because these late responses interface at the level of the spinal cord, they also provide valuable information about the physiology of the central nervous system (Fisher, 1992).

Since the latencies of F-waves and H-reflexes are similar, a clear distinction should be made between these late responses. Physiologic features of F-waves that distinguish them from H-reflexes include:

1. The F-wave is not a reflex. It is due to direct antidromic activation of spinal motor neurons; the same motor axon serves as the afferent and efferent arc.
2. F-waves are typically elicited by higher stimulus intensities than the H-reflex. Supramaximal stimulation for the direct motor response should be used to elicit the F-wave; this stimulus intensity abolishes the H-reflex.
3. The amplitude of F-waves is typically much lower than the H-reflex; F-wave amplitude is generally < 5% of the maximal CMAP amplitude.
4. F-wave responses are characterized by variability in amplitude, latency, and configuration (Figure 1-7), as a result of activation of different spinal motor neurons with each stimulus.
5. F-waves are ubiquitous and can be recorded from almost all skeletal muscles in an adult.

Physiologic features of the H-reflex include:

1. The H-reflex is a monosynaptic reflex elicited by electrical stimulation of large group Ia afferent fibers. In the lower limbs, it can be regarded as the electrical counterpart of the Achilles' reflex (in which a mechanical stretch activates the Ia afferents).
2. The H-reflex is elicited by a low-intensity stimulus that is often subthreshold for the direct motor response. With increases in stimulus intensity, a maximal H-reflex is elicited when the direct motor response is still submaximal. Further increases in intensity will increase the direct motor response while reducing the amplitude of the

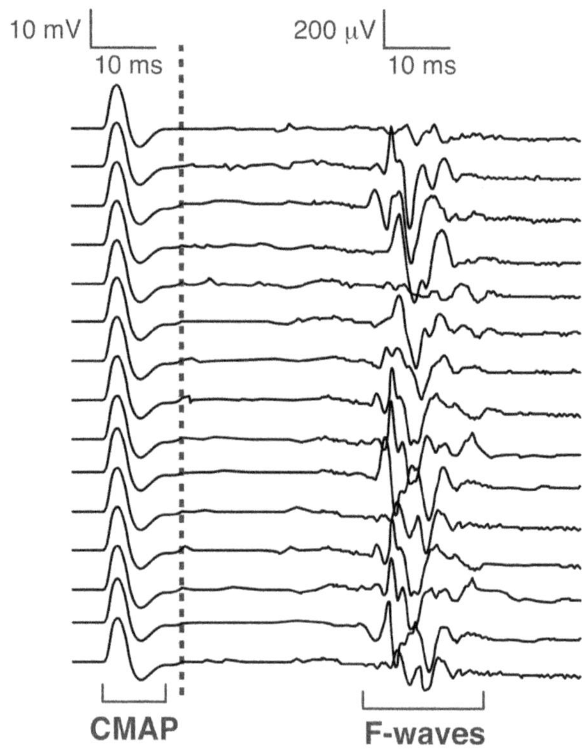

FIGURE 1-7 Consecutive tracings showing normal CMAP responses and F-waves recorded from abductor hallucis muscle following supramaximal stimulation to the tibial nerve at the medial malleolus. Note the variability in amplitude, latency, and configuration, as a result of antidromic activation of different spinal motor neurons with each stimulus.

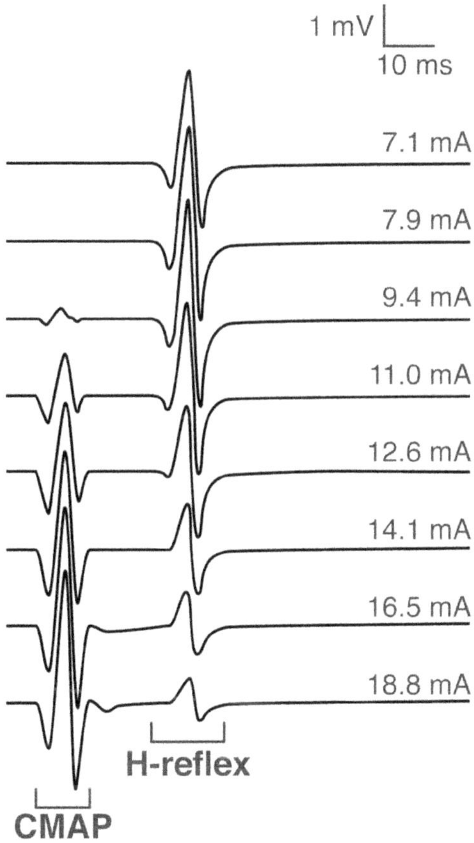

FIGURE 1-8 Consecutive tracings showing the contrasting behavior of normal CMAP and H-reflex responses recorded from the soleus muscle following increases in stimulus intensity to tibial nerve at the popliteal fossa. Initially, a low-intensity stimulus that is subthreshold for the direct CMAP elicits the H-reflex. With increases in stimulus intensity, the CMAP amplitude increases while the H-reflex amplitude decreases. Supramaximal stimulation for the CMAP abolishes the H-reflex.

H-reflex (Figure 1-8). With supramaximal stimulation for the direct motor response, the H-reflex is abolished and replaced by the F-wave.

3. The H-reflex latency is constant when recorded with surface electrodes and directly related to the length of the reflex arc.
4. The H-reflex is not ubiquitous. In adults, this response is routinely recorded from only calf muscles (gastrocnemius and soleus). Less commonly, an H-reflex can also be recorded from forearm flexors (flexor carpi radialis muscle). Slight voluntary contraction can also potentiate H-reflex responses in other muscles (e.g., intrinsic hand muscles).

Additional properties and clinical applications of F-waves and H-reflexes are discussed further in the respective chapters (see sections on median, ulnar, peroneal, and tibial F-waves, and tibial H-reflex).

TYPES OF NERVE INJURY

Historically, there are two major types of nerve injury that differently alter nerve conduction studies.

Neurapraxia

The mildest form of nerve injury is *neurapraxia* due to *demyelination* (Sunderland, 1978). In this form of nerve injury, there is loss of conduction due to loss of myelin without structural changes in the axon. After a neurapraxic injury, prognosis for recovery of function is favorable because remyelination usually occurs within days to a few weeks, provided that the source of injury is removed. Common clinical examples of acquired neurapraxic injury include acute entrapment neuropathies such as carpal tunnel syndrome, ulnar neuropathy at the elbow, Saturday night palsy of the radial nerve, common peroneal neuropathy at the fibular head due to habitual leg crossing, and mild traction injury to the brachial plexus.

On nerve conduction studies, the classic features of demyelination include: *(1)* the presence of conduction block; *(2)* marked slowing of conduction velocity; *(3)* marked prolongation of distal latency; or *(4)* temporal dispersion. In general, sensory or motor conduction velocities that are < 35 m/s in the upper limbs and < 30 m/s in the lower limbs imply demyelination. Focal demyelination gives rise to conduction block or slowing of conduction across the demyelinated segment, but not below the lesion. Consequently, there is preserved amplitude of the CMAP or SNAP with stimulation distal to the demyelinated segment. In contrast, the CMAP or SNAP is reduced in amplitude or absent with stimulation proximal to the demyelinated segment (Figure 1-9). By convention, a drop in the CMAP amplitude of ≥50% with proximal stimulation defines a conduction block, although smaller drops in amplitude between 20% and 50%, if reproducible and not due to technical factors, may reflect a partial conduction block. The clinical correlate of a focal conduction block is weakness or sensory loss in the distribution of the "blocked" nerve; without these clinical features, there can be no substantial conduction block. Focal and multifocal demyelination can also give rise to increased desynchronization of the volleys, so that individual nerve action potentials arrive at the recording electrodes at different times. This results in temporal dispersion of the CMAP, which appears irregular and drawn out (Figure 1-10). Distal demyelination gives rise to prolonged distal latencies. It can also lead to reduced CMAP amplitude because of distal conduction block. Relatively common clinical conditions characterized by multifocal demyelination include Guillain-Barré syndrome (acute inflammatory demyelinating polyneuropathy, AIDP) or chronic inflammatory demyelinating polyneuropathy (CIDP). In these two demyelinating neuropathies, nerve conduction studies often demonstrate all of the classic features of demyelination.

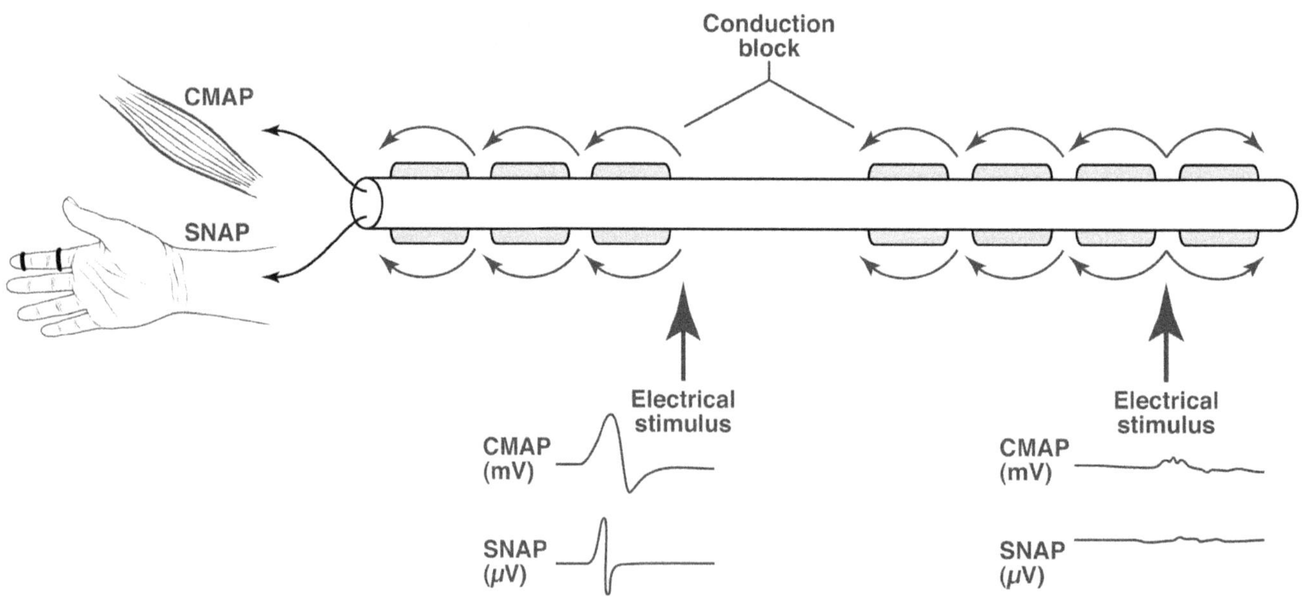

FIGURE 1-9 Conduction block due to focal demyelination. Saltatory conduction in motor and sensory fibers fails to propagate through structurally intact axons. The compound muscle action potential (CMAP) and sensory nerve action potential (SNAP) are reduced in amplitude or absent with stimulation proximal to the demyelinated segment. The clinical correlate of conduction block is focal weakness or sensory loss.

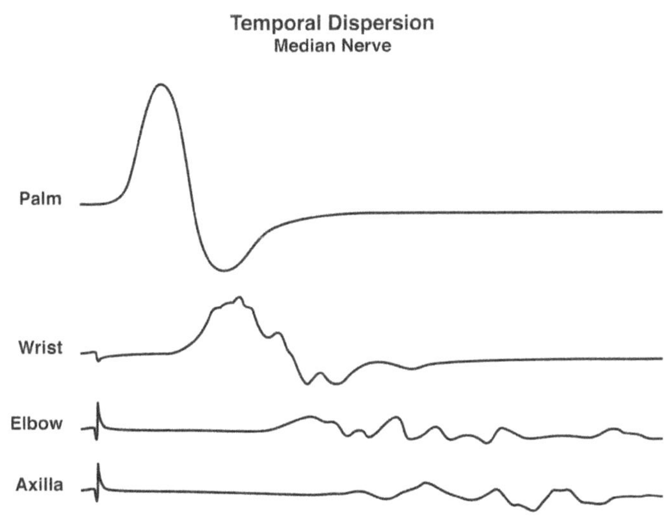

FIGURE 1-10 Temporal dispersion of the compound muscle action potential (CMAP) occurs when multifocal demyelination causes desynchronization of the motor volley, so that individual motor fiber action potentials arrive at the recording electrodes at different times.

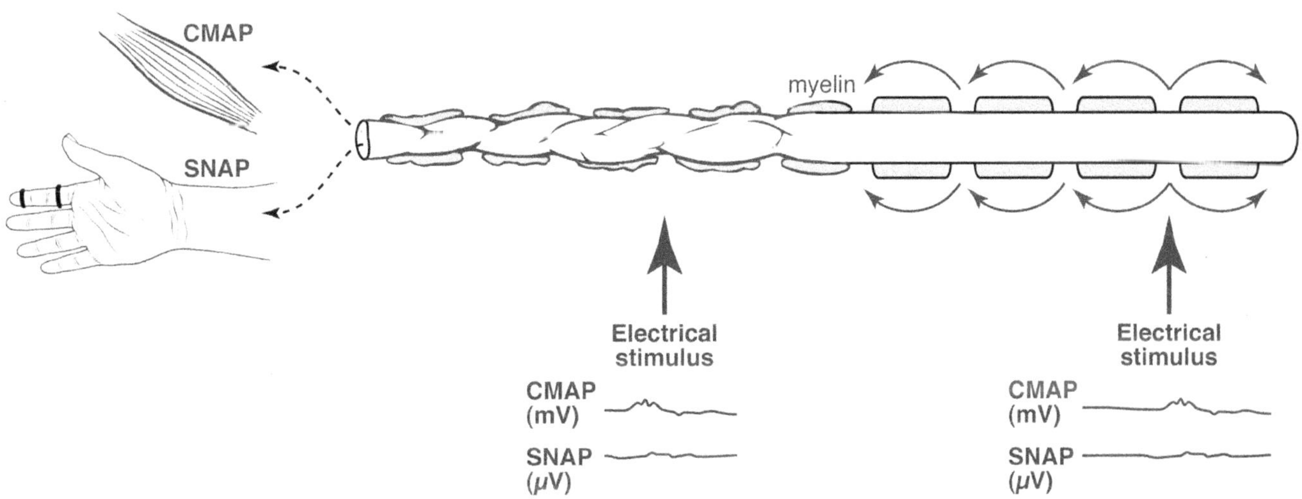

FIGURE 1-11 Axonal loss injury with Wallerian degeneration of the distal nerve segment and myelin sheath. Depending on the severity of the nerve injury, some or all axons will undergo Wallerian degeneration. On nerve conduction studies, compound muscle action potentials (CMAPs) and sensory nerve action potentials (SNAPs) are reduced or absent, irrespective of the site of stimulation.

Axonal Loss Injury

With more severe nerve injury, structural changes occur in the axon (Figure 1-11), leading to axonal loss. In this condition, axons lose continuity with subsequent *Wallerian degeneration* of the distal nerve segment, including myelin sheath (Sunderland, 1978). After an axonal loss injury, prognosis for recovery of function is less favorable or poor, depending on the degree of axonal loss. If the injury leads to complete loss of axons, it is termed *axonotmesis.* In the most severe form of nerve injury, termed *neurotmesis*, there is complete disruption of all axons, myelin sheath, and all supporting connective tissue structures. Recovery of function following an axonal loss injury will depend on the degree of reinnervation and regeneration, which may be slow (over months) and incomplete. During the first few days after an axonal loss injury, nerve conduction studies of the distal segment may remain normal, although all responses eventually disappear when Wallerian degeneration is complete. However, this may take one to two weeks. In addition, fibrillation potentials in denervated muscle typically develop 2 to 3 weeks after axonal loss injury. Accordingly, in some cases it may be prudent to defer nerve conduction studies and needle electromyography for 2 to 3 weeks after nerve injury. Features of axonal loss injury on nerve conduction studies include reduced or absent CMAPs or SNAPs irrespective of the site of stimulation, low-normal to mild slowing of conduction velocities (usually > 40 m/s in upper limbs and >30 m/s in lower limbs), and relatively normal or slightly delayed distal latencies. If the degree of axonal loss is mild, then nerve conduction studies are only minimally affected (Kimura, 1989). For example, in diffuse polyneuropathies, axonal loss commonly occurs. As the polyneuropathy progresses, additional loss of sensory and motor axons results in a length-dependent or distal symmetrical reduction in CMAPs and SNAPs, slowing of conduction velocities below the normal range, and relative delays in distal latencies.

In the attempt to physiologically classify nerve lesions into axonal loss versus demyelination, it should be understood that injury to axons and myelin are not mutually exclusive. Indeed, few cases fall precisely into one group or the other. Most cases of diffuse polyneuropathy will show electrodiagnostic features of both axonal loss and demyelination. Similarly, many cases exemplified by neurapraxic injury (e.g., carpal tunnel syndrome, Saturday night palsy) will frequently be accompanied by some axonal degeneration. Although physiological classification may seem a little arbitrary, it is still practical because the conduction abnormalities discussed above can be used in most cases to support a diagnosis of predominantly demyelinating neuropathy or predominantly axonal neuropathy. This serves as a useful aid in making a correct diagnosis and determining proper prognosis.

Ion Channel Disorders (Channelopathies)

In the past few years, a third category of nerve injury that differently alters nerve conduction studies has been recognized. This form of nerve injury is caused by dysfunctional ion channels and is associated with an expanding group of neurological disorders. The *ion channel disorders*, or *channelopathies*, cause paroxysmal or episodic disturbances of peripheral nerve or skeletal muscle function (Kullmann, 2010). Ion channels are responsible for the generation of electrical currents across excitable membranes, and channelopathies are characterized by increased or decreased excitability of nerve or muscle. Recognized causes include toxins, autoimmune conditions, and genetic mutations (England, 2002).

Toxins. The marine toxins tetrodotoxin, from eating puffer fish, and saxitoxin, from consuming shellfish, are potent sodium channel blockers that cause rapid onset of numbness, intense paresthesia and dysesthesia, and generalized muscle weakness. Death can result from respiratory failure. Nerve conduction studies show diffuse slowing of conduction velocities and decreased amplitudes in sensory and motor responses (Oda et al., 1989). However, these abnormalities are quickly reversible over a few days with no residual conduction defects. These findings are the direct result of the toxins blocking voltage-gated sodium channels in the axon. Ciguatera poisoning occurs from eating predatory reef fish containing ciguatoxin, a potent sodium channel toxin that causes prolonged activation of sodium channels (Cameron et al., 1991A, 1991B). This is the most common fish food poisoning encountered in man. Electrophysiological studies show slowing of motor and sensory conduction velocities and F-waves, and significantly reduced motor and sensory nerve amplitudes. The clinical presentation consists of vomiting and diarrhea followed by limb and perioral paresthesias, a sensation of loose teeth, myalgias, generalized weakness, and bradycardia or hypotension. As with other marine ion channel toxins, nerve conduction abnormalities are reversible. Tick paralysis is another condition in which ion channel toxins are thought to play a role. The very rapid reversal of clinical and physiologic deficits following removal of the tick implies ion channel dysfunction as opposed to axonal loss or demyelination as the primary disease mechanism (Vedanarayanan et al., 2004).

Autoimmune. Immune-mediated channelopathies include Lambert-Eaton myasthenic syndrome (LEMS), in which antibodies are directed against voltage-gated calcium channels in presynaptic motor nerve terminals. In LEMS, CMAP amplitudes are significantly reduced in amplitude. In the majority of patients with LEMS, a brief 10-second exercise of the tested muscle followed immediately by a second supramaximal stimulus will produce a marked incremental response in the CMAP of > 200%, due to calcium accumulation in the presynaptic nerve terminal with enhanced release of acetylcholine quanta. Rapid repetitive stimulation at 20 Hz to 50 Hz will also result in a striking incremental CMAP response. Antibodies to the skeletal muscle nicotinic acetylcholine receptor are the cause of acquired myasthenia gravis, the most intensely studied neuromuscular junction disorder. The electrodiagnosis of myasthenia gravis is well described in standard textbooks dealing with neuromuscular disorders. Myasthenia gravis is a ligand-gated (rather than voltage-gated) ion channelopathy, meaning that the ion channels are activated by binding of a *ligand* (from the Latin ligandum, *binding*) instead of a change in membrane potential. In the neuromuscular junction, acetylcholine is the ligand that binds to the postsynaptic acetylcholine receptor, causing a conformational change in the sodium ion channel, which allows sodium to enter the muscle cell to depolarize the sarcolemma. Hence, antibodies that bind, block, or modulate the acetylcholine receptor exert their deleterious effect by impairing the sodium channel. Antibodies to voltage-gated potassium channels in the peripheral nerve may result in hyperexcitability and abnormal firing of the peripheral nerve, giving rise to the condition known as *neuromyotonia*, or Isaac's syndrome. On needle electromyography (EMG), the hyperexcitability manifests as high-frequency neuromyotonic and myokymic discharges. Some of the neurophysiologic abnormalities seen in Guillain-Barré syndrome, traditionally regarded as the result of demyelination, may also reflect sodium channel dysfunction. In particular, the transient nature of some symptoms and the relatively rapid recovery seen in some Guillain-Barré syndrome patients favor a transient antibody-mediated channelopathy rather than a longer process of remyelination.

Genetic. Inherited channelopathies have now been described for all ion channels (sodium, potassium, chloride, calcium). In general, these channelopathies may cause an abnormal gain of function (such as myokymia or myotonia) or an abnormal loss of function (such as episodic attacks of weakness, paralysis, or numbness), depending on whether loss of channel function leads to excessive membrane excitability or to membrane inexcitability. The best described genetic channelopathies affect skeletal muscle, and result in either loss of muscle fiber excitability, which causes periodic paralysis, or excessive excitability, which manifests as myotonia. Mutations of potassium channels include Andersen-Tawil syndrome, which presents with attacks of periodic paralysis and cardiac arrhythmias, associated with subtle craniofacial, skeletal, or cognitive abnormalities. Other potassium mutations can give rise to hypokalemic periodic paralysis, or multisystem disorders that include episodic muscle weakness. Inherited disorders of skeletal muscle sodium channels underlie a spectrum of disorders ranging from myotonia to periodic paralysis, and include paramyotonia congenita, hyperkalemic or hypokalemic periodic paralysis, and potassium-aggravated myotonia. In addition, there are several rare congenital myasthenic syndromes due to mutations in the subunits of the postsynaptic acetylcholine receptor. These myasthenia syndromes may be considered to be genetic ligand-gated channelopathies. Inherited sodium ion channel disorders that alter sensory transduction and nociception in dorsal root ganglia (DRG), as well as sympathetic ganglia, have also emerged (Kullmann, 2010). These mutations give rise to distinct clinical syndromes. For example, primary erythromelalgia (PE) is characterized by episodes of burning pain and redness of the lower limbs or hands, often precipitated by high ambient temperatures. Paroxysmal extreme pain disorder (PEPD) presents in early childhood with autonomic instability (skin flushing, syncope) and attacks of severe deep burning pain in a perineal, periorbital, or mandibular distribution. Another mutation can manifest with complete insensitivity to pain. Calcium channel mutations account for most cases of hypokalemic periodic paralysis, which manifests with attacks of limb and neck muscle weakness associated with low serum potassium. Mutations of skeletal muscle chloride channel gene underlie myotonia congenita (Thomsen's and Becker's). Patients

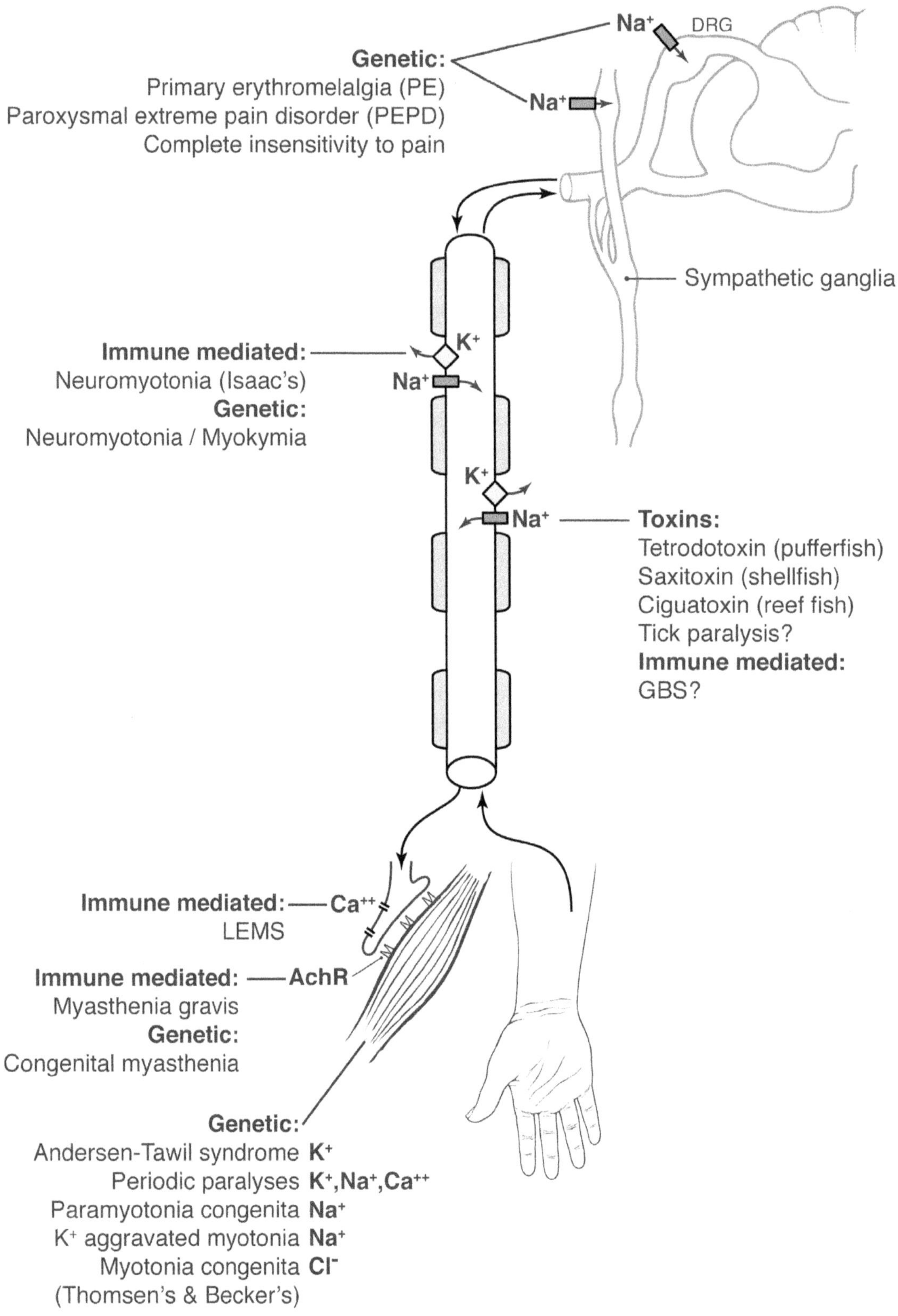

FIGURE 1-12 Summary of the major ion channel disorders (channelopathies) affecting skeletal muscle, neuromuscular junction, peripheral nerve, dorsal root ganglia (DRG), and sympathetic ganglia. Channelopathies cause paroxysmal or episodic disturbances of peripheral nerve or skeletal muscle function. Recognized causes include toxins, autoimmune conditions, and genetic mutations.

experience fluctuating stiffness of limb and facial muscles, with worsening in cold environments and improvement with muscle use.

Disorders of ion channels comprise a rapidly expanding subset of neuromuscular disorders. A common clinical feature of many channelopathies is that they cause paroxysmal attacks of dysfunction, often precipitated by a physiologic stress. During these attacks, nerve conduction studies and needle EMG examination may show abnormalities, although the electrodiagnostic and clinical findings typically normalize between attacks. However, discreet attacks may eventually give way to fixed or progressive impairment. Channelopathies can affect skeletal muscle, neuromuscular junction, peripheral nerve, dorsal root ganglia, and sympathetic ganglia (Figure 1-12). For a review of neurological channelopathies see Graves and Hanna, 2005, and Kullmann, 2010.

The nerve conduction study techniques used in individual electrodiagnostic laboratories should be consistent with those described in standard textbooks, journal articles, or publications of recognized organizations. Additional educational guidelines, practice aids, and other valuable resources for performing electrodiagnostic studies are available at the American Association of Neuromuscular and Electrodiagnostic Medicine (AANEM), American Clinical Neurophysiology Society (ACNS), and American Academy of Neurology (AAN).

REFERENCES

American Academy of Neurology. http://www.aan.com

American Association of Neuromuscular and Electrodiagnostic Medicine. https://www.aanem.org/

American Clinical Neurophysiology Society. https://www.acns.org/

Cameron J, Flowers AE, Capra MF. Effects of ciguatoxin on nerve excitability in rats (Part I). *J Neurol Sci* 1991;101:87–92.

Cameron J, Flowers AE, Capra MF. Electrophysiological studies on ciguatera poisoning in man (Part II). *J Neurol Sci* 1991;101:93–97.

Dawson GD. The relative excitability and conduction velocity of sensory and motor nerve fibres in man. *J Physiol* 1956;131(2): 436–451.

Denys EH. AAEM Minimonograph#14: The influence of temperature in clinical neurophysiology. *Muscle Nerve* 1991;14:795–811.

Dumitru D, Amato AA, Zwarts M. *Electrodiagnostic Medicine.* Ed 2. Hanley & Belfus, Inc., 2002.

England JD. Channelopathies. *CNI Review* 2002;13 (2). Available at: http://www.thecni.org/reviews/13-2-p02-england.htm

Fisher MA. AAEM Minimonograph#13: H reflexes and F waves: physiology and clinical indications. *Muscle Nerve* 1992;15(11):1223–1233. Review.

Graves TD, Hanna MG. Neurological channelopathies. *Postgrad Med J* 2005;81:20–32.

Kimura J. Electrodiagnosis. In *Diseases of Nerve and Muscle*, 2nd ed., FA Davis Co., Philadelphia, 1989.

Kullmann DM. Neurological channelopathies. *Annu Rev Neurosci* 2010;33:151–172.

Levin KH, Luders HO. *Comprehensive Clinical Neurophysiology.* W.B. Saunders Co., Philadelphia, 2000.

Long RR, Sargent JC, Hammer K. Paralytic shellfish poisoning: a case report and serial electrophysiologic observations. *Neurol* 1990;40:1310–1312.

Oda K, Araki K, Totoki T, Shibasaki H. Nerve conduction study of human tetrodotoxication. *Neurol* 1989;39:743–745.

Sunderland S. *Nerves and Nerve Injuries.* 2nd ed., Churchill Livingstone, New York, 1978

Vedanarayanan V, Sorey WH, Subramony SH. Tick paralysis. *Semin Neurol* 2004;24:181–184.

Wee AS, Leis AA, Kuhn AR, Gilbert RW. Anodal block: can this occur during routine nerve conduction studies? *Electromyogr Clin Neurophysiol* 2000;40:387–391.

2 OVERVIEW OF ELECTROMYOGRAPHY (EMG)

THE MOTOR UNIT

MUSCLE ACTION POTENTIALS can also be recorded by a n eedle electrode inserted into the muscle. The use of needle electrodes allows recording of individual *motor unit potentials* (MUPs) discharging within a narrow radius from the electrode tip (as opposed to surface electrodes that record summated activity from many muscle fibers). The origin of the MUPs is the *motor unit*, which consists of a motor neuron, its axon, and all the muscle fibers that it innervates (Figure 2-1; Levin and Luders, 2000). The muscle fibers belonging to one motor unit are typically dispersed or intermingled throughout part or most of the

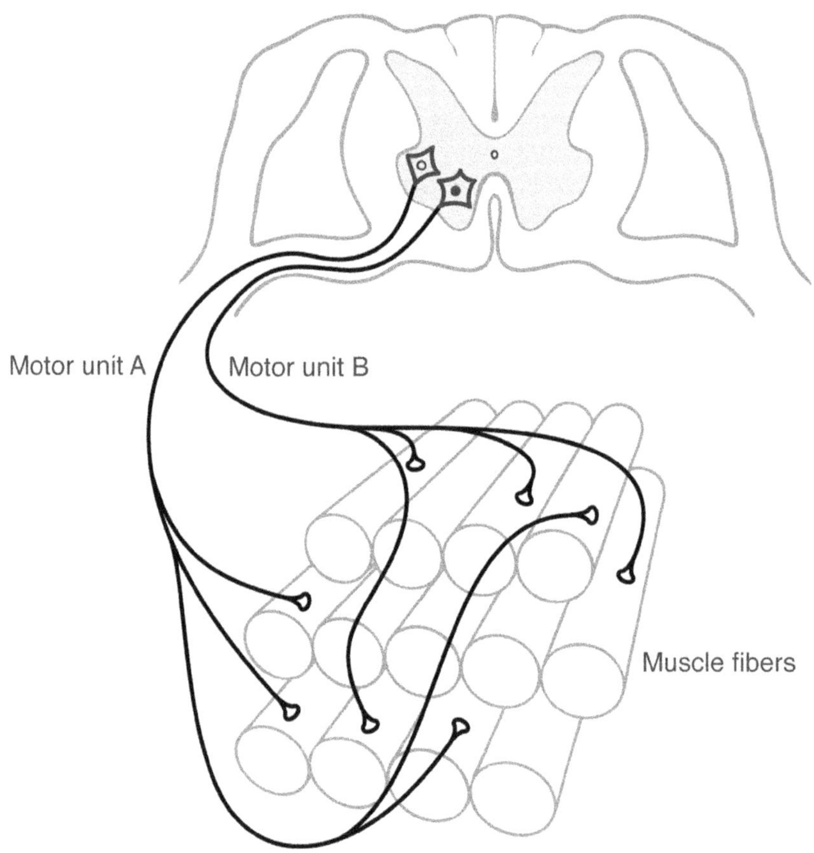

FIGURE 2-1 The motor unit consists of a single motor neuron and its motor axon (two motor units shown, A and B), which gives rise to branching axons, each of which terminates in a neuromuscular junction on a single muscle fiber. Nerve impulses passing down a single motor neuron will thus trigger a synchronous contraction in all muscle fibers supplied by that neuron. The motor unit is thus the minimum functional component of contraction.

entire muscle, depending on the number of fibers and size of the muscle. The *innervation ratio* (the number of muscle fibers innervated by one motor neuron) depends on the size and function of the muscle. Motor units may have ratios ranging from <1:10 to 1:1000. The closer the ratio approximates unity, the greater the finesse and specificity of the muscle action. For example, the innervation ratio of an extraocular muscle is about 10 muscle fibers to 1 motor neuron; that of an intrinsic hand muscle is about 100 muscle fibers to 1 motor neuron, and that of a large antigravity leg muscle may exceed 1000 muscle fibers to 1 motor neuron. A single discharge of the motor neuron gives rise to a synchronous contraction of all muscle fibers supplied by the axon, resulting in a weak but distributed muscle contraction. The activation of more motor neurons will result in more muscle fibers being activated, and therefore a stronger muscle contraction. Hence, the motor unit constitutes the smallest functional element of contraction. Electromyographers analyze the motor unit potentials on a visual display and the auditory characteristics associated with these waveforms.

NEEDLE ELECTRODES

For routine EMG, three types of needle electrodes are commonly used: standard concentric, bipolar concentric, or monopolar. The *standard concentric electrode* consists of a hollow stainless steel cannula containing an insulated, centrally located wire. The exposed distal tip of the wire on the bevel surface of the needle serves as the active electrode, while the barrel of the needle serves as the reference electrode. The *bipolar concentric electrode* consists of a hollow stainless steel cannula containing two insulated wires. The exposed distal tips of these wires on the bevel surface of the needle serve as the active and reference electrodes. The *monopolar electrode* consists of a solid stainless steel needle coated with insulation except for the distal coned tip, which serves as the active electrode. A surface electrode serves as the reference. In most EMG laboratories, commercially available disposable needles are used, although some special-purpose needles such as single-fiber needles are still commonly sterilized and reused.

MUSCLE SELECTION FOR NEEDLE EMG

The muscles selected for needle EMG depend on the clinical hypothesis (Daube and Rubin, 2009). For instance, proximal muscles are preferentially assessed if myopathy is suspected. Single limb muscles are studied if the clinical presentation favors isolated radiculopathy or entrapment neuropathy. In contrast, widely distributed muscles in different limbs and the tongue may be sampled in cases of suspected motor neuron disease.

THE NEEDLE EMG EXAMINATION

The needle examination of skeletal muscle consists of the assessment of: (1) *insertional activity* caused by movement of the needle electrode in the muscle; (2) *spontaneous activity* recorded with the muscle at rest; (3) *motor unit potentials* during minimal voluntary muscle contractions; and (4) *pattern of recruitment* during progressively increasing levels of muscle contraction (Kimura, 1989).

Assessment of Insertional Activity

Insertion of a needle electrode into skeletal muscle normally elicits a brief burst of activity. Movement of the needle within the muscle also triggers the same brief discharges, which appear as a cluster of high-frequency spikes accompanied by a crisp static sound. The insertional activity normally ceases with cessation of the needle movement or only slightly exceeds the movement of the needle. The discharges are regarded as injury potentials that arise from muscle fibers injured or mechanically irritated by the penetrating needle (Kimura, 1989). Typically, the needle is moved along a straight line through the muscle in short incremental steps (<1 mm), with a brief pause between each step (1 s or longer) to listen and watch for abnormal activity (Daube and Rubin, 2009). The needle is advanced from 5 to 20 such steps depending on muscle size, withdrawn to a subcutaneous position, and then redirected at a different angle in the same muscle. Two to three such passes usually suffice to adequately examine a muscle. Insertional activity is usually categorized as normal, increased, or decreased (Figure 2-2). This semi-quantitative analysis provides an important measure of muscle excitability. Insertional activity is *increased* when it persists after cessation of the needle movement. Typically, the bursts of activity continue in short runs or trains beyond cessation of the needle movement. Abnormally prolonged insertional activity indicates irritability or instability of the muscle membrane, and is typically seen in axonal lesions of peripheral nerve (neuropathy, trauma), diseases of the anterior horn cell (motor neuron disease, poliomyelitis), and certain myopathic disorders (myositis). In contrast, a decrease or absence of insertional activity suggests loss or absence of muscle fibers, as in fibrosis of muscle or severely atrophied muscle.

Assessment of Spontaneous Activity

Spontaneous activity is the electrical activity recorded from muscle at rest after insertional activity has subsided, and when there is no voluntary muscle contraction or external stimulus. Normal muscle fibers show no spontaneous activity outside of the end-plate region (Daube and Rubin, 2009). Hence, spontaneous activity, if reproducible in several muscle sites, is an unmistakable sign of abnormality and one of the most useful findings in clinical EMG. It is usually seen in lower motor neuron disorders, including anterior horn cell disease, radiculopathy, plexopathy, axonal mononeuropathy, and axonal polyneuropathy. All of these disorders cause denervation of muscle. In addition, spontaneous activity can also occur in certain myopathic disorders, including muscular dystrophies, dermatomyositis, or polymyositis. Less commonly, spontaneous activity can be seen in disorders of the neuromuscular junction. Because there is a latent period of 2 to 3 weeks after nerve injury until Wallerian degeneration has fully manifested and spontaneous activity is evident, the absence of spontaneous activity does not rule out denervation. This delay in the develop-

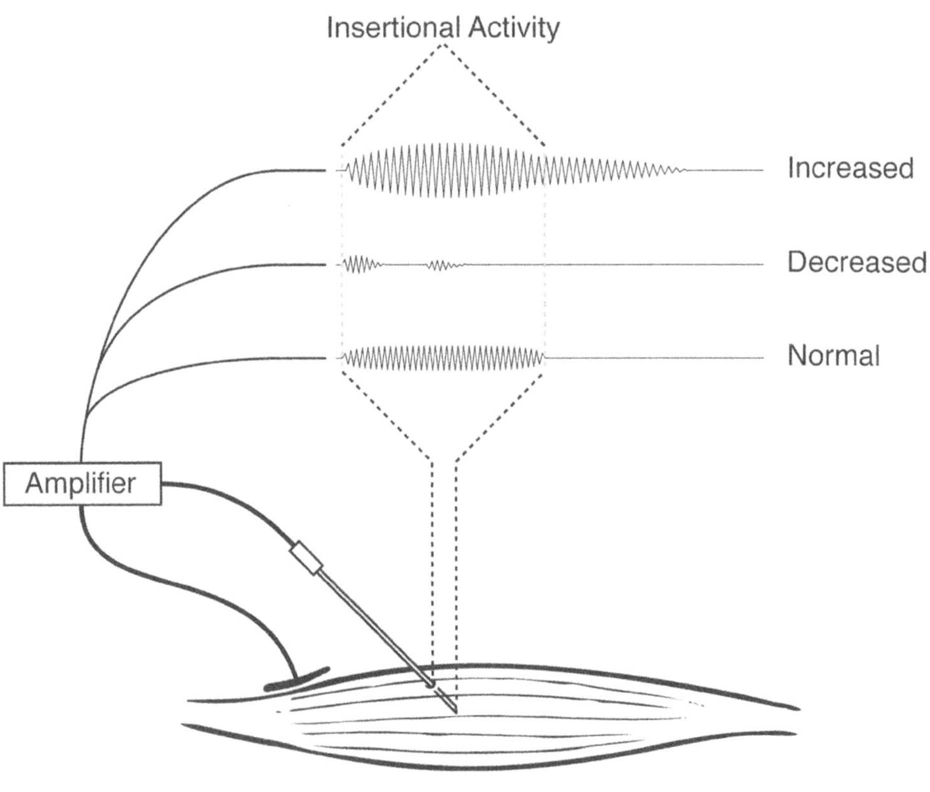

FIGURE 2-2 Insertional activity is classified as normal or increased, depending on whether the brief burst of activity associated with needle movement ceases with or outlasts the needle movement, respectively. It is classified as decreased when activity is absent or diminished despite the needle movement.

ment of spontaneous activity has given rise to a common myth that the EMG must be postponed 2 to 3 weeks following nerve injury before reliable information can be obtained. In fact, demonstrating preserved conduction in nerves of an injured limb may be of paramount importance immediately or soon after injury, since it can help to differentiate preserved nerves from damaged nerves. Moreover, in most cases of acute traumatic nerve injury, the documentation of preserved innervation to muscles supplied by an injured nerve obviates the need for nerve-related surgery. If there is substantial axonal or neurapraxic injury, the pattern of recruitment of motor unit potentials will immediately become abnormal (Feinberg, 2006), allowing a skilled electromyographer to approximate the degree of nerve injury and to determine future management. Nerve conduction studies across an injured segment of nerve will also be abnormal immediately after injury. However, the limitation of EMG and nerve conduction studies performed early after injury is that one cannot differentiate severe neurapraxic injury with complete conduction block from axonotmesis associated with severe axonal loss or nerve transection (Feinberg, 2006).

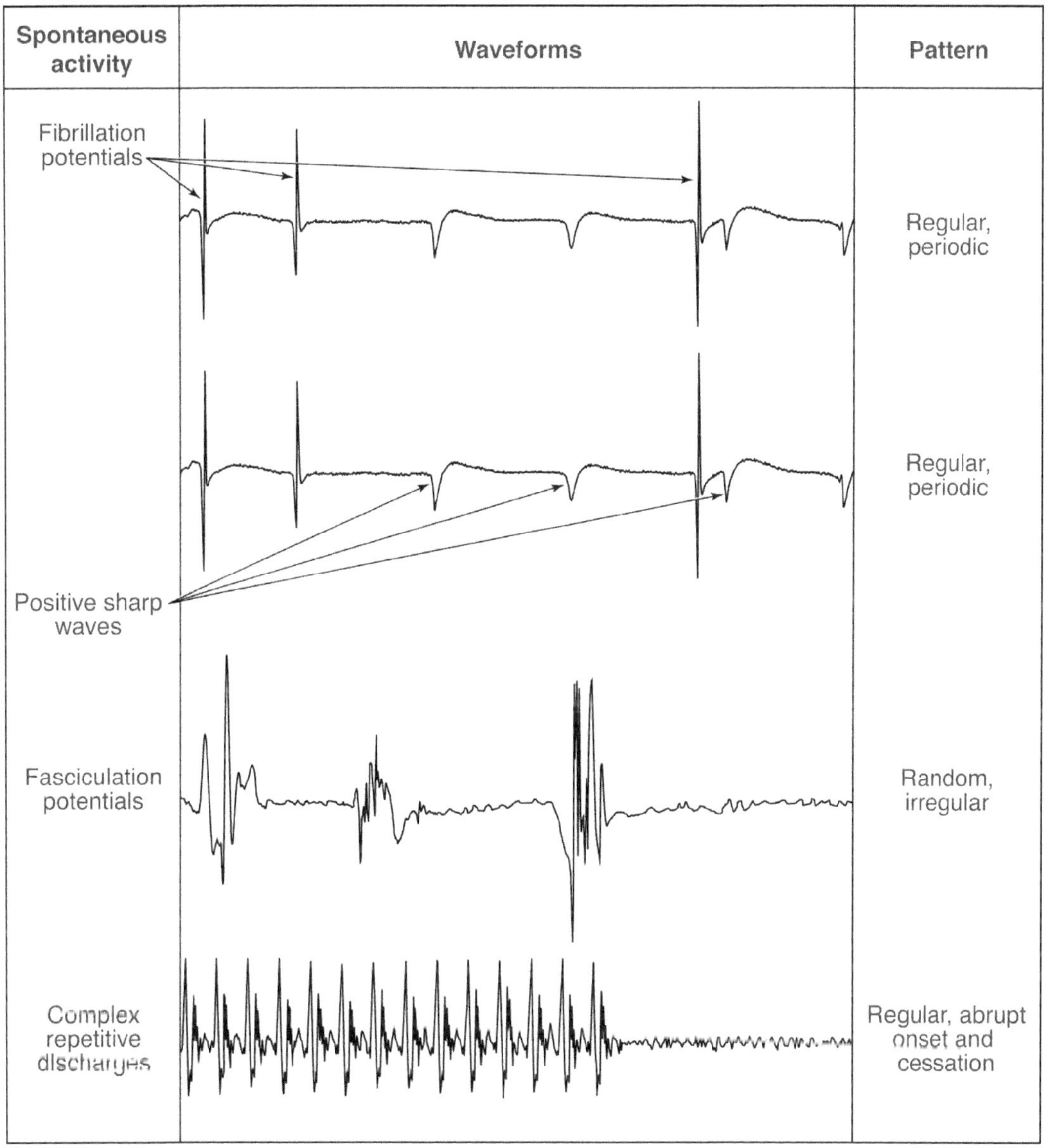

FIGURE 2-3 Examples of fibrillation potentials, positive sharp waves, fasciculation potentials, and complex repetitive discharges. These are the four most common and most basic types of spontaneous activity.

The basic types of spontaneous activity include fibrillation potentials, positive sharp waves, fasciculation potentials, and complex repetitive discharges (Figure 2-3).

Fibrillation potentials and *positive sharp waves* represent single muscle fiber activation that occurs in any muscle fiber that is not innervated, either due to neurogenic or myopathic processes. In neurogenic disorders such as mononeuropathies, plexopathies, radiculopathies, and motor neuron disease, loss of motor axons leads to denervation of muscle fibers. Conversely, in myopathic disorders, muscle fiber necrosis, fiber splitting, or inflammation may separate the muscle fibers from the motor axons or endplate zones, leading to denervation of muscle fibers. Both fibrillation potentials and positive sharp waves are usually seen together in denervated muscle, and both typically fire at a constant rate (i.e., in a regular or rhythmic pattern), although infrequently either can fire irregularly. In routine clinical practice, a numeric grading scale serves to semi-quantify fibrillation potentials and positive sharp waves on a scale of +1 to +4 (Figure 2-4; modified from Kimura, 1989).

Fasciculation potentials (Figure 2-3) are random isolated spontaneous discharges of a single motor unit or portion of a motor unit. The mechanical equivalent is the fasciculation, which is associated with spontaneous twitching of muscle fibers that may produce movement on the overlying skin or surface of the tongue. However, fasciculation potentials that lie deep in the muscle can only be documented with the needle examination. Fasciculation potentials can be observed in foot or gastrocnemius muscles of normal subjects, but they are usually more widespread or more frequent in the same pathological conditions that give rise to fibrillation potentials and positive sharp waves. Hence, the best way to evaluate fasciculation potentials is to analyze "the company that they keep" (Dumitru et al., 2002).

Complex repetitive discharges (CRDs; Figure 2-3) are spontaneous rapidly firing high-frequency discharges that form repetitive simple or complex patterns. They produce a distinct sound likened to a motorcycle or motorboat, but the hallmark of these waveforms is that they start and stop abruptly. Nerve blocks and curare do not abolish CRDs, suggesting that these discharges originate in muscle tissue (Dumitru et al., 2002) driven by ephaptic transmission of denervated muscle fibers and circular movements of currents

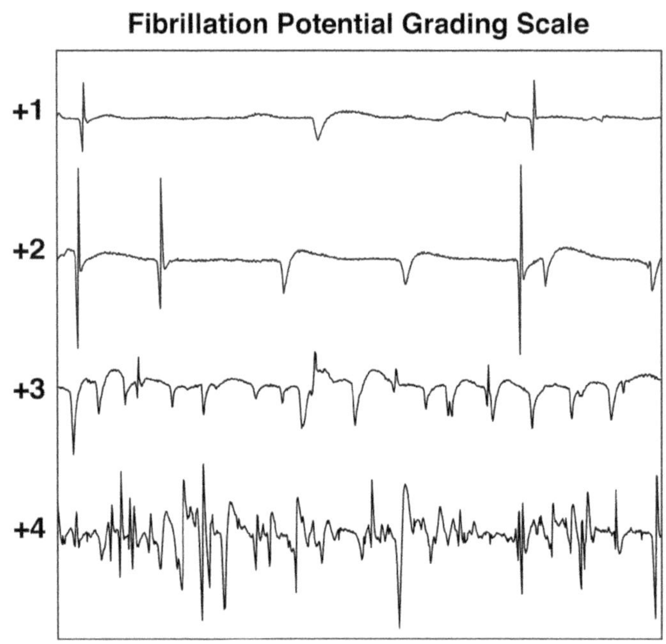

FIGURE 2-4 Numeric grading scale to semi-quantify fibrillation potentials and positive sharp waves. **+1:** Reproducible increased insertional activity or sparse fibrillation potentials or positive sharp waves. **+2:** More noticeable spontaneous activity in more than two different sites in a muscle. **+3:** Abundant spontaneous activity regardless of the position of the needle. **+4:** Marked fibrillation potentials and positive sharp waves that fill the screen.

among a group of muscle fibers (Kimura, 1989). When seen in lower motor neuron disorders, the distribution of spontaneous activity is an important aid in localizing lesions to the anterior horn cells, spinal roots, plexus, or peripheral nerve.

Less common forms of spontaneous activity include myotonic discharges, myokymic discharges, neuromyotonic discharges, and cramp discharges.

Myotonic discharges (Figure 2-5) are action potentials from single muscle fibers that fire in a prolonged fashion after mechanical irritation (Daube and Rubin, 2009). The discharges wax and wane in amplitude and frequency, giving rise to a characteristic "dive-bomber" sound. The classic disorders associated with myotonic discharges include myopathies with clinical features of myotonia (e.g., delayed relaxation of skeletal muscle following voluntary contraction) such as myotonic dystrophies, myotonia congenita, and paramyotonia congenita. However, myopathies without clinical myotonia can also give rise to myotonic discharges (hyperkalemic periodic paralysis, polymyositis, acid maltase deficiency, and occasionally toxic myopathies).

Myokymic discharges (Figure 2-5) are groups of recurrent spontaneously firing motor unit potentials (MUPs) that fire in characteristic regular, semirhythmic, or occasionally irregular repetitive bursts often described as sounding like "marching soldiers." Each burst

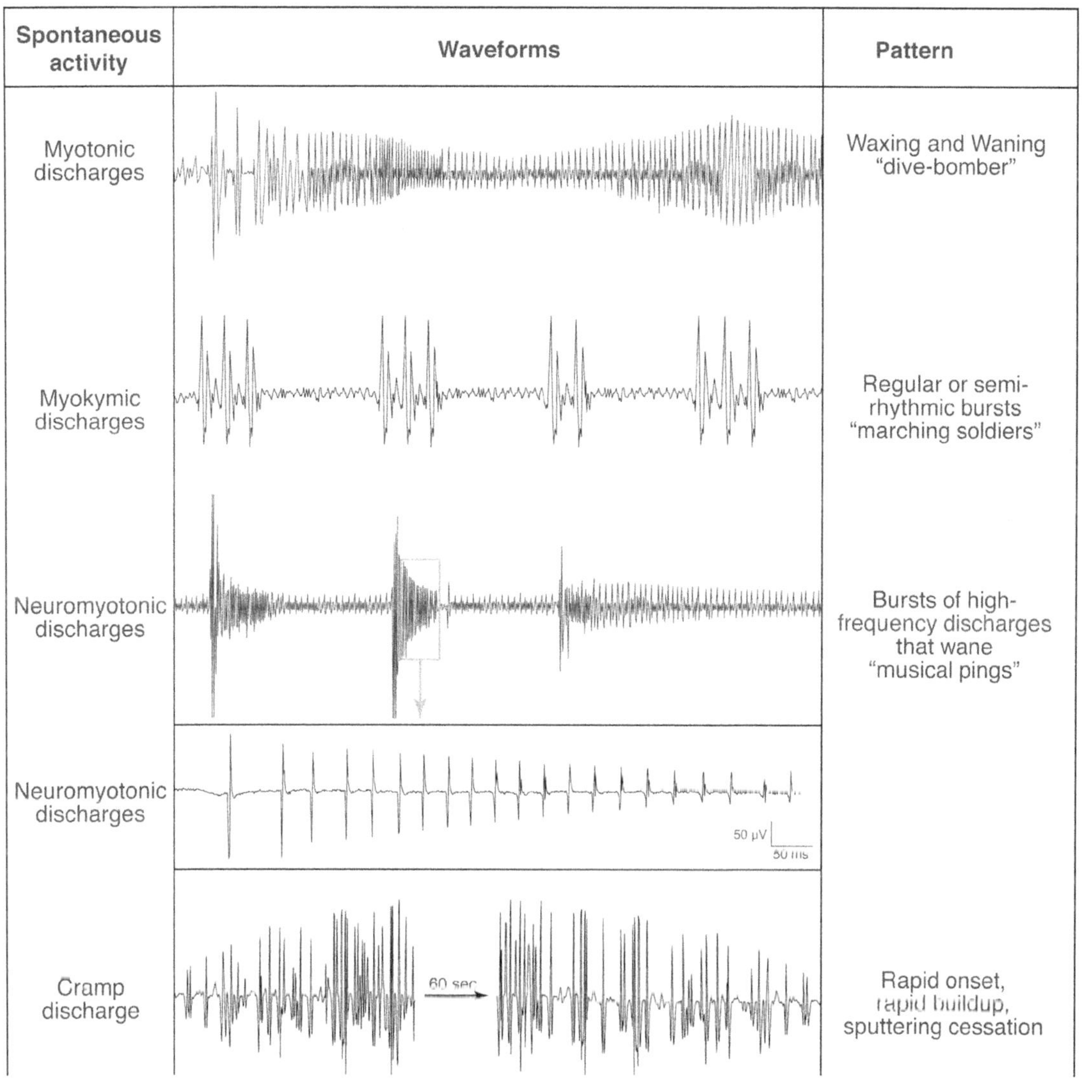

FIGURE 2-5 Examples of myotonic discharges, myokymic discharges, neuromyotonic discharges, and cramp discharges.

may be composed of from 2 to 10 MUPs (Daube and Rubin, 2009). Myokymic discharges may be associated with clinical myokymia, which appears as fine, "worm-like" quivering muscle twitches. Clinically, myokymia is often observed in facial muscles, although myokymic discharges are more commonly recorded in limb muscles. Disorders associated with facial myokymic discharges include multiple sclerosis, brainstem tumors (glioma, schwannoma), Bell's palsy, radiation therapy to head, and occasionally Guillain-Barré syndrome. The disorder that is typically associated with limb myokymic discharges is radiation plexopathy, although many disorders of peripheral nerve hyperexcitability (Isaac's syndrome, cramp-fasciculation syndrome), toxins (rattlesnake, herbicides, insecticides), systemic conditions (hypocalcemia, thyroid disease), and focal nerve lesions can also give rise to myokymic discharges (http://neuromuscular.wustl.edu/).

Neuromyotonic discharges (Figure 2-5) are bursts of motor unit potentials that originate in the motor axons and fire at high rates (100 to 300 Hz). The discharges often last several seconds and can start abruptly, although the amplitude of the discharges typically decreases or wanes because muscle fibers cannot maintain discharge rates > 100 Hz. The high-frequency decrementing nature of the discharges can produce unique musical sounds described as "pings," which distinguish these discharges from complex repetitive discharges or myotonic discharges (Kimura, 1989). Neuromyotonic discharges can occur spontaneously or be precipitated by needle movement, percussion of the nerve, ischemia, or voluntary muscle contraction or exercise. The classic disorder associated with these discharges is Isaac's syndrome (also known as neuromyotonia or continuous muscle fiber activity syndrome), in which there is hyperexcitability or continuous firing of motor axons that activate muscle fibers. Symptoms include progressive muscle stiffness that is most prominent in limb and trunk muscles, continuous contraction or twitching of muscles, cramps, increased sweating, and delayed muscle relaxation (NINDS information sheet on Isaac's syndrome). Isaac's syndrome is now considered to be an acquired form of the *peripheral nerve hyperexcitability* (PNH) syndrome, a heterogeneous disorder involving peripheral nerves in patients with a high propensity for developing autoimmunity (Rubio-Agusti et al., 2011). Associated neuromuscular diseases include myositis, nonspecific myopathic changes, myasthenia gravis, and antibodies to voltage-gated potassium channels on the motor nerve. There is also an association with paraneoplastic syndromes (thymoma, thyroid carcinoma, other cancers).

Cramp discharges (Figure 2-5) are involuntary repetitive firing of MUPs at a relatively high frequency (40 Hz to 60 Hz) usually associated with painful and palpable muscle contraction. Typically, potentials in a cramp have a rapid onset and rapid buildup characterized by an increase in the discharge frequency and the number of recruited MUPs. This is followed by a gradual or "sputtering" decrease in discharge frequency and number of MUPs as the cramp subsides. Cramps in gastrocnemius muscles occurring after voluntary contraction, and nocturnal cramps limited to the anatomical leg or foot, are usually considered normal. However, cramps in other muscles are often associated with other neuromuscular disorders of motor neurons, roots, nerves, or muscle, and in disorders of peripheral nerve hyperexcitability, such as Isaac's syndrome or cramp-fasciculation syndrome. In addition, systemic disorders associated with cramps include dehydration, metabolic abnormalities such as low sodium, magnesium, or calcium, thyroid disease (hyper- or hypo-), and pregnancy (http://neuromuscular.wustl.edu/).

Muscle fibers show spontaneous activity when the needle electrode is positioned near the region of the end-plate. This *end-plate activity* is normal and has no clinical significance (Daube and Rubin, 2009). The end-plate activity may present as either end-plate noise or end-plate spikes. End-plate noise reflects the normally occurring, spontaneous release of individual quanta of acetylcholine at the neuromuscular junction that produces miniature end-plate potentials (MEPPs). These MEPPs are recorded as low-amplitude, usually monophasic potentials that occur in a dense, steady pattern that gives rise to the characteristic "sea-shell sound" or "sea-shell roar" (Figure 2-6). End-plate spikes are moderate-amplitude, short duration spikes generated by muscle fibers that are activated follow-

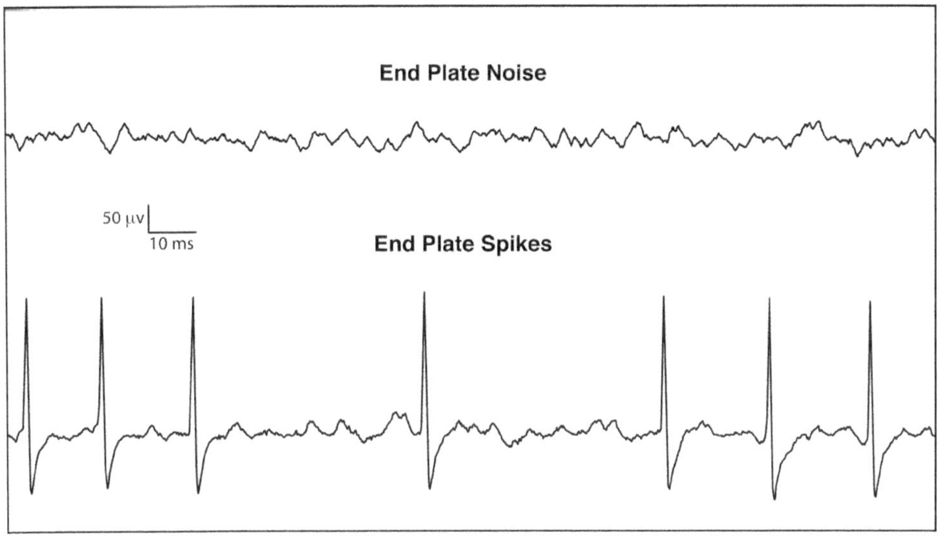

FIGURE 2-6 End-plate activity.

ing mechanical irritation of the nerve terminal by the needle. End-plate spikes often occur in the presence of end-plate noise and characteristically fire in a very irregular pattern, producing a crispy sound like "sputtering fat in a frying pan" or "slowly ripping Velcro." The irregular firing and the underlying end-plate noise distinguish end-plate activity from fibrillation potentials or voluntarily recruited motor unit potentials. Needle placement near an end-plate usually evokes more pain. Accordingly, the needle should be quickly repositioned away from this region.

Assessment of Motor Unit Potentials

All voluntary muscle activity is controlled by the motor unit (motor neurons and corresponding innervated muscle fibers, Figure 2-1) and recorded electrically as the motor unit potential (MUP). Hence, the MUP reflects the sum of all individual muscle fiber potentials from a single motor unit that occur almost synchronously within the recording radius of the needle electrode. Many factors affect or alter the morphology of the MUP. The spatial relationship between the needle and the muscle fibers is vital, and slight repositioning of the needle will often redefine the MUP. The needle electrode is positioned to minimize the *rise time*, which is the time lag between the initial positive peak of the MUP and the subsequent negative peak (Figure 2-7). By convention, only MUPs with a rise time of < 0.5 ms, preferably < 0.2 ms, are analyzed (Kimura, 1989). An MUP with a rise time of 0.2 ms will produce a crisp sound, whereas one with a rise time of >0.5 ms will produce a dull or "thuddy" sound.

In routine clinical EMG practice, the assessment of MUPs is accomplished primarily by visual inspection and semi-quantitative analysis during a low-level voluntary contraction. The MUP is usually categorized by its duration, amplitude, number of phases (biphasic, triphasic, polyphasic) or number of turns, and pattern of recruitment (normal, neurogenic, myopathic; Figure 2-7). The *duration* of an MUP is the time from the initial deflection away from the baseline to the final return to baseline (Daube and Rubin, 2009). It reflects the area of the motor unit, since even relatively distant muscle fibers may contribute to the initial and terminal low-amplitude portions of the MUP. The duration normally varies from 5 ms to 15 ms, with values gradually increasing with age (Kimura, 1989). The *amplitude* of the MUP is measured from the peak-to-peak of the potential. The amplitude is determined from the action potentials of muscle fibers that are in the vicinity of the tip of the needle electrode. It is estimated that in the normal state, only about 20 muscle fibers contribute to the major spike of the MUP. Distant

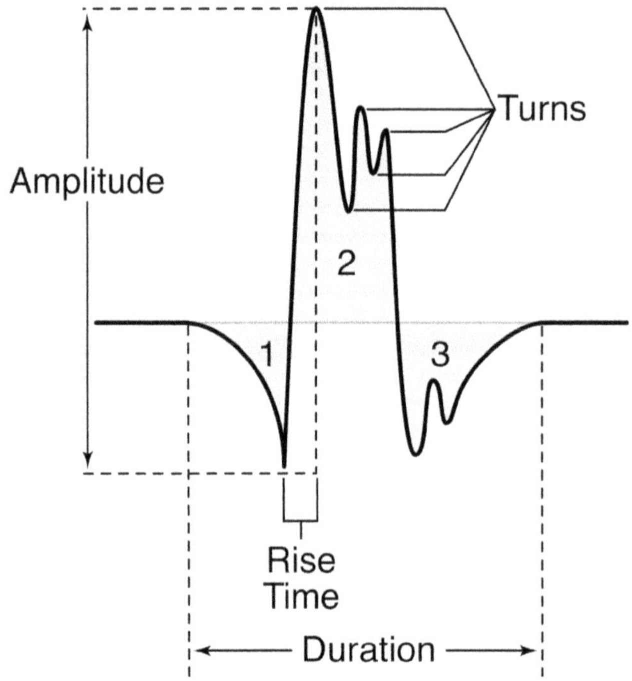

FIGURE 2-7 Motor unit potential (MUP) parameters. The gray areas numbered 1–3 reflect the three phases of the MUP. The evaluation of MUPs is critically important in the interpretation of EMG studies, and the majority of the time spent performing the needle examination involves the assessment of voluntarily recruited MUPs.

muscle fibers contribute little to the amplitude, despite the fact that all muscle fibers in a motor unit discharge in near synchrony. The MUP amplitude normally ranges from about 500 μV to about 2 mV, although nonphysiologic factors also play a role, including type of needle electrode, amplifier properties, filter settings, and display sensitivity and sweep. Both MUP duration and amplitude also vary with the muscle being sampled, patient's age, and intramuscular temperature; cooling increases the duration and amplitude of an MUP.

The number of *phases* of an MUP is defined as the number of times that the potential crosses the baseline plus one (i.e., phases = baseline crossings + 1). Normally, MUPs have four or fewer phases (Kimura, 1989), and are typically biphasic or triphasic. The configuration depends on the synchrony of firing of the muscle fibers in the vicinity of the needle. MUPs with more than four phases are termed *polyphasic*, and are usually less than 15% of analyzed MUPs in most muscles. However, some MUPs also show several *turns* or directional changes without crossing the baseline. These serrated MUPs, with excessive turns and polyphasic MUPs, reflect excessive desynchronization of the action potentials of muscle fibers near the needle.

Assessment of Firing Pattern and Recruitment

MUPs are further characterized by their firing pattern and recruitment. All MUPs under voluntary control fire in a semi-rhythmic (nearly regular) pattern. MUP recruitment reflects the progressive activation of a muscle by successive recruitment of motor units (motor neurons) to accomplish a motor task. Hence, MUP recruitment reflects how many motor neurons are activated for a particular muscle, and is therefore a measure of how many muscle fibers of that muscle are activated; the higher the recruitment, the stronger the muscle contraction. Motor units (and MUPs) are generally recruited in order of smallest to largest as contraction increases; i.e., smallest motor neurons with fewest muscle fibers to largest motor neurons with most muscle fibers. This orderly pattern of recruitment is known as *Henneman's Size Principle* (Henneman et al., 1965; Henneman, 1990), and is a useful concept for understanding the control of muscle contraction (Figure 2-8).

The morphology of the MUP in conjunction with the pattern of MUP recruitment usually make it possible to determine if an abnormality reflects a disorder of nerve origin or a disorder of muscle origin. The terms *neurogenic* or *neuropathic* have often been used to refer to disorders of nerve, while the term *myopathic* has been used to refer to disorders of muscle (Figure 2-9). Although such terms have been discouraged in favor of more descriptive features of the MUP (Kimura, 1989), the concept of inferring the underlying disease process based on the MUP characteristics is fundamental to the practice of EMG. In *neurogenic* disorders associated with focal demyelination (conduction block) or acute loss of motor axons, there are fewer MUPs available to accomplish the motor task. Consequently, there is a reduced pattern of recruitment reflecting the reduced number of MUPs. The limited number of remaining MUPs must fire at higher frequencies to accomplish the motor task; the more severe the loss of nerve fibers or the block in conduction, the fewer the MUPs. In extreme cases, there may be a single MUP on the screen firing at very high frequency (≥50 Hz, see bottom of Figure 2-9). The MUPs in neurogenic disorders due to conduction block or acute axonal loss are normal in morphology (phases, duration, and amplitude). In contrast, in neurogenic disorders associated with chronic axonal loss, MUPs are typically polyphasic, long duration, and high amplitude (Figure 2-9), reflecting reinnervation (the addition of muscle fibers by reinnervation will make an MUP larger). However, there is still reduced recruitment because of the reduced number of MUPs, and the rate of firing will still be excessively fast. Such disorders include motor neuron disease, radiculopathy, plexopathy, axonal mononeuropathy, and axonal polyneuropathy.

In *myopathic* disorders due to injury or damage of muscle fibers, there are relatively normal numbers of MUPs available to accomplish the motor task. However, the MUPs are typically short duration and low amplitude, reflecting damaged muscle fibers (loss of muscle fibers in a myopathy will make an MUP smaller). Because the injured muscle fibers produce less force, more MUPs need to be recruited to accomplish the motor task. This results in the characteristic "early" recruitment, in which an excessive number of small MUPs are recruited relative to the force of contraction (see top of Figure 2-9). In cases of

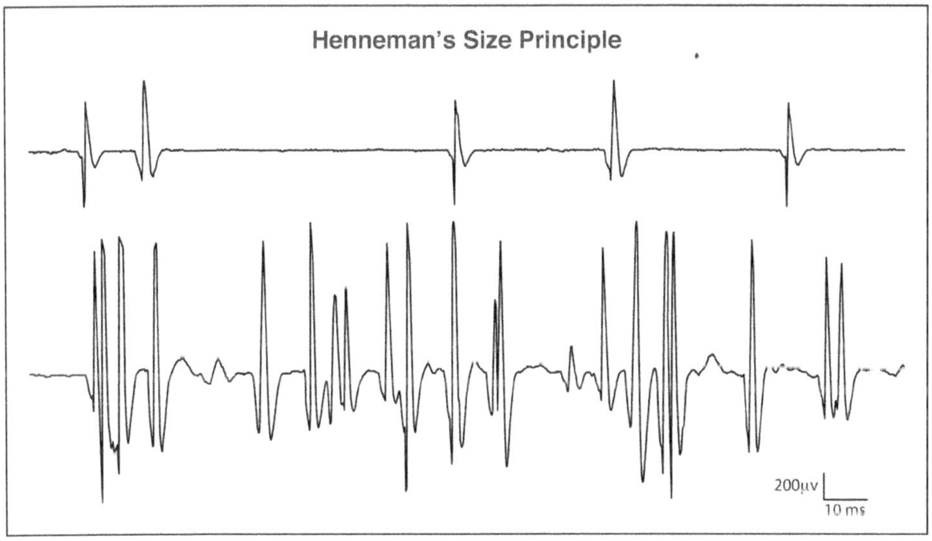

FIGURE 2-8 According to Henneman's Size Principle, smaller motor neurons innervating smaller motor units discharge initially with minimal effort. These smaller motor units give rise to smaller motor unit potentials, MUPs (top tracing). With greater effort of contraction, larger motor neurons innervating larger motor units are activated, giving rise to larger MUPs (bottom tracing).

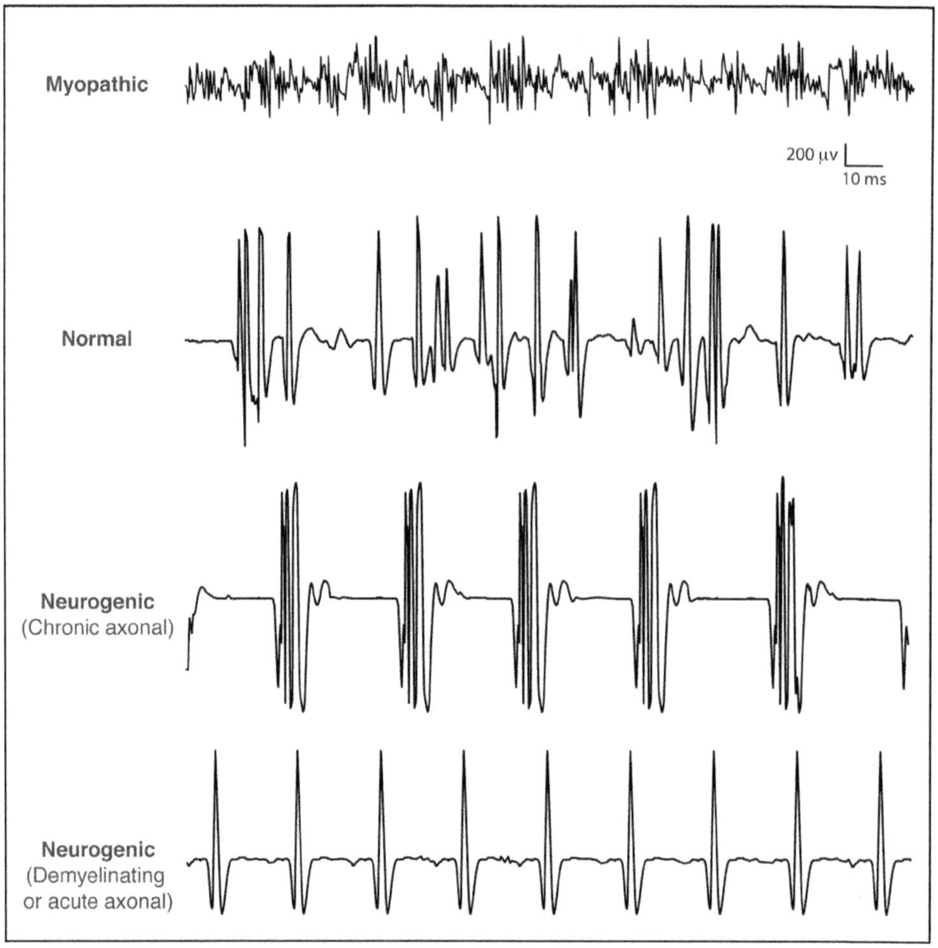

FIGURE 2-9 Examples of myopathic, normal, and neurogenic recruitment of motor unit potentials (MUPs). In myopathic disorders, there is full recruitment of small MUPs relative to force of contraction. In neurogenic disorders, there is a loss of motor units in a muscle, either because of loss of motor axons or conduction block, such that the reduced number of MUPs must fire at higher frequencies to accomplish the motor task.

severe muscle injury, a full pattern of small MUPs may flood the screen during minimal muscle contractions. This type of recruitment is the hallmark of myopathic disorders.

COMPLICATIONS RELATED TO NEEDLE ELECTROMYOGRAPHY

Complications related to needle EMG are rare (Al-Shekhlee et al., 2003). In patients taking anticoagulant or antiplatelet medications, hematoma formation from a standard needle EMG is rare (Lynch et al., 2008). Moreover, when hematomas do occur, they are usually small and subclinical. However, there are anecdotal reports of paraspinal or lower limb hematomas following needle examination in patients on anticoagulants (Daube and Rubin, 2009). Accordingly, when needle EMG is performed on fully anticoagulated patients, it is prudent to define the minimal number of muscles necessary to confirm or exclude a suspected diagnosis. Firm pressure should also be placed on the puncture site for about 1 minute following the examination. In addition, deep muscles (e.g., paraspinal muscles) should probably be avoided, particularly in obese subjects, since visual identification of hematoma will be lost. In patients with thrombocytopenia, if the platelet count is > 30, 000/mm^2, the needle examination can usually be performed safely (Daube and Rubin, 2009). If the platelet count is < 30, 000/mm^2, the needle examination should be rescheduled. In patients with hemophilia or other inherited bleeding disorders, hematoma formation associated with clinical deficits may be more common than reported (personal experience of the author AAL). For this reason, the patient's internist or hematologist should be consulted prior to the needle examination.

In patients with transmissible diseases, including human immunodeficiency virus (HIV), viral hepatitis, or rapidly progressive dementia suggesting Creutzfeldt-Jacob disease, universal precautions should be taken when performing the EMG (see universal precautions fact sheet, CDC Home Page). It is therefore imperative that patients be questioned about transmissible diseases prior to the needle examination.

In patients with skin infections (e.g., cellulitis), the needle should not be inserted into the area of infection (AANEM Position Statement, 2009). In patients with severe lymphedema, stagnant flow of tissue fluid through the limb may predispose to infections that are difficult to treat. Accordingly, caution should be exercised in performing needle examinations in lymphedematous regions to avoid complications (AANEM Position Statement, 2009). In contrast, there is no contraindication to performing a needle examination in a patient with a cardiac pacemaker or valvular heart disease or prosthetic valves. Needle EMG is not listed in American Heart Association guidelines as a procedure requiring prophylactic antibiotic treatment to prevent endocarditis in patients with valvular heart disease (AANEM Position Statement, 2009).

REFERENCES

Al-Shekhlee A, Shapiro BE, Preston DC. Iatrogenic complications and risks of nerve conduction studies and needle electromyography. *Muscle Nerve* 2003;27:517–526.

American Association of Neuromuscular & Electrodiagnostic Medicine. http://www.aanem.org/.

AANEM Position Statement. *Risks in Electrodiagnostic Medicine*. 2009. Available at: http://www.aanem.org/getmedia/2034191e-583b-4c55-b725-fc38ea8262e2/risksinEDX.pdf.aspx

American Clinical Neurophysiology Society. http://www.acns.org/.

Centers for Disease Control and Prevention (CDC) Home Page. Universal precautions fact sheet. Available at: http://www.cdc.gov/niosh/topics/bbp/universal.html.

Daube JR, Rubin DI. Needle electromyography. AANEM monograph. *Muscle Nerve* 2009;39:244–270.

Dumitru D, Amato AA, Zwarts M. *Electrodiagnostic Medicine*. 2nd ed. Hanley & Belfus, Inc., 2002.

Feinberg J. EMG: myths and facts. *HSS Journal*. 2006;2(1):19–21.

Henneman E, Somjen G, Carpenter DO. Functional significance of cell size in spinal motoneurons. *J Neurophysiol* 1965;28:560–580.

Henneman E. Comments on the logical basis of muscle control. In: *The Segmental Motor System*, edited by Binder MD and Mendell LM. New York: Oxford University Press, 1990, pp. 7–10.

Kimura J. Electrodiagnosis. In: *Diseases of Nerve and Muscle*. 2nd ed. FA Davis Co., Philadelphia, 1989.

Levin KH, Luders HO. *Comprehensive Clinical Neurophysiology*. WB Saunders Co., Philadelphia, 2000.

Lynch SL, Boon AJ, Smith J, Harper CM Jr, Tanaka EM. Complications of needle electromyography: hematoma risk and correlation with anticoagulation and antiplatelet therapy. *Muscle Nerve* 2008;38:1225–1230.

Rubio-Agusti I, Perez-Miralles F, Bataller L, et al. Peripheral nerve hyperexcitability. A clinical and immunologic study of 38 patients. *Neurology* 2011;76:172–178.

Sunderland S. *Nerves and Nerve Injuries*. 2nd ed. Churchill Livingstone, New York, 1978.

Washington University, St. Louis, Neuromuscular Disease Center. http://neuromuscular.wustl.edu/.

3 BRACHIAL PLEXUS

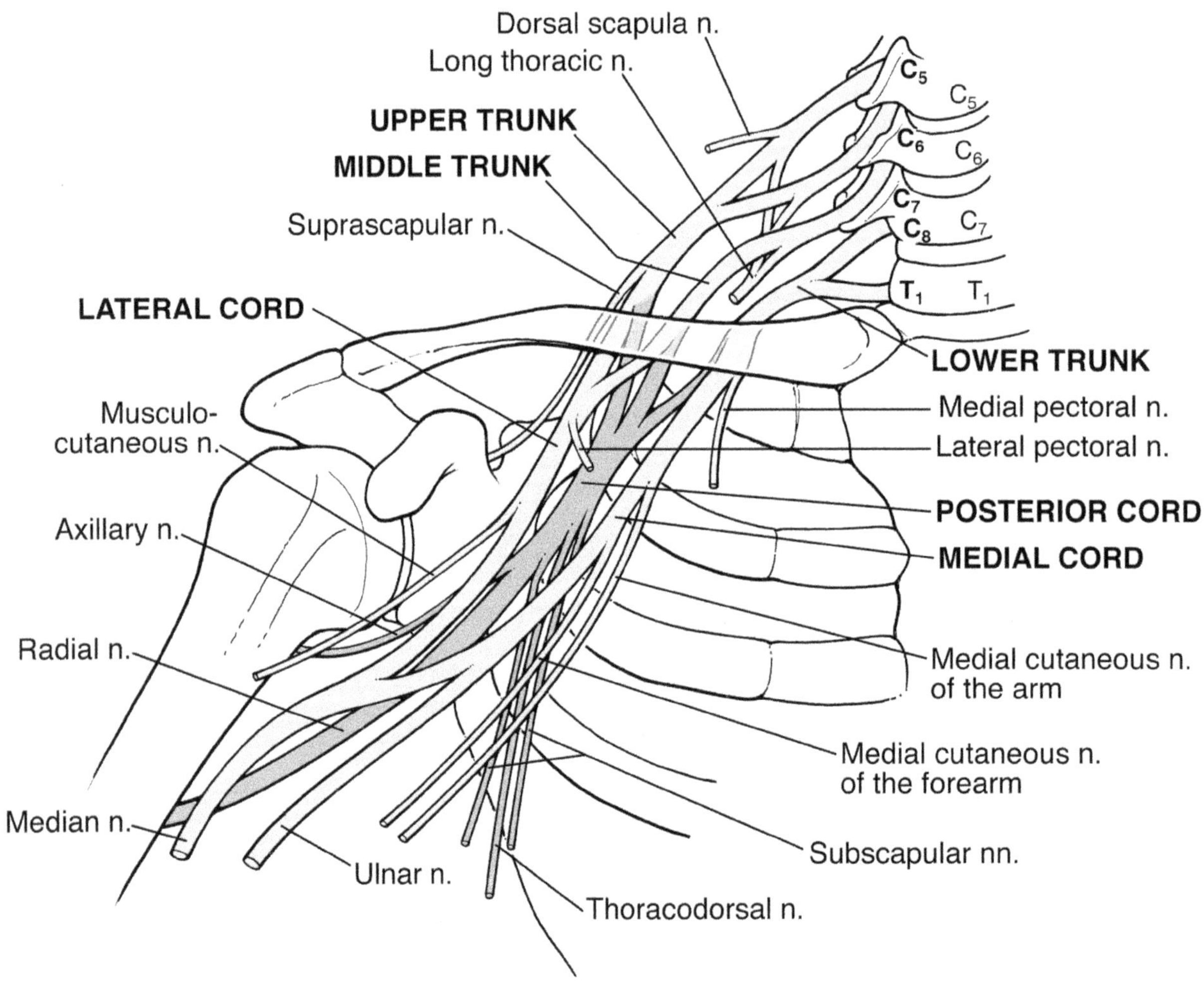

FIGURE 3-1 Brachial plexus and its branches, anterior view. See color insert

The brachial plexus (Figure 3-1) is formed by the union of the fifth, sixth, seventh, and eighth cervical ventral rami and the first thoracic ventral ramus (*Gray's Anatomy,* 1995). Contributions to the plexus from C_4 and T_2 vary. In a *prefixed* plexus, the contribution from C_4 is large and the branch from T_1 is reduced. In a *postfixed* plexus, the contribution from T_2 is large and the branch from C_5 is reduced. In the most common arrangement, the C_5 and C_6 rami unite at the lateral border of the scalenus medius to form the *upper trunk*, C_7 gives rise to the *middle trunk*, and C_8 and T_1 join behind the scalenus anterior as the *lower trunk*. The three trunks descend laterally; at the level of the clavicle, each trunk bifurcates into anterior and posterior divisions. The anterior divisions of the upper and middle trunks form the *lateral cord*, lateral to the axillary artery. The anterior division of the lower trunk emerges medial to the axillary artery to form the *medial cord*, which may also receive a branch from the C_7 ramus. Posterior divisions of all three trunks form the *posterior cord*, posterior to the axillary artery.

Brachial plexus lesions may involve the entire plexus or be confined to a particular part of it; the degree of nerve injury is seldom uniform. Acute lesions of the brachial plexus may be due to open or closed injury. In open injuries, wounding is commonly due to gunshot or sharp penetrating objects, and involves the more superficial part of the plexus. Wounding involving the lower plexus is more likely to be fatal because of simultaneous damage to the lung and great vessels at the root of the neck (Sunderland, 1968). In closed injuries the causative agent is commonly traction or compression of the plexus. Neuralgic amyotrophy, also known as idiopathic brachial plexopathy, Parsonage-Turner syndrome, shoulder girdle neuritis, or acute brachial neuropathy, ranks first in incidence among nontraumatic conditions (Beghi et al., 1985), and most commonly affects the upper plexus and shoulder girdle muscles (Subramony, 1988).

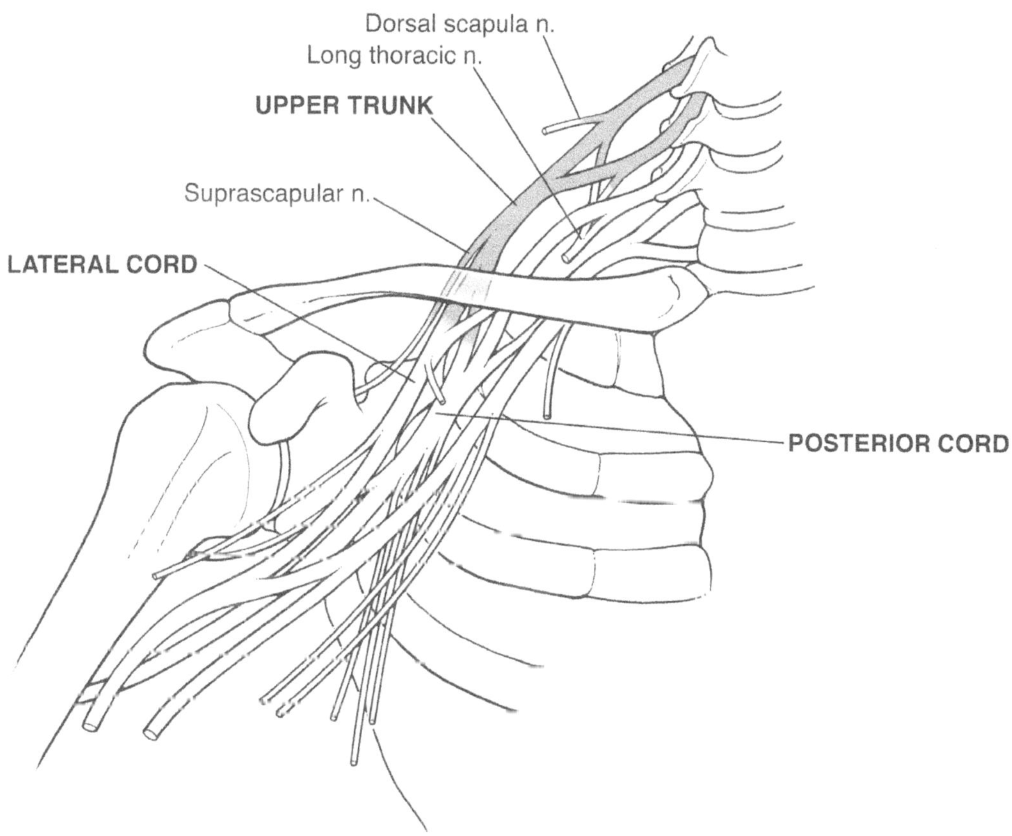

FIGURE 3-2 Upper trunk of brachial plexus.

UPPER TRUNK LESION (FIGURE 3-2)

Etiology

Neuralgic amyotrophy, also known as Parsonage-Turner syndrome or idiopathic brachial plexus neuritis, is the most common nontraumatic condition and usually affects the upper trunk and shoulder girdle muscles (Subramony, 1988; Sumner, 2009).

Trauma, including stab or gunshot wounds.

Stretch injuries occur when the neck and shoulder are violently forced apart, when a blow or heavy weight depresses the shoulder, or when an adducted limb is forced violently downward (Sunderland, 1968). Stretch injuries include traction injury during difficult delivery (birth palsy), "rucksack" or "pack palsy" due to lifting a heavy backpack, and the football injury known as a "stinger" (Kimura, 1989).

General Comments

Stretch injuries to the upper trunk may be combined with C_5, C_6 root avulsion (Erb's palsy).

Clinical Features

The distribution of weakness is similar to that of Erb's palsy, with involvement of the shoulder and upper arm and sparing of hand function.

There is gross wasting of shoulder girdle muscles with a complete inability to abduct or externally rotate the arm and marked weakness of elbow flexion and radial wrist extension.

Numbness occurs over the lateral aspects of the arm, forearm, and hand.

The biceps stretch reflex is absent or reduced.

Electrodiagnostic Strategy

Use nerve conduction studies to confirm a lesion of the upper trunk (low amplitude or unelicitable sensory responses from superficial radial, lateral cutaneous nerve of forearm and median nerve recording from thumb or index finger; low amplitude or unelicitable motor responses from biceps and deltoid). In a predominantly demyelinating lesion, routine nerve conduction studies may be normal; search for local demyelinating block or slowing of conduction across the site of injury. Note: Sensory responses are normal in radiculopathies because the lesion is proximal to the dorsal root ganglion (preganglionic lesion) and the cell bodies in the ganglion maintain viability of the peripheral sensory fibers.

Demonstrate neurogenic electromyography (EMG) needle examination (i.e., spontaneous activity, abnormal motor unit potentials, abnormal recruitment) in muscles supplied by the upper trunk.

Use needle EMG to exclude C_5,C_6 radiculopathies. Radiculopathies may produce neurogenic findings in paraspinal muscles as well as limb muscles; plexopathies never do so because the plexus is formed by *ventral rami*, whereas paraspinal muscles are innervated by *posterior rami* (Wilbourn, 1985).

MIDDLE TRUNK LESION (FIGURE 3-3)

Etiology

Neuralgic amyotrophy is a nontraumatic cause.

Isolated injury to the middle trunk is rare.

With lateral traction on the arm, the middle trunk may be the first to be injured (Sunderland, 1968).

General Comments

The middle trunk occupies a position between upper and lower trunks, being at times damaged with either the upper plexus or the lower plexus.

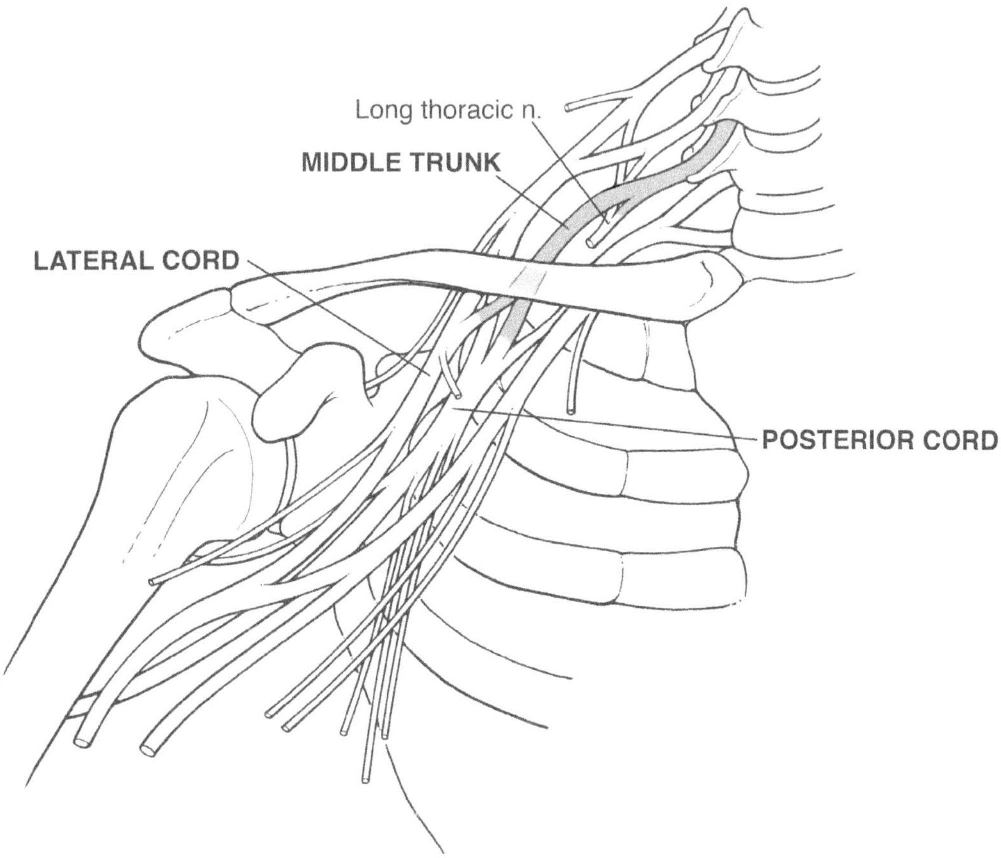

FIGURE 3-3 Middle trunk of brachial plexus.

Clinical Features

Weakness occurs in the general territory of the radial nerve, with partial involvement of the triceps and other C_7-innervated muscles and sparing of brachioradialis.

Numbness or loss of sensation occurs in the middle finger and sometimes the index finger.

The triceps stretch reflex may be reduced.

Electrodiagnostic Strategy

Nerve conduction studies may suggest a lesion of the middle trunk (low amplitude or unelicitable sensory responses from median nerve–innervated middle finger and possibly index finger; the remaining studies are normal). In a demyelinating lesion, routine nerve conduction studies may be normal; search for local demyelinating block or slowing of conduction across the site of injury. *Note*: Sensory responses are normal in a C_7 radiculopathy because the lesion is proximal to the dorsal root ganglion (preganglionic lesion) and the cell bodies in the ganglion maintain viability of the peripheral sensory fibers.

Demonstrate neurogenic EMG needle examination (i.e., spontaneous activity, abnormal motor unit potentials, abnormal recruitment) in muscles supplied by the middle trunk.

Use needle EMG to exclude C_7 radiculopathy. Radiculopathies may produce neurogenic EMG in paraspinal muscles as well as limb muscles; plexopathies never do so, because the plexus is formed by *ventral rami*, whereas paraspinal muscles are innervated by *posterior rami* (Wilbourn, 1985).

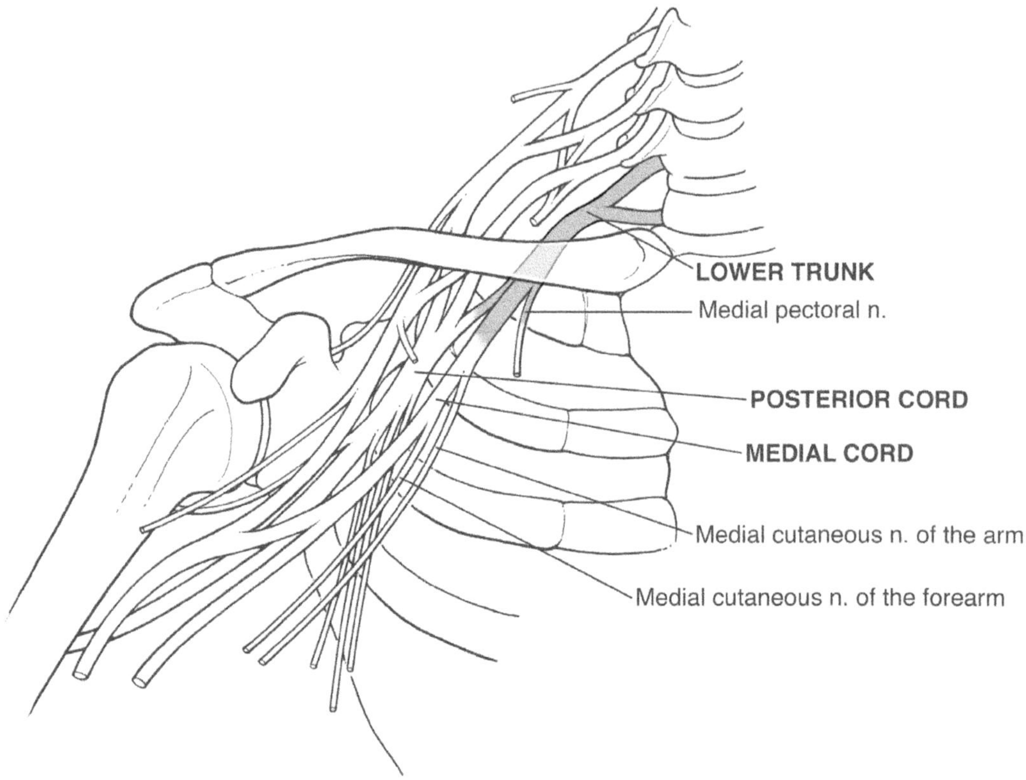

FIGURE 3-4 Lower trunk of brachial plexus.

LOWER TRUNK LESION (FIGURE 3-4)

Etiology

Metastasis (lymph node infiltration in axilla) or direct invasion (Pancoast's tumor in apex of lung) can cause a lower trunk lesion.

Neuralgic amyotrophy is a nontraumatic cause.

Neurogenic thoracic outlet syndrome (TOS) is a rare cause.

Traumatic causes include stab wounds and bullet wounds.

Traction applied to the fully abducted arm (i.e., subject jerked upward by the outstretched arm) can cause a lower trunk lesion.

General Comments

True neurogenic TOS is rare (1 per 1,000,000) and results from lower trunk fibers being stretched over a fibrous band extending from the first rib to the C_7 transverse process or a rudimentary cervical rib (Wilbourn, 1988).

When traction is applied to the fully abducted arm, it is the lower roots and trunk of the plexus that suffer most (Sunderland, 1968).

Stretch injuries to the lower trunk may be combined with C_8, T_1 root avulsion (Klumpke's palsy).

Clinical Features

The distribution of weakness is similar to that of Klumpke's palsy, with involvement of all intrinsic hand muscles and sparing of shoulder and upper arm muscles.

In addition to intrinsic hand muscles, finger flexors and extensors in the forearm are weak.

Numbness or loss of sensation occurs in the medial aspect of the arm, medial forearm, and medial hand, including fourth and fifth digits.

Electrodiagnostic Strategy

Use nerve conduction studies to localize a lesion to the lower trunk or medial cord (low amplitude or unelicitable sensory responses from little finger and medial cutaneous nerve of forearm; low amplitude or unelicitable motor responses from median and ulnar hand muscles). In a demyelinating lesion, special nerve conduction studies may be needed to demonstrate demyelinating block or slowing of conduction across the site of injury. *Note*: Sensory responses are normal in radiculopathies because the lesion is proximal to the dorsal root ganglion.

Demonstrate neurogenic EMG needle examination (i.e., spontaneous activity, abnormal motor unit potentials, abnormal recruitment) in muscles supplied by the lower trunk.

Exclude C_8, T_1 radiculopathies by needle EMG. Radiculopathies may produce neurogenic EMG in paraspinal muscles as well as limb muscles; plexopathies never do so, because the plexus is formed by *ventral rami*, whereas paraspinal muscles are innervated by *posterior rami* (Wilbourn, 1985).

PLEXUS CORD LESIONS

General Comments

The consequences of lesions affecting the lateral, medial, or posterior cords of the brachial plexus may be determined by combining the effects following injury to the individual nerves that originate from the respective cords (Sunderland, 1968).

REFERENCES

Beghi E, Kurland LT, Mulder D W, Nicolosi A. Brachial plexus neuropathy in the population of Rochester, Minnesota, 1970–1981. *Ann Neurol* 1985;18:320–323.

Gray's Anatomy. 38th Edition. Churchill Livingstone, New York, 1995, pp. 1266–1274.

Kimura J. *Electrodiagnosis in Diseases of Nerve And Muscle*. 2nd Edition. FA Davis, Philadelphia, 1989, pp 447–461.

Subramony SH. AAEE case report # 14: Neuralgic amyotrophy (acute brachial neuropathy). *Muscle Nerve* 1988; 11:39–44.

Sumner AJ. Idiopathic brachial neuritis. *Neurosurgery* 2009;65(4 Suppl):A150-152.

Sunderland S. *Nerves and Nerve Injuries*. Williams & Wilkins, Baltimore, 1968, pp. 953–1011.

Wilbourn AJ. Electrodiagnosis of plexopathies. *Neurol Clin* 1985;3:511–529.

Wilbourn AJ. Thoracic outlet syndrome surgery causing severe brachial plexopathy. *Muscle Nerve* 1988;11:66–74.

4 MEDIAN NERVE

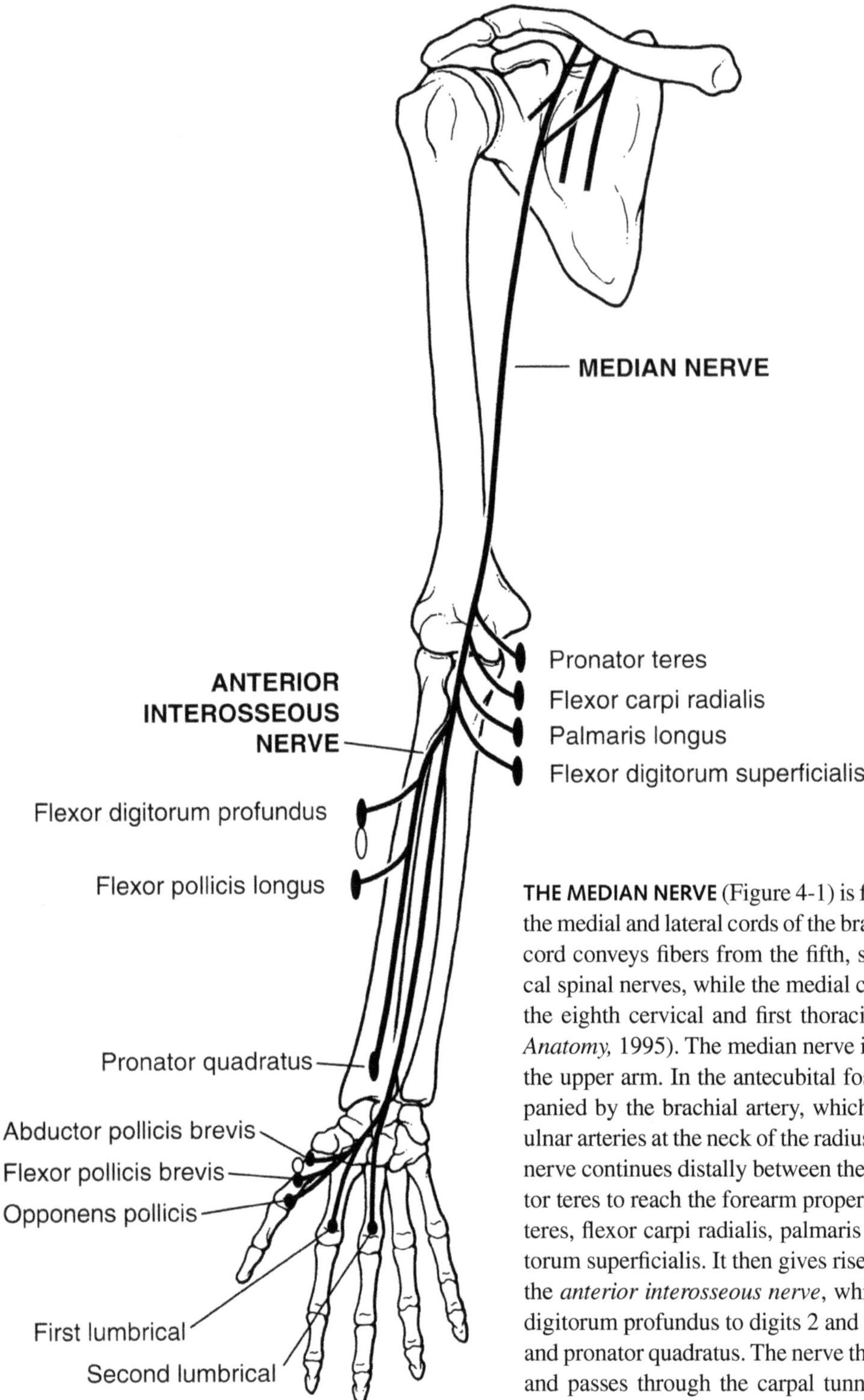

FIGURE 4-1 Diagram of the median nerve and the muscles that it supplies. Note: The white oval signifies that a muscle receives a part of its innervation from another peripheral nerve.

THE MEDIAN NERVE (Figure 4-1) is formed in the axilla from the medial and lateral cords of the brachial plexus. The lateral cord conveys fibers from the fifth, sixth, and seventh cervical spinal nerves, while the medial cord supplies fibers from the eighth cervical and first thoracic spinal nerves (*Gray's Anatomy,* 1995). The median nerve innervates no muscles in the upper arm. In the antecubital fossa, the nerve is accompanied by the brachial artery, which divides into radial and ulnar arteries at the neck of the radius. From this position, the nerve continues distally between the two heads of the pronator teres to reach the forearm proper. It supplies the pronator teres, flexor carpi radialis, palmaris longus, and flexor digitorum superficialis. It then gives rise to a pure motor branch, the *anterior interosseous nerve*, which innervates the flexor digitorum profundus to digits 2 and 3, flexor pollicis longus, and pronator quadratus. The nerve then descends the forearm and passes through the carpal tunnel as it enters the palm (Figure 4-2). It supplies the first and second lumbricals, and gives off the recurrent thenar branch to the abductor pollicis brevis, flexor pollicis brevis (superficial head), and opponens pollicis. The median nerve also subserves sensation to the

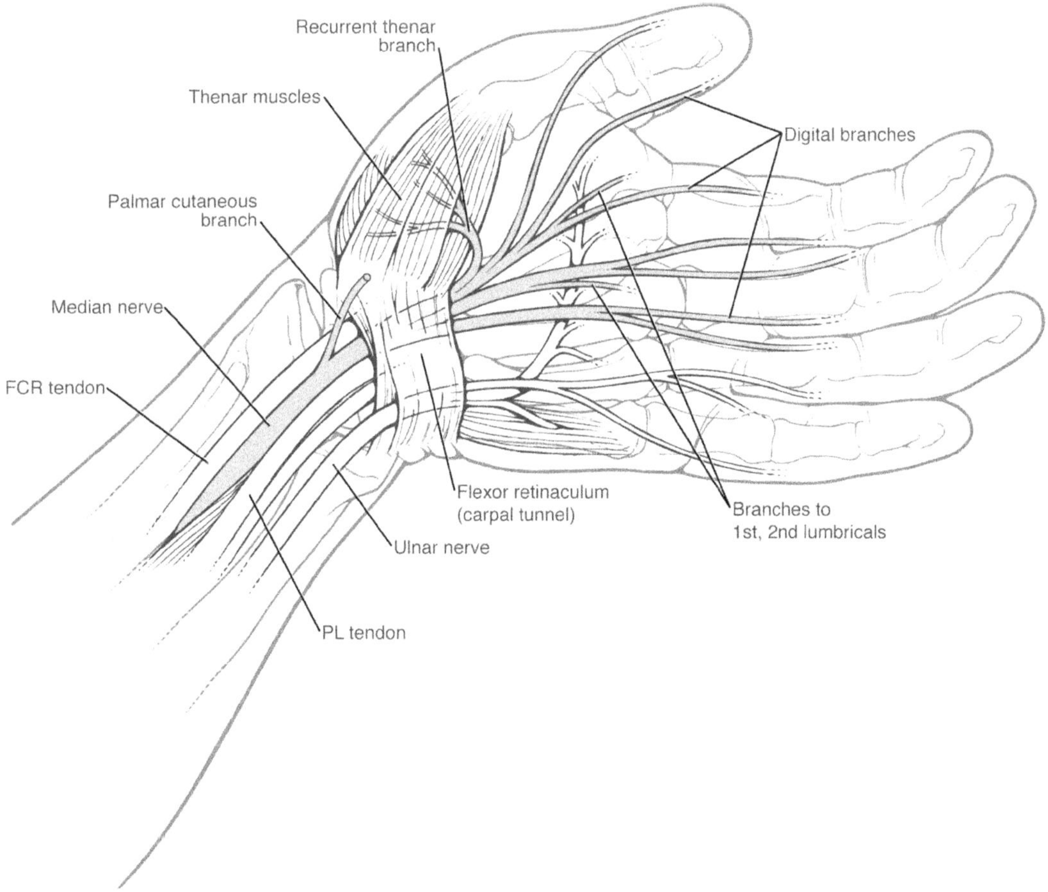

FIGURE 4-2 Anatomy of the median nerve at the wrist and palm.

skin overlying the lateral aspect of the palm, dorsal surface of the distal phalanges, volar surface of the thumb, index, and middle fingers, and half of the ring finger.

Although the median nerve, or its branches, may be affected by penetrating injuries at any level, there are certain sites where the nerve is prone to injury (Sunderland, 1968). In the upper arm, the nerve is closely bound to the axillary artery and then to the brachial artery as far as the cubital fossa. This close relationship explains why combined nerve–arterial injury is common in this region, and why the nerve is subject to compression from aneurysms. In the lower arm, a spur of bone may rarely project from the anteromedial aspect of the supracondylar surface of the humerus and be joined to the medial epicondyle by a strong ligament (Struthers' ligament). This ligament may compress the median nerve proximal to the innervation to the pronator teres. In the pronator teres syndrome, the median nerve is injured in the upper forearm due to trauma, fracture, or, under exceptional circumstances, compression between the two heads of the pronator teres or a fibrous band as it emerges from this muscle. More distally in the forearm, the anterior interosseous branch may be injured by trauma or as a consequence of neuralgic amyotrophy. Entrapment of the anterior interosseous nerve may also result from fibrous bands or anomalous muscles (Wertsch, 1992). At the wrist, damage to the median nerve is commonly due to compression of the nerve in the carpal tunnel. This results in *carpal tunnel syndrome*, the most common entrapment neuropathy in humans.

CARPAL TUNNEL SYNDROME

Etiology

Carpal tunnel syndrome is caused by compression of the nerve in the carpal tunnel.

General Comments

Carpal tunnel syndrome is the most common entrapment neuropathy.

Women are affected more often than men.

Symptoms usually involve the dominant hand, with a higher incidence in persons who use their hands occupationally.

Predisposing conditions include obesity, pregnancy, polyneuropathy, diabetes, amyloidosis, acromegaly, rheumatoid arthritis, hypothyroidism with myxedema, and lupus erythematosus.

Clinical Features

Hand pain may be perceived more proximally in the forearm, arm, or shoulder, mimicking cervical radiculopathy.

Numbness usually involves the lateral four digits, but all digits may be affected or sensory loss may be confined to one digit.

Pain and paresthesia are aggravated by repetitive use of the hand.

Patients characteristically awaken at night with symptoms (nocturnal paresthesia).

In severe cases, there is weakness and atrophy of thenar muscles.

Onset is insidious in most cases.

Electrodiagnostic Strategy

Use nerve conduction studies to confirm a focal lesion of median sensory and motor fibers in the carpal tunnel. Many techniques have been developed for identifying conduction abnormalities within the carpal tunnel (Ross and Kimura, 1995).

Perform EMG needle examination in thenar muscles. In carpal tunnel syndrome associated with loss of motor fibers, EMG will show neurogenic changes (i.e., spontaneous activity, abnormal motor unit potentials, abnormal recruitment).

If EMG of thenar muscles is abnormal, study proximal median-innervated muscles to exclude median nerve lesion above the wrist. Also, study C_8, T_1 muscles innervated by ulnar or radial nerves to exclude C_8, T_1 radiculopathy.

If clinical symptoms or signs suggest cervical radiculopathy, study muscles supplied by C_6 and C_7 roots to exclude C_6 or C_7 radiculopathy. The differential diagnosis for carpal tunnel syndrome includes C_6 and C_7 radiculopathies due to overlap of dermatomes with median sensory distribution.

ANTERIOR INTEROSSEOUS NERVE SYNDROME

Etiology

Neuralgic amyotrophy (idiopathic brachial plexopathy) may exclusively affect the anterior interosseous nerve (AIN).

Trauma, including stab wounds and gunshot wounds, can cause AIN syndrome.

Entrapment may rarely result from fibrous bands or anomalous muscles (Wertsch, 1992).

General Comments

The AIN is the largest branch of the median nerve.

It is a "pure" motor nerve because it lacks a cutaneous representation. However, sensory fibers from wrist and hand joints travel in the AIN.

The AIN innervates three muscles: flexor digitorum profundus (digits 2 and 3), flexor pollicis longus, and pronator quadratus.

Fifty percent of Martin-Gruber anastomoses arise from the AIN.

Clinical Features (Figure 4-3)

A typical symptom is acute onset of thumb and index finger weakness.

Numbness and tingling do not occur.

A dull, aching pain may be present in the volar wrist or forearm.

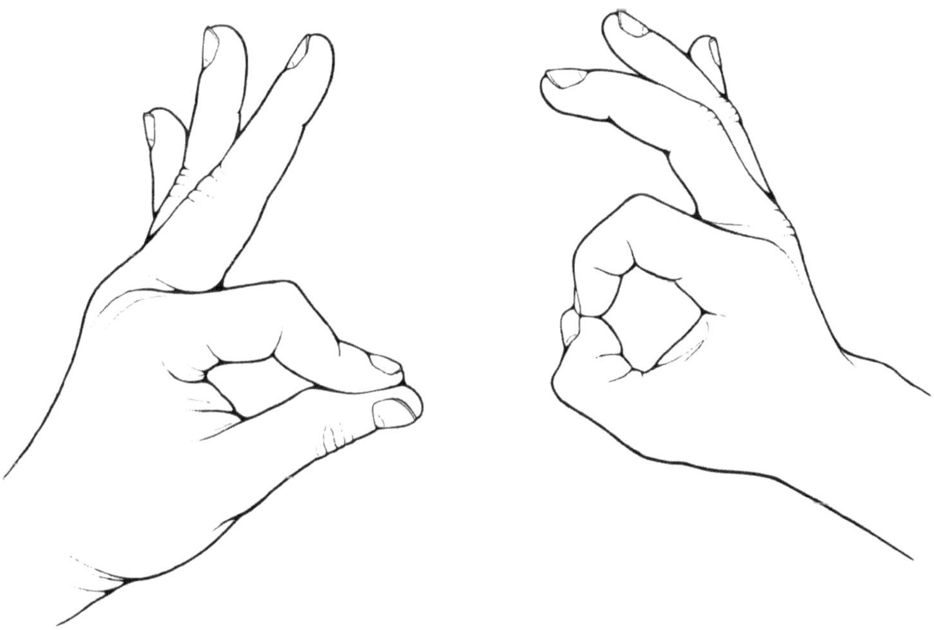

FIGURE 4-3 Clinical features of anterior interosseous nerve syndrome. Weakness of flexor pollicis longus and flexor digitorum profundus to digits 2 and 3 produces the characteristic inability to form an "O" with the thumb and index finger.

The patient is unable to form an "O" with the thumb and index finger (Figure 4-3), due to weak flexion of terminal phalanges of the thumb and index finger.

Weakness in the pronator quadratus may be difficult to detect.

In a person with Martin-Gruber anastomosis and AIN syndrome, there may be additional weakness or atrophy of intrinsic hand muscles supplied by the crossing fibers (Wertsch, 1992).

The cutaneous sensory examination is normal.

Electrodiagnostic Strategy

Routine nerve conduction studies are normal.

Perform EMG needle examination in multiple muscles, including proximal and scapular muscles. EMG is crucial for identifying the possibility that AIN syndrome is a manifestation of neuralgic amyotrophy.

In AIN syndrome, EMG will show neurogenic changes (spontaneous activity, abnormal motor unit potentials, abnormal recruitment) in the flexor digitorum profundus to digits 2 and 3, flexor pollicis longus, and pronator quadratus.

In a person with Martin-Gruber anastomosis and AIN syndrome, EMG may show neurogenic changes in muscles supplied by the crossing fibers (usually dorsal interossei, adductor pollicis, or abductor digiti minimi).

PRONATOR TERES SYNDROME

Etiology

Trauma, usually deep penetrating wounds, is causative.

Entrapment may rarely occur between the two heads of the pronator teres or by a fibrous band connecting the pronator teres with the tendinous arch of the flexor digitorum superficialis.

General Comments

Most investigators have never encountered a true entrapment of the median nerve as it passes through the pronator teres; there is some doubt as to whether such an entrapment exists.

Clinical Features

Pain and tenderness occur over the pronator teres.

Numbness or tingling can occur in the median sensory distribution of the hand, including over the proximal palm and thenar eminence. (Note: The palmar cutaneous branch is spared in carpal tunnel syndrome because it passes superficial to the carpal tunnel. Sensory deficits in the palm and thenar eminence can help to differentiate a proximal median neuropathy from carpal tunnel syndrome.)

In severe cases, there is weakness and atrophy of the median innervated muscles distal to the pronator teres.

Electrodiagnostic Strategy

Nerve conduction studies may show reduced conduction velocity or conduction block in the median nerve in the elbow to wrist segment.

EMG may show a neurogenic pattern in median-innervated muscles distal to the pronator teres.

LIGAMENT OF STRUTHERS' SYNDROME

Etiology

Entrapment is caused by Struthers' ligament (Figure 4-4), which is a fibrous band joining the supracondylar process (bony spur) on the anteromedial aspect of the lower humerus with the medial epicondyle of the humerus.

General Comments

A supracondylar process is present in only 0.3%–2.7% of humans (Pecina et al., 1997). When the supracondylar process is present, the median nerve, and sometimes the brachial artery, deviates medially to pass under Struthers' ligament.

Clinical Features

Pain and paresthesia occur in the median sensory distribution of the hand, including the palm and thenar eminence (Note: The palmar cutaneous branch is spared in the carpal tunnel syndrome because it passes superficial to the carpal tunnel.)

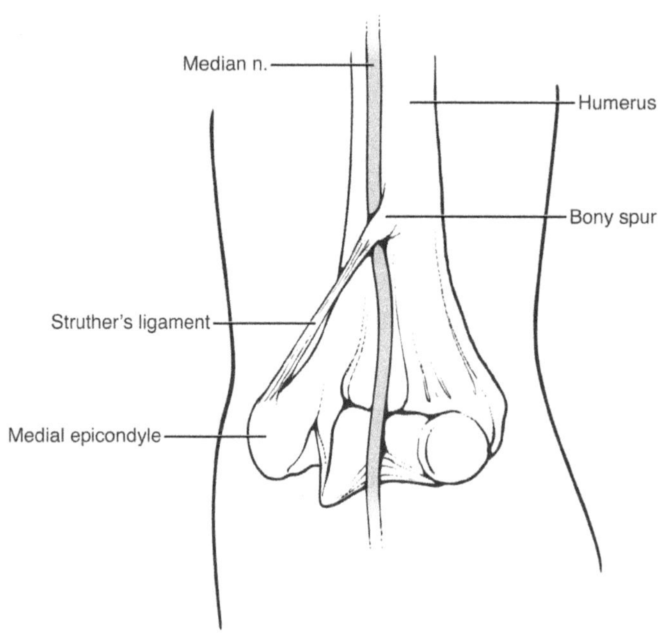

FIGURE 4-4 Anatomy of the ligament of Struthers' syndrome, anterior view of left arm.

In severe cases, there is weakness and atrophy of all median-innervated muscles, including the pronator teres. Weakness of pronation differentiates this condition from pronator teres syndrome.

Radiographic studies (plain films) show the supracondylar bony spur.

Electrodiagnostic Strategy

Nerve conduction studies may show reduced conduction velocity or conduction block in the median nerve in the upper arm to elbow segment.

Demonstrate neurogenic EMG in the median-innervated muscles, including the pronator teres.

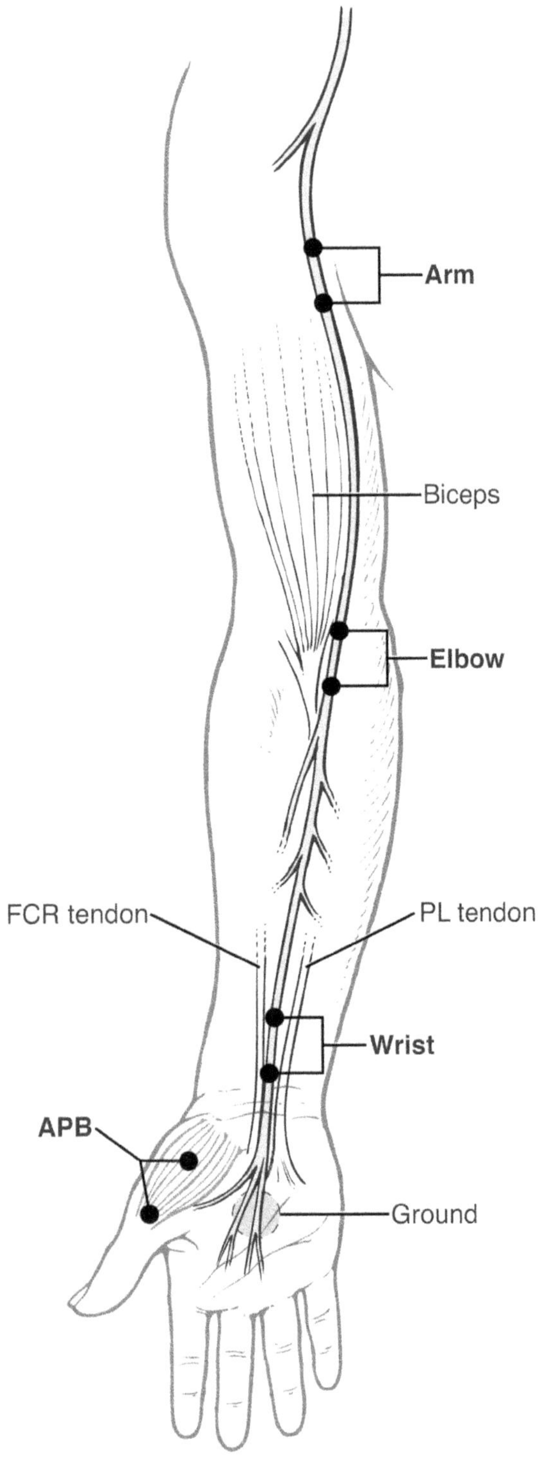

FIGURE 4-5 Median motor nerve conduction study.

MEDIAN NERVE CONDUCTION STUDIES

Median Motor Nerve Conduction Study

Recording (Figure 4-5)

Active electrode: position over the belly of the abductor pollicis brevis (APB) or opponens pollicis muscles.

Reference electrode: place over the tendon of the APB at the base of the proximal phalanx of the thumb (belly-tendon recording).

Ground electrode: place on the dorsum of the hand, between stimulating and recording electrodes.

Stimulation

Wrist: place cathode 2 to 3 cm proximal to the distal crease between the flexor carpi radialis (FCR) tendon and the palmaris longus (PL) tendon. Anode is 3 cm proximal to cathode. In an average size hand, this usually results in a distance of about 7 cm between cathode and active electrode.

Elbow: place cathode at the antecubital fossa over the brachial artery pulse, just medial to the biceps tendon. Anode is proximal to cathode.

Arm: place cathode at the upper arm just below the belly of the biceps muscle. Anode is proximal to cathode.

Normal Values

Distal latency (ms) ≤ 4.2

Amplitude (mV) ≥ 5.0

Conduction velocity (m/s) in wrist to elbow and elbow to arm segments > 50 m/s

Normal values differ depending on the distance used, size of the hand, and different recording techniques. The normal amplitude of the thenar CMAP has a very large range and standard deviation (Felsenthal, 1978). Therefore, nerve conduction studies should ideally be performed bilaterally because side-to-side comparisons are more useful than normal value tables that may not apply to your patient.

Stimulation (alternative technique)

Palm: the median nerve can be stimulated at the palm, although care should be taken to avoid coactivation of the deep ulnar motor branch. This technique is useful when wrist stimulation produces a low-amplitude CMAP, because it can identify conduction block at the carpal tunnel due to focal demyelination (neurapraxia) and distinguish it from loss of motor axons. In conduction block, the CMAP amplitude will normalize with stimulation distal to the carpal tunnel. In axonal loss, the CMAP elicited with stimulation across the carpal tunnel will remain absent or reduced.

Erb's point: stimulation at this proximal site can be performed in median or ulnar nerves, but is technically difficult, particularly in large or obese subjects. In many subjects, even maximal stimulation may not depolarize median or ulnar nerve fibers that lie deep within the lower trunk.

Short Segment Stimulation across the Palm ("inching technique")

Recording (Figure 4-6)

Identical recording technique as that used to elicit the CMAP during routine median motor conduction studies.

Stimulation

Stimulate at 1 cm or 2 cm intervals across the wrist (Kimura, 1989). An abrupt change in CMAP waveform indicates the point of localized conduction delay. In Figure 4-6, stimulation at 1 cm increments results in a motor conduction velocity of < 2 m/s across the carpal tunnel. An abrupt change in SNAP recording from digits can also localize the site of conduction delay.

Comments

In carpal tunnel syndrome (CTS), sensory responses are usually the first to show abnormality, so standard motor distal latency may be normal, borderline normal, or prolonged. When motor distal latency approaches borderline values (about 4.0 ms), comparative nerve conduction studies for the diagnosis of CTS should be performed.

CMAP abnormalities document motor fiber involvement and can be used to localize a lesion when SNAPs are absent (Stevens 1997).

Median (or ulnar) motor conduction studies are commonly used as a distal nerve in repetitive stimulation studies to look for a defect in neuromuscular transmission. Patients

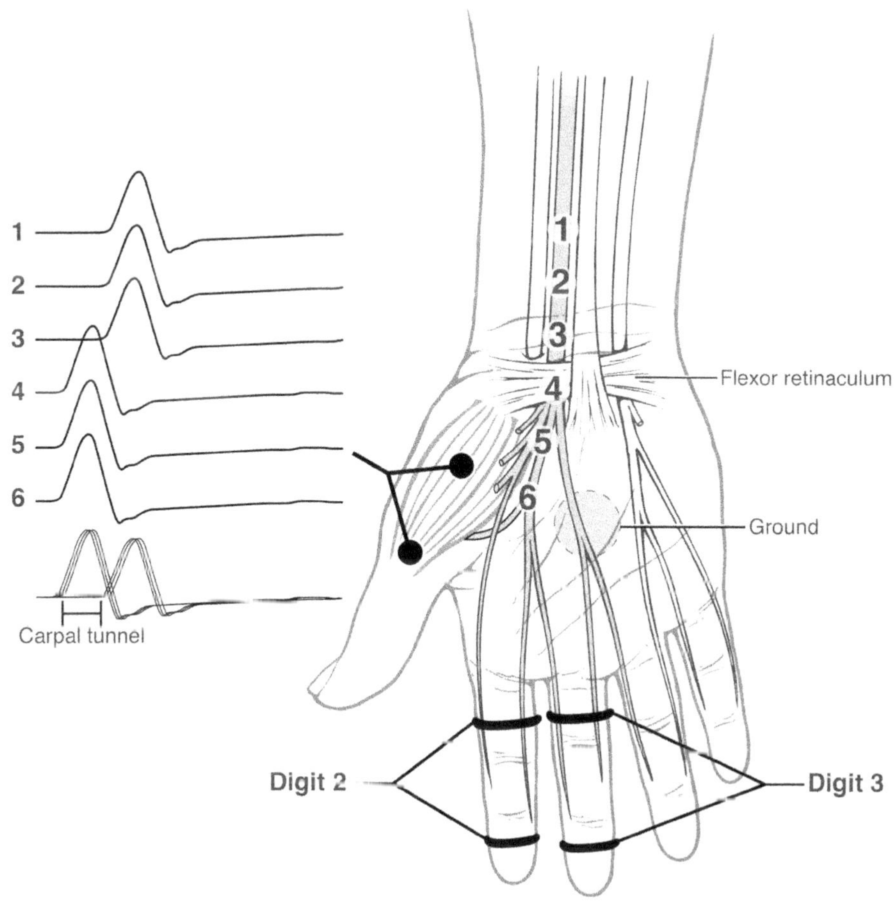

FIGURE 4-6 Short segment stimulation across the palm (inching technique).

with myasthenia gravis may demonstrate a decrement in the CMAP on repetitive stimulation studies of the median (or ulnar) nerves, particularly if intrinsic hand muscles are clinically weak. The setup for repetitive stimulation studies of the median (or ulnar) nerves is identical to the routine motor conduction study, although repetitive stimulation (5 stimuli at 3 Hz) is delivered instead of single shocks. Immobilization of the hand is *not* usually needed and only complicates the recording, although recording electrodes and stimulator should be secured with tape. Exercise is performed by instructing the patient to perform a brief (10-second) maximum contraction of the muscle, and the train of stimuli are repeated immediately upon cessation of exercise to look for repair of the decrement (post-tetanic repair) or an increment in the CMAP (post-tetanic potentiation). A marked increment ≥ 200 % suggests a presynaptic defect in neuromuscular transmission, specifically Lambert-Eaton myasthenic syndrome (LEMS), although lesser magnitudes of potentiation can be seen in other presynaptic disorders, most notably botulism. Repetitive stimulation studies are then repeated at 1, 2, 3, and 4 minutes after one minute of sustained maximum voluntary contraction, because some patients with myasthenia gravis may only demonstrate a significant decrement (greater than 10%) several minutes after sustained exercise.

Pitfalls

A common source of technical error arises when inappropriately high stimulus intensities are used. Overstimulation at the wrist causes the current to spread to the adjacent ulnar nerve, which may confound interpretation of latencies and CMAP morphology.

Temperature has a profound effect on nerve conduction studies. Lower temperatures prolong distal latencies, slow conduction velocity, and increase action potential amplitudes (see Chapter 1). Lower temperatures can also mask a defect in neuromuscular transmission. Skin temperature should be maintained at 34° C or higher.

Failure to recognize the Martin-Gruber anastomosis (see Figure 4-8) is a common source of error in clinical electrophysiology.

Median F-waves

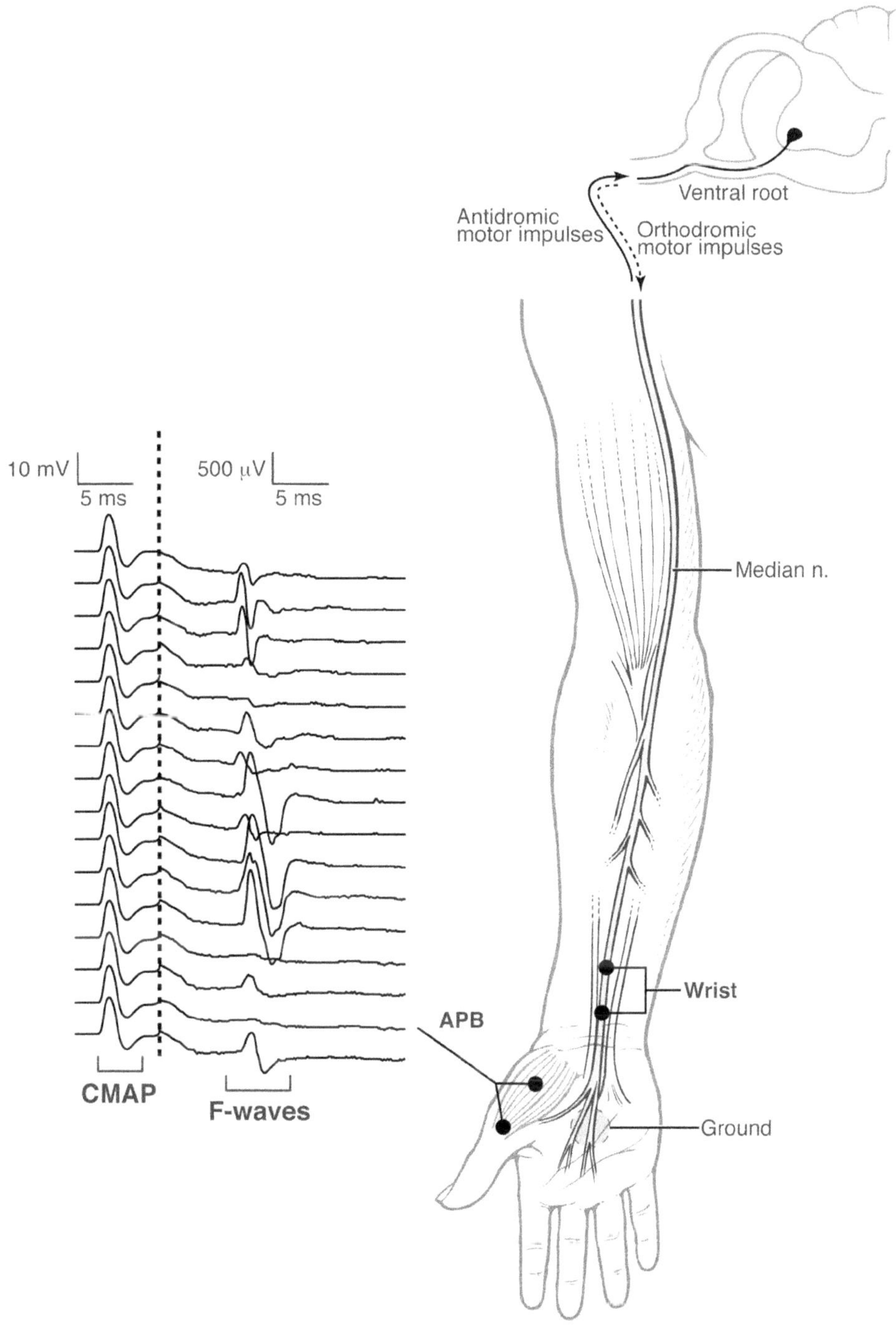

FIGURE 4-7 Median F-waves.

Recording F-waves (Figure 4-7)

Identical recording technique as that utilized to elicit the CMAP during routine median motor conduction studies, except that the gain is set to 200 μV and sweep speed 5 ms/division to allow visualization of this late response. At least 10 to 20 F-wave responses are recorded.

Stimulation

Identical stimulation technique as that utilized for distal stimulation at the wrist (place cathode in the same site and deliver supramaximal stimuli). By convention, the anode is rotated 180 degrees from its original position to avoid the theoretical possibility of nerve hyperpolarization under the anode (anodal conduction block). However, in routine clinical practice, anodal block is not observed (Wee et al., 2000).

F-wave Measurements and Normal Values

Minimum F-wave latency is the most commonly obtained measurement. This is the shortest onset latency of all recorded F-waves. Since F-wave latency varies with height, most laboratories define the upper limits of normal for different ranges of height. In hand muscles, typical upper limits of minimum F-wave latency are 25 ms for height 4'11" (150 cm), 28 ms for height 5'7" (170 cm) and 32 ms for height 6'3" (190 cm). A right–left asymmetry of minimal F-wave latency >2.0 ms in hand muscles is considered abnormal (Kimura, 1989; Fisher, 1992; Puksa et al. 2003).

Mean F-wave latency is calculated by adding all individual F-wave latencies and dividing this sum by the number of F-waves recorded. Some investigators endorse this value as the optimal practical measure (Fisher, 1992), because it minimizes the error inherent in a single latency measurement. The upper limits of this value will be approximately 2 ms longer than minimum F-wave latency for the corresponding heights (Nobrega, et al. 2004).

Maximum F-wave latency is the longest onset latency of all recorded F-waves. The upper limits of this value will be about 4 ms longer than minimum F-wave latency for the corresponding heights (Nobrega, et al. 2004).

F-wave dispersion (also known as chronodispersion) provides a measure of the range of conductions and is calculated as the difference between minimum and maximum F-wave latencies. In hand muscles, a typical upper limit of normal F-wave dispersion is <5 ms (Puksa et al. 2003). Excessive chronodispersion suggests temporal dispersion and demyelination.

F-wave amplitude usually measures <5% of the maximal CMAP or M-wave amplitude (F/M amplitude ratio). This is a measure of the proportion of the motor neuron pool activated by antidromic stimulation. F-wave amplitude may be increased in upper motor neuron dysfunction, especially when spasticity is present.

F-wave persistence is the percentage of F-waves obtained following a series of stimulations (i.e., the number of measureable F-waves divided by the number of stimuli). This reflects the antidromic excitability of a particular motor neuron pool (Fisher, 1992). F-wave persistence in median, ulnar, and tibial nerves is normally >50%, although in the peroneal nerve it can be <25%. F-wave persistence is typically decreased in lower motor neuron dysfunction and increased in upper motor neuron dysfunction, particularly when spasticity is present.

Comments Regarding F-waves

In patients with entrapment neuropathies, the minimum, mean, and maximum F-wave latencies are proportionately prolonged.

In radiculopathy, F-waves are of limited value and less sensitive than needle EMG examination in assessing motor fiber involvement.

F-waves are commonly abnormal in a variety of axonal and demyelinating polyneuropathies. In Guillain-Barré syndrome, F-waves may be absent or delayed during the acute stages when other nerve conduction studies are normal. Increased F-wave dispersion suggests temporal dispersion and demyelination.

F-waves provide a means of assessing motor neuron excitability (Fisher, 1992). F-waves are typically absent or decreased in spinal shock (Leis et al., 1996) and early after acute stroke, compatible with a decreased central excitability state. In contrast, F-waves are typically increased in patients with established spasticity.

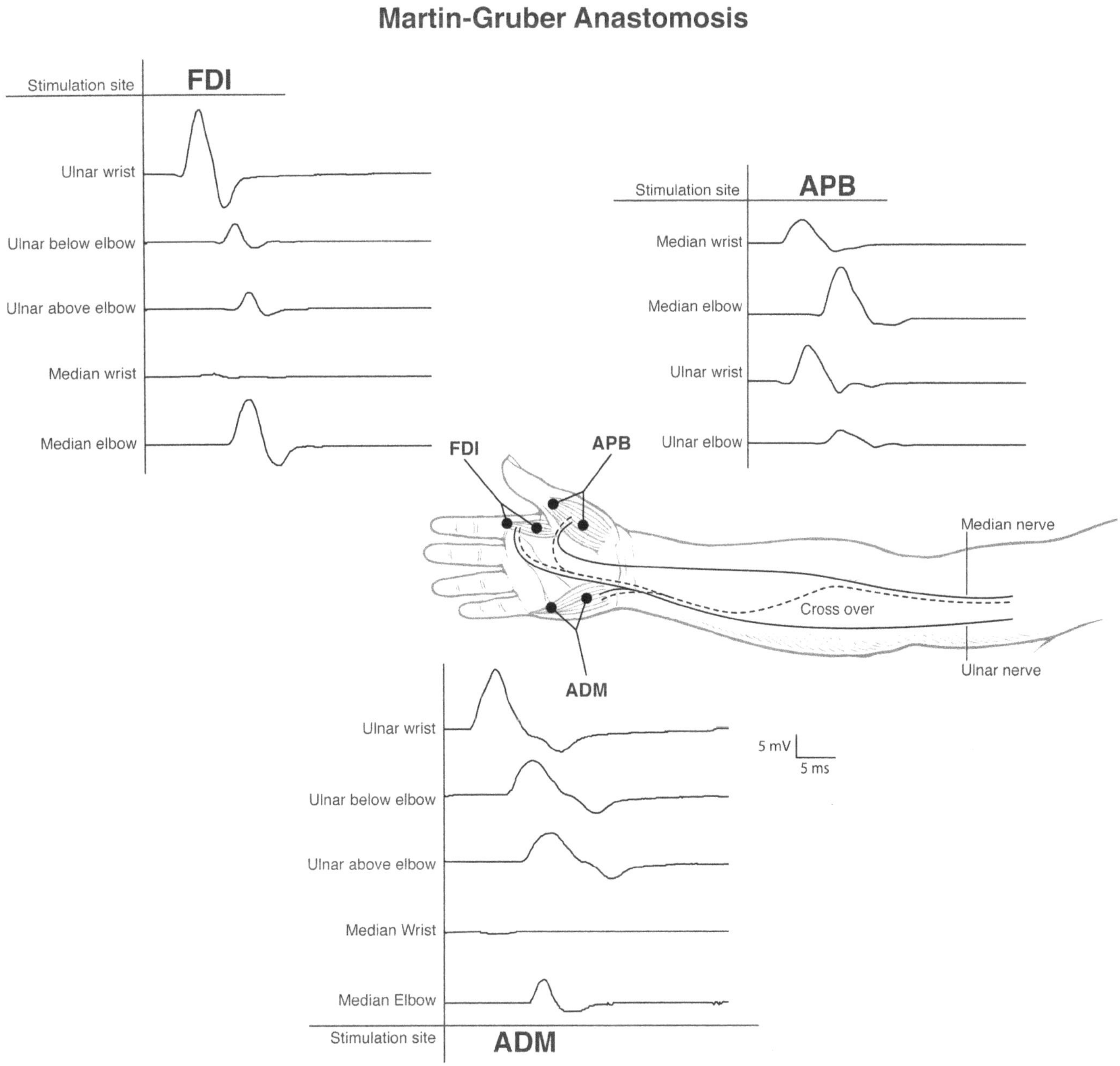

FIGURE 4-8 Martin-Gruber anastomosis.

Martin-Gruber anastomosis (MGA) is a median to ulnar nerve "crossover" in the mid forearm that involves motor fibers (Figure 4-8). It is the most common clinically relevant anomaly, occurring in about one-third of median nerves (Rosenbaum and Ochoa, 2002). When present, it tends to be bilateral. The MGA often arises from the anterior interosseous nerve, although other branching patterns occur. MGA fibers typically supply intrinsic hand muscles normally innervated by the ulnar nerve (first dorsal interosseous, adductor pollicis, deep head of flexor pollicis brevis, abductor digiti minimi), although less commonly they can also supply thenar muscles innervated by the median nerve. Standard median nerve conduction studies with CMAP recordings solely over thenar muscles will detect less than 14% of MGA cases (Amoiridis and Vlachonikolis, 2003). When present, the MGA can lead to unusual sparing of muscles after severe proximal ulnar nerve injury or CTS. This occurs because the fibers contributing to the MGA traverse the antecubital fossa with the median nerve and then traverse the wrist with the ulnar nerve, avoiding the two most common entrapment neuropathies: CTS and ulnar neuropathy at the elbow. Conversely, a proximal median nerve injury can lead to unexpectedly widespread denervation in the presence of the MGA (Rosenbaum and Ochoa, 2002).

During routine median nerve conduction studies, the MGA can be recognized by a CMAP that is larger with stimulation of the median nerve at the antecubital fossa than at the wrist. In such cases, the CMAP from the APB muscle will be smaller with stimulation of the ulnar nerve at the elbow compared with ulnar nerve stimulation the wrist. In a patient with CTS and MGA, stimulation of the median nerve at the wrist will evoke a delayed CMAP from APB, whereas stimulation at the antecubital fossa will evoke a CMAP with normal latency (since MGA fibers bypass the carpal tunnel). This discrepancy between proximal and distal stimulation leads to an unreasonably fast conduction velocity in the forearm segment (Figure 4-9). In severe CTS and MGA, the latency of the median CMAP after wrist stimulation may even exceed that of the anomalous MGA response elicited with elbow stimulation. In patients with CTS and MGA, avoid the temptation to overstimulate at the wrist, since this can activate MGA fibers adjacent to the ulnar nerve and confound interpretation.

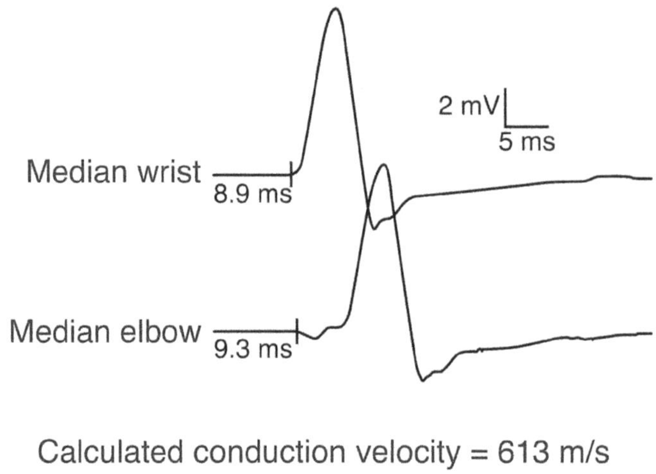

FIGURE 4-9 Carpal tunnel syndrome (CTS) and Martin-Gruber anastomosis (MGA). In patients with CTS and MGA, stimulation of the median nerve at the wrist evokes a delayed CMAP from APB (top tracing), whereas stimulation at the antecubital fossa evokes a CMAP with normal latency (bottom tracing) because MGA fibers bypass the carpal tunnel. The discrepancy between proximal and distal stimulation leads to an unreasonably fast conduction velocity in the forearm segment.

Median Sensory Nerve Conduction Study

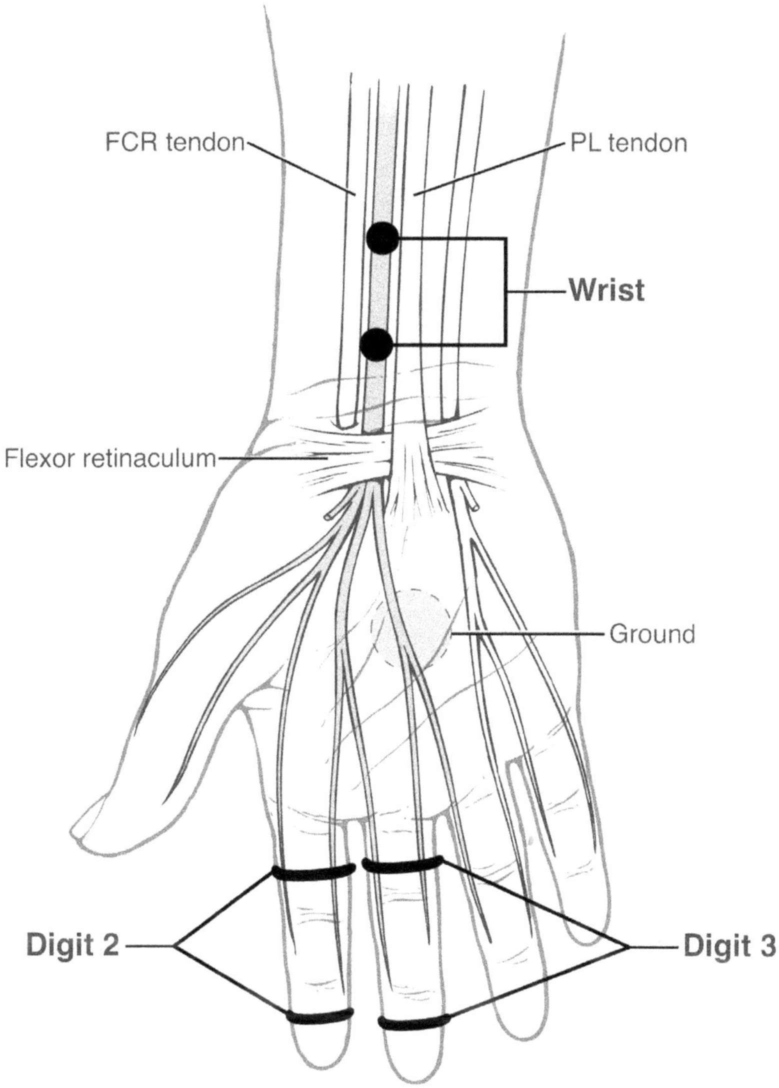

FIGURE 4-10 Median sensory nerve conduction study (antidromic).

Recording (with ring electrodes, Figure 4-10)

Active electrode: position around the mid-portion of the proximal phalanx of the second or third digits (just proximal to the proximal interphalangeal joint). Additional recording sites include ring electrodes placed around the first digit and fourth digit.

Reference electrode: position around the mid-portion of the distal phalanx (just distal to the distal interphalangeal joint).

Ground electrode: place on the dorsum of the hand, between the stimulating and recording electrodes.

Stimulation

Wrist: place cathode over the median nerve between the flexor carpi radialis (FCR) tendon and the palmaris longus (PL) tendon, 14 cm proximal to the recording electrode. In most hands, this distance is sufficient to include the segment from carpal tunnel to digits. Anode is 3 cm proximal to cathode.

Comments

This is the standard median sensory nerve conduction study for evaluating a variety of peripheral nerve abnormalities ranging from CTS to peripheral neuropathy.

Normal Values

Latency (ms) ≤ 2.8 (onset latency); ≤ 3.5 (peak latency)

Amplitude (μV) ≥ 20

Conduction velocity (m/s) in wrist to digit segment ≥ 50 m/s

The normal amplitude of the median sensory response has a large range and standard deviation. Therefore, nerve conduction studies should ideally be performed bilaterally because side-to-side comparisons are more useful than normal value tables that may not apply to your patient. When latency and conduction velocity approach borderline values, comparative nerve conduction studies for the diagnosis of CTS should be performed.

Median and Ulnar Palmar Comparative Study for the Diagnosis of CTS

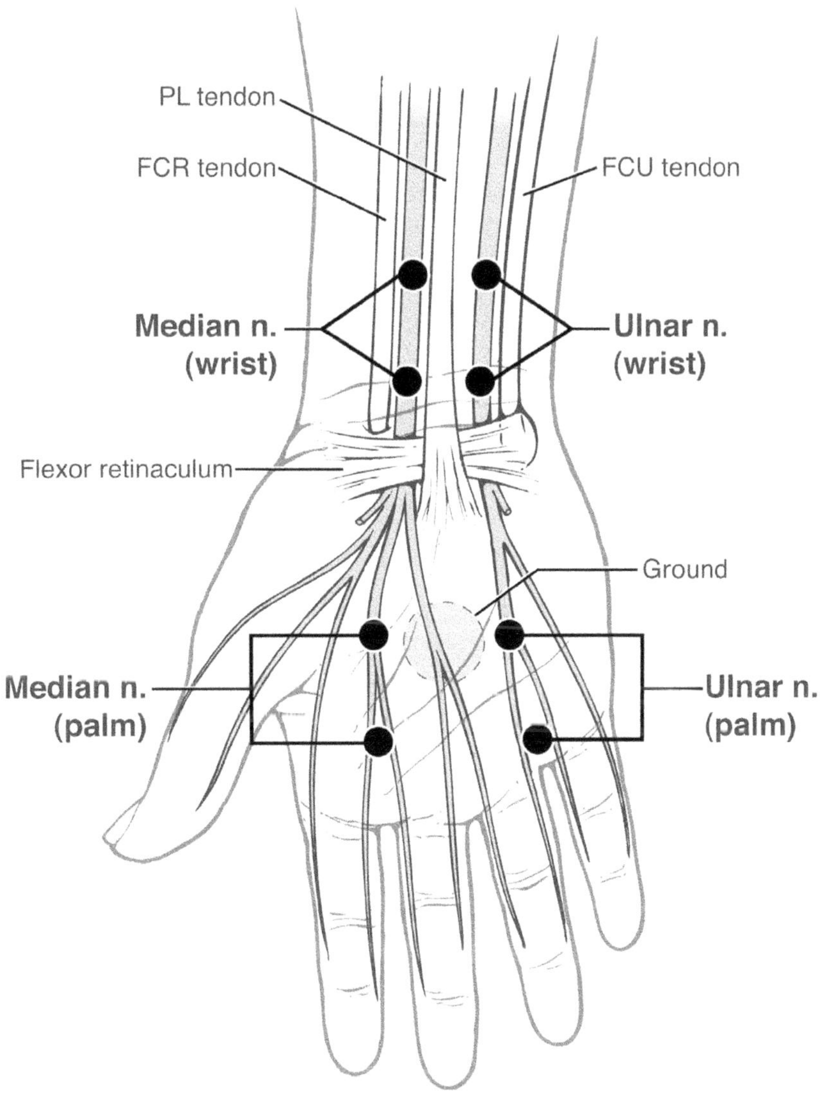

FIGURE 4-11 Median and ulnar palmar comparative study (transcarpal mixed nerve technique).

Recording (Figure 4-11)

Median nerve active electrode: Place 2 cm proximal to the distal wrist crease between the flexor carpi radialis (FCR) tendon and the palmaris longus (PL) tendon.

Ulnar nerve active electrode: Place 2 cm proximal to the distal wrist crease just lateral to the flexor carpi ulnaris (FCU) tendon.

Reference electrode: Place 3 cm proximal to the active electrode along the median or ulnar nerves, respectively.

Ground electrode: Place on the dorsum of the hand, between stimulating and recording electrodes.

Stimulation

Median nerve palm: Place cathode 7 or 8 cm distal to the active recording electrode between the second and third metacarpal interspace in the palm (cathode is positioned proximal to the anode). Anode is 3 cm distally.

Ulnar nerve palm: Place cathode 7 or 8 cm distal to the active recording electrode between the fourth and fifth metacarpal interspace in the palm (cathode is positioned proximal to anode). Anode is 3 cm distally.

Normal values

The major useful value is the peak difference between the median and ulnar responses.
Latency peak difference (ms) ≤ 0.3.

Comments

This is the most commonly used comparative study to diagnose CTS. As with all comparative studies, careful distance measurements are crucial. The selected distance (7 or 8 cm) should be consistently used to improve reproducibility.

Median and Ulnar Digit 4 (ring finger) Comparative Study

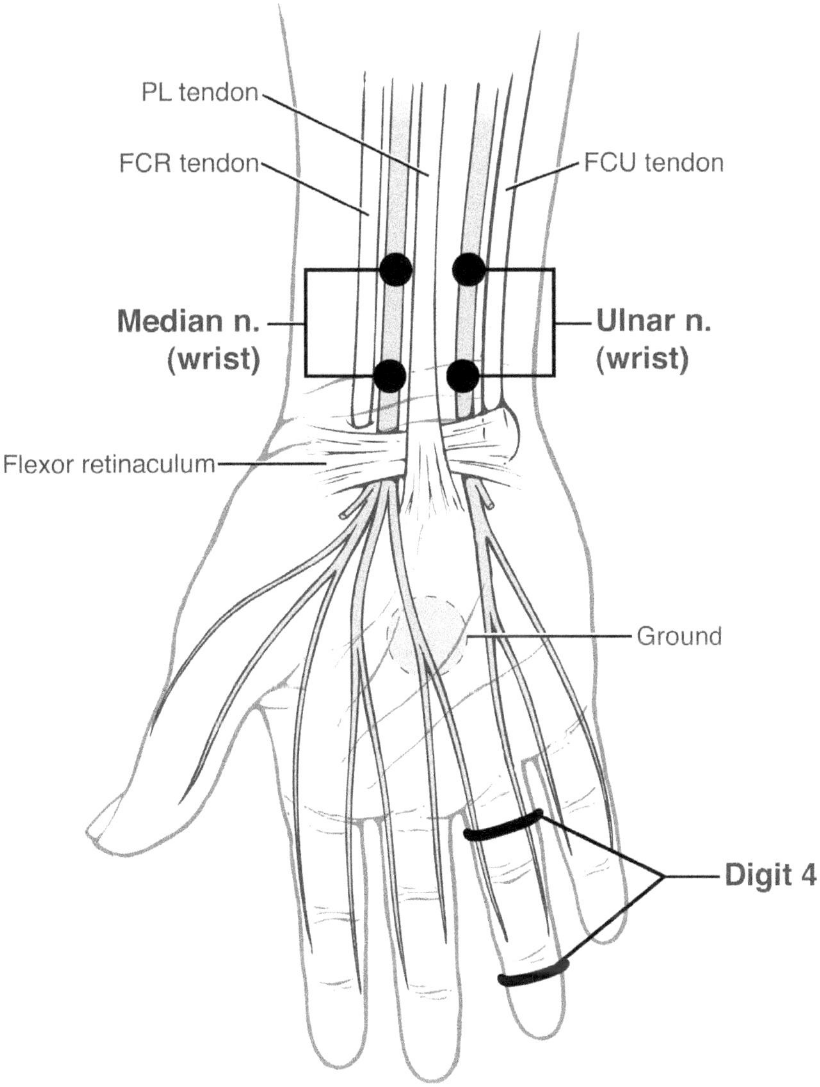

FIGURE 4-12 Median and ulnar digit 4 (ring finger) comparative study (antidromic).

Recording (with ring electrodes, Figure 4-12)

Active electrode: Position around the mid-portion of the proximal phalanx of the fourth digit (just proximal to the proximal interphalangeal joint)

Reference electrode: Position around the mid-portion of the distal phalanx (just distal to the distal interphalangeal joint).

Ground electrode: Place on the dorsum of the hand, between the stimulating and recording electrodes.

Stimulation

Median nerve wrist: Place cathode over the median nerve at the wrist between the flexor carpi radialis (FCR) tendon and the palmaris longus (PL) tendon, 14 cm proximal to the recording electrode. Anode is 3 cm proximal to cathode.

Ulnar nerve wrist: Place cathode over the ulnar nerve at the wrist just lateral to the flexor carpi ulnaris (FCU) tendon, 14 cm proximal to the recording electrode. Anode is 3 cm proximal to cathode.

Normal values

The major useful value is the peak latency difference between median and ulnar digit 4 responses. Normal values vary between laboratories, with latency peak difference ≤ 0.3 ms to ≤ 0.4 ms.

Comments

This is a commonly used comparative study to diagnose CTS. However, a disadvantage of this technique is the lower amplitude of the ring finger SNAP, particularly for the ulnar nerve, compared with the amplitudes from other digits (Rosenbaum and Ochoa, 2002). In addition, anomalous sensory innervation to ring finger (exclusively or predominantly median or ulnar) may rarely confound interpretation.

Median and Superficial Radial Digit 1 (thumb) Comparative Study

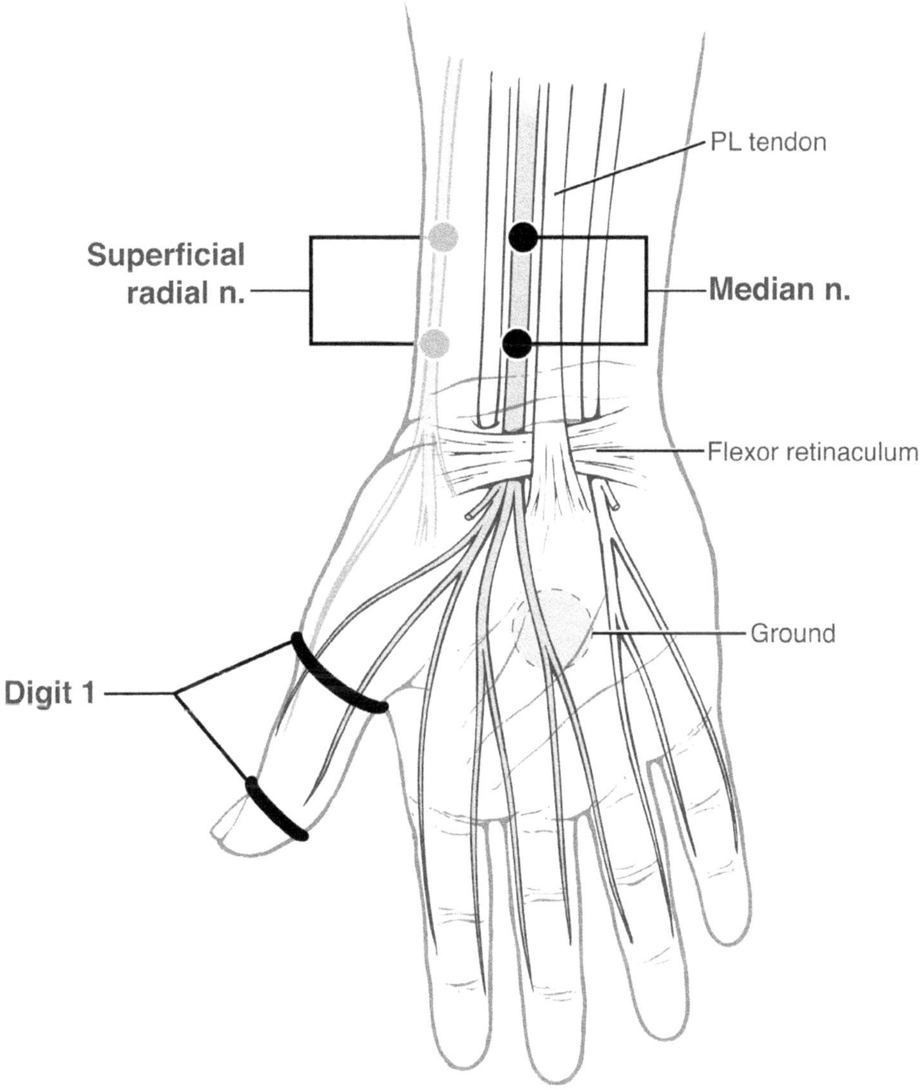

FIGURE 4-13 Median and superficial radial digit 1 (thumb) comparative study (antidromic).

Recording (with ring electrodes, Figure 4-13)

Active electrode: Position around the mid-portion of the proximal phalanx of the thumb.
Reference electrode: Position around the mid-portion of the distal phalanx of the thumb.
Ground electrode: Place on the dorsum of the hand, between the stimulating and recording electrodes.

Stimulation

Median nerve wrist: Place cathode over the median nerve at the wrist between the flexor carpi radialis (FCR) tendon and the palmaris longus (PL) tendon, 10 cm proximal to the recording electrode. Anode is 3 cm proximal to cathode.
Superficial radial nerve distal forearm: Place cathode over the lateral wrist (dorsolateral aspect of the radius), 10 cm proximal to the recording electrode. Anode is 3 cm proximal to cathode.

Normal Values

The major useful value is the peak latency difference between the median and superficial radial thumb responses. Normal values vary between laboratories, with latency peak difference ≤ 0.4 ms to ≤ 0.5 ms.

Comments

This is a commonly used comparative study to diagnose CTS (Stevens, 1997). However, it is more difficult to make an accurate distance measurement because of the potentially variable course of median sensory branches to thumb.

Combined Sensory Index (CSI)

The CSI is the sum of the three comparative latency differences from: (1) median and ulnar palmar (transcarpal) study (8 cm); (2) median and ulnar digit 4 study (14 cm); and (3) median and superficial radial digit 1 study (10 cm) (Robinson et al. 1998). The CSI has better specificity and sensitivity for the diagnosis of CTS than an individual comparison latency, and better reliability than a single test result. It is particularly useful when standard median nerve conduction studies are borderline. The lower limit of normal is 1.0 ms. For example:

Median and ulnar palmar difference	=	0.3 ms
Median and ulnar digit 4 difference	=	0.4 ms
Median and radial digit 1 difference	=	0.4 ms
CSI	=	1.1 ms (>1.0 indicates physiologic CTS)

Standards for Severity of Carpal Tunnel Syndrome

There is no universally agreed upon standard for grading the severity of CTS. However, classification schemes for grading the severity of CTS by electrodiagnostic criteria are still useful when writing a consultation. One such scheme is provided below (modified from Stevens 1997):

- Mild CTS – sensory or mixed nerve latencies (antidromic, orthodromic, or palmar) are relatively or absolutely prolonged; SNAP amplitude is normal or reduced (relative or absolute decrease); median motor distal latency is normal or slightly prolonged (relative or absolute; e.g., 4.0 to <4.5 ms).
- Moderate CTS – above mild abnormalities plus more prolonged median motor distal latency (e.g., ≥ 4.5 ms). Motor amplitude (CMAP) remains normal.
- Severe CTS – above moderate abnormalities plus markedly reduced or absent sensory and mixed nerve responses, and reduced or absent CMAP. Needle EMG examination of thenar muscles typically reveals fibrillations, reduced recruitment, and neuropathic MUP changes.

Nerve conduction studies performed after carpal tunnel surgery usually show significant improvement, correlating with symptomatic improvement. However, conduction abnormalities in moderate to severe cases of CTS may not return to normal, even when symptoms are relieved (Stevens, 1997). In addition, although nerve conduction studies provide objective evidence of the severity of a neuropathic condition, the degree of physiologic dysfunction may not correlate with symptom severity.

Digital Branch Injury

Sensory responses recorded from individual digits are useful to identify a digital branch injury, which is a pure sensory neuropathy of a digital nerve caused by acute or chronic local trauma or pressure (Dobyns, 1992; Goldwirth and Goodwin, 1999). Acute digital branch injury can result from a variety of risk factors, including home, occupational, and avocational situations. For example, *plastic bag digital neuropathy* occurs when pressure on the neurovascular bundle of a digit by commercial plastic bags causes temporary ischemia in the finger and neurapraxia of the digital nerve (Goldwirth and Goodwin, 1999). In severe or repetitive cases, axonal loss may occur. Chronic widespread digital branch injury is usually associated with occupations where there is persistent or repetitive pressure on the digits (e.g., automobile mechanics, construction workers, assembly line workers, fish packers, etc). In such patients, median and ulnar digital SNAPs are often disproportionately reduced in amplitude compared to normal proximal SNAPs (e.g., superficial radial, dorsal ulnar cutaneous, medial and lateral cutaneous nerves of the forearm). Treatment of digital neuropathy is best accomplished by identifying and avoiding risk activities whenever possible. Rarely, surgery may be of benefit (Dobyns 1992). Digital neuropathy may also accompany systemic illnesses such as rheumatoid arthritis, diabetes mellitus, leprosy, or monoclonal gammopathies.

REFERENCES

Amoiridis G, Vlachonikolis IG. Verification of the median-to-ulnar and ulnar-to-median nerve motor fiber anastomosis in the forearm: an electrophysiological study. *Clin Neurophysiol* 2003;114:94–98.

Bergman RA, Thompson SA, Afifi AK. *Catalog of Human Variation*, Urban & Schwarzenberg, Baltimore, 1984, pp.31–32.

Dobyns JH. Digital nerve compression. *Hand Clinics* 1992;8:359–367.

Felsenthal G. Median and ulnar muscle and sensory evoked potentials. *Am J Phys Med* 1978;57:167–182.

Fisher MA. AAEM Minimonograph #13: H reflexes and F waves: physiology and clinical indications. *Muscle Nerve* 1992;15(11):1223–1233. Review.

Goldwirth M, Goodwin DR. The "Plastic Bag Syndrome." Compression of the digital neurovascular bundles by commercial plastic bags. *J Hand Surg Br* 1999;24:116–117.

Gray's Anatomy. 38th edition, Churchill Livingstone, New York, 1995, pp.1266–1274.

Kimura J. *Electrodiagnosis in Diseases of Nerve and Muscle*. 2nd ed., FA Davis Co., Philadelphia, 1989.

Leis AA, Kronenberg MF, Stetkarova I, Paske WC, Stokic DS. Spinal motoneuron excitability after acute spinal cord injury in man. *Neurology* 1996;47:231–237.

Nobrega JAM, Pinhiero DS, Manzano GM, Kimura J. Various aspects of F-wave values in a healthy population. *Clin Neurophysiol* 2004;115:2336–2342.

Pecina MM, Krmpotic-Nemanic J, Markiewitz AD. *Tunnel Syndromes: Peripheral Nerve Compression Syndromes,* 2nd ed., CRC Press, New York, 1997, pp.73–76.

Puksa L, Stalberg E, Falck B. Reference values of F wave parameters in healthy subjects. *Clin Neurophysiol* 2003;114:1079–1090.

Robinson LR, Micklesen PJ, Wang L. Strategies for analyzing nerve conduction data: superiority of a summary index over single tests. *Muscle Nerve* 1998;21:1166–1171.

Rosenbaum RB, Ochoa JL, eds. *Carpal tunnel syndrome and other disorders of the median nerve*. Butterworth Heinemann, Boston, 2002.

Ross MA, Kimura J. AAEM case report #2: The carpal tunnel syndrome. *Muscle Nerve* 1995;18: 567–573.

Stevens JC. AAEM minimonograph #26: The electrodiagnosis of carpal tunnel syndrome. *Muscle Nerve* 1997;20:1477–1486.

Sunderland S. *Nerves and Nerve Injuries*. Williams and Wilkins, Baltimore, 1968, pp.781–807.

Sunderland S. *Nerves and Nerve Injuries*. 2nd ed., Churchill Livingstone, New York, 1978.

Wee AS, Leis AA, Kuhn AR, Gilbert RW. Anodal block: can this occur during routine nerve conduction studies? *Electromyogr Clin Neurophysiol* 2000;40:387–391.

Wertsch JJ. AAEM case report #25: Anterior interosseous nerve syndrome. *Muscle Nerve* 1992;15:977–983.

Abductor Pollicis Brevis

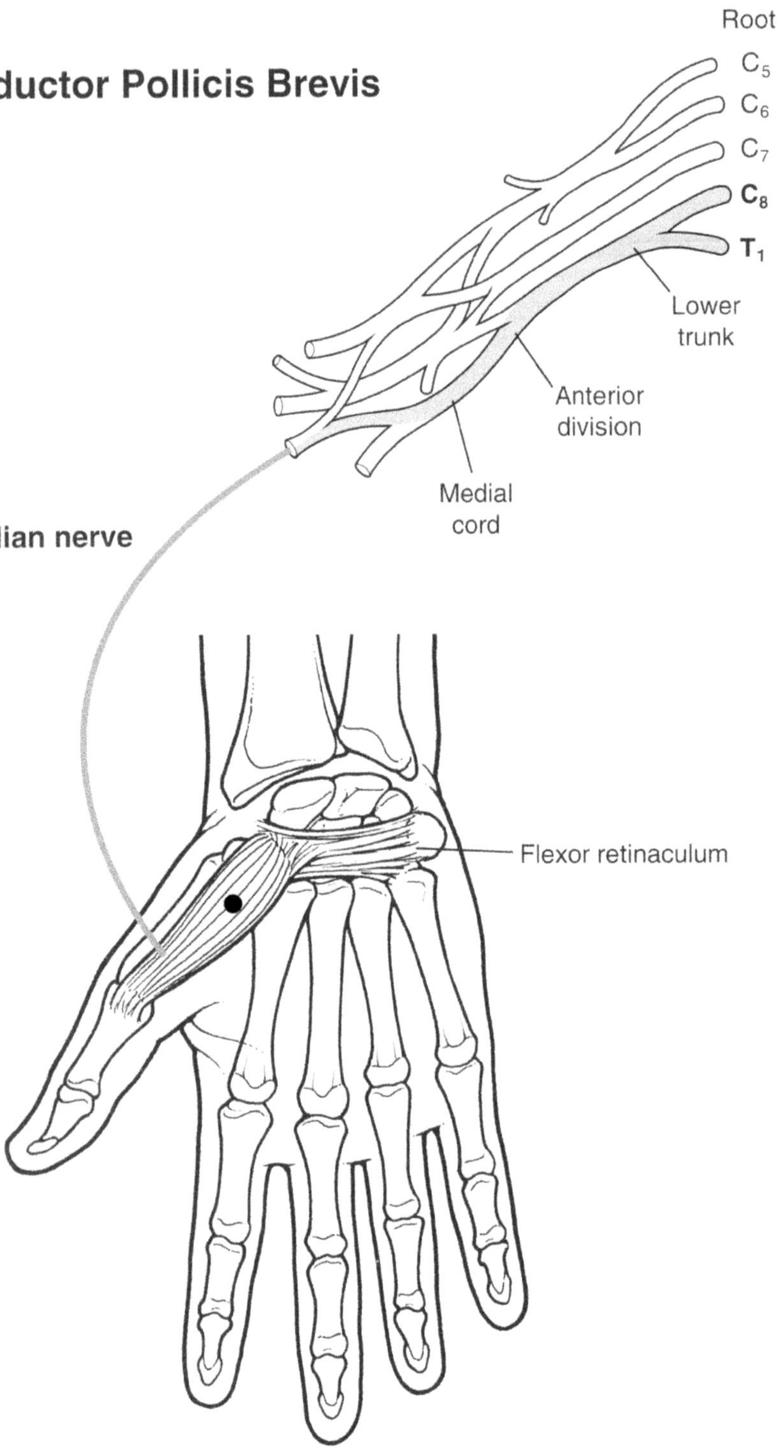

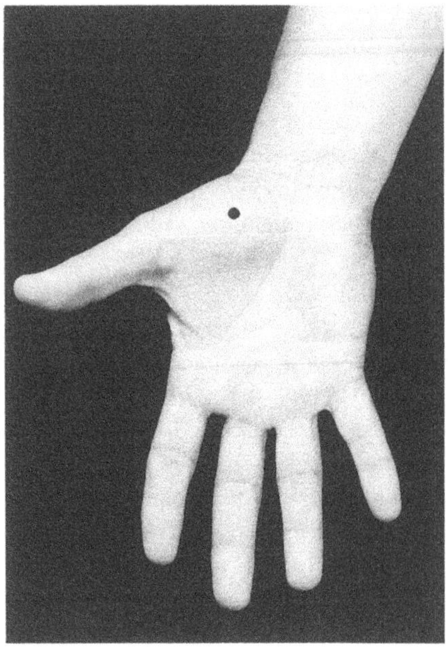

Innervation

Innervation is via the median nerve, medial cord, lower trunk, and roots C_8, T_1.

Origin

The muscle originates in the palmar retinaculum and the tubercle of the scaphoid and trapezium.

Insertion

The muscle is inserted at the base of the proximal phalanx of the thumb.

Activation Maneuver

Abduction of the thumb (movement of the thumb out of the plane of the palm) activates the muscle.

EMG Needle Insertion

Insert the needle obliquely near the muscle origin. Assess abnormal EMG activity by directing the needle distally along the muscle.

Pitfalls

If the needle is inserted too medially, it may penetrate the flexor pollicis brevis, which receives dual innervation from the median and ulnar nerves.

If the needle is inserted too deeply, it may penetrate the adductor pollicis, which receives innervation from the ulnar nerve.

Clinical Comments

Needle examination may show neurogenic changes with axonal loss lesions of the median nerve due to carpal tunnel syndrome, pronator teres syndrome, ligament of Struther's syndrome, medial cord lesions, C_8, T_1 radiculopathy, Klumpke's palsy (C_8, T_1 root avulsion), and anterior horn cell disease.

EMG will be normal in the anterior interosseous nerve syndrome.

Opponens Pollicis

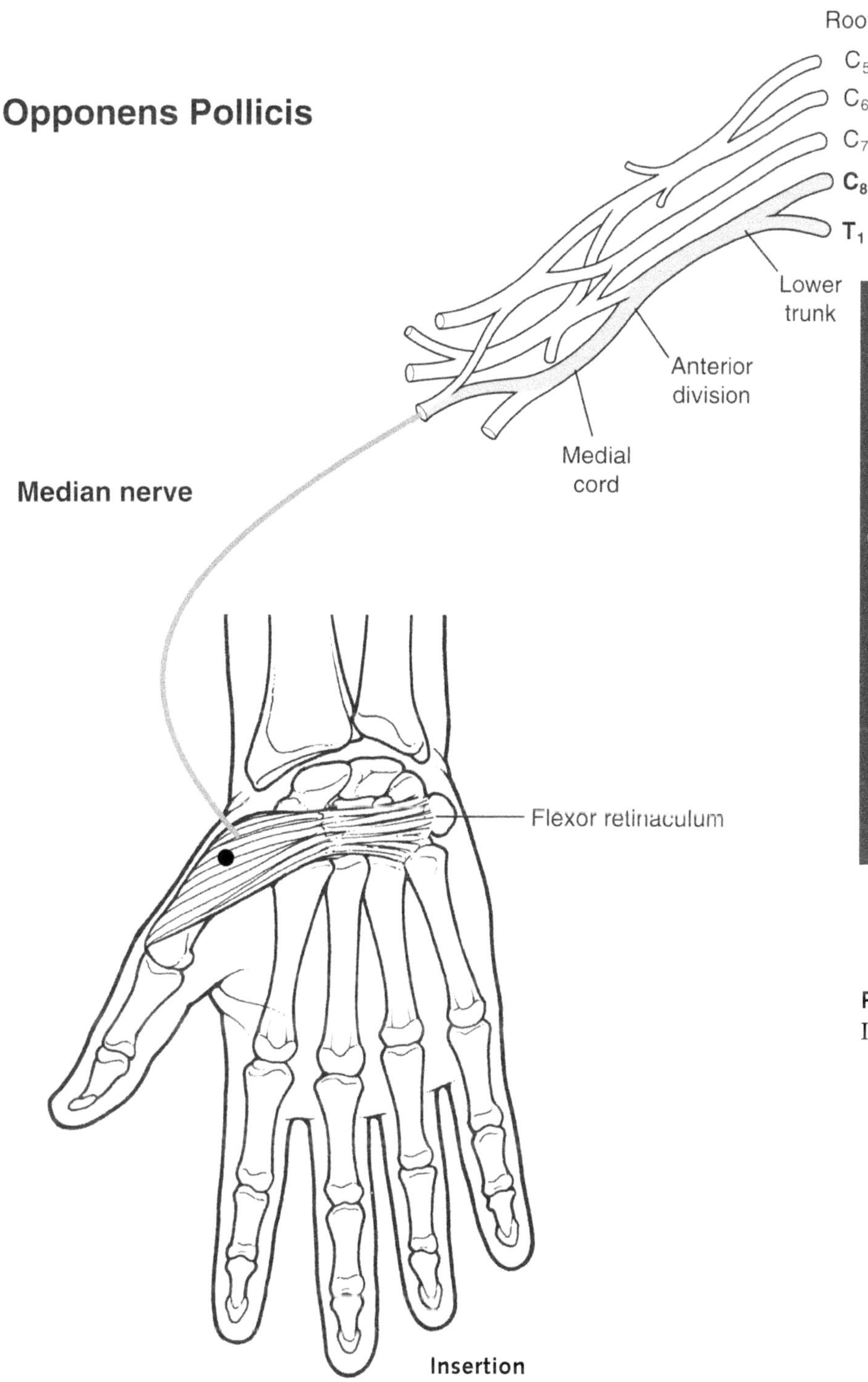

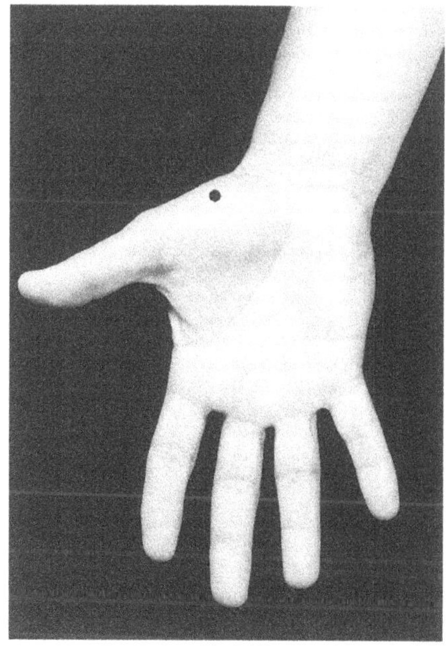

Innervation
Innervation is via the median nerve, medial cord, lower trunk, and roots C_8, T_1.

Origin
The muscle originates in the palmar retinaculum, and the tubercle of the trapezium.

Insertion
The muscle is inserted at the palmar surface of the first metacarpal bone.

Activation Maneuver
Opposition of the thumb to the little finger activates the muscle.

EMG Needle Insertion
Insert the needle obliquely at the midpoint of the first metacarpal shaft just lateral to the abductor pollicis brevis muscle.

Pitfalls
If the needle is inserted too medially, it will be in the abductor pollicis brevis, which still receives innervation from the median nerve. If inserted even more medially, it may be in the flexor pollicis brevis, which receives dual innervation from the median and ulnar nerves. If the needle is inserted too deeply, it may penetrate the adductor pollicis, which receives innervation from the ulnar nerve.

Clinical Comments
EMG may show neurogenic changes in the carpal tunnel syndrome, pronator teres syndrome, ligament of Struthers' syndrome, medial cord lesions, C_8, T_1 radiculopathy, Klumpke's palsy (C_8, T_1 root avulsion), and anterior horn cell disease.

EMG will be normal in the anterior interosseous nerve syndrome.

Flexor Pollicis Brevis

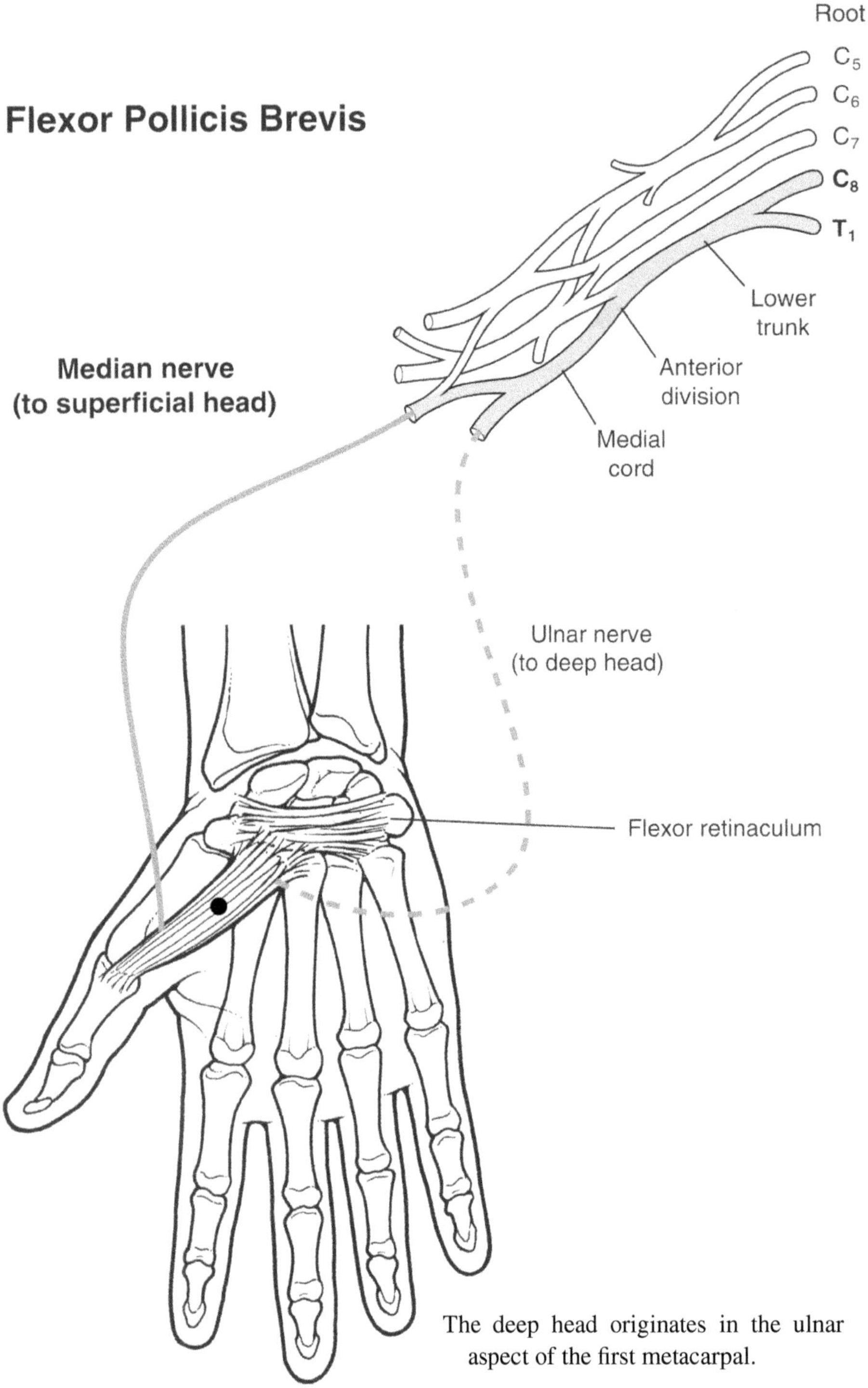

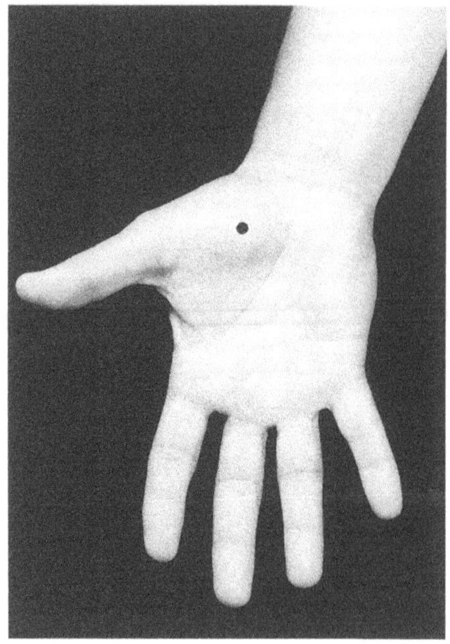

Innervation

Superficial head: Innervation is via the median nerve, medial cord, lower trunk, and roots C_8, T_1.

Deep head: Innervation is via the ulnar nerve, medial cord, lower trunk, and roots C_8, T_1.

Origin

The superficial head originates in the flexor retinaculum and trapezium.

The deep head originates in the ulnar aspect of the first metacarpal.

Insertion

The superficial head is inserted at the radial aspect of the base of the proximal phalanx of the thumb.

The deep head is inserted at the ulnar aspect of the base of the proximal phalanx of the thumb.

Activation Maneuver

Flexing of the metacarpophalangeal joint of the thumb activates the muscle.

EMG Needle Insertion

Superficial head: Insert the needle obliquely at a depth of 0.5–1 cm at the midpoint of a line drawn between the metacarpophalangeal joint and the pisiform. Assess abnormal EMG activity by directing the needle distally along the muscle.

Deep head: The procedure is the same as that for the superficial head, but insert the needle to a depth of 1–2 cm.

Pitfalls

If the needle is inserted too deeply, it may penetrate the opponens pollicis, which is innervated by the median nerve; if inserted still deeper, it may be in the adductor pollicis, which receives innervation from the ulnar nerve.

If the needle is inserted too laterally, it will be in the abductor pollicis brevis, which receives innervation from the median nerve.

Clinical Comments

Testing of the flexor pollicis brevis is rarely of benefit in a routine EMG needle evaluation (in general, muscles that receive dual innervation should be avoided).

The superficial head will show neurogenic changes in lesions of the median nerve.

The deep head will show neurogenic changes in lesions of the ulnar nerve.

Both heads may show neurogenic changes in C_8, T_1 radiculopathy, Klumpke's palsy (C_8, T_1 root avulsion), and anterior horn cell disease.

1st, 2nd Lumbricals

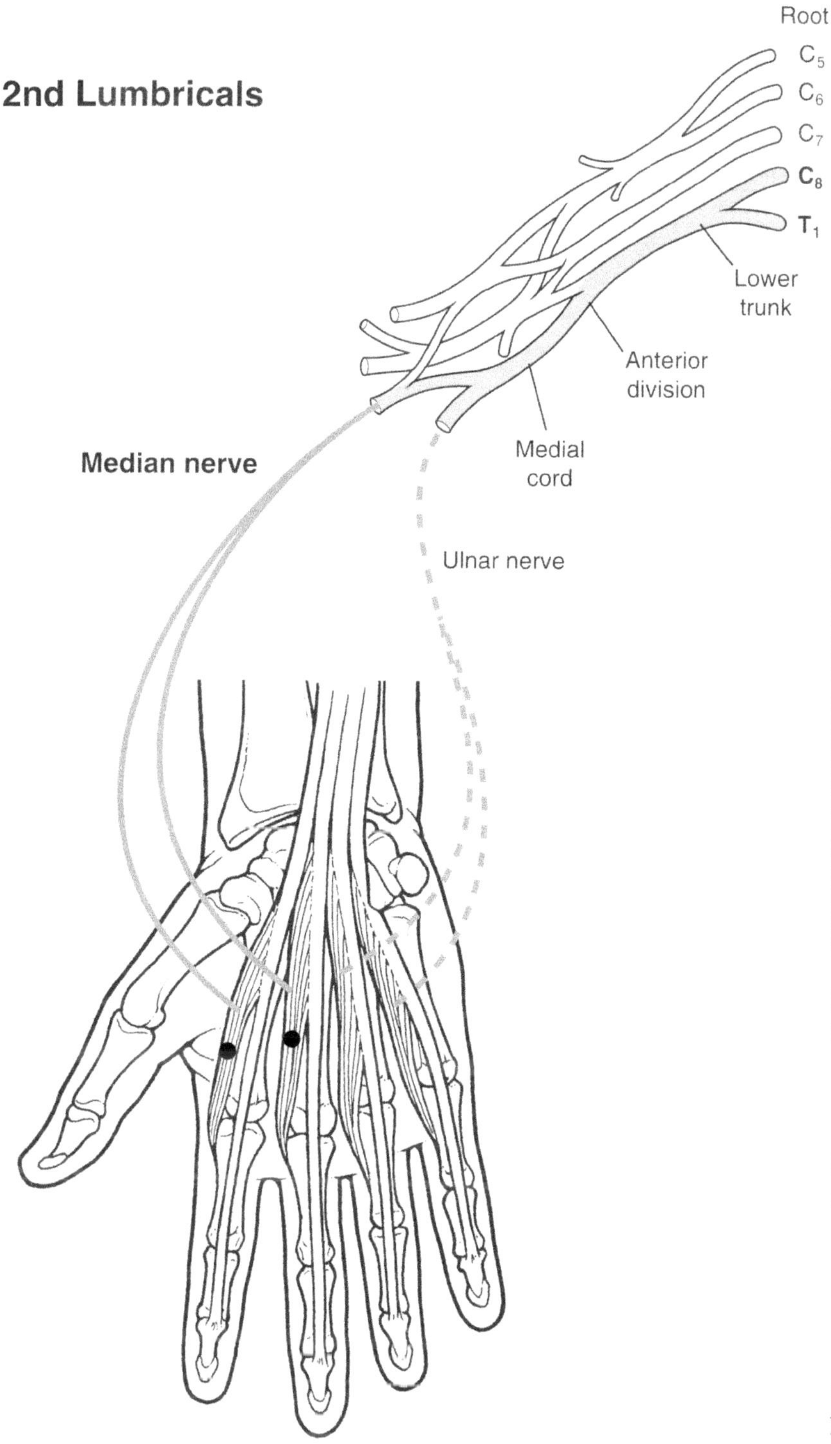

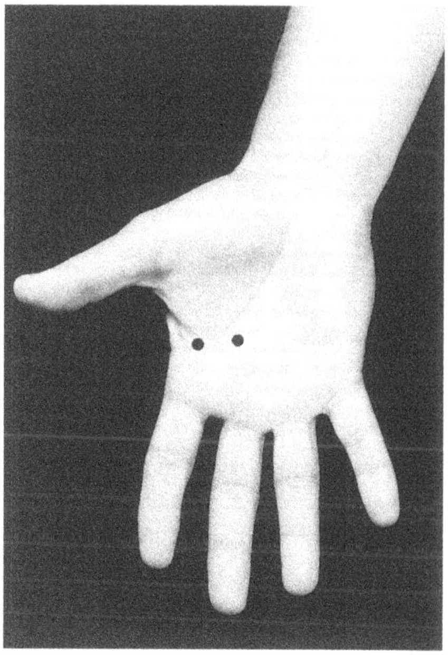

Innervation
Innervation is via the median nerve, medial cord, lower trunk, and roots C_8, T_1.

Origin
The first and second lumbricals originate in the radial aspect of the tendon sheath of the flexor digitorum profundus.

Insertion
The muscles are inserted at the radial lateral band of the dorsal digital expansion.

Activation Maneuver
Extension of the finger at the proximal interphalangeal joint with the metacarpophalangeal joint extended and fixed activates the first and second lumbricals.

EMG Needle Insertion
Insert the needle just proximal to the metacarpophalangeal joint and radial to the flexor tendon.

Pitfalls
All muscles surrounding the first and second lumbricals receive innervation from the ulnar nerve. It is therefore easy to erroneously access ulnar intrinsic hand muscles.

Clinical Comments
Lumbrical examination causes pain. It is rarely of benefit in a routine EMG needle evaluation.

Needle examination will show neurogenic changes with axonal loss lesions of median nerve due to carpal tunnel syndrome, pronator teres syndrome, ligament of Struthers' syndrome, C_8, T_1 radiculopathy, Klumpke's palsy (C_8, T_1 root avulsion), and anterior horn cell disease.

Pronator Quadratus

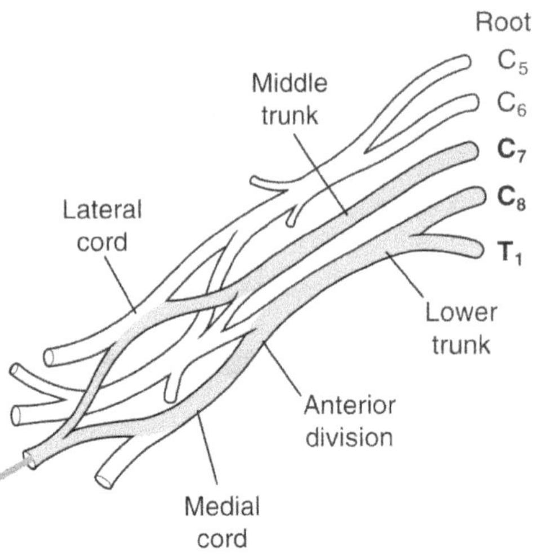

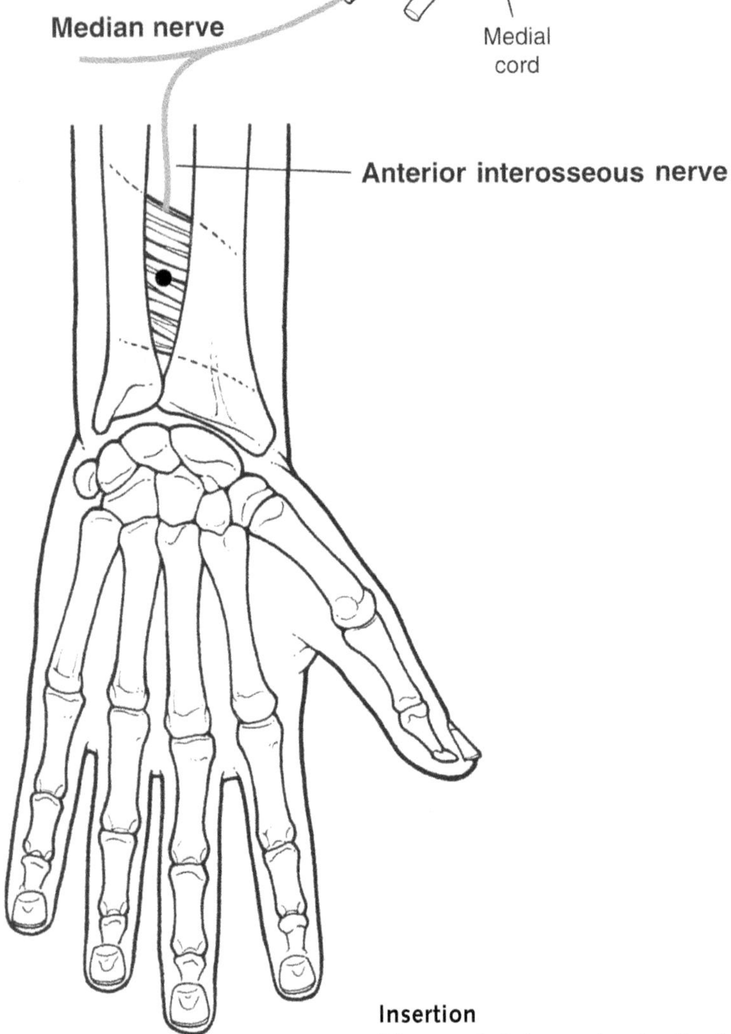

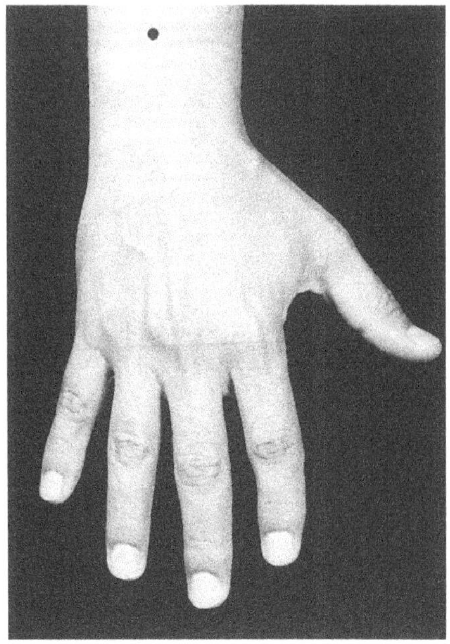

Innervation

Innervation is via the anterior interosseous branch, median nerve, lateral and medial cords, middle and lower trunks, and roots C_7, C_8, T_1.

Origin

The pronator quadratus originates in the distal fourth of the volar surface of the ulna.

Insertion

The muscle is inserted at the distal fourth of the lateral border and the volar surface of the radius.

Activation Maneuver

Pronation of the forearm activates the muscle.

EMG Needle Insertion

Place the forearm in a neutral position to full supination (this opens up the area between the ulna and the radius). Insert the needle dorsally 2–3 cm proximal to the ulnar styloid just lateral (in the radial direction) to the ulna to a depth of 2–2.5 cm. Slant the needle slightly toward the shaft of the radius to penetrate the interosseous membrane.

Pitfalls

If the needle is inserted too deeply, it may penetrate the flexor digitorum superficialis, which receives innervation from the median nerve.

Clinical Comments

EMG needle examination will be normal in the carpal tunnel syndrome.

EMG may show neurogenic changes in lesions of the anterior interosseous nerve, producing axonal loss.

EMG may show neurogenic changes in more proximal lesions affecting median nerve fibers (pronator teres syndrome, ligament of Struthers' syndrome, C_7, C_8, T_1 radiculopathy, root avulsion, and anterior horn cell disease).

Flexor Pollicis Longus

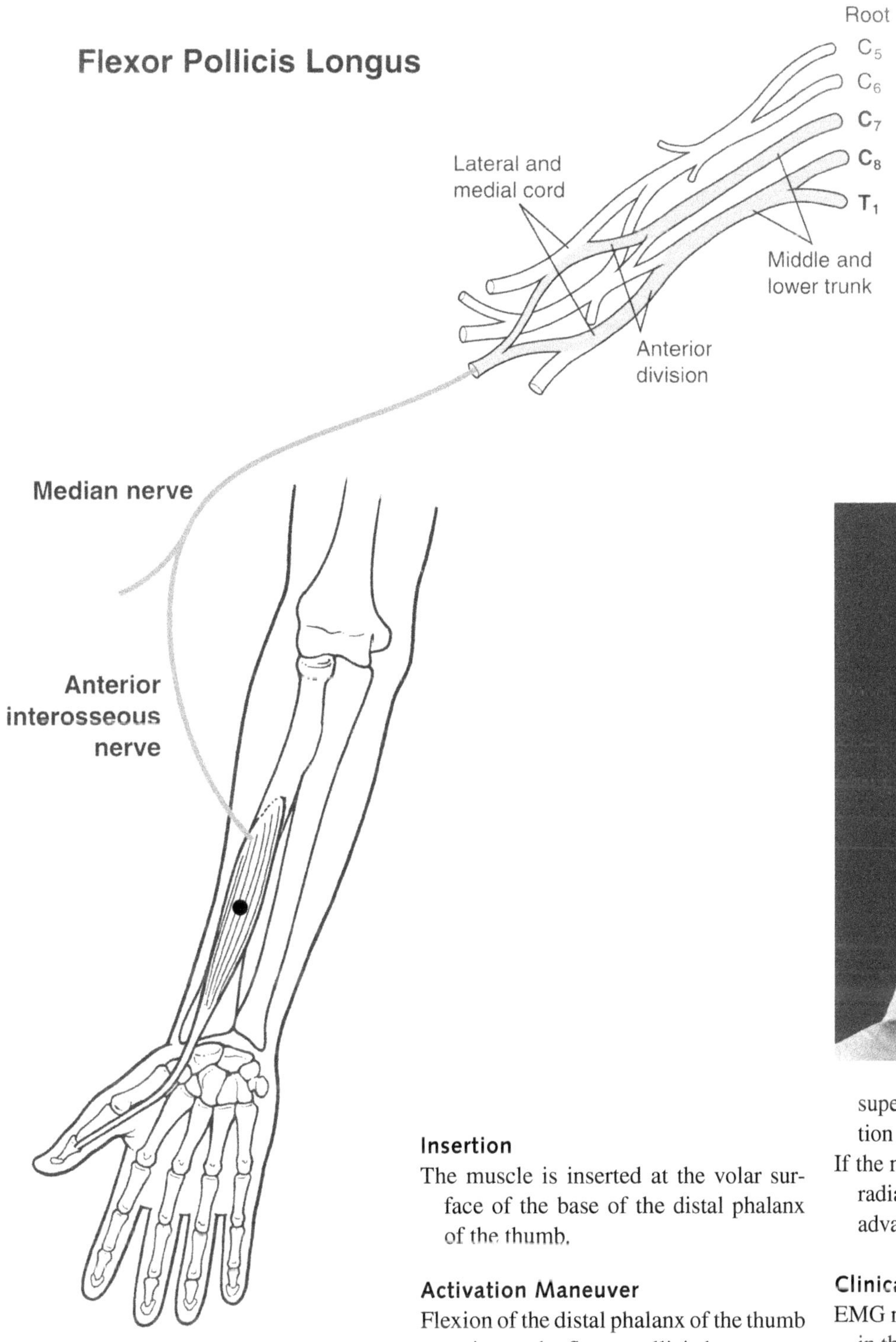

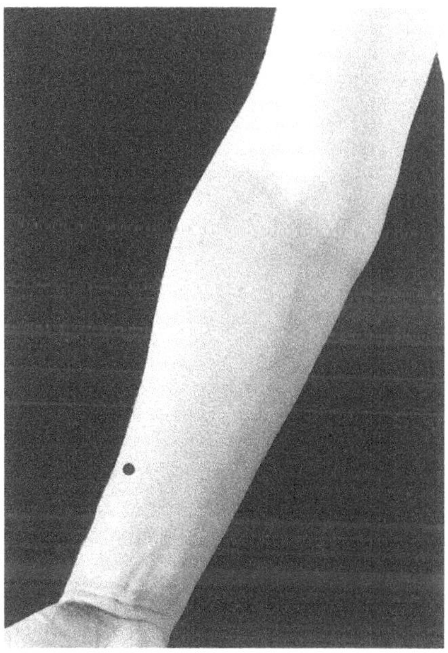

Innervation

Innervation is via the anterior interosseous branch, median nerve, lateral and medial cords, middle and lower trunks, and roots C_7, C_8, T_1.

Origin

The flexor pollicis longus originates in the volar surface of the radius.

Insertion

The muscle is inserted at the volar surface of the base of the distal phalanx of the thumb.

Activation Maneuver

Flexion of the distal phalanx of the thumb activates the flexor pollicis longus.

EMG Needle Insertion

Palpate the radial artery. Insert the needle 5–7 cm proximal and 1–1.5 cm lateral to the radial artery pulse.

Pitfalls

If the needle is inserted too superficially, it may lie in the flexor digitorum superficialis, which receives innervation from the median nerve.

If the needle is inserted too medially, the radial artery will lie in the path of the advancing needle.

Clinical Comments

EMG needle examination will be normal in the carpal tunnel syndrome.

EMG may show neurogenic changes in lesions of the anterior interosseous nerve, producing axonal loss.

EMG may show neurogenic changes in more proximal lesions affecting median nerve fibers (pronator teres syndrome, ligament of Struthers' syndrome, C_7, C_8, T_1 radiculopathy, root avulsion, and anterior horn cell disease).

Flexor Digitorum Profundus Digits 2 and 3

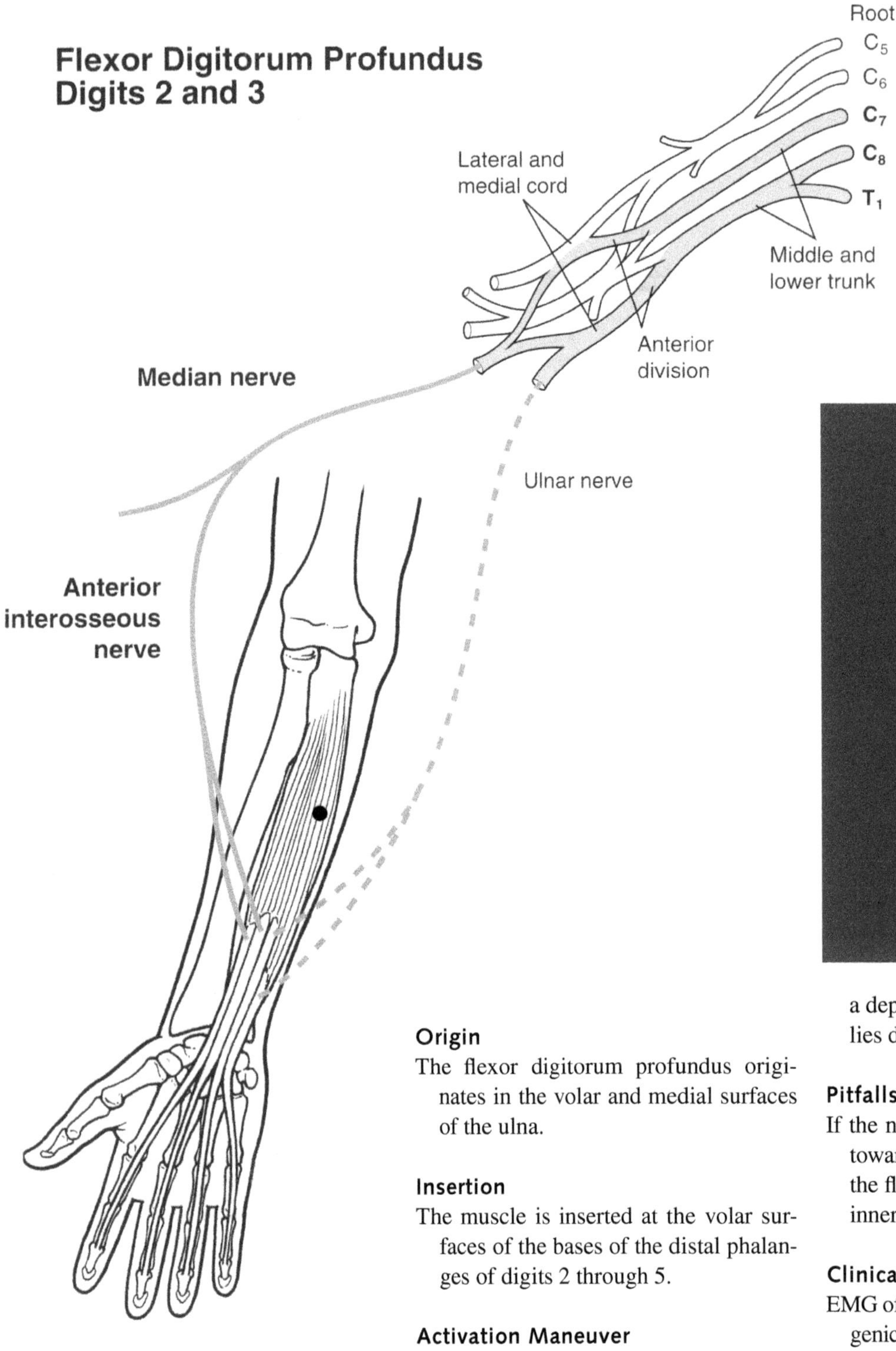

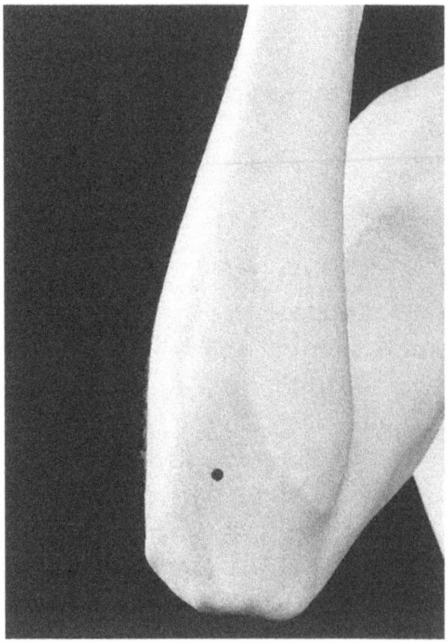

Innervation

Digits two and three: Innervation is via the anterior interosseous branch, median nerve, lateral and medial cords, middle and lower trunks, and roots C_7, C_8.

Digits four and five: Innervation is via the ulnar nerve, medial cord, lower trunk, and roots C_8, T_1.

Origin

The flexor digitorum profundus originates in the volar and medial surfaces of the ulna.

Insertion

The muscle is inserted at the volar surfaces of the bases of the distal phalanges of digits 2 through 5.

Activation Maneuver

Flexion of the distal phalanges of digits 2 through 5 activates the flexor digitorum profundus.

EMG Needle Insertion

Insert the needle 5–7 cm distal to the olecranon process and 1–1.5 cm medial to the shaft of the ulna. The ulnar innervated portion lies superficially at a depth of 1–2 cm; the median portion lies deep at a depth of 3–4 cm.

Pitfalls

If the needle is inserted too volarly (i.e., toward the palmar surface), it may lie in the flexor carpi ulnaris, which receives innervation from the ulnar nerve.

Clinical Comments

EMG of the deep portion may show neurogenic changes in the anterior interosseous nerve syndrome and in proximal lesions affecting median nerve fibers (pronator teres syndrome, ligament of Struthers' syndrome, C_7, C_8 radiculopathy, avulsion, and anterior horn cell disease).

EMG of the superficial portion may show neurogenic changes in axonal loss lesions of the ulnar nerve at the elbow (cubital tunnel or retrocondylar groove).

Flexor Digitorum Superficialis (sublimis)

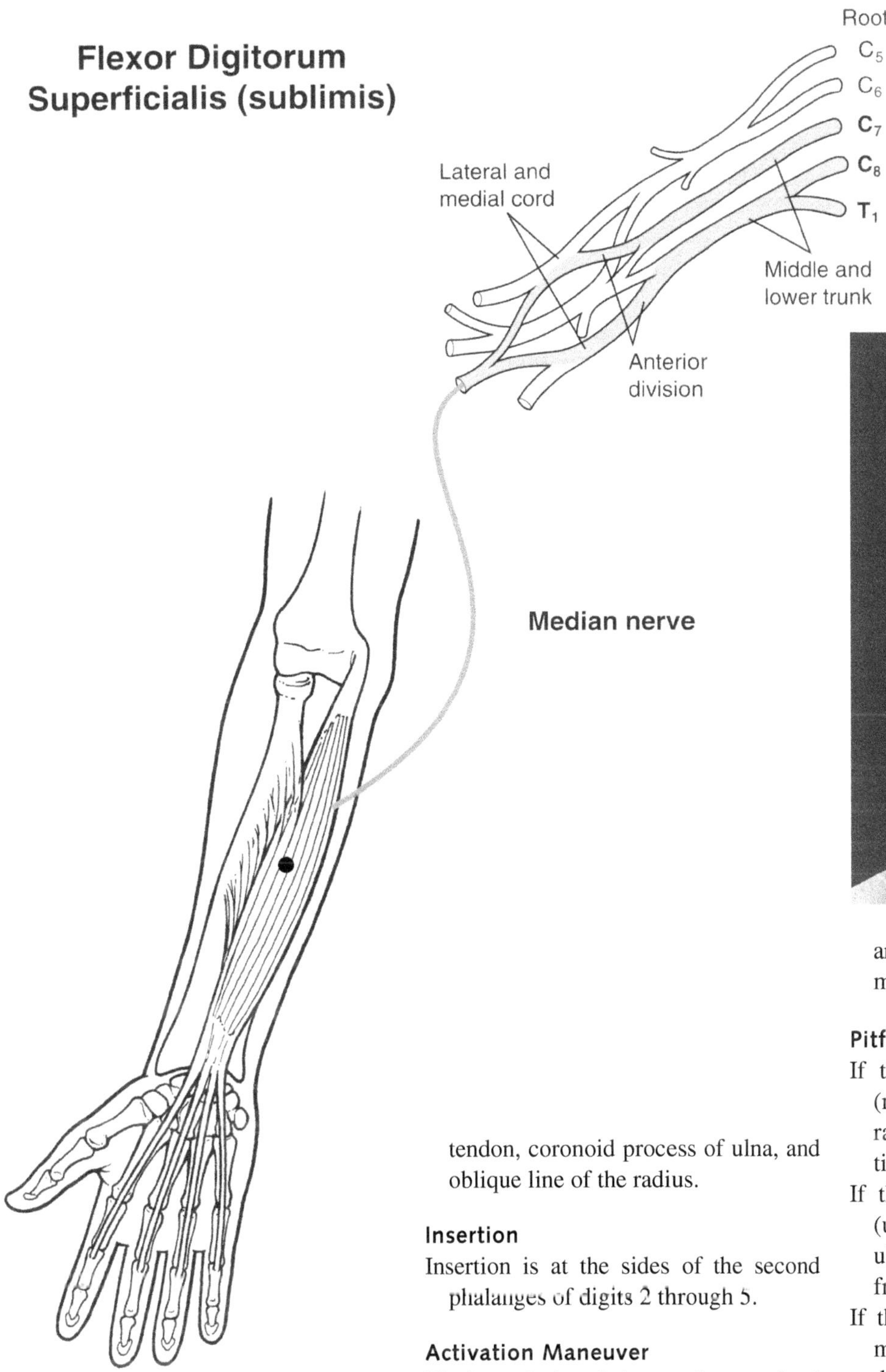

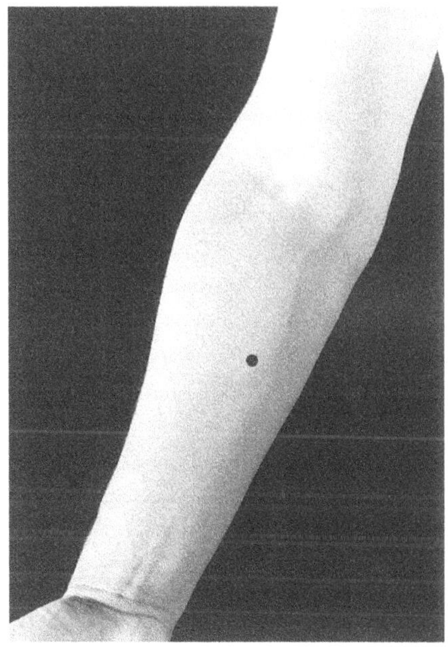

Innervation

Innervation is via the median nerve, lateral and medial cords, middle and lower trunks, and roots C_7, C_8, T_1.

Origin

The flexor digitorum superficialis (sublimis) originates in the medial epicondyle of the humerus by the common tendon, coronoid process of ulna, and oblique line of the radius.

Insertion

Insertion is at the sides of the second phalanges of digits 2 through 5.

Activation Maneuver

Flexion of the digits at the proximal interphalangeal joint, with the proximal phalanx fixed and the distal interphalangeal joint in hyperextension, activates the muscle.

EMG Needle Insertion

Insert the needle into the volar surface of the forearm approximately 7–9 cm distal to the biceps tendon (midforearm) and 2–3 cm medial to the ventral midline.

Pitfalls

If the needle is inserted too laterally (radially), it may lie in the flexor carpi radialis, which also receives innervation from the median nerve.

If the needle is inserted too medially (ulnarly), it may be in the flexor carpi ulnaris, which receives innervation from the ulnar nerve.

If the needle is inserted too deeply, it may be in the flexor digitorum profundus (median innervated portion).

Clinical Comments

Needle examination may show neurogenic changes with axonal loss lesions of the median nerve due to pronator teres syndrome, ligament of Struthers' syndrome, brachial plexopathy, C_7, C_8, or T_1 radiculopathies, and anterior horn cell disease.

Palmaris Longus

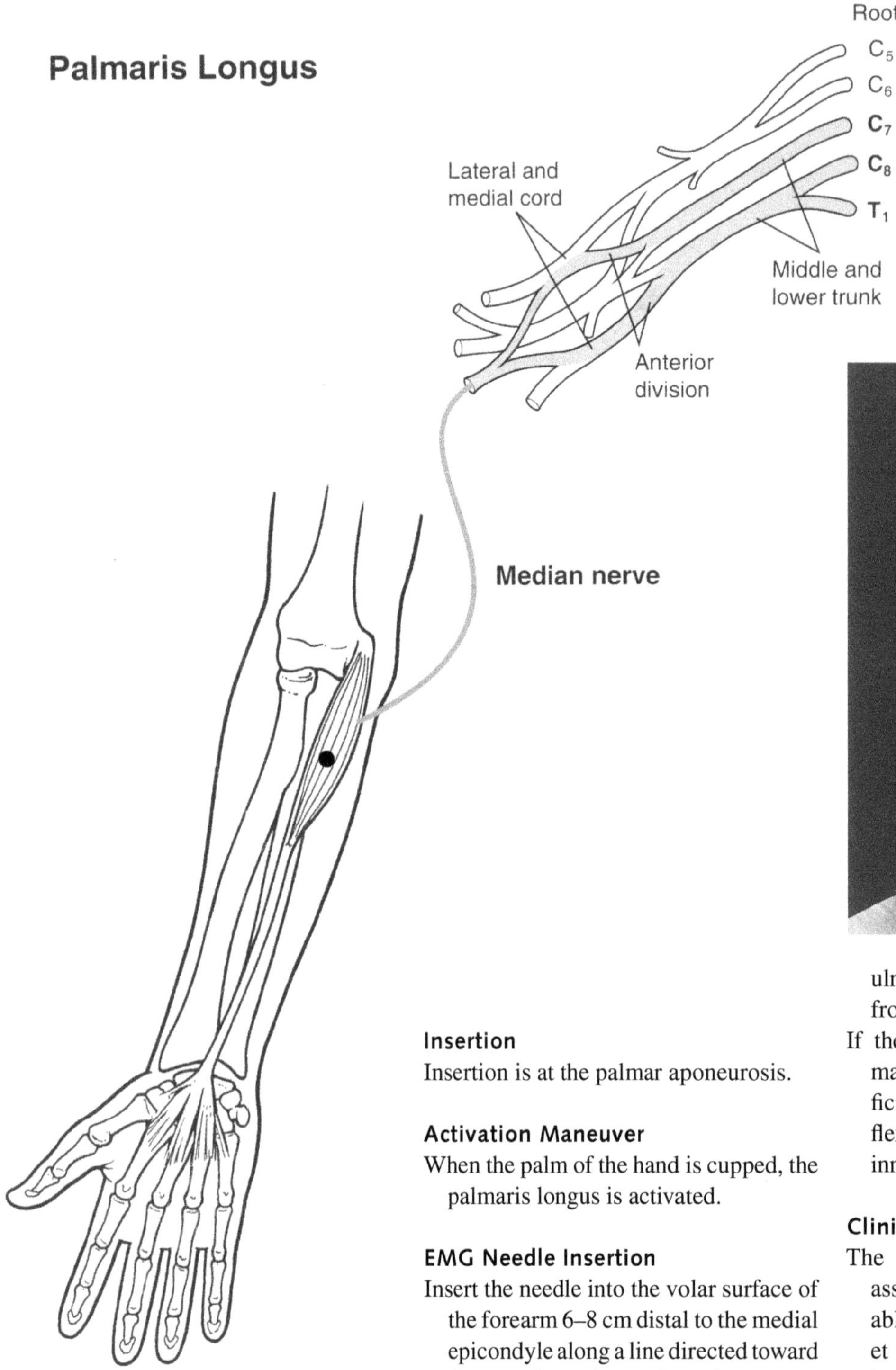

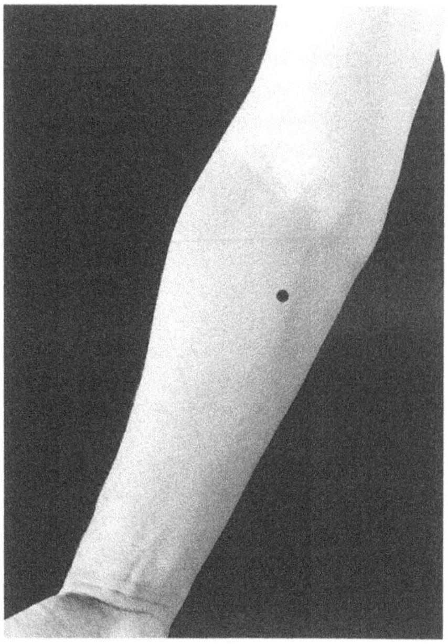

Innervation

Innervation is via the median nerve, lateral and medial cords, middle and lower trunks, and roots C_7, C_8, T_1.

Origin

The palmaris longus originates in the medial epicondyle of the humerus.

Insertion

Insertion is at the palmar aponeurosis.

Activation Maneuver

When the palm of the hand is cupped, the palmaris longus is activated.

EMG Needle Insertion

Insert the needle into the volar surface of the forearm 6–8 cm distal to the medial epicondyle along a line directed toward the muscle tendon at the wrist.

Pitfalls

If the needle is inserted too laterally (radially), it may lie in the flexor carpi radialis, which receives innervation from the median nerve.

If the needle is inserted too medially (ulnarly), it may be in the flexor carpi ulnaris, which receives innervation from the ulnar nerve.

If the needle is inserted too deeply, it may be in the flexor digitorum superficialis (median nerve innervation) or flexor digitorum profundus (median-innervated portion).

Clinical Comments

The palmaris longus is not routinely assessed. This muscle is the most variable muscle of the body (Bergman, et al., 1984). It is absent in 11% of humans (both arms in 8%; right arms, 4%; left arms, 5%).

Needle examination may show neurogenic changes with loss of axons in the median nerve due to pronator teres syndrome, ligament of Struthers' syndrome, brachial plexopathy, C_7, C_8, or T_1 radiculopathies, and anterior horn cell disease.

Flexor Carpi Radialis

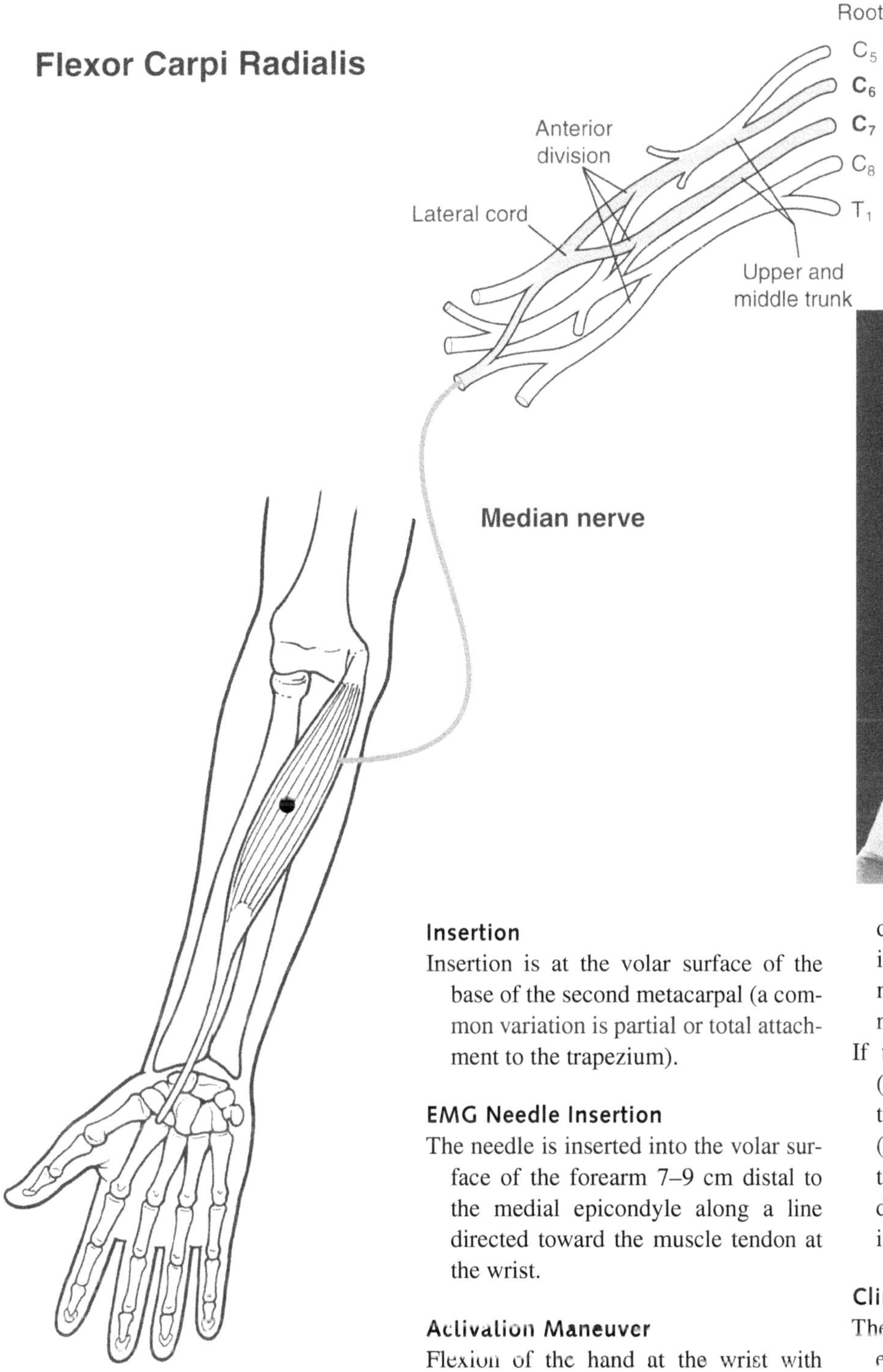

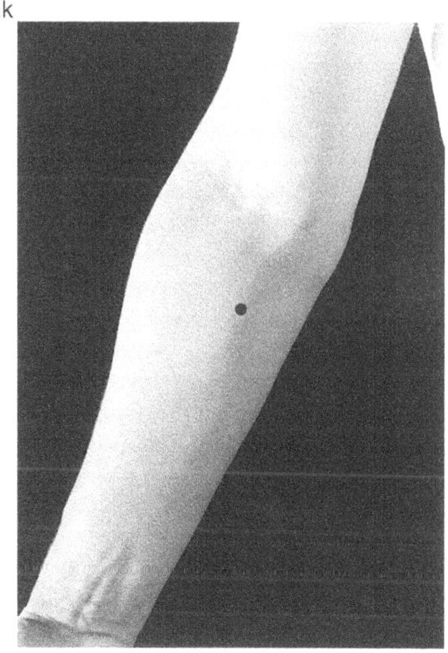

Innervation

Innervation is via the median nerve, lateral cord, upper and middle trunks, and roots C_6, C_7.

Origin

The flexor carpi radialis originates in the medial epicondyle of the humerus.

Insertion

Insertion is at the volar surface of the base of the second metacarpal (a common variation is partial or total attachment to the trapezium).

EMG Needle Insertion

The needle is inserted into the volar surface of the forearm 7–9 cm distal to the medial epicondyle along a line directed toward the muscle tendon at the wrist.

Activation Maneuver

Flexion of the hand at the wrist with radial deviation activates the muscle. Hint: Avoid coactivation of the flexor digitorum superficialis or the pronator teres when performing the activation maneuver.

Pitfalls

If the needle is inserted too laterally (radially), it may be in the brachioradialis (radial nerve innervation); if it is inserted too lateral and proximal, it may be in the pronator teres (median nerve innervation).

If the needle is inserted too medially (ulnarly), it may be in the flexor digitorum superficialis or palmaris longus (median nerve innervation); if inserted too deeply, it will be in the flexor digitorum superficialis (median nerve innervation).

Clinical Comments

The flexor carpi radialis is routinely examined after carpal tunnel syndrome is diagnosed to exclude coexisting proximal median nerve injury (double lesion).

Needle examination may show neurogenic changes with loss of axons in the median nerve due to pronator teres syndrome, ligament of Struthers' syndrome, lateral cord lesion, C_6, C_7 radiculopathy, and anterior horn cell disease.

Pronator Teres

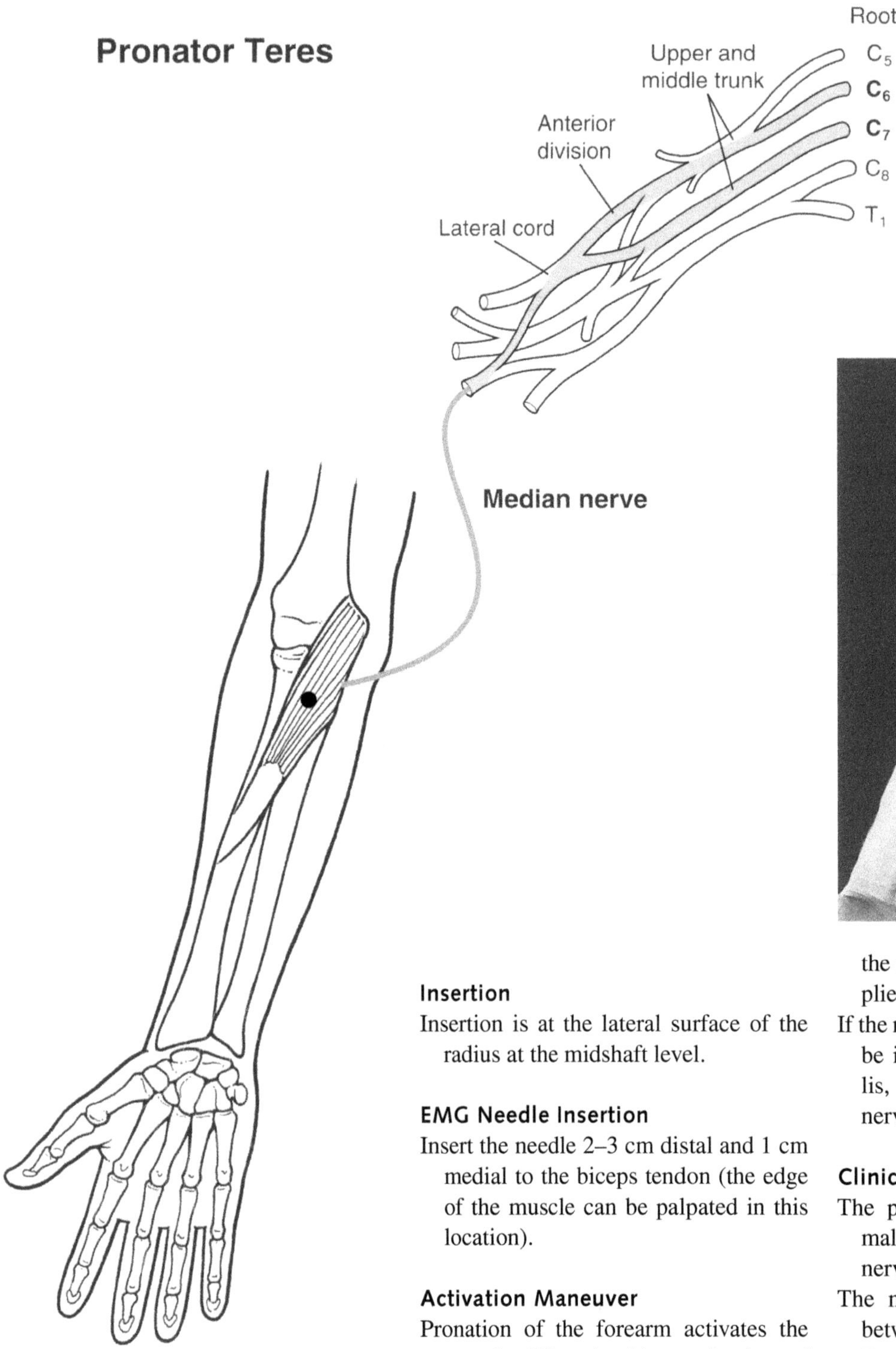

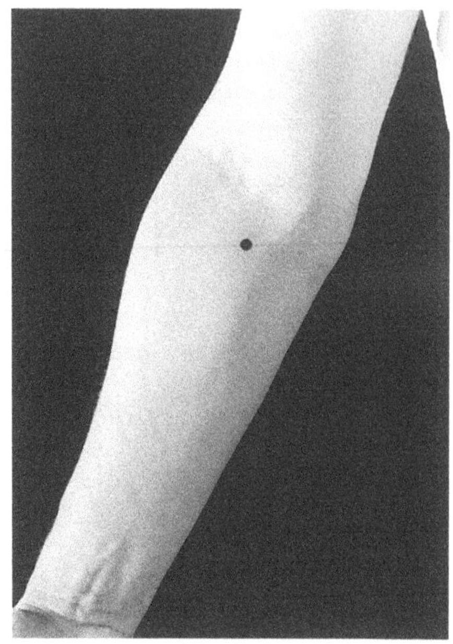

Innervation

Innervation is via the median nerve, lateral cord, upper and middle trunks, and roots C_6, C_7.

Origin

The pronator teres arises as two heads, one from the medial epicondyle of the humerus and the other from the coronoid process of the ulna.

Insertion

Insertion is at the lateral surface of the radius at the midshaft level.

EMG Needle Insertion

Insert the needle 2–3 cm distal and 1 cm medial to the biceps tendon (the edge of the muscle can be palpated in this location).

Activation Maneuver

Pronation of the forearm activates the muscle. Hint: Avoid coactivation of the flexor carpi radialis when performing the activation maneuver.

Pitfalls

If the needle is inserted too laterally (radially), it may be in the brachioradialis, which is supplied by the radial nerve.

If the needle is inserted too medially (ulnarly) or too distally, it may be in the flexor carpi radialis, which is supplied by the median nerve.

If the needle is inserted too deeply, it will be in the flexor digitorum superficialis, which is supplied by the median nerve.

Clinical Comments

The pronator teres is the most proximal muscle innervated by the median nerve.

The median nerve enters the forearm between the two heads of this muscle. Entrapment produces the pronator teres syndrome.

EMG may show neurogenic changes with loss of axons in the median nerve due to ligament of Struthers' syndrome, lateral cord lesion, C_6, C_7 radiculopathy, and anterior horn cell disease.

EMG is usually normal in the pronator teres syndrome. Note: The muscle naming a syndrome is usually spared in that syndrome.

ULNAR NERVE

5

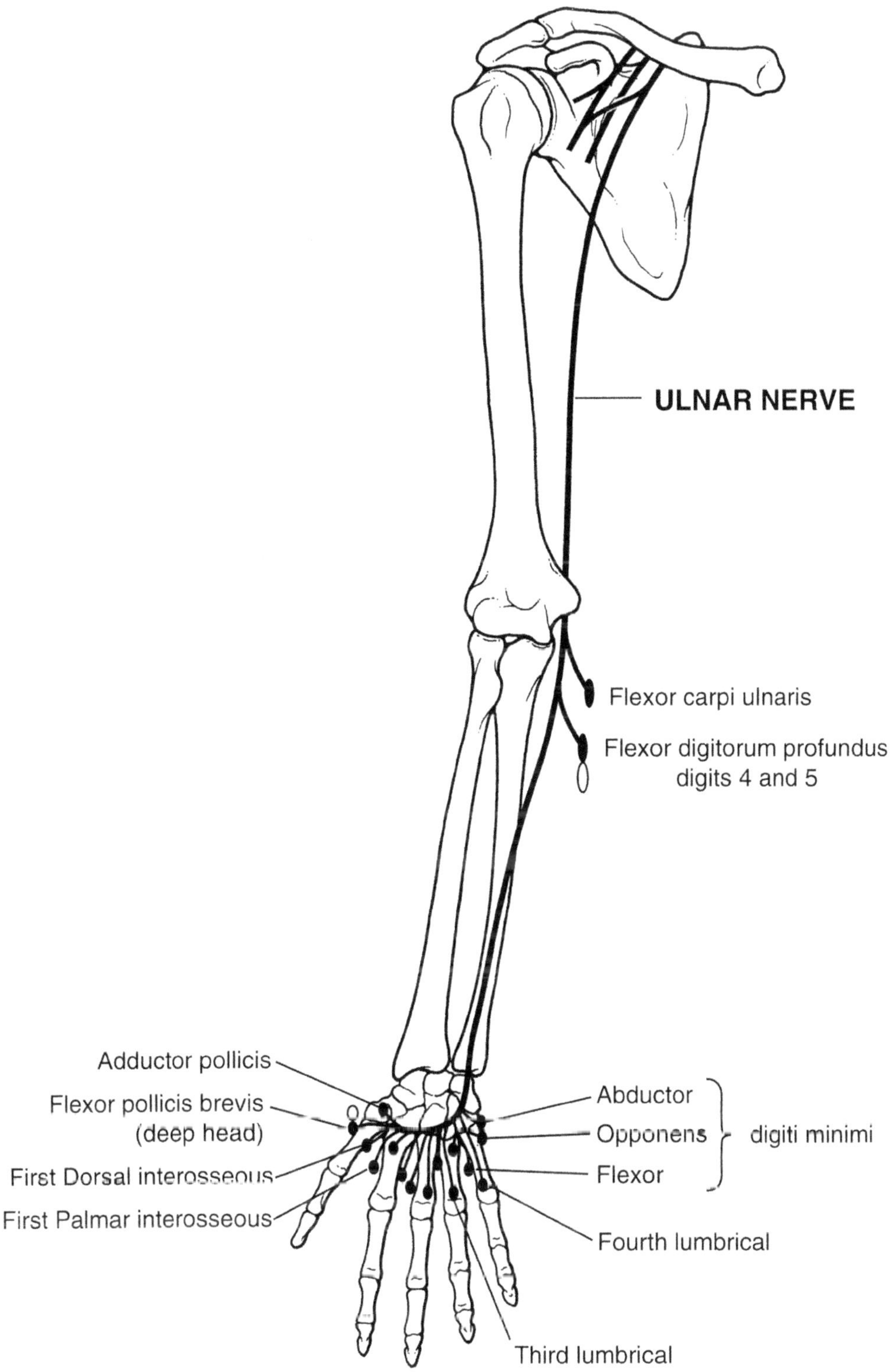

FIGURE 5-1 Diagram of the ulnar nerve and the muscles that it supplies. Note: The white oval signifies that a muscle receives a part of its innervation from another peripheral nerve.

THE ULNAR NERVE (Figure 5-1) is the main continuation of the medial cord of the brachial plexus. Its fibers are usually derived from the eighth cervical and first thoracic roots, although occasionally the seventh cervical root makes a contribution via the lateral cord (*Gray's Anatomy,* 1995). In the axilla, the nerve runs between the axillary artery and vein. In the arm, it stays between the brachial artery and vein, sharing the neurovascular bundle with the median nerve. At the mid-arm, it leaves the neurovascular bundle and passes posteriorly through the medial intermuscular septum to descend on the medial aspect of the medial head of the triceps. The nerve is superficial throughout this course and innervates no muscles in the arm.

At the elbow, the nerve lies in a groove formed by the medial epicondyle of the humerus and the olecranon process of the ulna (the retrocondylar groove). It enters the forearm through an aponeurotic arcade (the cubital tunnel) joining the two heads of the flexor carpi ulnaris, which it innervates. The arcade typically lies about 1.5 cm distal to the medial epicondyle (Campbell, 1989). The nerve travels through the belly of the flexor carpi ulnaris and then exits by piercing the aponeurosis on the undersurface of the muscle. It then lies in the plane between the flexor carpi ulnaris and the flexor digitorum profundus (to digits 4 and 5), which it innervates.

The nerve is joined by the ulnar artery in the upper forearm to form a neurovascular bundle. About the middle of the forearm, the ulnar nerve gives rise to the palmar cutaneous branch, which descends to provide sensory innervation to the medial aspect of the proximal palm. About 7 cm proximal to the wrist it also gives off a dorsal cutaneous branch, which provides innervation to the medial aspect of the dorsum of the hand and the dorsoproximal aspect of the fifth and medial fourth digits. The ulnar nerve provides no sensory innervation above the wrist. Hence, sensory loss in the forearm or arm is not a feature of an ulnar nerve lesion.

At the wrist, the ulnar nerve and artery lie in a canal formed by the pisiform medially and the hook of the hamate laterally (Guyon's canal). In this region the nerve divides into superficial and deep branches. Although the superficial branch is generally considered a sensory branch, it supplies the palmaris brevis, a thin muscle beneath the skin of the proximal medial palm, which cannot be studied electromyographically. It then provides sensory innervation to the distal palm and terminates in two digital branches that are distributed to the ulnar side of the fifth digit and the adjoining sides of the fourth and fifth digits. The deep muscular branch gives off a hypothenar branch to innervate the abductor, opponens, and flexor digit minimi. It then follows the course of the deep palmar arch across the hand. As it crosses, it supplies dorsal and palmar interossei and the third and fourth lumbricals. At its termination between the thumb and index fingers, it supplies the flexor pollicis brevis (deep head) and adductor pollicis.

Although the ulnar nerve, or its branches, may be involved by penetrating injuries at any level, there are certain sites where the nerve is prone to injury (Sunderland, 1968). Compression neuropathies of the ulnar nerve at the elbow are common and widely recognized. In the retrocondylar groove, the nerve lies on bone covered only by a thin layer of skin, and is subject to chronic compression from multiple etiologies (Figure 5-2). At 1–2 cm distally, the nerve may be entrapped at the cubital tunnel. Compression at either site may result in the clinical presentation known as *ulnar neuropathy at the elbow*. Rarely, the nerve may be entrapped in the proximal forearm as it pierces the deep aponeurosis investing the undersurface of the flexor carpi ulnaris (Amadio and Beckenbaugh, 1986; Campbell et al., 1988) or in the distal forearm by a fibrovascular band or hypertrophied flexor carpi ulnaris tendon (Campbell, 1989). Entrapment at the wrist (Guyon's canal) may present with different patterns of sensorimotor deficits, depending on the degree of involvement of the superficial (sensory), deep (motor) or hypothenar (motor) branches.

ULNAR NEUROPATHY AT THE ELBOW (RETROCONDYLAR GROOVE)

Etiology

Ulnar neuropathy at the elbow can be caused by compression at the retrocondylar groove due to repeated trauma (habitual leaning on the elbows, sustained hyperflexion at the elbows), traumatic joint deformity, distal humerus fractures, elbow dislocations, callus formation, rheumatic and degenerative joint disease, congenital anomalies of the elbow, valgus deformity, and immobilization during surgery.

General Comments

Originally, the term *tardy ulnar palsy* referred to antecedent traumatic joint deformity or recurrent subluxation of the nerve out of the retrocondylar groove. However, it is not clear that recurrent subluxation is a risk factor for ulnar neuropathy (personal observation) and many clinicians now use the term for any entrapment of the ulnar nerve at the elbow.

The appearance of ulnar mononeuropathy may herald the onset of a more generalized neuropathy.

Ulnar neuropathy at the retrocondylar groove should be distinguished electrodiagnostically from cubital tunnel syndrome. The distinction can be important in surgical management; the former generally requires surgical transposition of the nerve, whereas the latter may warrant simple decompression of the nerve in the tunnel, without transposition (Miller, 1991).

Clinical Features

Paresthesia, pain, or numbness occurs in the sensory distribution of the ulnar nerve, including the dorsum of the hand.

There is pain or tenderness at the elbow.

Weakness and wasting of the first dorsal interosseous and other ulnar-innervated hand muscles may occur in severe cases. Clinical evidence of weakness may preferentially involve the first dorsal interosseous (Stewart, 1987).

Weakness of the flexor carpi ulnaris and flexor digitorum profundus (to digits 4 and 5) may be variable.

Radiographic studies may visualize rheumatic, arthritic, or post-traumatic changes around the elbow.

Electrodiagnostic Strategy

Use routine motor nerve conduction studies to demonstrate slowing of conduction velocity or conduction block to the retrocondylar region.

Use routine sensory nerve conduction studies to demonstrate an absent or reduced superficial sensory response (from fifth digit) and dorsal ulnar cutaneous response.

Use special nerve conduction studies ("inching technique") to precisely localize the conduction abnormality (focal slowing, conduction block) to the retrocondylar region.

Demonstrate neurogenic EMG abnormalities in the first dorsal interosseous and other ulnar-innervated hand muscles.

EMG abnormalities in the flexor carpi ulnaris and flexor digitorum profundus (superficial head) localize the lesion to the elbow. In many patients, however, these muscles may be normal, particularly in mild ulnar neuropathy (Kincaid, 1988; Campbell et al., 1989).

ULNAR NEUROPATHY AT THE ELBOW (CUBITAL TUNNEL SYNDROME)

Etiology

Entrapment of the ulnar nerve occurs in the tunnel formed by the tendinous arch connecting the humeral and ulnar heads of the flexor carpi ulnaris 1–2 cm distal to the medial epicondyle. Variations in the anatomy of the cubital tunnel may predispose to ulnar neuropathy (O'Driscoll et al., 1991).

General Comments

When the elbow is flexed, the cubital tunnel narrows and the ulnar nerve is pulled tightly across the retrocondylar groove. Sustained hyperflexion at the elbow (e.g., using hand

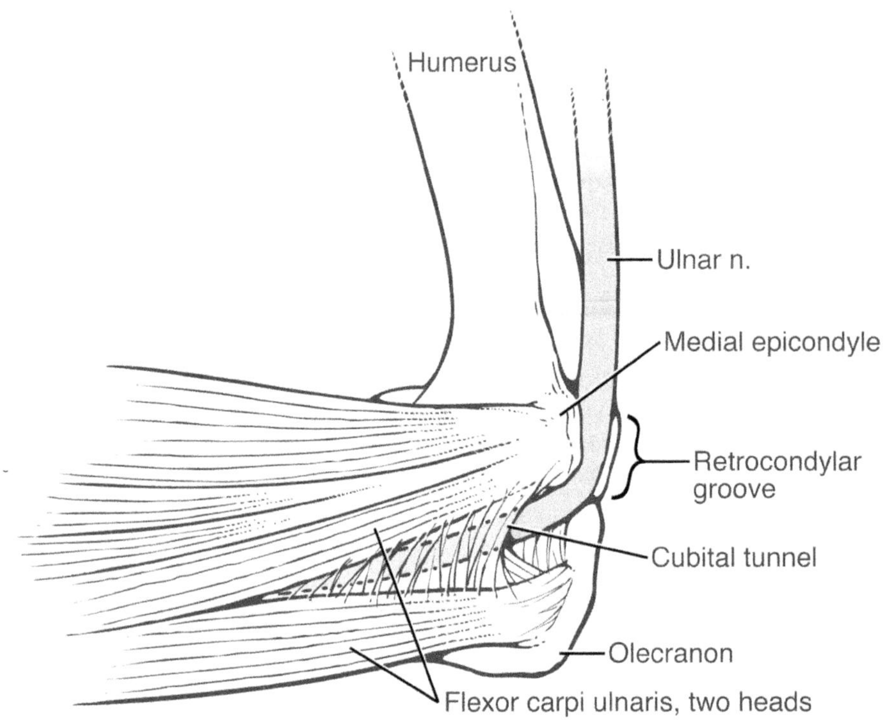

FIGURE 5-2 Anatomy of the ulnar nerve at the elbow.

as a pillow, prolonged talking on cell phone, placing elbow on a firm surface) is important in the development of cubital tunnel syndrome and ulnar neuropathy at the retrocondylar groove.

There may be no predisposing joint deformity or prior trauma to the elbow.

Bilateral ulnar neuropathy occurs commonly.

Ulnar neuropathy at the retrocondylar groove should be distinguished electrodiagnostically from cubital tunnel syndrome. The former generally requires surgical transposition of the nerve, whereas the latter may warrant simple decompression in the tunnel, without transposition (Miller, 1991).

Clinical Features

Paresthesia, pain, or numbness occurs in the sensory distribution of the ulnar nerve, including the dorsum of the hand.

There is pain or tenderness at or slightly distal to the elbow.

In severe cases, weakness and wasting of the first dorsal interosseous and other ulnar-innervated hand muscles may occur. Clinical evidence of weakness may preferentially involve the first dorsal interosseous (Stewart, 1987).

Weakness of the flexor carpi ulnaris and flexor digitorum profundus (to digits 4 and 5) may be variable.

Radiographic studies are usually normal.

Electrodiagnostic Strategy

Use routine motor nerve conduction studies to demonstrate slowing of conduction velocity or conduction block at the elbow.

Use routine sensory nerve conduction studies to demonstrate an absent or reduced superficial sensory response (from fifth digit) and dorsal ulnar cutaneous response.

Use special nerve conduction studies ("inching technique") to precisely localize the conduction abnormality (focal slowing, conduction block) to the cubital tunnel.

Demonstrate neurogenic EMG abnormalities in the first dorsal interosseous and other ulnar-innervated hand muscles.

EMG abnormalities in the flexor carpi ulnaris and flexor digitorum profundus (superficial head) localize the lesion to the elbow. These muscles may be normal, however, particularly in mild ulnar neuropathy (Kincaid, 1988; Campbell et al., 1989).

ULNAR NEUROPATHY AT THE WRIST (GUYON'S CANAL)

Etiology

Entrapment of the ulnar nerve occurs in the tunnel formed by the pisiform bone medially and the hook of the hamate laterally (Figure 5-3). The firm floor consists of the thick transverse carpal ligament and subjacent bone. The distal roof is rigidly bound by the pisohamate ligament.

Entrapment may be associated with a lipoma, ganglion cyst, aneurysm, other mass lesion, or chronic compression to the hypothenar region (bicycle bars, crutches, occupation).

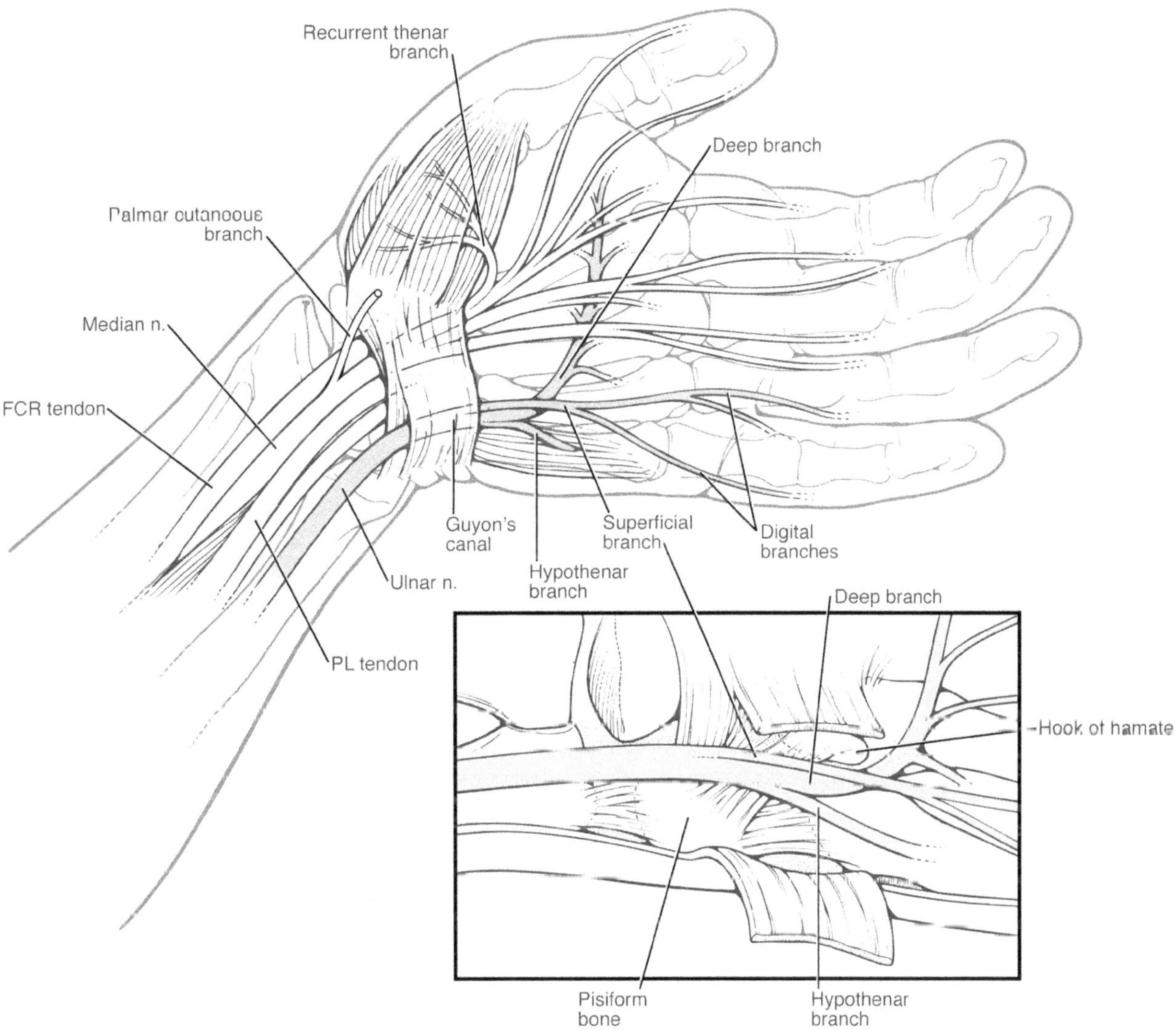

FIGURE 5-3 Anatomy of the ulnar nerve at the wrist and palm.

General Comments

Within the canal, the nerve divides into superficial (sensory), deep (muscular), and hypothenar (muscular) branches.

Clinical Features

Compression within Guyon's canal may predominantly affect certain fascicles or branches of the ulnar nerve to produce distinctive patterns of symptoms and signs (Olney and Hanson, 1988). *Pattern 1*: A lesion primarily involving the deep branch will produce weakness in interossei and lumbricals but not hypothenar muscles; there are no sensory deficits. *Pattern 2*: A lesion involving deep branch and hypothenar motor branch will produce weakness in interossei, lumbricals, and hypothenar muscles; there are no sensory deficits. *Pattern 3*: A lesion at or proximal to the bifurcation into deep and superficial branches will produce weakness in interossei, lumbricals, and hypothenar muscles, and sensory deficits in the distal palm, fifth digit, and ulnar side of the fourth digit. *Pattern 4*: A lesion primarily involving the superficial sensory branch will produce only sensory deficits in the distal palm, fifth digit, and ulnar side of the fourth digit.

Lesions that compress the deep and hypothenar motor branches (patterns 1 and 2) are the most common and may be confused with focal onset of amyotrophic lateral sclerosis, particularly in the all-ulnar hand (Riches-Cannieu anastomosis).

Lesions that compress the superficial branch (patterns 3 and 4) do not produce loss of sensation over the ulnar dorsal surface of the hand (dorsal ulnar cutaneous distribution).

Electrodiagnostic Strategy

Use nerve conduction studies to localize the conduction abnormality (prolonged distal latencies in motor or sensory responses, reduced amplitudes) to the wrist. Motor conduction studies should record over the first dorsal interosseous as well as hypothenar muscles. This allows detection of distal deep branch lesions.

Elicit normal sensory nerve conduction studies of the ulnar dorsal cutaneous branch.

Demonstrate neurogenic EMG abnormalities in the first dorsal interosseous and other ulnar-innervated hand muscles.

Perform EMG in additional muscles to exclude anterior horn cell disease and C_8, T_1 radiculopathy.

Ulnar Motor Nerve Conduction Study from Abductor Digiti Minimi (ADM)

Recording

Active electrode: Position over the belly of the ADM.

Reference electrode: Place over the tendon of the ADM at the base of the proximal phalanx of the little finger (belly-tendon recording).

Ground electrode: Place on the dorsum of the hand, between stimulating and recording electrodes.

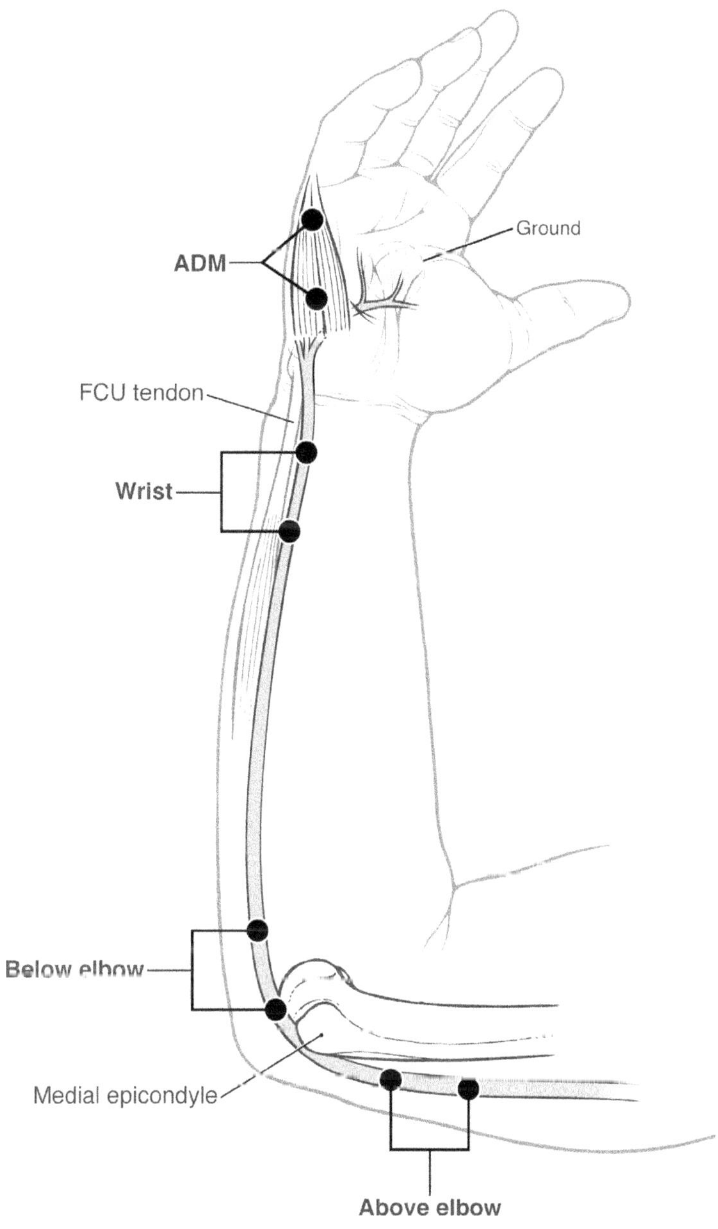

FIGURE 5-4 Ulnar motor nerve conduction study from abductor digiti minimi (ADM).

Stimulation

Wrist: Place cathode 2 to 3 cm proximal to the distal crease just lateral to the flexor carpi ulnaris (FCU) tendon. Anode is 3 cm proximal to cathode. In an average size hand, this usually results in a distance of about 7 cm between cathode and active electrode.

Below elbow: Place cathode 3 to 4 cm distal to the medial epicondyle and retrocondylar groove. Anode is 3 cm proximal to cathode.

Above elbow: Place cathode 4 to 5 cm proximal to the medial epicondyle and retrocondylar groove between the biceps and triceps muscles. This site lies approximately 8 to 10 cm proximal to the below-elbow site. Anode is proximal to cathode.

Normal Values

Distal latency (ms) ≤ 3.0

Amplitude (mV) ≥ 5.0

Conduction velocity (m/s) in wrist to below-elbow segment and below-elbow to above-elbow segment ≥ 50 m/s

Normal values differ depending on the distance used, size of the hand, and different recording techniques. The normal amplitude of the hypothenar CMAP has a large range and standard deviation. Therefore, nerve conduction studies should ideally be performed bilaterally, because side-to-side comparisons are more useful than normal value tables that may not apply to your patient.

Pitfalls

When performing ulnar motor studies, the flexed elbow position should be used because measurements must follow the curved path of the nerve. Imprecise measurements over this relatively short segment are a common source of technical error.

A proximal site of stimulation in the upper arm or near the axilla can be performed, but tends to coactivate the median nerve.

Failure to recognize the Martin-Gruber anastomosis (see Figure 5-8) is a common source of error in clinical electrophysiology.

Ulnar Motor Nerve Conduction Study from First Dorsal Interosseous (FDI)

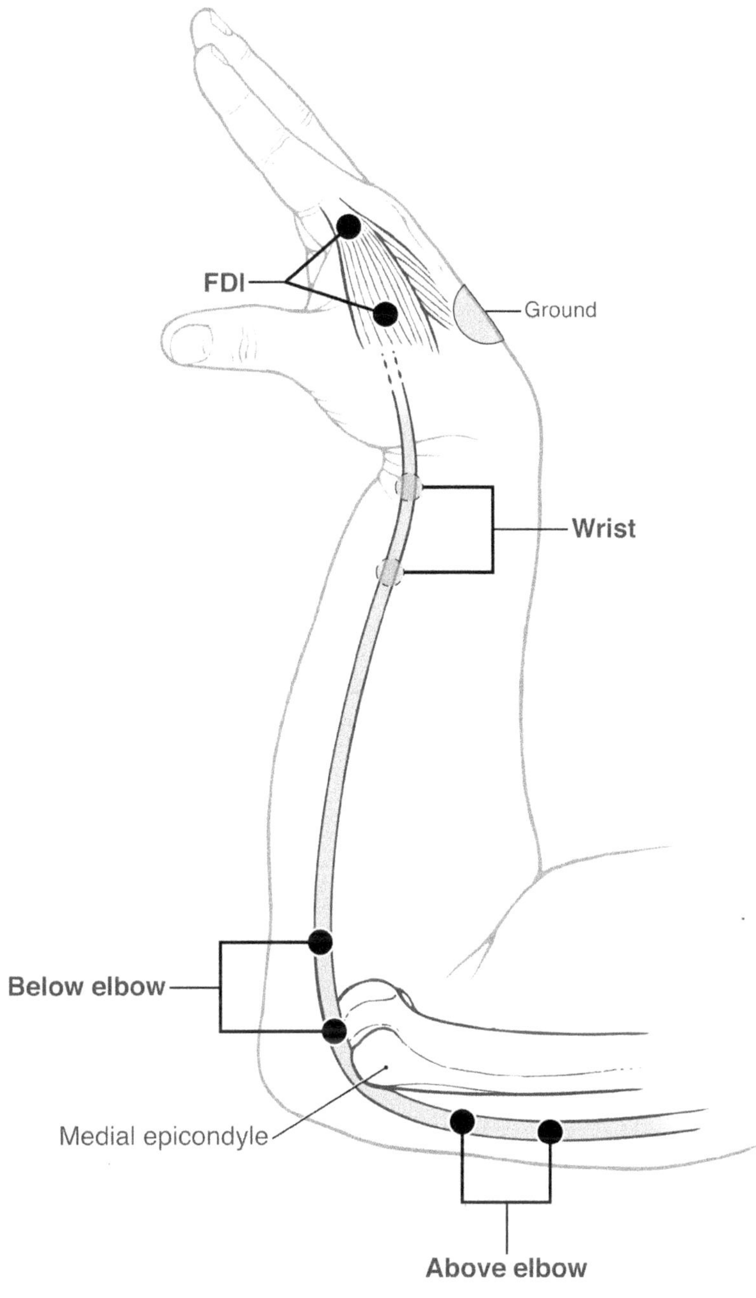

FIGURE 5-5 Ulnar motor nerve conduction study from first dorsal interosseous (FDI)

Recording

Active electrode: Position over the belly of the FDI.

Reference electrode: Place over the tendon of the FDI at the base of the proximal phalanx of the index finger (belly-tendon recording).

Ground electrode: Place on the dorsum of the hand, between stimulating and recording electrodes.

Stimulation

Wrist: Place cathode 2 to 3 cm proximal to the distal crease just lateral to the flexor carpi ulnaris (FCU) tendon. Anode is 3 cm proximal to cathode.

Below elbow: Place cathode 3 to 4 cm distal to the medial epicondyle and retrocondylar groove. Anode is 3 cm proximal to cathode.

Above elbow: Place cathode 4 to 5 cm proximal to the medial epicondyle and retrocondylar groove between the biceps and triceps muscles. This site lies approximately 8 to 10 cm proximal to the below-elbow site. Anode is proximal to cathode.

Normal Values

Distal latency (ms) ≤ 4.0

Amplitude (mV) ≥ 7.0

Conduction velocity (m/s) in wrist to below-elbow segment and below-elbow to above-elbow segment ≥ 50 m/s

Normal values differ depending on the distance used, size of the hand, and different recording techniques. The normal amplitude of the CMAP from FDI has a large range and standard deviation. Therefore, nerve conduction studies should ideally be performed bilaterally because side-to-side comparisons are more useful than normal value tables.

Pitfalls

When performing ulnar motor studies, the flexed elbow position should be used because measurements must follow the curved path of the nerve. Imprecise measurements over this relatively short segment are a common source of technical error.

A proximal site of stimulation in the upper arm or near the axilla can be performed, but tends to coactivate the median nerve.

Failure to recognize the Martin-Gruber anastomosis (see Figure 5-8) is a common source of error in clinical electrophysiology.

Short Segment Stimulation across the Elbow ("inching technique")

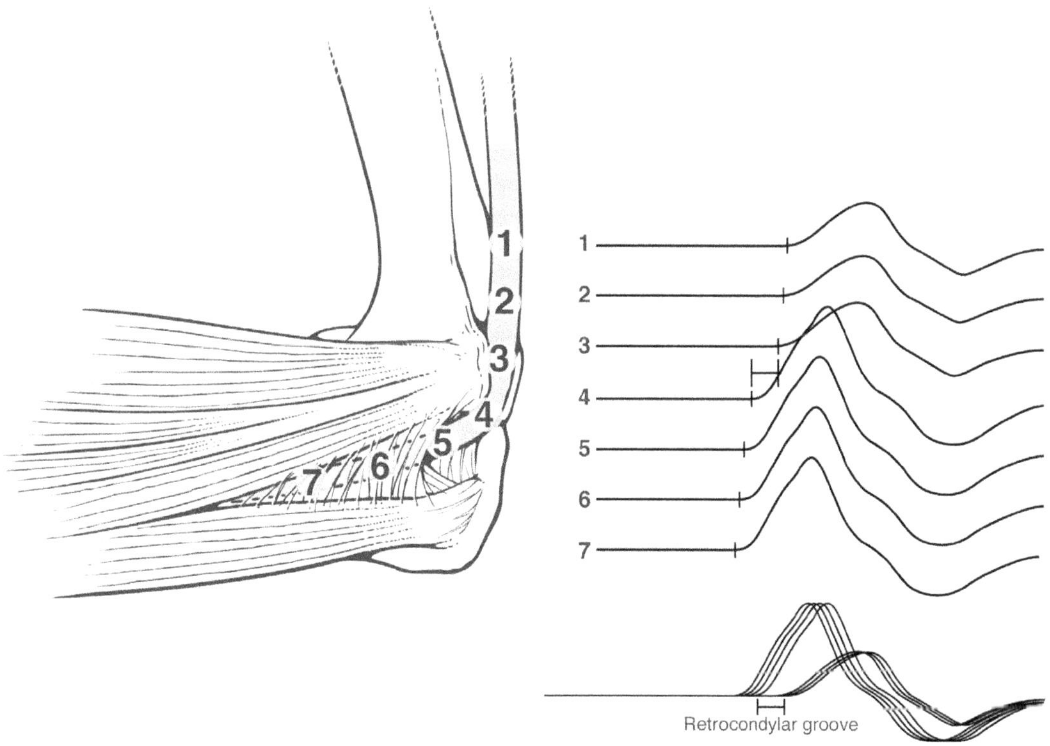

FIGURE 5-6 Short segment stimulation across the elbow ("inching technique").

Recording

Identical recording technique to that used to elicit the CMAP from the ADM or FDI during routine ulnar motor conduction studies.

Stimulation

Stimulate at 1 or 2 cm intervals across the elbow (Kimura, 1989). An abrupt change in CMAP waveform indicates the point of localized conduction delay or conduction block. In Figure 5-6, stimulation at 1 cm increments results in a motor conduction velocity of <20 m/s localized to the retrocondylar groove associated with a partial conduction block (focal demyelination). An abrupt change in SNAP recording from the fifth digit can also be used to aid in the localization of a conduction abnormality at the elbow. However, this technique is confounded by the substantial reduction in SNAP amplitude that occurs even in normal subjects with proximal stimulation compared with distal stimulation (see Chapter 1).

Ulnar F-waves

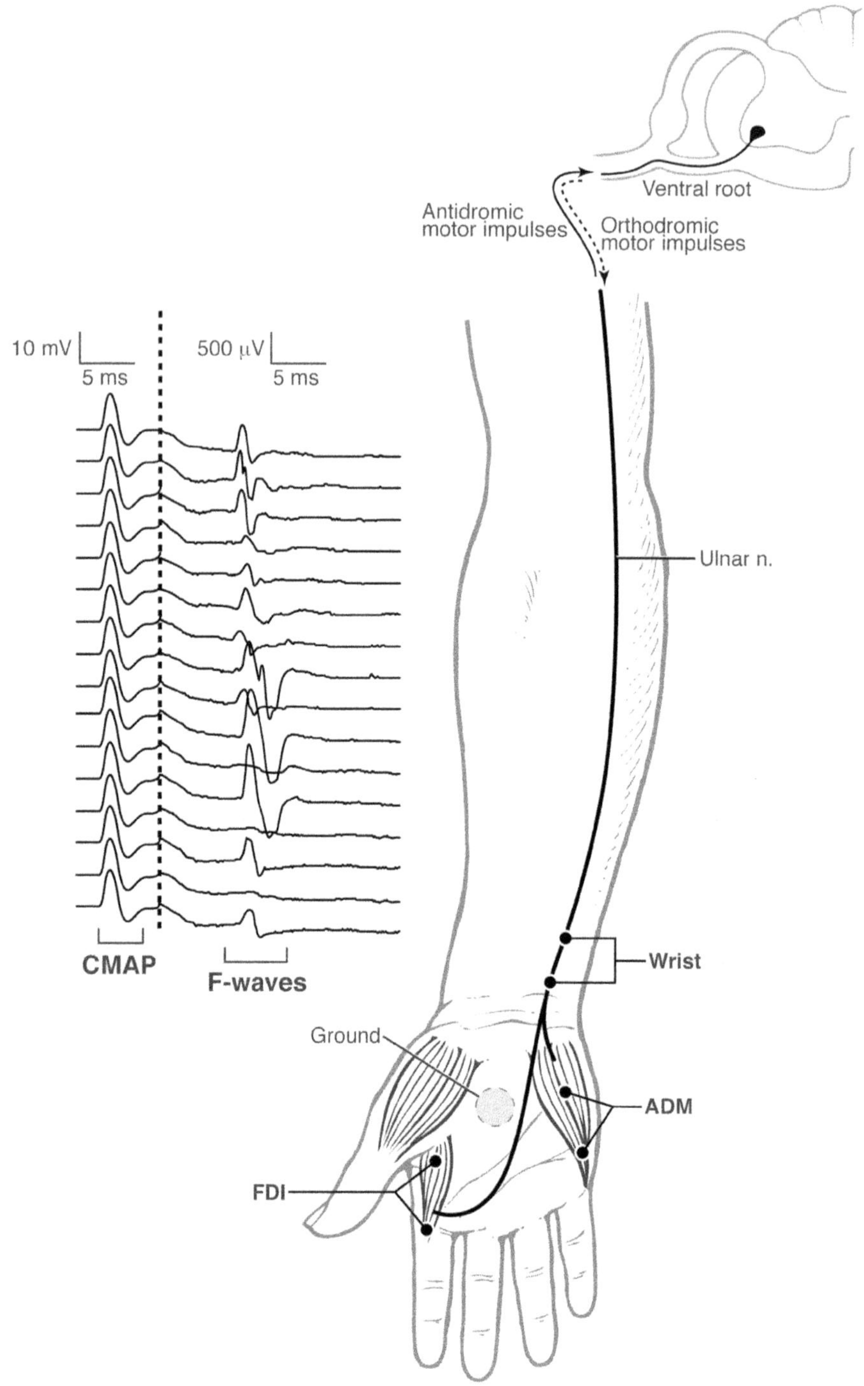

FIGURE 5-7 Ulnar F-waves.

Recording F-waves

Identical recording technique to that utilized to elicit the CMAP from ADM or FDI during routine ulnar motor conduction studies, except that the gain is set to 200 μV to 500 μV and sweep speed 5 ms/division to allow visualization of this late response. At least 10 to 20 F-wave responses are recorded.

Stimulation

Identical stimulation technique to that utilized for distal stimulation at the wrist (place cathode in the same site and deliver supramaximal stimuli). By convention, the anode is rotated 180 degrees from its original position to avoid the theoretical possibility of nerve hyperpolarization under the anode (anodal conduction block). However, in routine clinical practice, anodal block is not observed (Wee et al., 2000).

F-wave Measurements and Normal Values

Minimum F-wave latency is the most commonly obtained measurement. In hand muscles, upper limits of minimum F-wave latency are 25 ms for height 4'11" (150 cm), 28 ms for height 5'7" (170 cm) and 32 ms for height 6'3" (190 cm). A right–left asymmetry of minimal F-wave latency >2.0 ms in hand muscles is considered abnormal (Kimura, 1989; Fisher, 1992; Puksa et al. 2003).

Mean F-wave latency is calculated by adding all individual F-wave latencies and dividing this sum by the number of F-waves recorded (Fisher, 1992). The upper limits of normal for this value will be approximately 2 ms longer than minimum F-wave latency for the corresponding heights (Nobrega, et al. 2004).

Maximum F-wave latency is the longest onset latency of all recorded F-waves. The upper limits of this value will be about 4 ms longer than minimum F-wave latency for the corresponding heights (Nobrega, et al. 2004).

F-wave dispersion (or chronodispersion) provides a measure of the range of conductions, and is calculated as the difference between minimum and maximum F-wave latencies. In hand muscles, a typical upper limit of normal F-wave dispersion is <5 ms (Puksa et al. 2003). Excessive chronodispersion suggests temporal dispersion and demyelination.

F-wave amplitude usually measures <5% of the maximal CMAP or M-wave amplitude (F/M amplitude ratio). This is a measure of the proportion of the motor neuron pool activated by antidromic stimulation. F-wave amplitude may be increased in upper motor neuron dysfunction, especially when spasticity is present.

F-wave persistence is the percentage of F-waves obtained following a series of stimulations (i.e., the number of measureable F-waves divided by the number of stimuli). This reflects the antidromic excitability of a particular motor neuron pool (Fisher, 1992). F-wave persistence in median, ulnar, and tibial nerves is normally >50%, although in the peroneal nerve it can be <25%. F-wave persistence is often decreased in lower motor neuron dysfunction and increased in upper motor neuron dysfunction, particularly when spasticity is present.

Comments

In patients with entrapment neuropathies, the minimum, mean, and maximum F-wave latencies are proportionately prolonged.

In radiculopathy, F-waves are of limited value and less sensitive than needle EMG examination in assessing motor fiber involvement

F-waves are commonly abnormal in a variety of axonal and demyelinating polyneuropathies. In Guillain-Barré syndrome, F-waves may be absent or delayed during the acute stages when other nerve conduction studies are normal. Increased F-wave dispersion suggests temporal dispersion and demyelination.

F-waves provide a means of assessing motor neuron excitability (Fisher, 1992). F-waves are typically absent or decreased in spinal shock (Leis et al., 1996) and early after acute stroke, compatible with a decreased central excitability state. In contrast, F-waves are typically increased in patients with established spasticity.

Martin-Gruber Anastomosis

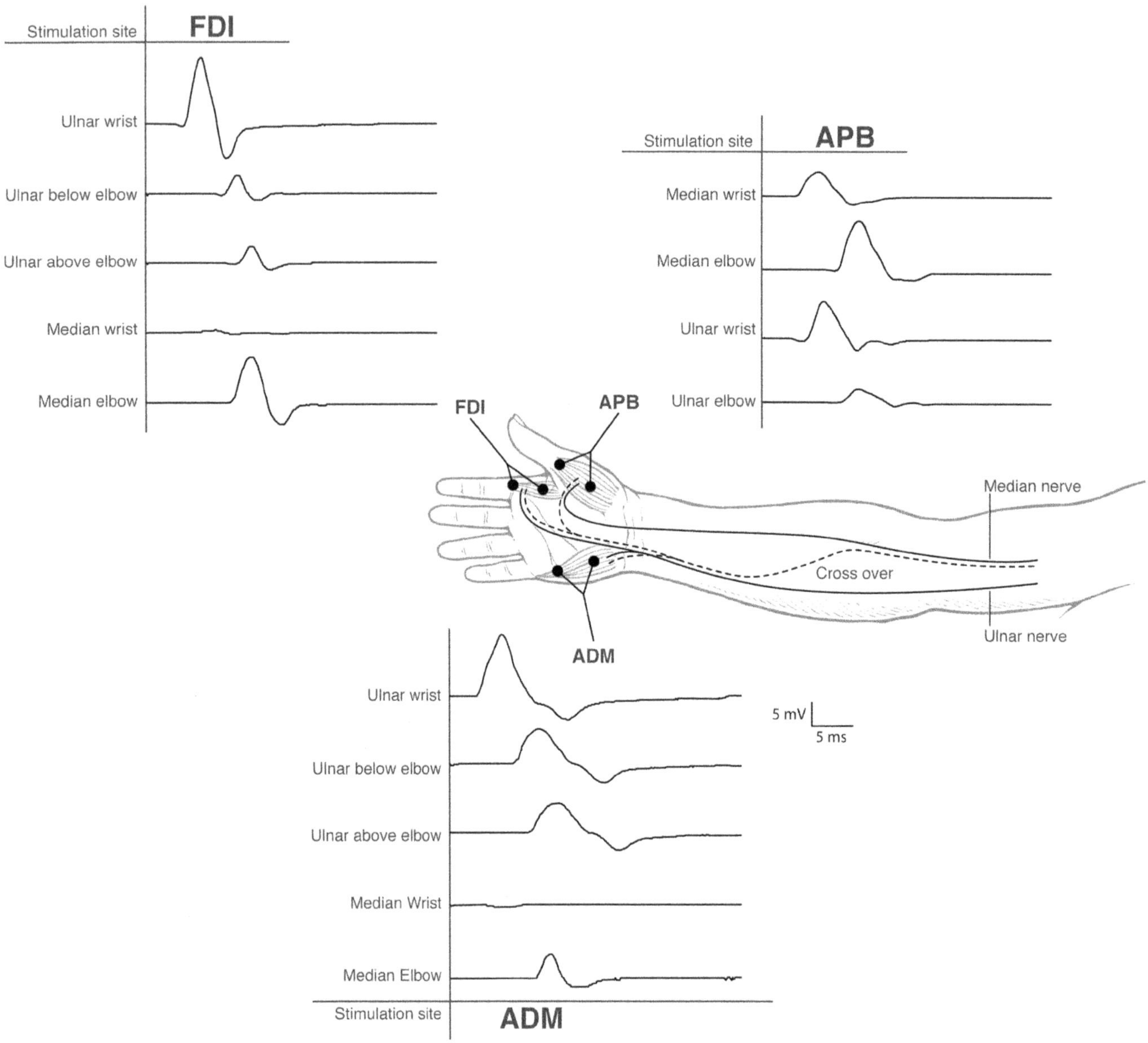

FIGURE 5-8 Martin-Gruber anastomosis.

Martin-Gruber anastomosis (MGA) is a median to ulnar nerve "crossover" in the mid-forearm that involves motor fibers. It is the most common clinically relevant anomaly, occurring in approximately one-third of median nerves (Rosenbaum and Ochoa, 2002). When present, it tends to be bilateral. The MGA often arises from the anterior interosseous nerve, although other branching patterns occur. MGA fibers typically supply ordinarily ulnar intrinsic hand muscles (first dorsal interosseous, adductor pollicis, deep head of flexor pollicis brevis, abductor digiti minimi), although less commonly they can also supply thenar muscles normally innervated by the median nerve (Amoiridis and Vlachonikolis, 2003). The MGA can lead to unusual sparing of muscles after severe proximal ulnar nerve injury or CTS. This occurs because the fibers contributing to the MGA traverse the antecubital fossa with the median nerve, and then traverse the wrist with the ulnar nerve, avoiding the two most common entrapment neuropathies: CTS and ulnar neuropathy at the elbow. Conversely, a proximal median nerve injury can lead to unexpectedly widespread denervation in the presence of the MGA (Rosenbaum and Ochoa, 2002).

During routine ulnar nerve conduction studies, the MGA can be recognized by a CMAP that is smaller with stimulation of the ulnar nerve below the elbow than at the wrist. This produces a "pseudo-conduction block" in the forearm (Preston and Shapiro, 2005), which is usually more apparent when recording from the FDI muscle because the MGA fibers innervate the FDI more commonly than hypothenar or thenar muscles (Wilbourn and Lambert, 1976). In such cases, the CMAP from the FDI (or ADM) muscle will be larger with stimulation of the median nerve at the elbow (antecubital fossa) compared with median nerve stimulation at the wrist. This documents that the CMAPs from the FDI and ADM are derived from the stimulated fibers lying in the ulnar nerve at the wrist and median nerve at the elbow.

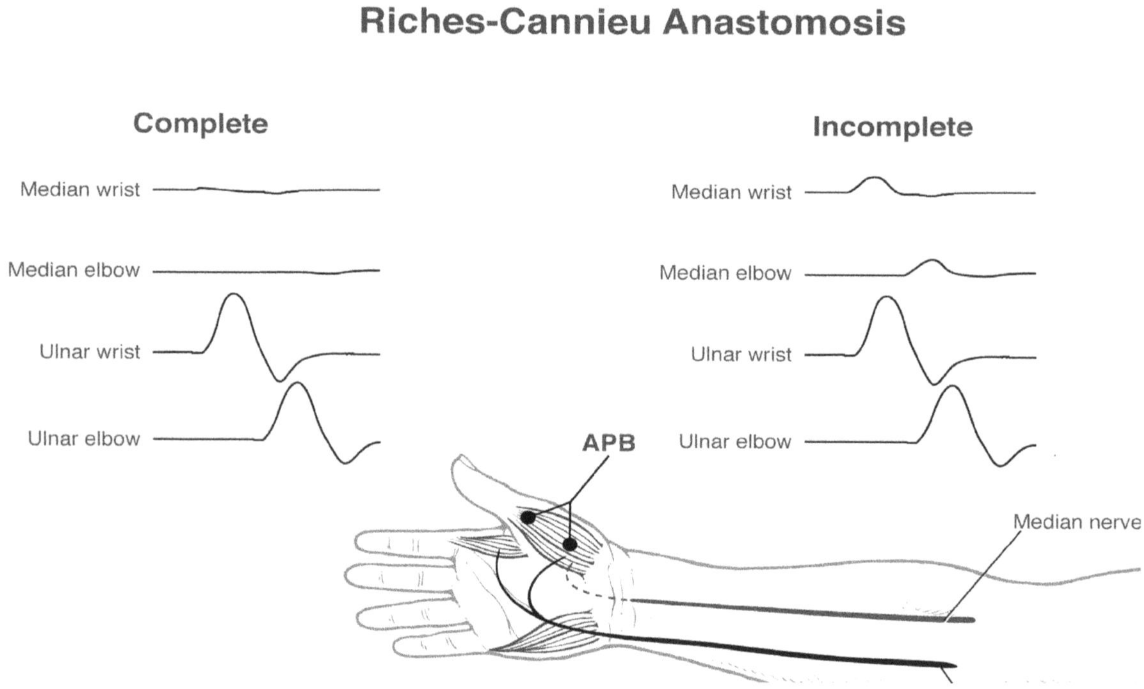

FIGURE 5-9 Riches-Cannieu anastomosis (RCA) "all ulnar hand."

In this anomaly, the ulnar nerve supplies thenar muscles ordinarily innervated by the median nerve. It is usually described as an anastomosis in the palm between the ulnar deep branch and median muscular branch, although RCA likely has a proximal source that is rerouted in the palm to the original destination. RCA is relatively rare compared with Martin-Gruber anastomosis. These cases usually come to light after severe median nerve injury in the forearm or arm (e.g., complete transaction of the nerve) is associated with profound weakness and denervation of forearm flexor muscles and paradoxical sparing of thenar muscles. In contrast, severe ulnar nerve injury in the forearm or elbow may cause unexpectedly profound weakness and denervation of all intrinsic hand muscles, including thenar (Preston and Shapiro, 2005).

Miscellaneous Anatomic Variations

The ulnar to median anastomosis in the forearm ("reverse MGA") is rare. In 303 unselected subjects, Kimura (1989) found no cases of this anomaly. Amoirides (1992) also found no cases in 100 left arms, whereas MGA was present in 32% of cases.

Ulnar Sensory Nerve Conduction Study

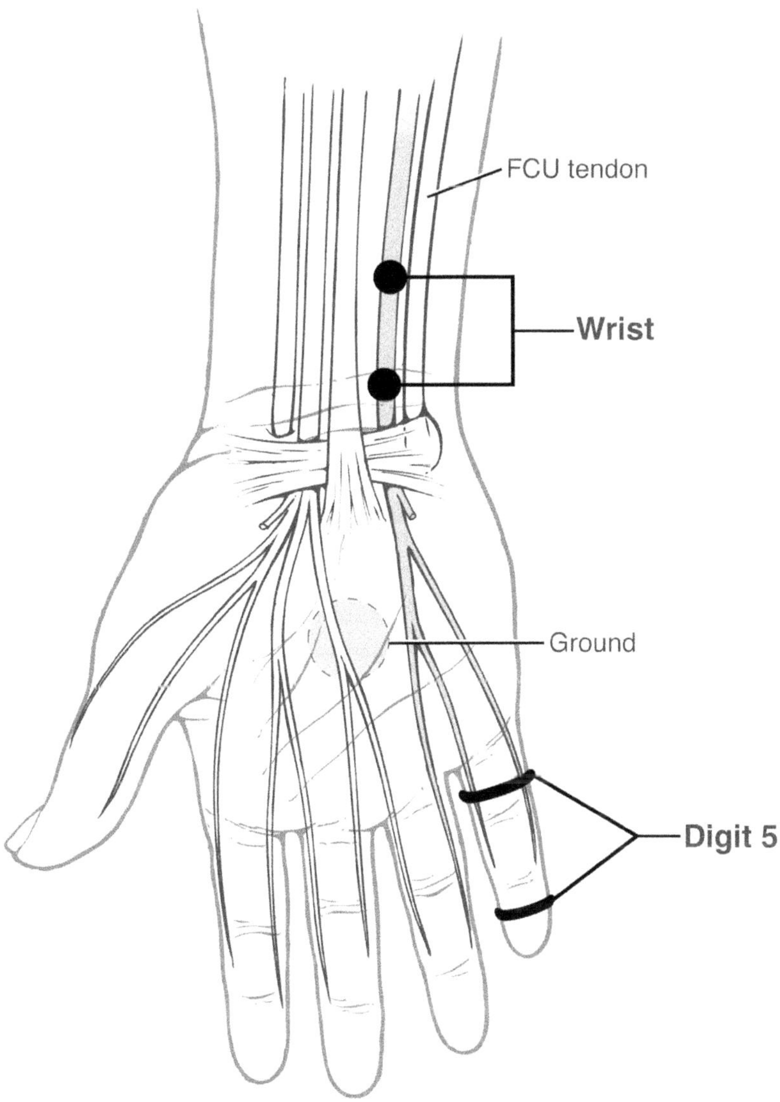

FIGURE 5-10 Ulnar sensory nerve conduction study (antidromic).

Recording (with ring electrodes)

Active electrode: Position around the mid-portion of the proximal phalanx of the fifth digit (just proximal to the proximal interphalangeal joint).

Reference electrode: Position around the mid-portion of the distal phalanx (just distal to the distal interphalangeal joint).

Ground electrode: Place on the dorsum of the hand, between the stimulating and recording electrodes.

Ring electrodes can also be placed around the fourth digit (see median and ulnar ring finger comparative study, Chapter 4).

Stimulation

Wrist: Place cathode over the ulnar nerve just lateral to the flexor carpi ulnaris (FCU) tendon, 14 cm proximal to the recording electrode. In smaller hands, shorter distances may be needed (11 to 13 cm). Anode is 3 cm proximal to cathode.

Comments

This is the standard ulnar sensory nerve conduction study for evaluating a variety of peripheral nerve abnormalities ranging from ulnar neuropathy to diffuse polyneuropathy.

Normal Values

Latency (ms) ≤ 2.8 (onset latency); ≤ 3.5 (peak latency)
Amplitude (μV) ≥ 16
Conduction velocity (m/s) in wrist to digit segment ≥ 50 m/s

The normal latency depends on the distal distance, which varies in different laboratories from 11 cm to 14 cm. Accordingly, the calculated conduction velocity is the preferred value to determine abnormality. In addition, the amplitude of the ulnar sensory response has a large range and standard deviation. Therefore, nerve conduction studies should ideally be performed bilaterally, because side-to-side comparisons are more useful than normal value tables that may not apply to your patient.

Dorsal Ulnar Cutaneous (DUC) Nerve Conduction Study

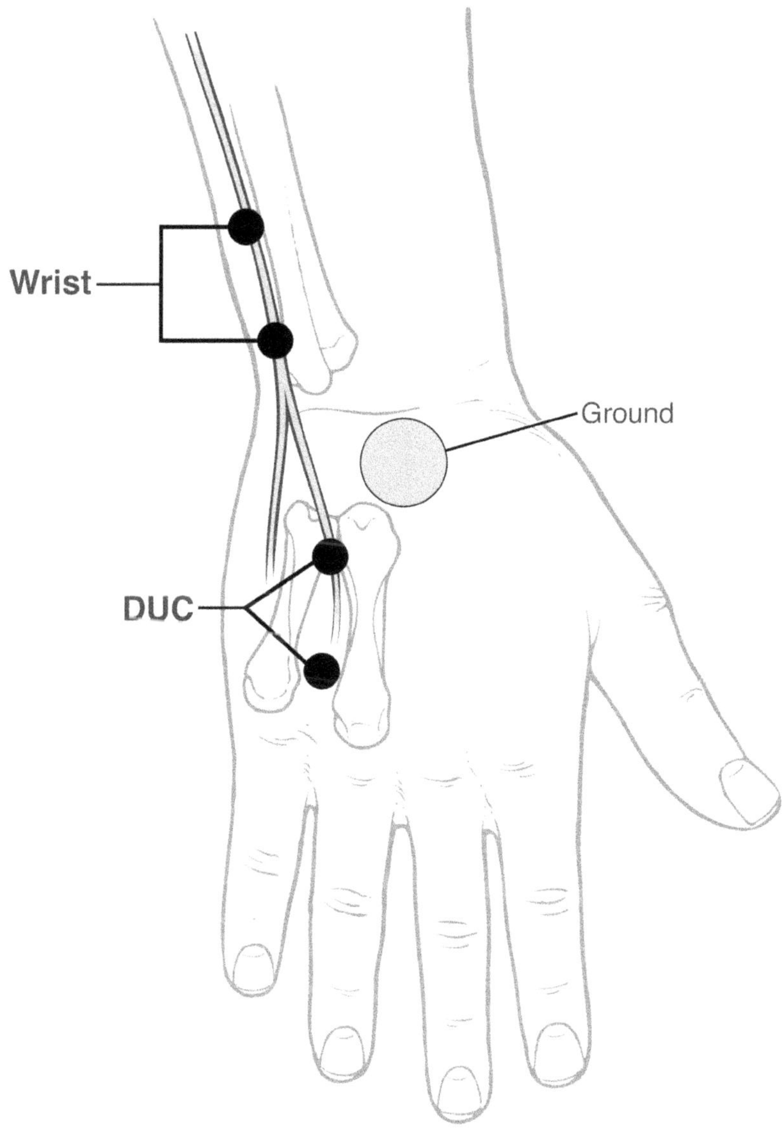

FIGURE 5-11 Dorsal ulnar cutaneous (DUC) nerve conduction study (antidromic).

Recording (modified from Jabre, 1980)

Active electrode: Place on the ulnar dorsum of hand at the apex of the "V" formed by the fourth and fifth metacarpal bones.

Reference electrode: Position 3 cm distally over the web space between the little and ring fingers.

Ground electrode: Place on the dorsum of the hand, between the stimulating and recording electrodes.

Stimulation

Wrist: Place cathode proximal to the ulnar styloid along the inferior border of the ulna, about 7 to 8 cm proximal to the recording electrode. Anode is 3 cm proximal to cathode. The nerve is quite superficial, so supramaximal stimulation is achieved at low stimulus intensities (e.g., 10 to 15 mA). Higher stimulation intensities may produce stimulus artifact that can obscure the onset SNAP latency, although peak latency usually remains well defined.

Normal Values

Latency (ms) ≤ 1.8 (onset latency); ≤ 2.5 (peak latency)
Amplitude (μV) ≥ 15
Conduction velocity (m/s) ≥ 50 m/s

Normal latency values depend on the distal distance, which varies in different laboratories from 7 to 10 cm. Amplitude of the DUC response has a large range and standard deviation. Therefore, nerve conduction studies should be performed bilaterally, particularly when uncommon nerve conduction studies are performed (Preston and Shapiro, 2005).

Comments

In chronic axonal loss lesions of the ulnar nerve at the elbow (e.g., ulnar neuropathy at the elbow), the DUC sensory response will usually be absent or reduced in amplitude, in union with the abnormal superficial branch SNAP from the little or ring fingers. However, if the lesion of the ulnar nerve at the elbow is acute (too early for Wallerian degeneration to fully manifest) or purely demyelinating (neurapraxia), then both DUC and superficial branch SNAP may be spared. Conversely, in a chronic axonal loss lesion of the ulnar nerve at the wrist (e.g., ulnar neuropathy at Guyon's canal), the superficial branch SNAP will be abnormal, while the DUC response will be spared because it arises proximal to the wrist. Accordingly, although an abnormal DUC response indicates that the lesion is proximal to the wrist (and implies ulnar neuropathy at the elbow), the examiner must be aware of two conditions that may confound interpretation: the first is the anomalous superficial radial innervation to ulnar dorsum of hand, a relatively common but under-recognized normal variant (Figure 5-12; Leis and Wells, 2008), and the second is preferential fascicular involvement or sparing that may occur with an ulnar nerve lesion at the elbow (Campbell et al., 1989). Hence, the combination of superficial and DUC sensory responses should not be used alone to localize an ulnar neuropathy (Preston and Shapiro, 2005).

Anomalous Superficial Radial Innervation to Ulnar Dorsum of Hand

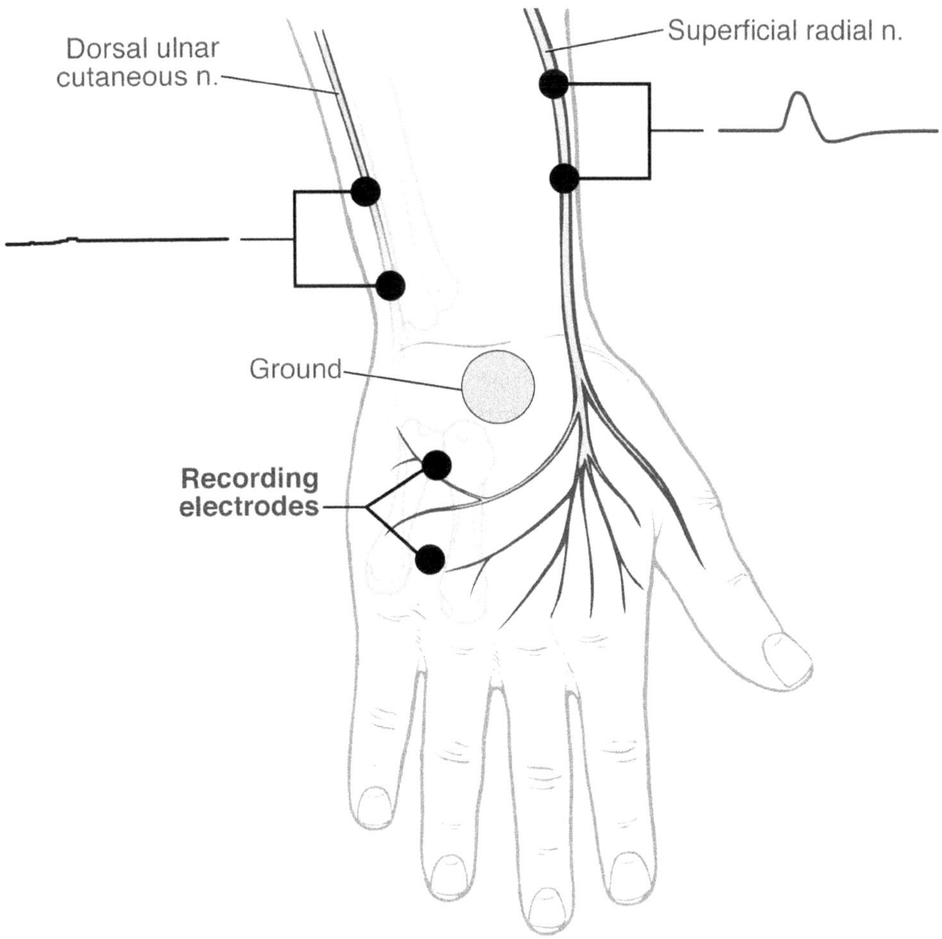

FIGURE 5-12 Anomalous superficial radial innervation to ulnar dorsum of hand.

Anomalous superficial radial innervation to the ulnar dorsum of the hand is the most common cause of an absent DUC response in the population at large (Leis and Wells, 2008). In 100 subjects examined without radial or ulnar neuropathy, 16 had this anomaly. Only 3 subjects had an absent DUC response without this variant. The anomaly was unilateral in 14 subjects and bilateral in 2, manifesting in 18 of 200 hands (9%). In 71 patients with various ulnar neuropathies, failure to recognize this anomaly confounded the clinical and electrodiagnostic impression. For this reason, it is important to recognize this variant to avoid erroneous diagnoses and inappropriate treatment.

The coexistence of Martin-Gruber anastomosis (MGA) and anomalous superficial radial innervation to the ulnar dorsum of the hand introduces a potentially common, yet rarely recognized, pitfall in nerve conduction studies (Leis et. al., 2010). During routine ulnar nerve conduction studies, the MGA produces an apparent conduction block ("pseudo-conduction block") in ulnar motor fibers in the forearm, whereas the anomalous superficial radial innervation to ulnar dorsum of the hand produces an apparently absent DUC response. Failure to recognize the coexistence of these two common variants may lead to the misdiagnosis of ulnar neuropathy in the forearm, and inappropriate treatment.

Infrequently, MGA may occur in the high proximal forearm or elbow (Rosenbaum and Ochoa, 2002), giving rise to an apparent conduction block at or near the elbow. In the setting of an apparently absent DUC response, this combination of variants may be more likely to be misinterpreted as ulnar neuropathy at the elbow (Leis et. al., 2010).

REFERENCES

Amadio PC, Beckenbaugh RD. Entrapment of the ulnar nerve by the deep flexor pronator aponeurosis. *J Hand Surg* 1986;11A:83–87.

Amoiridis G. Median–ulnar nerve communications and anomalous innervation of the intrinsic hand muscles: An electrophysiological study. *Muscle Nerve* 1992;15:576–579.

Amoiridis G, Vlachonikolis IG. Verification of the median-to-ulnar and ulnar-to-median nerve motor fiber anastomosis in the forearm: an electrophysiological study. *Clin Neurophysiol* 2003;114:94–98.

Campbell WW. AAEE case report #18: Entrapment neuropathy in the distal forearm. *Muscle Nerve* 1989;12:347–352.

Campbell WW, Pridgeon RM, Ria G, Crostic EG, et. al. Sparing of the flexor carpi ulnaris in ulnar neuropathy at the elbow. *Muscle Nerve* 1989;12:965–967.

Campbell WW, Pridgeon RM, Sahni KS. Entrapment neuropathy of the ulnar nerve at its point of exit from the flexor carpi ulnaris muscle. *Muscle Nerve* 1988;11:467–470.

Fisher MA. AAEM Minimonograph#13: H reflexes and F waves: physiology and clinical indications. *Muscle Nerve* 1992;15(11):1223–1233. Review.

Gray's Anatomy. 38th edition, Churchill Livingstone, New York, 1995, pp.1266–1274.

Jabre JF. Ulnar nerve lesions at the wrist: new technique for recording from the sensory dorsal branch of the ulnar nerve. *Neurology* 1980;30:873–876.

Kimura J. *Electrodiagnosis in Diseases of Nerve and Muscle.* 2nd ed., FA Davis Co., Philadelphia, 1989.

Kincaid JC. AAEE minimonograph #31: The electrodiagnosis of ulnar neuropathy at the elbow. *Muscle Nerve* 1988;11:1005–1015.

Leis AA, Kronenberg MF, Stetkarova I, Paske WC, Stokic DS. Spinal motoneuron excitability following acute spinal cord injury in man. *Neurology* 1996;47:231–237.

Leis AA, Wells KJ. Radial nerve cutaneous innervation to the ulnar dorsum of the hand. *Clin Neurophysiol* 2008;119:662–666.

Leis AA, Stetkarova I, Wells KJ. Martin-Gruber anastomosis with anomalous superficial radial innervation to ulnar dorsum of hand: A pitfall when common variants coexist. *Muscle Nerve* 2010;41:313–317.

Nobrega JAM, Pinhiero DS, Manzano GM, Kimura J. Various aspects of F-wave values in a healthy population. *Clin Neurophysiol* 2004;115:2336–2342.

Miller RG. AAEM case report #1: Ulnar neuropathy at the elbow. *Muscle Nerve* 1991;14:97–101.

Olney RK, Hanson M. AAEE case report #15: Ulnar neuropathy at or distal to the wrist. *Muscle Nerve* 1988;11:828–832.

O'Driscoll SW, Horii E, Carmichael SW, Morrey BF. The cubital tunnel and ulnar neuropathy. J Bone Joint Surg [Br] 1991;73-B:613-617.

Preston DC, Shapiro BE. Electromyography and neuromuscular disorders. Clinical-electrophysiologic correlations. 2nd ed., Philadelphia, Elsevier Butterworth Heinemann, 2005.

Puksa L, Stalberg E, Falck B. Reference values of F-wave parameters in healthy subjects. *Clin Neurophysiol* 2003;114:1079–1090.

Rosenbaum RB, Ochoa JL, eds. *Carpal tunnel syndrome and other disorders of the median nerve.* Butterworth Heinemann, Boston, 2002.

Stewart JD. The variable clinical manifestations of ulnar neuropathies at the elbow. *J Neurol Neurosurg Psychiatry* 1987;50:252–258.

Sunderland S. *Nerves and Nerve Injuries.* Williams and Wilkins, Baltimore, 1968, pp. 808–885.

Sunderland S. *Nerves and Nerve Injuries.* 2nd ed., Churchill Livingstone, New York, 1978.

Wee AS, Leis AA, Kuhn AR, Gilbert RW. Anodal block: can this occur during routine nerve conduction studies? *Electromyogr Clin Neurophysiol* 2000;40:387–391.

Wilbourn AJ, Lambert EH. The forearm median-to-ulnar nerve communication; electrodiagnostic aspects. *Neurology* 1976;26:368.

Adductor Pollicis

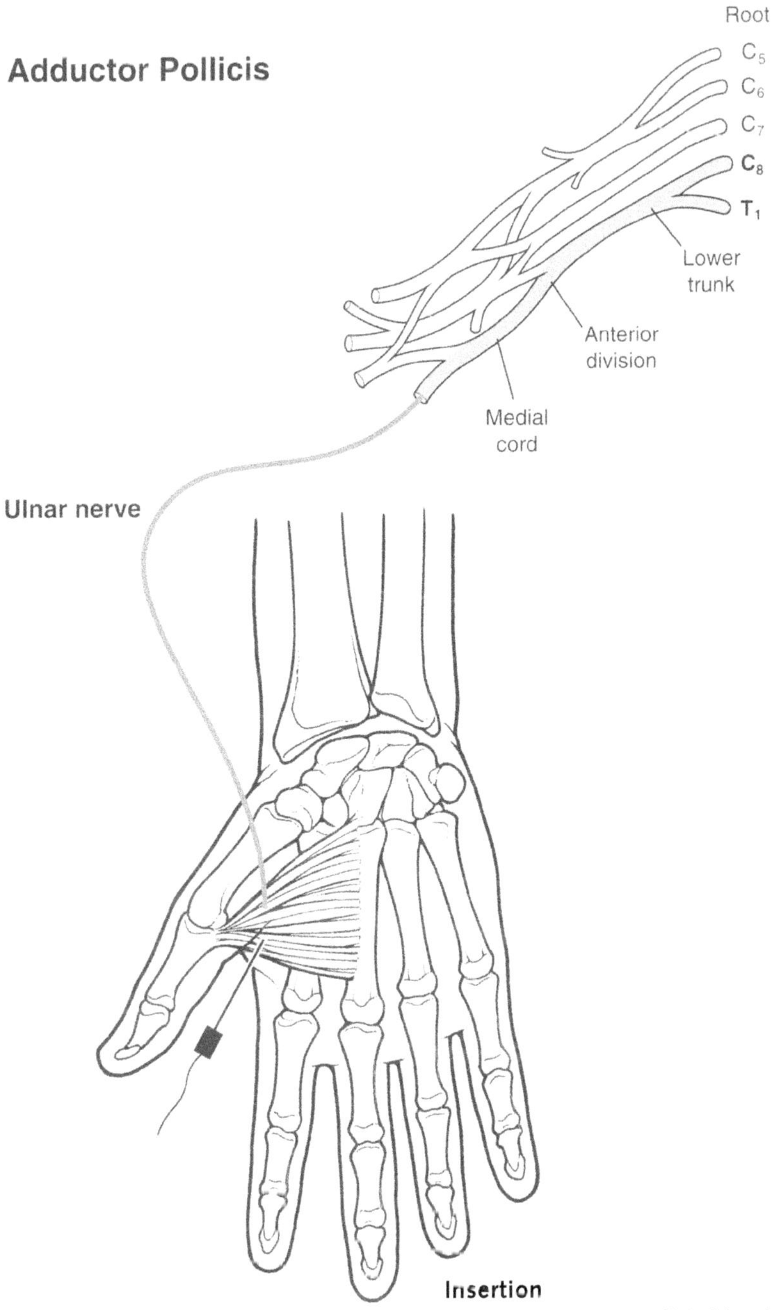

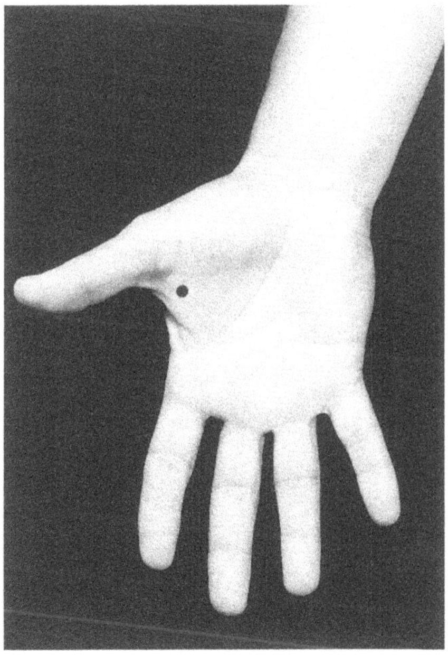

Innervation
Innervation is via the ulnar nerve, medial cord, lower trunk, and roots C_8, T_1

Origin
Oblique fibers arise from the capitate bone and bases of the second and third metacarpal bones; transverse fibers arise from the distal two-thirds of the metacarpal bone of the middle finger.

Insertion
Insertion is at the medial side of the base of the proximal phalanx of the thumb.

Activation Maneuver
Adduction of the thumb activates the adductor pollicis.

EMG Needle Insertion
Insert the needle into the first web space just anterior (volar) to the edge of the first dorsal interosseous and proximal to the first metacarpophalangeal joint.

Pitfalls
If the needle is inserted too posteriorly (dorsally), it will be in the first dorsal interosseous, which is also supplied by the ulnar nerve.

If the needle is inserted too anteriorly (volarly) and proximally, it may be in thenar muscles innervated by the median nerve.

Clinical Comments
This is the most distal muscle innervated by the ulnar nerve.

If ulnar-innervated muscles are atrophied, the needle is more likely to enter median-innervated thenar muscles.

In ulnar neuropathy at the wrist (Guyon's canal) or elbow (cubital tunnel, retrocondylar groove), the needle examination may show neurogenic changes when compression produces axonal loss (i.e., in moderate to severe entrapment).

In C_8, T_1 radiculopathy, the needle examination may show neurogenic changes when root pathology produces axonal loss (i.e., in moderate to severe radiculopathy).

In Klumpke's palsy (C_8, T_1 root avulsion), needle examination will show neurogenic changes.

Flexor Pollicis Brevis

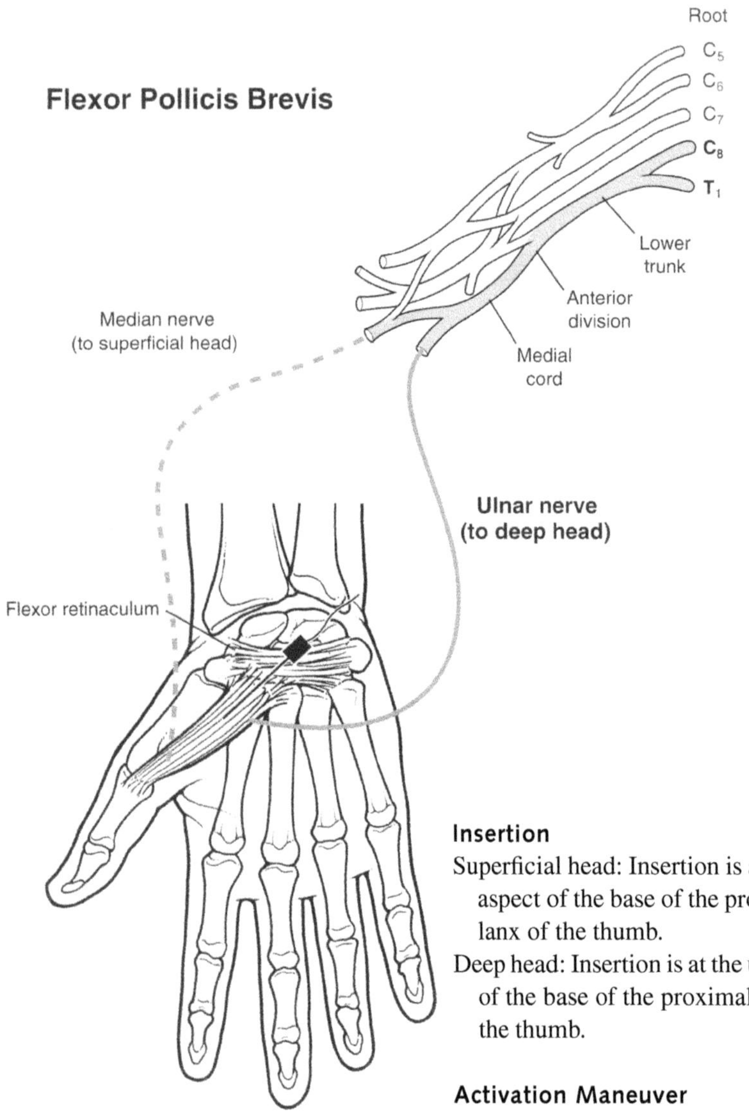

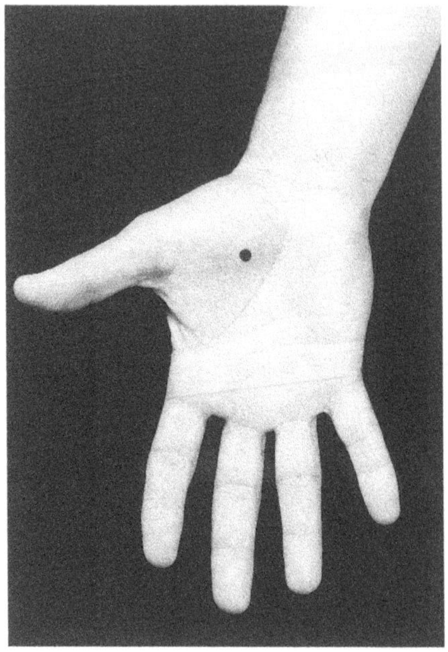

Innervation

Superficial head: Innervation is via the median nerve, medial cord, lower trunk, and roots C_8, T_1.

Deep head: Innervation is via the ulnar nerve, medial cord, lower trunk, and roots C_8, T_1.

Origin

The superficial head of the flexor pollicis brevis originates in the flexor retinaculum and trapezium.

The deep head of the flexor pollicis brevis originates in the ulnar aspect of the first metacarpal.

Insertion

Superficial head: Insertion is at the radial aspect of the base of the proximal phalanx of the thumb.

Deep head: Insertion is at the ulnar aspect of the base of the proximal phalanx of the thumb.

Activation Maneuver

Flexion of the metacarpophalangeal joint of the thumb activates the muscle.

EMG Needle Insertion

Superficial head: Insert the needle obliquely to a depth of 0.5–1 cm at the midpoint of a line drawn between the metacarpophalangeal joint and the pisiform. Assess abnormal EMG activity by directing the needle distally along the muscle.

Deep head: The procedure is the same as that for the superficial head, except that the needle is inserted to a depth of 1–2 cm.

Pitfalls

If the needle is inserted too deeply, it may penetrate the opponens pollicis, which is innervated by the median nerve; if it is inserted even deeper, it may penetrate the adductor pollicis, which receives innervation from the ulnar nerve.

If the needle is inserted too laterally, it will be in the abductor pollicis brevis, which receives innervation from the median nerve.

Clinical Comments

Examination of the flexor pollicis brevis is rarely of benefit in a routine EMG needle evaluation (in general, muscles that receive dual innervation should be avoided).

The superficial head will show neurogenic changes in lesions of the median nerve.

The deep head will show neurogenic changes in lesions of the ulnar nerve.

In C_8, T_1 radiculopathy, needle examination will show neurogenic changes if root pathology has resulted in axonal loss in motor fibers (i.e., in moderate to severe radiculopathy).

In Klumpke's palsy (C_8, T_1 root avulsion), needle examination will show neurogenic changes.

First Dorsal Interosseous

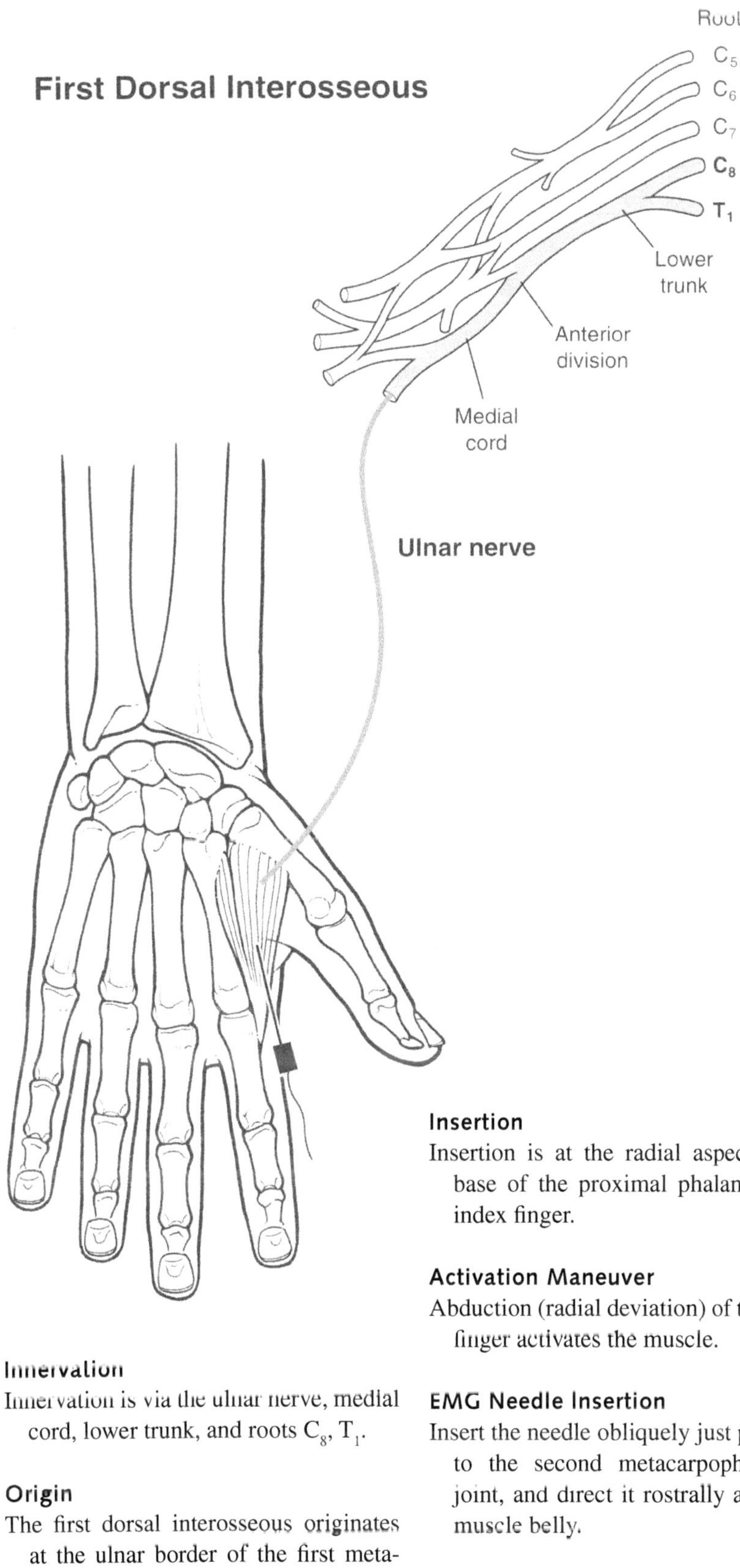

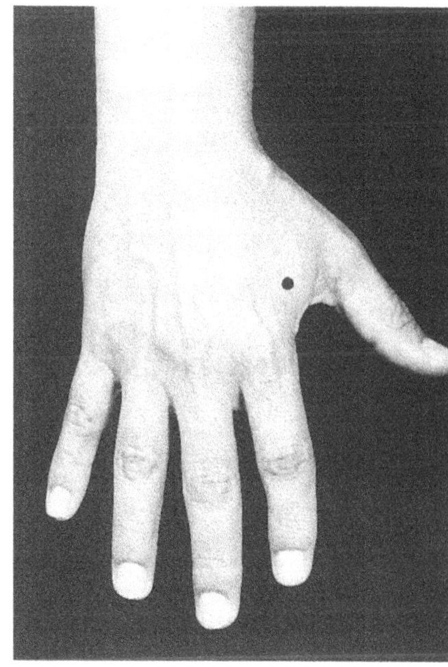

Innervation
Innervation is via the ulnar nerve, medial cord, lower trunk, and roots C_8, T_1.

Origin
The first dorsal interosseous originates at the ulnar border of the first metacarpal bone (outer head) and the radial border of the second metacarpal bone (inner head).

Insertion
Insertion is at the radial aspect of the base of the proximal phalanx of the index finger.

Activation Maneuver
Abduction (radial deviation) of the index finger activates the muscle.

EMG Needle Insertion
Insert the needle obliquely just proximal to the second metacarpophalangeal joint, and direct it rostrally along the muscle belly.

Pitfalls
There are no pitfalls. If the needle is inserted too deeply, it will still be in C_8, T_1 muscles innervated by the ulnar nerve.

Clinical Comments
In ulnar neuropathy at the wrist (Guyon's canal), needle examination may show neurogenic changes when compression produces axonal loss (i.e., in moderate to severe entrapment).

In ulnar neuropathy at the elbow (cubital tunnel, retrocondylar groove), needle examination may show neurogenic changes when compression produces axonal loss.

In C_8, T_1 radiculopathy, needle examination may show neurogenic changes when root pathology produces axonal loss (i.e., in moderate to severe radiculopathy).

In Klumpke's palsy (C_8, T_1 root avulsion), needle examination will show neurogenic changes.

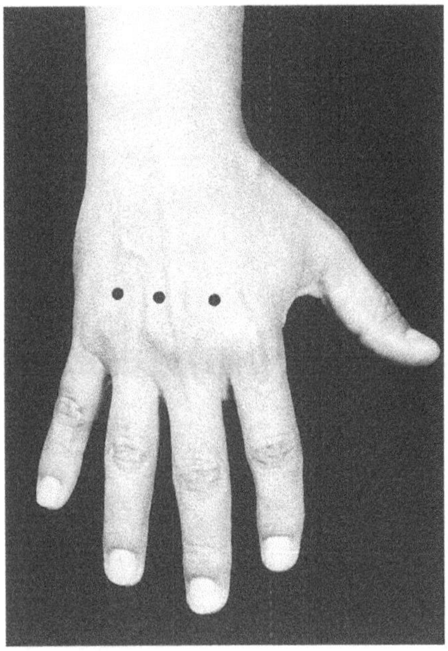

2nd, 3rd, 4th Dorsal Interossei

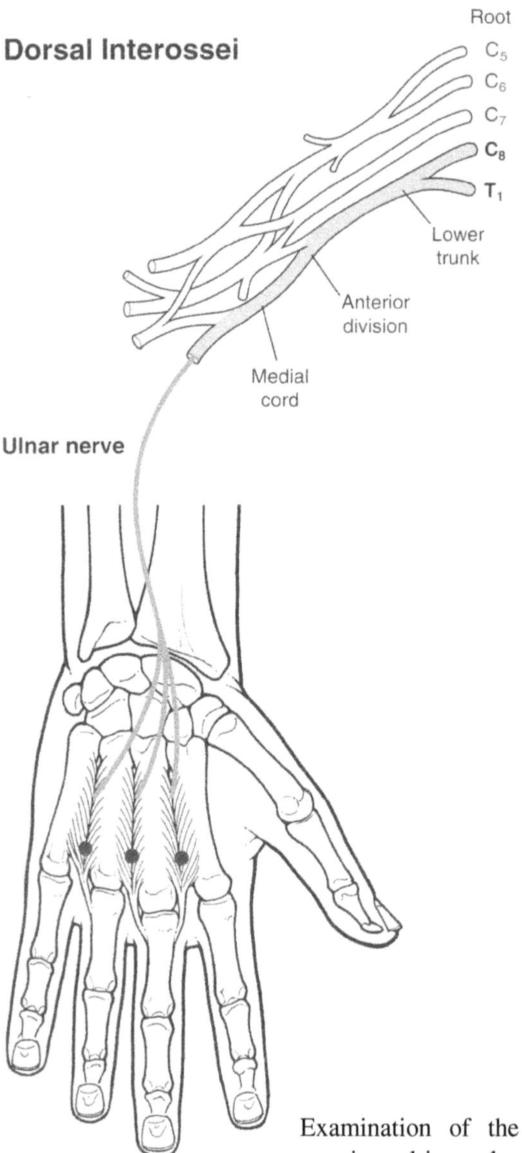

Innervation

Innervation is via the ulnar nerve, medial cord, lower trunk, and roots C_8, T_1.

Origin

The second dorsal interosseous originates at the radial border of the third metacarpal bone and the ulnar border of the second metacarpal bone.

The third and fourth dorsal interossei originate at the ulnar border of the third and fourth metacarpal bones and the radial border of the fourth and fifth metacarpal bones, respectively.

Insertion

Second: Insertion is at the radial aspect of the base of the proximal phalanx of the third digit.

Third and fourth: Insertion is at the ulnar aspect of the base of the proximal phalanx of the third and fourth digit, respectively.

Activation Maneuver

Second: Abduction (radial deviation) of the third digit activates the muscle.

Third and fourth: Adduction (ulnar deviation) of the third and fourth digit, respectively, activates the muscle.

EMG Needle Insertion

Second: Insert the needle just radial to the third metacarpal bone.

Third and fourth: Insert the needle just ulnar to the third and fourth metacarpal bones, respectively.

Pitfalls

There are no pitfalls. If the needle is inserted too deeply, it will still be in C_8, T_1 muscles innervated by the ulnar nerve.

Clinical Comments

The interossei are occasionally doubled in one or more spaces, or they may be absent in one or more spaces.

There may be variable innervation to these muscles from the median nerve.

Examination of the interossei causes pain and is rarely of benefit in a routine EMG needle evaluation.

In ulnar neuropathy at the wrist (Guyon's canal), needle examination may show neurogenic changes when compression produces axonal loss (i.e., in moderate to severe entrapment).

In ulnar neuropathy at the elbow (cubital tunnel, retrocondylar groove), needle examination may show neurogenic changes when compression produces axonal loss.

In C_8, T_1 radiculopathy, needle examination may show neurogenic changes when root pathology produces axonal loss (i.e., in moderate to severe radiculopathy).

In Klumpke's palsy (C_8, T_1 root avulsion), needle examination will show neurogenic changes.

Palmar Interossei

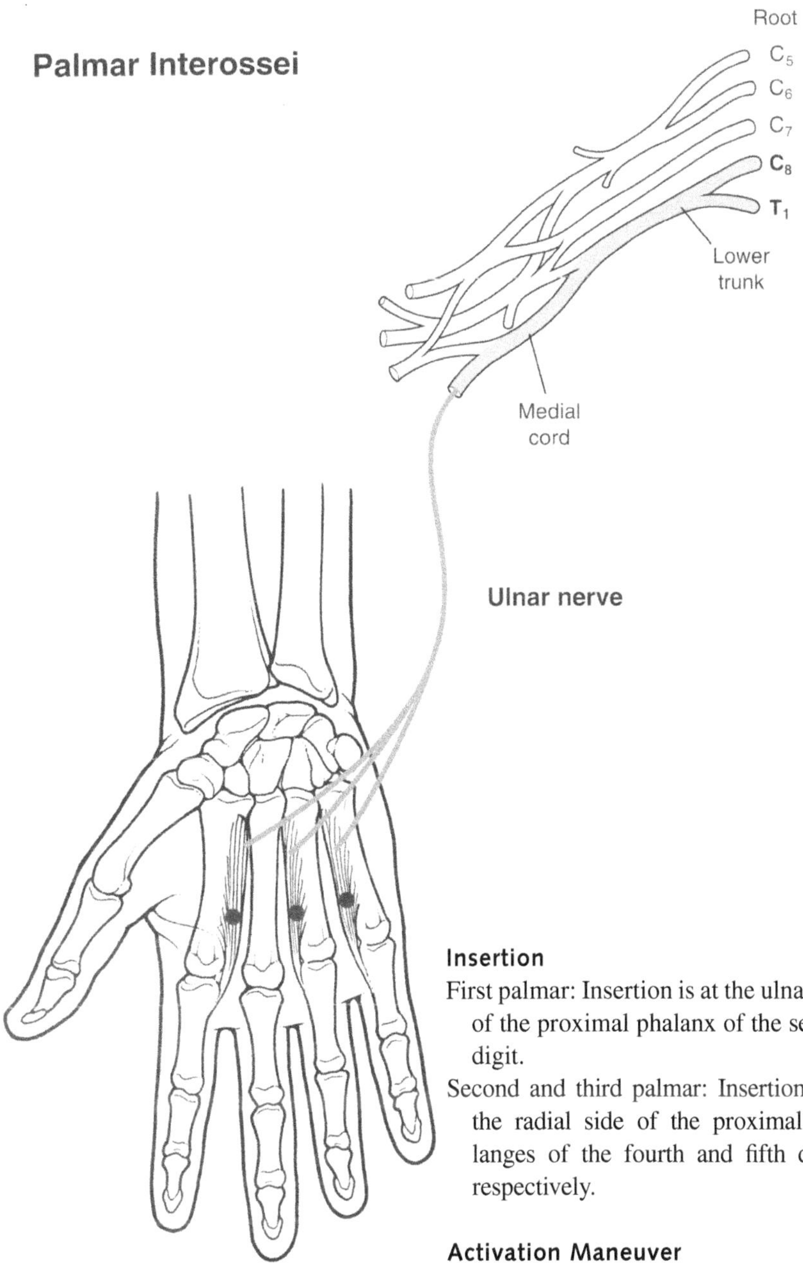

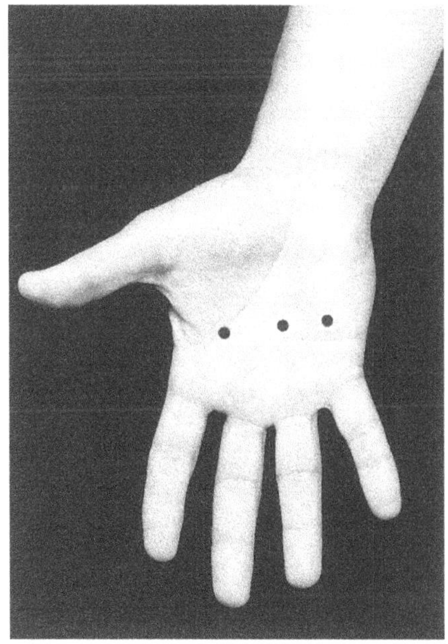

Innervation
Innervation is via the ulnar nerve, medial cord, lower trunk, and roots C_8, T_1.

Origin
The first palmar interosseous originates at the ulnar aspect of the second metacarpal bone.

The second and third palmar interossei originate at the radial aspect of the fourth and fifth metacarpal bones, respectively.

Insertion
First palmar: Insertion is at the ulnar side of the proximal phalanx of the second digit.

Second and third palmar: Insertion is at the radial side of the proximal phalanges of the fourth and fifth digits, respectively.

Activation Maneuver
The palmar interossei adduct the fingers to an imaginary line drawn longitudinally through the center of the third digit (middle finger). The first palmar performs ulnar deviation of the second digit; the second and third palmars perform radial deviation of the fourth and fifth digits, respectively.

EMG Needle Insertion
First palmar: Insert the needle just ulnar to the second metacarpal bone.

Second and third palmars: Insert the needle just radial to the fourth and fifth metacarpal bones, respectively.

Pitfalls
There are no pitfalls. If the needle is inserted too deeply, it will still be in C_8, T_1 muscles innervated by the ulnar nerve.

Clinical Comments
The interossei are occasionally doubled in one or more spaces, or they may be absent in one or more spaces.

There may be variable innervation to these muscles from the median nerve.

Examination of the palmar interossei causes pain and is rarely of benefit in a routine EMG needle evaluation.

In ulnar neuropathy at the wrist (Guyon's canal), needle examination may show neurogenic changes when compression produces axonal loss (i.e., in moderate to severe entrapment).

In ulnar neuropathy at the elbow (cubital tunnel, retrocondylar groove), needle examination may show neurogenic changes when compression produces axonal loss.

In C_8, T_1 radiculopathy, needle examination may show neurogenic changes when root pathology produces axonal loss (i.e., in moderate to severe radiculopathy).

In Klumpke's palsy (C_8, T_1 root avulsion), needle examination will show neurogenic changes.

3rd, 4th Lumbricals

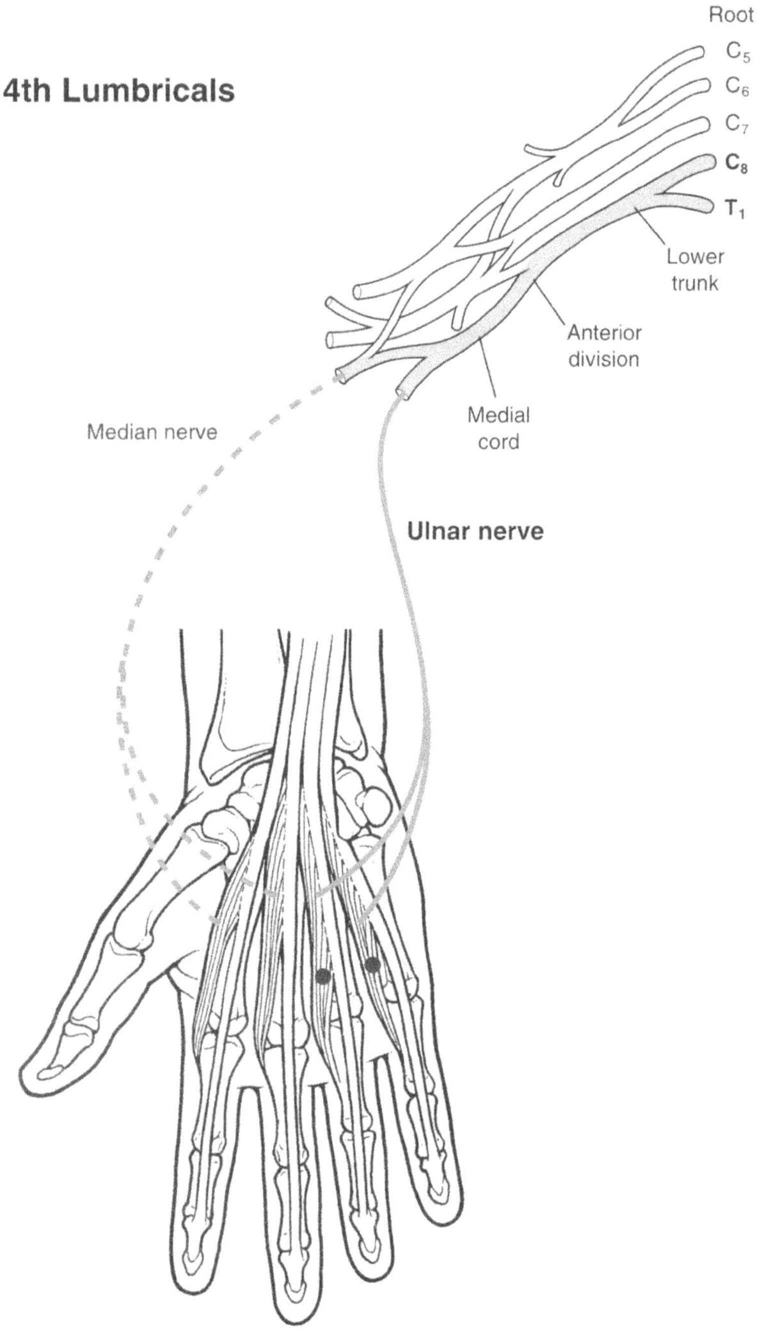

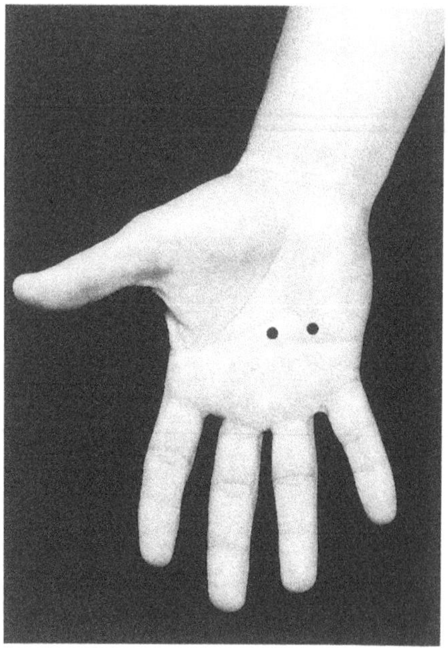

Innervation

Innervation is via the ulnar nerve, medial cord, lower trunk, and roots C_8, T_1.

Origin

The third and fourth lumbricals originate at the radial aspect of the tendon sheath of the flexor digitorum profundus.

Insertion

Insertion is at the radial lateral band of the dorsal digital expansion (tendinous expansion of the extensor digitorum communis).

Activation Maneuver

Extension of the finger at the proximal interphalangeal joint, with the metacarpophalangeal joint extended and fixed, activates the muscles.

EMG Needle Insertion

Insert the needle just proximal to the metacarpophalangeal joint and radial to the flexor tendon.

Pitfalls

There are no pitfalls. All muscles surrounding the third and fourth lumbricals receive innervation from the ulnar nerve.

Clinical Comments

Examination of the third and fourth lumbricals causes pain and is rarely of benefit in a routine EMG needle evaluation.

In ulnar neuropathy at the wrist (Guyon's canal), needle examination may show neurogenic changes when compression produces axonal loss (i.e., in moderate to severe entrapment.

In ulnar neuropathy at the elbow (cubital tunnel, retrocondylar groove), needle examination may show neurogenic changes when compression produces axonal loss.

In C_8, T_1 radiculopathy, needle examination may show neurogenic changes when root pathology produces axonal loss (i.e., in moderate to severe radiculopathy).

In Klumpke's palsy (C_8, T_1 root avulsion), needle examination will show neurogenic changes.

Abductor Digiti Minimi

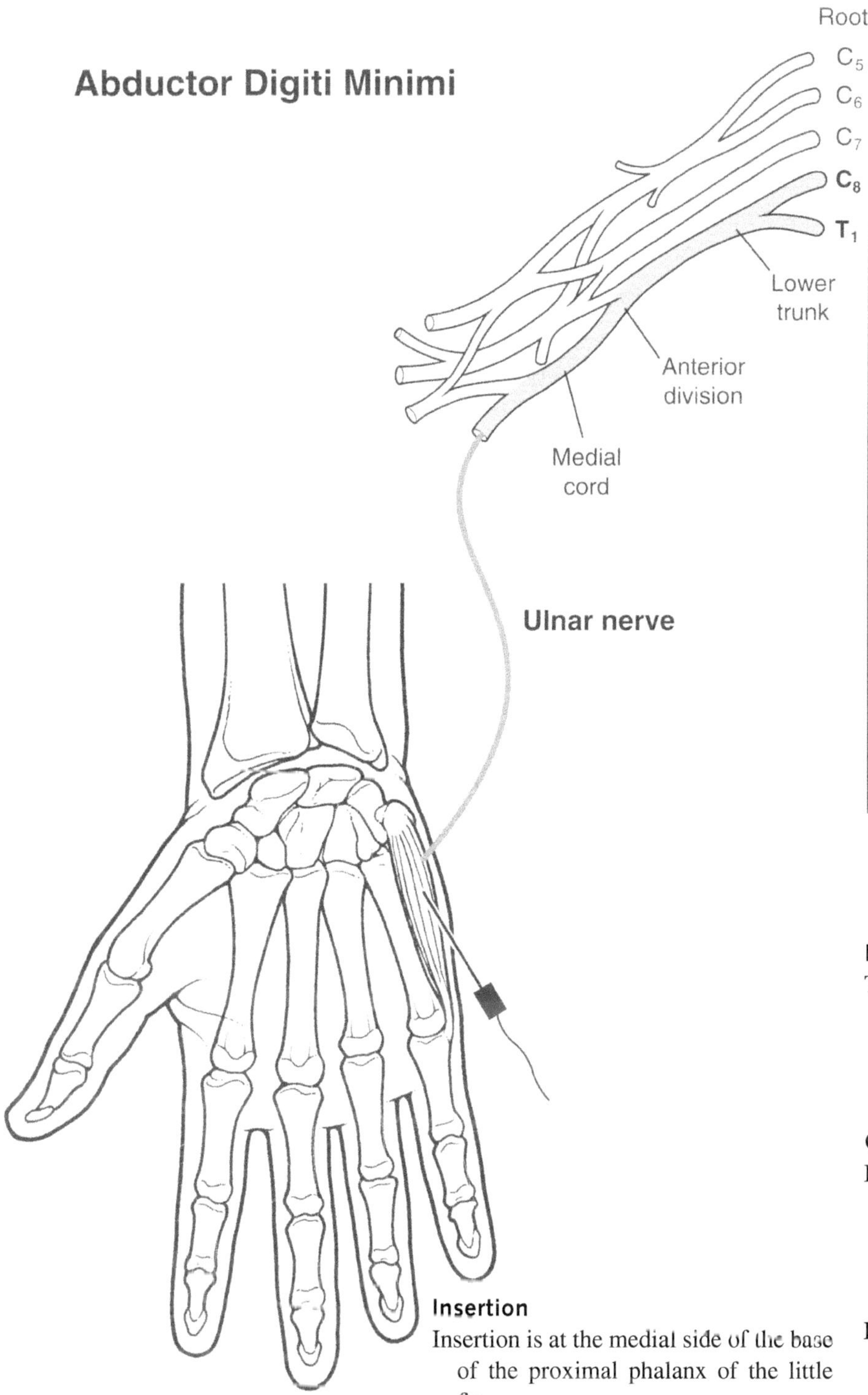

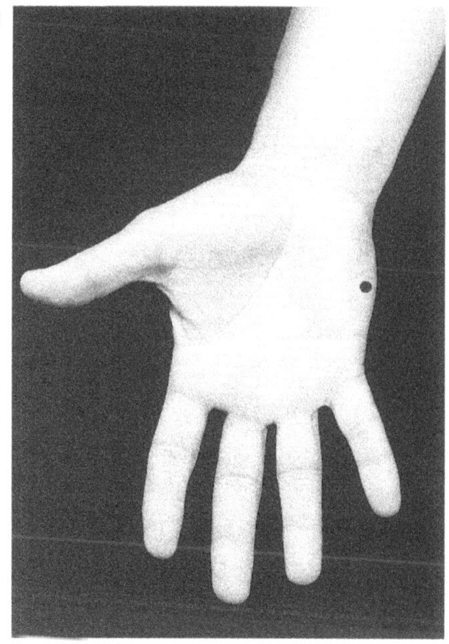

Innervation
Innervation is via the ulnar nerve, medial cord, lower trunk, and roots C_8, T_1.

Origin
The abductor digit minimi originate at the pisiform bone.

Insertion
Insertion is at the medial side of the base of the proximal phalanx of the little finger.

Activation Maneuver
Abduction of the little finger activates the muscles.

EMG Needle Insertion
Insert the needle obliquely at the midpoint between the fifth metacarpophalangeal joint (metacarpophalangeal crease) and the ulnar aspect of the pisiform (distal wrist crease).

Pitfalls
There are no pitfalls. If the needle is inserted too deeply or laterally, it will still be in C_8, T_1 muscles innervated by the ulnar nerve.

Clinical Comments
In ulnar neuropathy at the wrist (Guyon's canal), needle examination may show neurogenic changes when compression produces axonal loss (i.e., in moderate to severe entrapment).

In ulnar neuropathy at the elbow (cubital tunnel, retrocondylar groove), needle examination may show neurogenic changes when compression produces axonal loss.

In C_8, T_1 radiculopathy, needle examination may show neurogenic changes when root pathology produces axonal loss (i.e., in moderate to severe radiculopathy).

In Klumpke's palsy (C_8, T_1 root avulsion), needle examination will show neurogenic changes.

Opponens Digiti Minimi

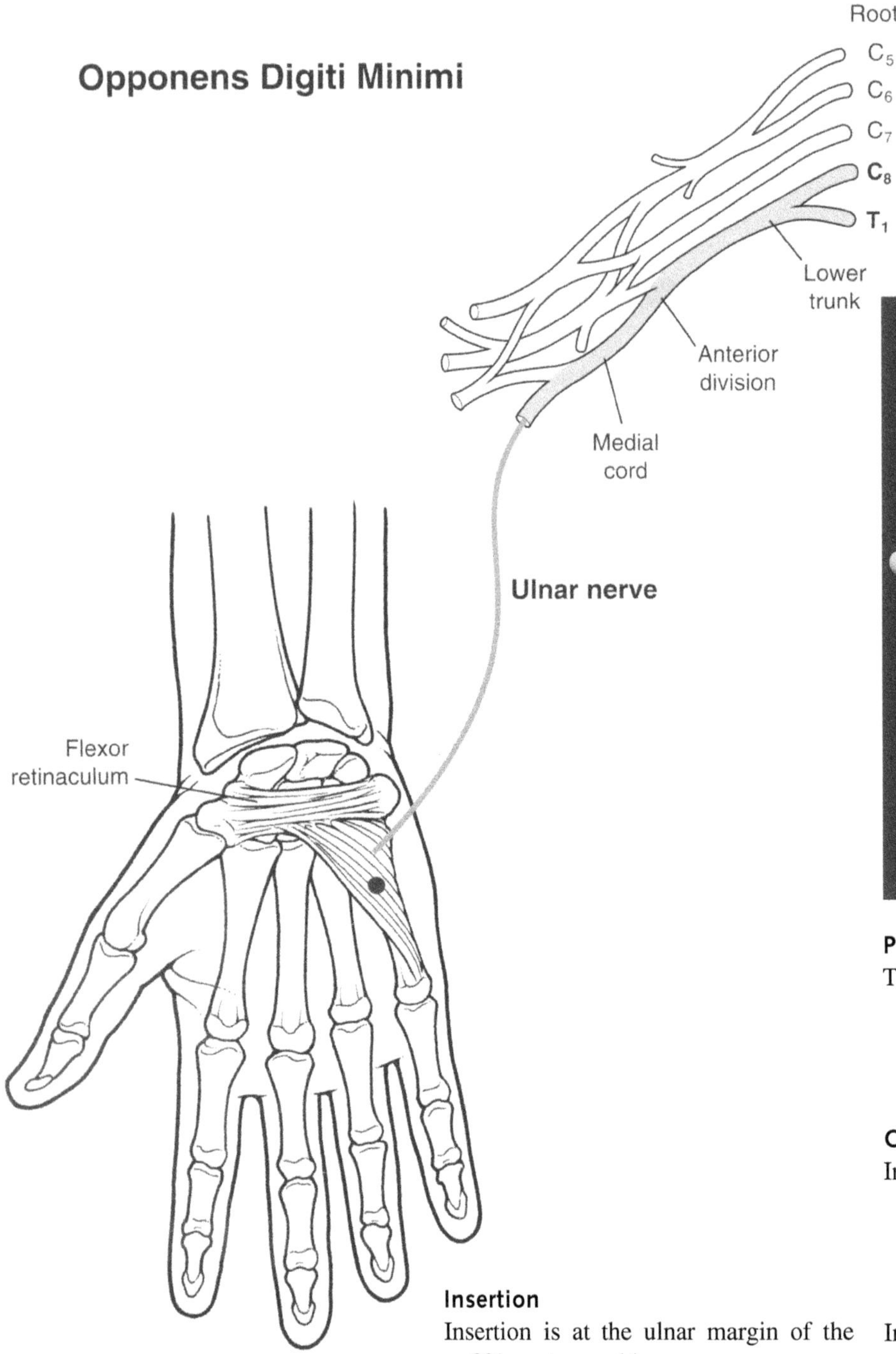

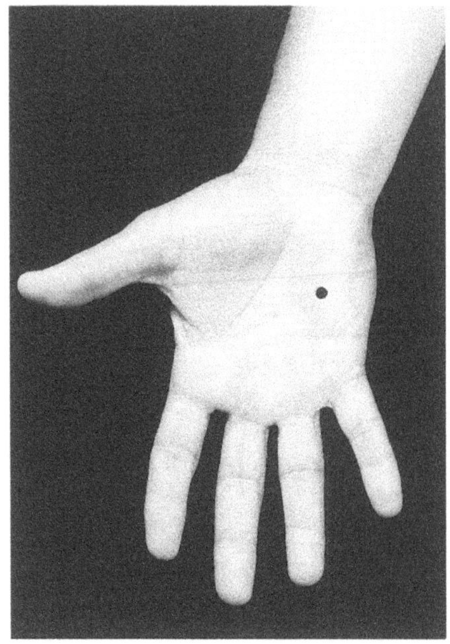

Innervation
Innervation is via the ulnar nerve, medial cord, lower trunk, and roots C_8, T_1.

Origin
The opponens digiti minimi originate at the flexor retinaculum and the hook of the hamate.

Insertion
Insertion is at the ulnar margin of the fifth metacarpal bone.

Activation Maneuver
Opposition of the little finger to the thumb activates the muscles.

EMG Needle Insertion
Insert the needle at the midpoint between the fifth metacarpophalangeal joint (metacarpophalangeal crease) and the pisiform (distal wrist crease), just radial to the abductor digiti minimi.

Pitfalls
There are no pitfalls. If the needle is inserted too deeply or laterally, it will still be in C_8, T_1 muscles innervated by the ulnar nerve.

Clinical Comments
In ulnar neuropathy at the wrist (Guyon's canal), needle examination may show neurogenic changes when compression produces axonal loss (i.e., in moderate to severe entrapment).

In ulnar neuropathy at the elbow (cubital tunnel, retrocondylar groove), needle examination may show neurogenic changes when compression produces axonal loss.

In C_8, T_1 radiculopathy, needle examination may show neurogenic changes when root pathology produces axonal loss (i.e., in moderate to severe radiculopathy).

In Klumpke's palsy (C_8, T_1 root avulsion), needle examination will show neurogenic changes.

Flexor Digiti Minimi

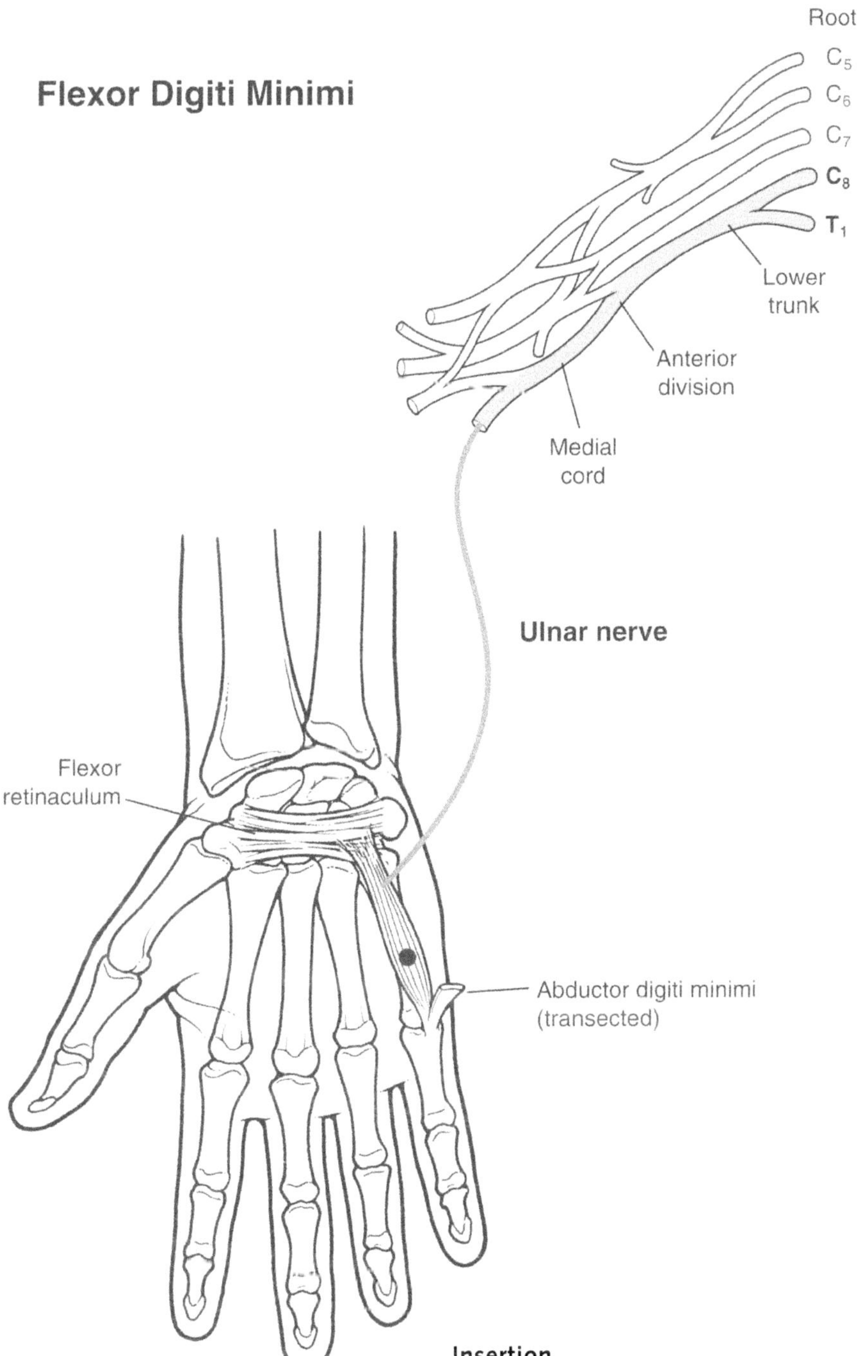

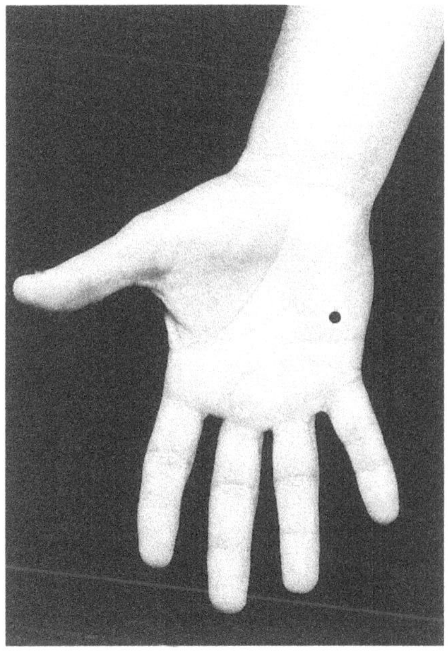

Innervation

Innervation is via the ulnar nerve, medial cord, lower trunk, and roots C_8, T_1.

Origin

The flexor digiti minimi originate at the hook of the hamate and the flexor retinaculum.

Insertion

Insertion is at the ulnar side of the base of the proximal phalanx of the little finger.

Activation Maneuver

Flexion of the proximal phalanx of the fifth digit activates the muscles.

EMG Needle Insertion

Insert the needle at the midpoint between the fifth metacarpophalangeal joint (metacarpophalangeal crease) and the ulnar aspect of the pisiform (distal wrist crease), just radial to the abductor digiti minimi.

Pitfalls

There are no pitfalls. If the needle is inserted too deeply, it will be in the opponens digiti minimi, which is still innervated by the ulnar nerve.

Clinical Comments

In ulnar neuropathy at the wrist (Guyon's canal), needle examination may show neurogenic changes when compression produces axonal loss (i.e., in moderate to severe entrapment).

In ulnar neuropathy at the elbow (cubital tunnel, retrocondylar groove), needle examination may show neurogenic changes when compression produces axonal loss.

In C_8, T_1 radiculopathy, needle examination may show neurogenic changes when root pathology produces axonal loss (i.e., in moderate to severe radiculopathy).

In Klumpke's palsy (C_8, T_1 root avulsion), needle examination will show neurogenic changes.

Flexor Digitorum Profundus Digits 4 and 5

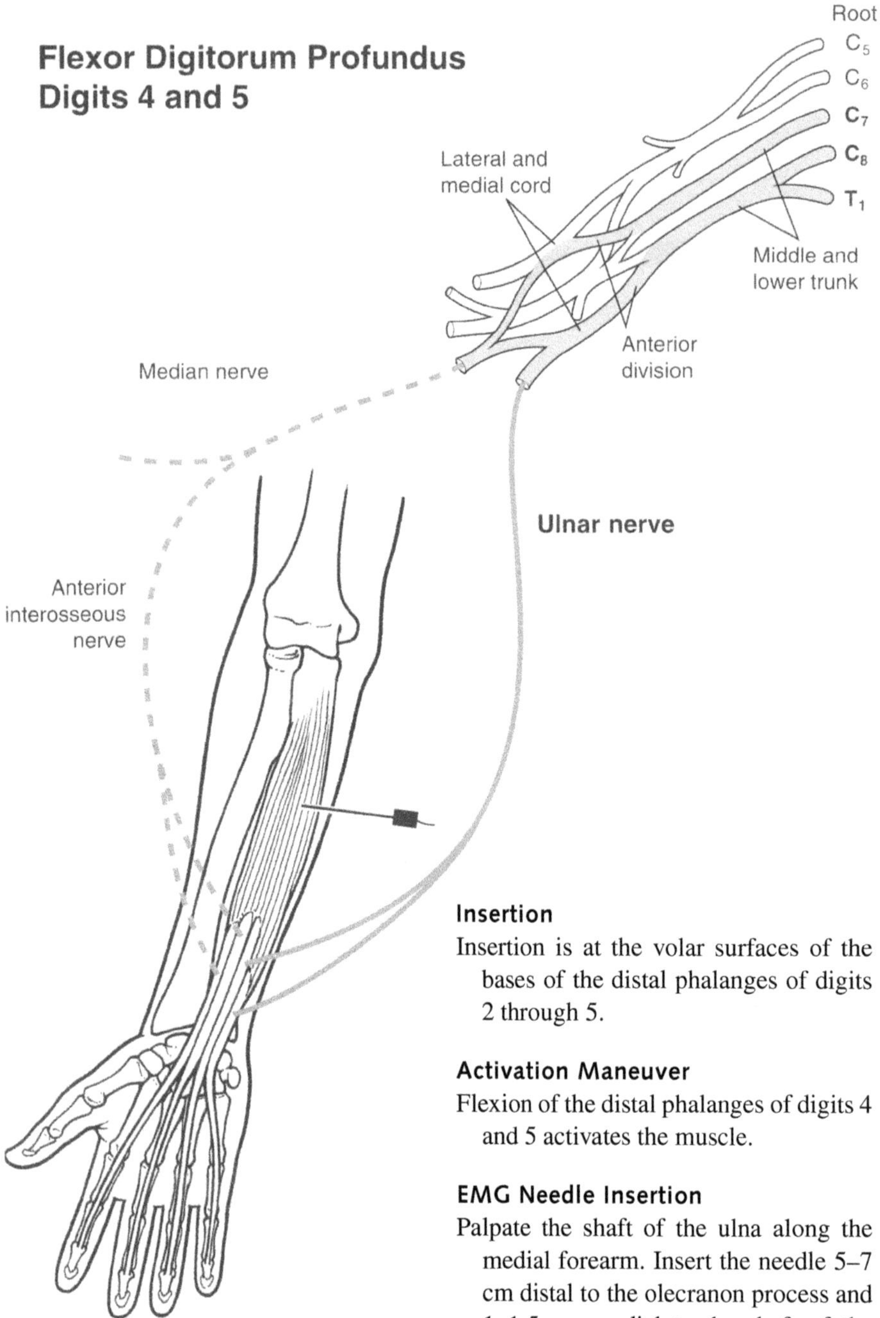

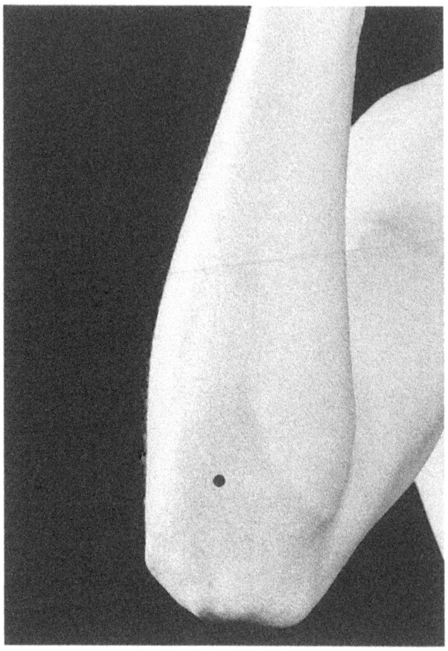

Innervation

Digits four and five: Innervation is via the ulnar nerve, medial cord, lower trunk, and roots C_8, T_1.

Digits two and three: Innervation is via the anterior interosseous branch, median nerve, lateral and medial cords, middle and lower trunks, and roots C_7, C_8.

Origin

The flexor digitorum profundus originates at the volar and medial surfaces of the shaft of the ulna.

Insertion

Insertion is at the volar surfaces of the bases of the distal phalanges of digits 2 through 5.

Activation Maneuver

Flexion of the distal phalanges of digits 4 and 5 activates the muscle.

EMG Needle Insertion

Palpate the shaft of the ulna along the medial forearm. Insert the needle 5–7 cm distal to the olecranon process and 1–1.5 cm medial to the shaft of the ulna. The ulnar-innervated portion lies superficially at a depth of 1–2 cm; the median portion lies deep at a depth of 3–4 cm. Note: The easiest approach to this muscle is for the subject to place the forearm perpendicular to the table with the hand and wrist relaxed. The shaft of the ulna and the adjacent belly of the muscle can easily be palpated (see photograph).

Pitfalls

If the needle is inserted too volarly (i.e., toward the palmar surface), it may lie in the flexor carpi ulnaris, which also receives innervation from the ulnar nerve.

Clinical Comments

Needle examination of the superficial portion may show neurogenic changes in axonal loss lesions of the ulnar nerve at the elbow (cubital tunnel or retrocondylar groove).

Needle examination of the deep portion may show neurogenic changes if a lesion of the anterior interosseous nerve produces axonal loss and in axonal loss lesions of the median nerve at the elbow (pronator teres syndrome) or above the elbow (ligament of Struthers' syndrome).

In C_8, T_1 radiculopathy, the needle examination may show neurogenic changes when root pathology has resulted in axonal loss (i.e., in moderate to severe radiculopathy).

In Klumpke's palsy (C_8, T_1 root avulsion), needle examination will show neurogenic changes.

Flexor Carpi Ulnaris

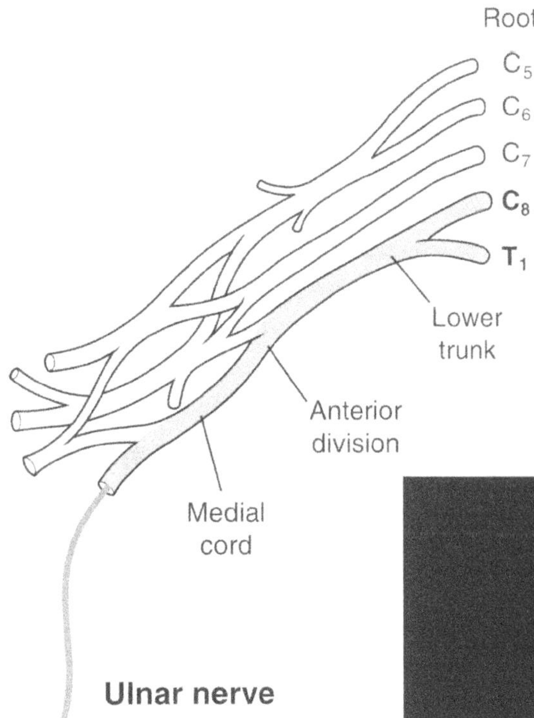

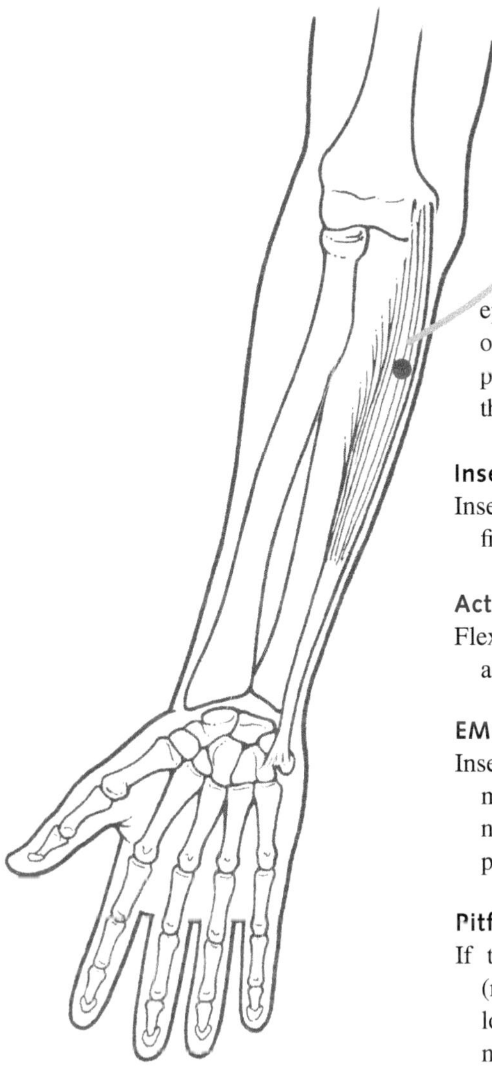

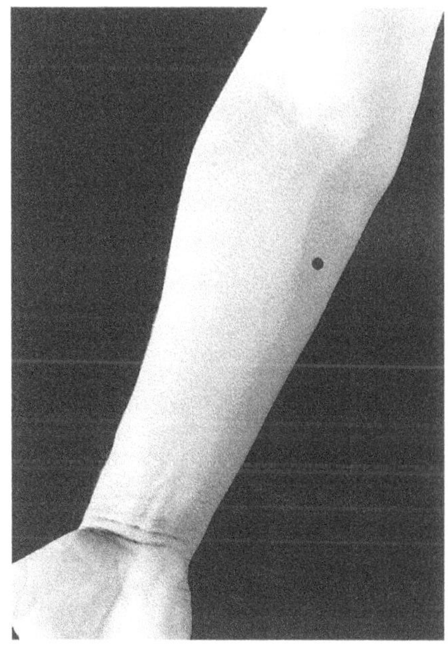

Innervation

Innervation is via the ulnar nerve, medial cord, lower trunk, and roots C_8, T_1.

Origin

The flexor carpi ulnaris arises by two heads. One head is from the medial epicondyle of the humerus, and the other head is from the olecranon process and the upper two thirds of the posterior border of the ulna.

Insertion

Insertion is at the pisiform, hamate, and fifth metacarpal bones.

Activation Maneuver

Flexion at the wrist with ulnar deviation activates the muscles.

EMG Needle Insertion

Insert the needle 5–8 cm distal to the medial epicondyle along a line connecting the medial epicondyle and pisiform bone.

Pitfalls

If the needle is inserted too laterally (radially), it may be in the palmaris longus or the flexor carpi radialis, both muscles innervated by the median nerve.

If the needle is inserted too deeply, it may be in the flexor digitorum superficialis (supplied by median nerve), or, if still deeper, it may penetrate the flexor digitorum profundus (supplied by median and ulnar nerves).

Clinical Comments

The two heads are connected by a tendinous arch that forms the cubital tunnel 1–2 cm distal to the medial epicondyle, through which passes the ulnar nerve. Entrapment at this site produces ulnar neuropathy at the elbow (cubital tunnel).

Needle examination of this muscle is usually normal in cubital tunnel entrapment. It may also be normal in ulnar neuropathy due to compression at the retrocondylar groove.

In C_8, T_1 radiculopathy, needle examination may show neurogenic changes when root pathology produces axonal loss (i.e., in moderate to severe radiculopathy).

In Klumpke's palsy (C_8, T_1 root avulsion), needle examination will show neurogenic changes.

6 RADIAL NERVE

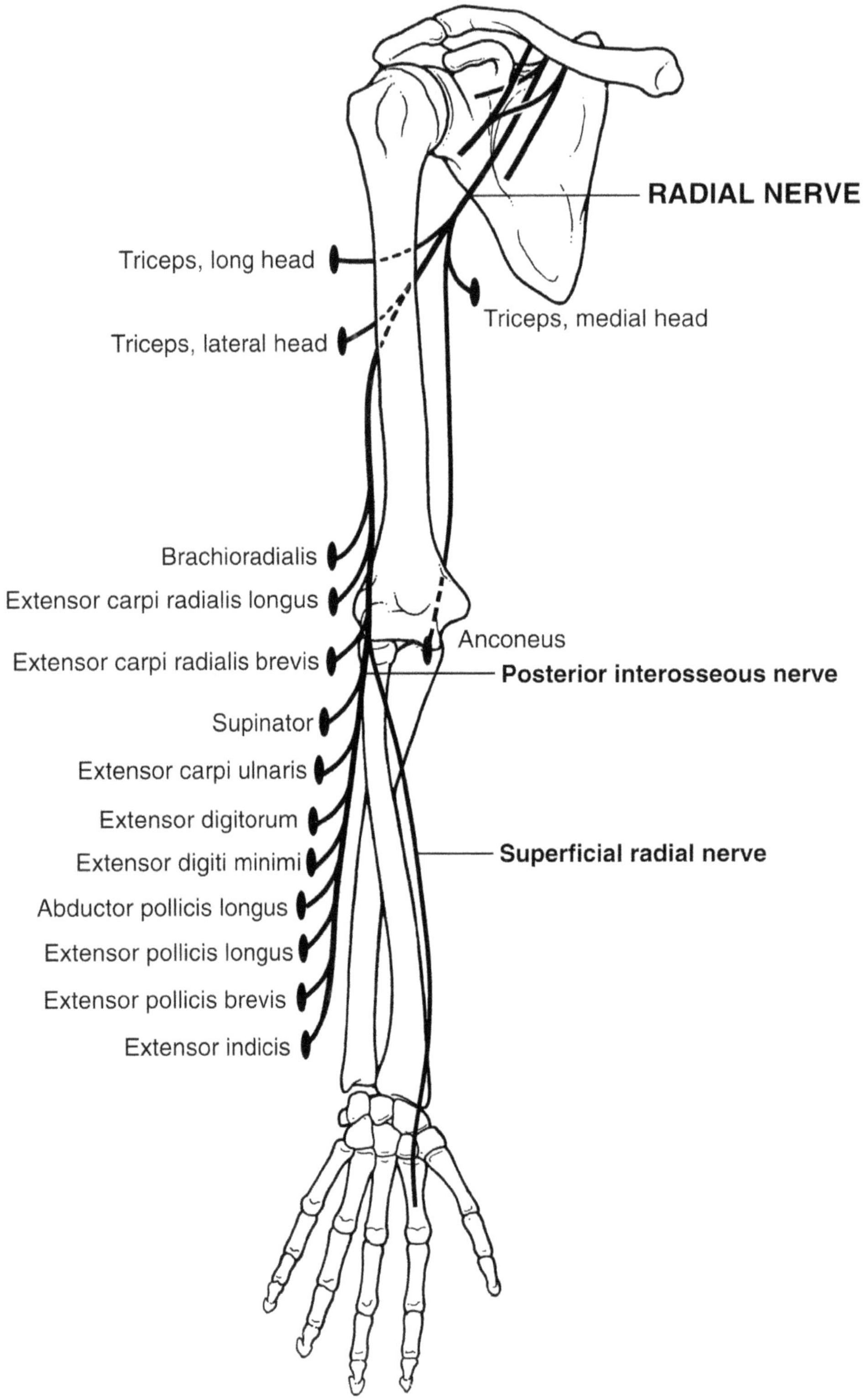

FIGURE 6-1 Diagram of the radial nerve and the muscles that it supplies.

THE RADIAL NERVE (Figure 6-1) is the largest branch of the brachial plexus, arising from the posterior cord and the fifth, sixth, seventh, and eighth cervical roots, with occasional contribution from the first thoracic root (*Gray's Anatomy,* 1995). From its origin on the posterior axillary wall, it descends behind the axillary artery to reach the angle between the medial aspect of the arm and the posterior wall of the axilla (brachio-axillary angle). Branches to the heads of the triceps and anconeus arise in the axilla and brachio-axillary angle. The radial nerve also gives off several sensory branches, including the posterior cutaneous nerve of the arm, the inferior lateral cutaneous nerve of the arm, and the posterior cutaneous nerve of the forearm, which supply cutaneous innervation to the posterior arm, inferolateral arm, and posterior forearm, respectively.

With the profunda brachii artery, the radial nerve inclines downward between the long and medial heads of the triceps, after which it passes obliquely along the back of the humerus in the spiral groove (also known as the *radial groove*). Here it is in direct contact with bone. On reaching the lateral side of the humerus, the nerve pierces the lateral intermuscular septum to enter the anterior compartment. It then descends in the furrow between the brachialis medially and brachioradialis laterally. The nerve gives off branches to the brachialis (this muscle is supplied primarily by the musculocutaneous nerve) and brachioradialis. The nerve is overlapped, in turn, by the extensor carpi radialis longus and extensor carpi radialis brevis. The radial nerve supplies both muscles, although the extensor carpi radialis brevis may receive its nerve supply from the posterior interosseous nerve (Sunderland, 1968).

Anterior to the lateral epicondyle, the radial nerve divides into its two terminal branches: the posterior interosseous nerve and the superficial radial nerve. The former is a pure muscular nerve that innervates the supinator before passing through the arcade formed by the superficial and deep heads of this muscle (arcade of Fröhse). On the dorsum of the forearm, the posterior interosseous nerve divides in a variable manner to innervate the extensor carpi ulnaris, extensor digitorum communis, extensor digiti minimi, abductor pollicis longus, extensor pollicis longus and brevis, and extensor indicis. The superficial radial branch is primarily a sensory nerve. It provides cutaneous innervation to the dorsum of the hand lateral to the ring finger, dorsum of the thumb, radial aspect of the thenar eminence, and dorsum of the index, middle, and radial half of the ring fingers as far distally as the middle phalanx.

Although the radial nerve, or its branches, may be involved in penetrating injuries at any level, there are certain sites where the nerve is more prone to injury (Sunderland, 1968). In the brachio-axillary angle, compression may result from a misused crutch or from fractures of the upper third of the humerus. In the region of the spiral groove and lateral intermuscular septum, compression neuropathies of the radial nerve are common and widely recognized. The nerve is most commonly damaged by fractures of the humerus or during deep intoxication with the arm draped over the edge of a bed, chair, or bench (Saturday night palsy). In its course through the supinator (arcade of Fröhse), the posterior interosseous nerve is prone to damage from fractures of the upper third of the radius, and less commonly from entrapment. Injury to the superficial radial branch may result from tight handcuffs (handcuff neuropathy) or carelessly administered intravenous infusions.

RADIAL NERVE LESION IN THE ARM

Etiology

Compression of the nerve in the spiral groove (radial groove) of the humerus can cause a radial nerve lesion in the arm (Figure 6-2).

The condition is called "Saturday night palsy" when sedatives or alcohol produce deep sleep in someone, and an arm is draped over the edge of a bed, chair, or bench.

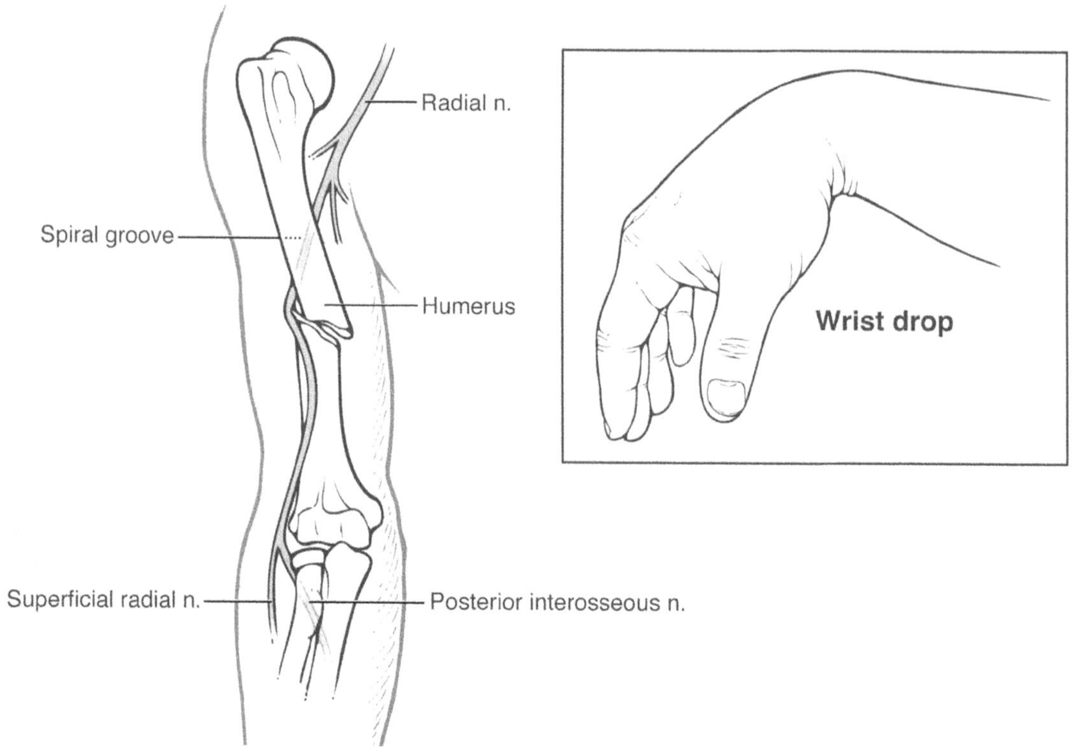

FIGURE 6-2 Radial nerve lesion in the arm. In the region of the spiral groove, the nerve lies on bone and is commonly injured by a fracture of the humerus. It is also commonly injured by external pressure applied to the region of the spiral groove ("Saturday night palsy").

The condition is called "honeymooner's palsy" when compression results from the weight of a partner's head lying on the arm.

A radial nerve lesion can occur secondary to a fracture of the humerus, prolonged or excessive muscle contraction (as in masons, carpenters, or athletes in throwing sports), anatomical anomalies of the triceps, and deep intramuscular injections.

General Comments

A radial nerve lesion in the arm is a common compression neuropathy.

Predisposing factors include diabetes, malnutrition, alcohol or sedative use, and hereditary susceptibility to pressure palsies (Brown and Watson, 1993).

The differential diagnosis includes lead poisoning, porphyria, diabetes, and periarteritis nodosa.

Clinical Features

Wrist drop occurs with a radial nerve lesion in the arm.

There is normal function of the triceps (extension of forearm at elbow).

There is weakness of the brachioradialis and all other muscles supplied by the radial nerve beyond the spiral groove.

Pain is not a typical feature, but it may be perceived in the area of the lateral epicondyle, radial styloid, or dorsum of hand.

Numbness can occur in the distribution of the superficial radial nerve and occasionally in the territory of the posterior cutaneous nerve of the forearm.

Most cases of "Saturday night palsy" fully resolve in days to a few weeks, which is consistent with a demyelinating lesion. Delayed or incomplete recovery implies a greater degree of axonal loss.

Electrodiagnostic Strategy

Use nerve conduction studies to confirm a focal lesion (conduction block, slowing of conduction velocity) at the spiral groove and to obtain information on severity and prognosis. Cases characterized by conduction block resolve quickly; those with axonal loss and Wallerian degeneration show a reduction of motor or sensory amplitudes and resolve slowly or incompletely.

In cases of axonal loss, EMG may show neurogenic changes (spontaneous activity, abnormal motor unit potentials, and abnormal recruitment) in the brachioradialis and other muscles supplied by the radial nerve distal to the spiral groove.

EMG is normal in cases of demyelination and in the early stages of axonal loss in which Wallerian degeneration has not yet occurred.

EMG of the triceps and anconeus is normal.

The superficial radial sensory response is reduced in amplitude or absent in cases of axonal loss (normal in cases of demyelination and in the early stages of axonal loss).

EMG of nonradial innervated C_7 muscles may be necessary to exclude C_7 radiculopathy.

RADIAL NERVE LESION IN THE AXILLA

Etiology

Compression of the nerve in the axilla by high-riding crutches can cause the condition called *crutch palsy* or *crutch neuropathy* (Figure 6-3). Most cases of crutch neuropathy involve the posterior cord of the brachial plexus (Sunderland, 1978; Raikin and Froimson, 1997), although other cords and individual nerves may also be affected.

A radial nerve lesion can occur secondary to shoulder trauma, humerus fractures, tumor, or anatomical anomalies of the coracobrachialis or triceps.

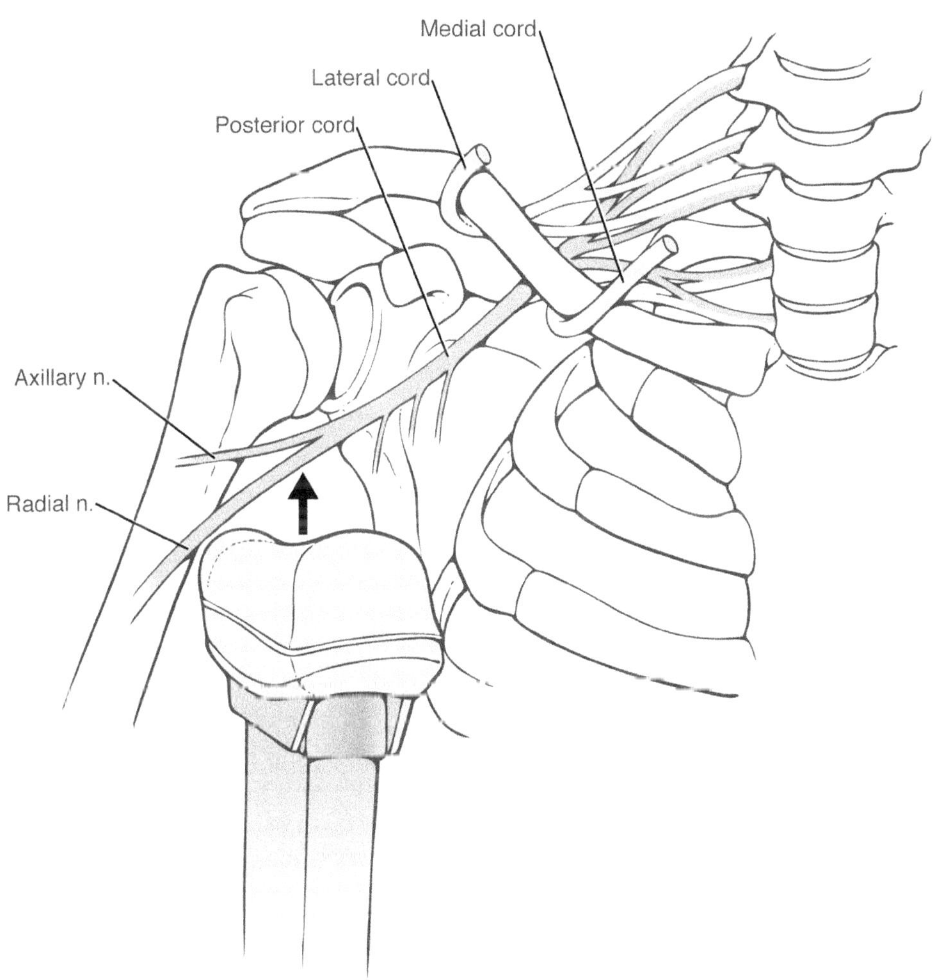

FIGURE 6-3 Radial nerve lesion in the axilla following the use of crutches ("crutch palsy").

Clinical Features

Wrist drop occurs with a radial nerve lesion in the axilla.

Weakness occurs in all muscles supplied by the radial nerve, including the triceps.

The triceps reflex is absent.

Numbness occurs in the distribution of the superficial radial nerve, and occasionally in the territories of the posterior cutaneous nerves of the forearm or arm and inferior lateral cutaneous nerve of the arm.

Most cases fully resolve in days to a few weeks, which is consistent primarily with a demyelinating lesion. Delayed or incomplete recovery implies a greater degree of axonal loss.

Electrodiagnostic Strategy

Use electrodiagnostic evaluation to obtain information on severity and prognosis. Cases associated with axonal loss and Wallerian degeneration show a reduction of motor or sensory amplitudes and resolve slowly or incompletely.

In cases of axonal loss, EMG may show neurogenic changes in the triceps and all other muscles supplied by the radial nerve.

EMG is normal in cases of demyelination and in the early stages of axonal loss in which Wallerian degeneration has not yet occurred.

The superficial radial sensory response is reduced in amplitude or absent in cases of axonal loss (normal in cases of demyelination and in the early stages of axonal loss).

EMG of nonradial innervated C_7 muscles may be necessary to exclude C_7 radiculopathy.

POSTERIOR INTEROSSEOUS NERVE SYNDROME

Etiology

Compression of the nerve as it passes between the two layers of the supinator muscle in the arcade of Fröhse can cause posterior interosseous nerve syndrome (Figure 6-4).

Posterior interosseous nerve syndrome can occur secondary to radial subluxation, a fracture of the proximal radius, prolonged or repeated pronation–supination movements, tumors (lipoma), neuralgic amyotrophy, and compression by the extensor carpi radialis brevis.

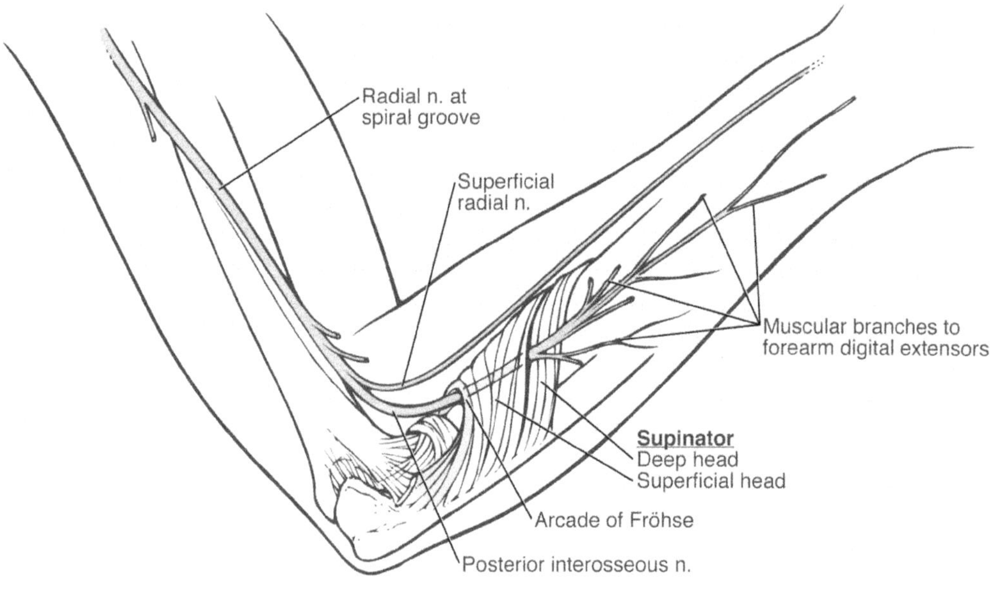

FIGURE 6-4 Anatomy of the posterior interosseous nerve in relation to the arcade of Fröhse and supinator muscle.

General Comments

Posterior interosseous nerve syndrome is also known as the *supinator syndrome*.

Injury to the posterior interosseous nerve is usually associated with trauma (fractures, gunshot wounds, lacerations) rather than with true entrapment.

Clinical Features

There is normal supination of the forearm and radial wrist extension (supinator and extensor carpi radialis are normal).

Weakness occurs in the extensor carpi ulnaris; attempted wrist extension results in characteristic radial deviation of the wrist.

Weakness occurs during finger extension and thumb extension. Thumb abduction may be normal because the abductor pollicis brevis (median nerve) is unaffected.

There is pain in the lateral upper forearm (usually 5–8 cm distal to the lateral epicondyle).

There is no sensory impairment because the superficial radial nerve arises above the arcade of Fröhse.

Electrodiagnostic Strategy

The superficial radial sensory response is normal.

Motor studies may reveal a focal lesion (conduction block, slowing of conduction velocity) across the entrapment (Kimura, 1989). Cases characterized by conduction block resolve quickly; those associated with Wallerian degeneration show a reduction of motor amplitude and resolve slowly or incompletely.

EMG may show neurogenic changes (spontaneous activity, abnormal motor unit potentials, and abnormal recruitment) in all muscles supplied by the posterior interosseous nerve below the supinator.

EMG of radial innervated muscles (triceps, anconeus, brachioradialis, and extensor carpi radialis longus) is normal.

SUPERFICIAL RADIAL NERVE LESION

Etiology

Compression of the sensory branch of the radial nerve at the wrist or distal forearm can cause a superficial radial nerve lesion.

The condition is called *cheiralgia paresthetica* when tight-fitting watches, bracelets, or bands compress the superficial radial nerve.

The condition is also referred to as *handcuff neuropathy* when tight handcuffs compress the superficial radial nerve.

A superficial radial nerve lesion can occur secondary to a fracture of the distal radius because the nerve lies adjacent to the bone.

General Comments

A superficial radial nerve lesion at the wrist or distal forearm is a common cutaneous neuropathy.

Clinical Features

Sensory disturbance occurs in the radial dorsum of the hand (Figure 6-5). In most cases, sensation is blunted but not lost, and limited to a portion of the radial dorsum of the hand, usually maximal in the interspace between thumb and index finger (Sunderland, 1978). In some cases, profound sensory deficits may occur.

In cases of anomalous superficial radial nerve innervation to the ulnar dorsum of the hand, superficial radial nerve injury may result in more extensive sensory deficits over the entire dorsum of the hand (see figure 5-12; Leis and Wells, 2008).

Occasionally, pain or dysesthesia in the radial dorsum of hand is the chief complaint.

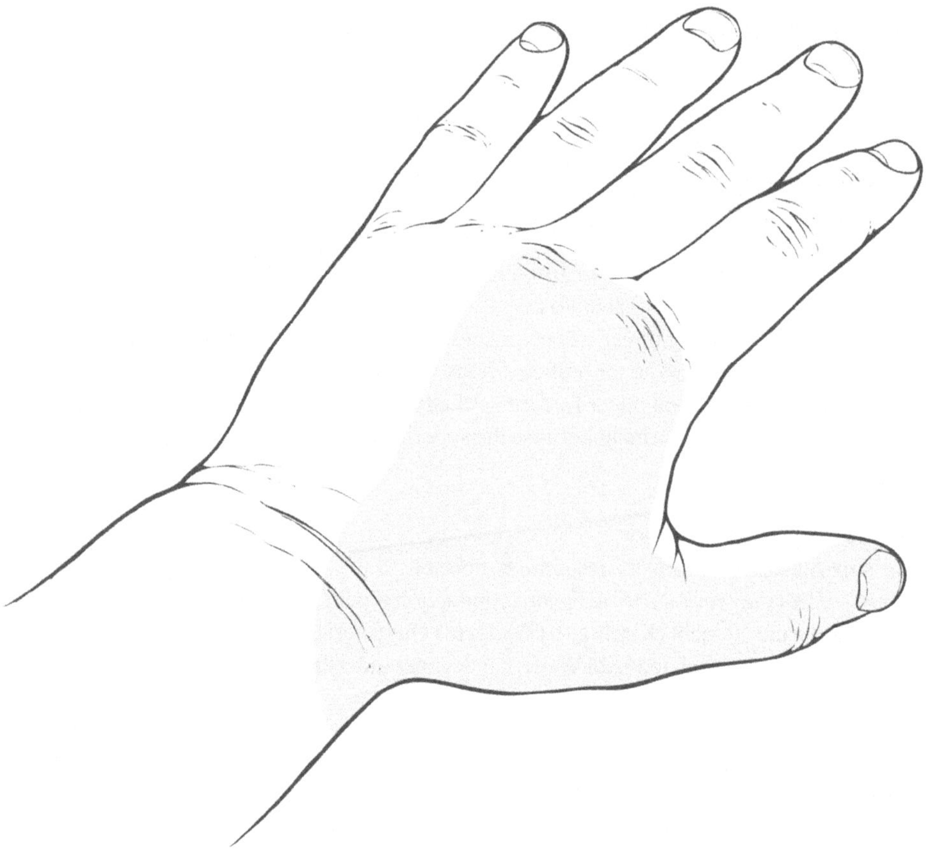

FIGURE 6-5 Distribution of sensory deficits in a lesion of the superficial radial nerve. In most cases, sensation is blunted or altered, but not lost.

There is no wrist drop or muscle weakness, since the superficial radial nerve is a pure sensory branch.

Electrodiagnostic Strategy

In a superficial radial nerve lesion characterized by neurapraxia (demyelination) the superficial radial sensory response will be preserved. These patients typically recover quickly.

Superficial radial sensory response will be reduced or absent in more severe cases associated with axonal loss (Wallerian degeneration). These cases recover slowly or incompletely.

Radial motor studies are normal.

EMG is normal in all muscles supplied by the posterior interosseous nerve and the radial nerve.

Radial Motor Nerve Conduction Study

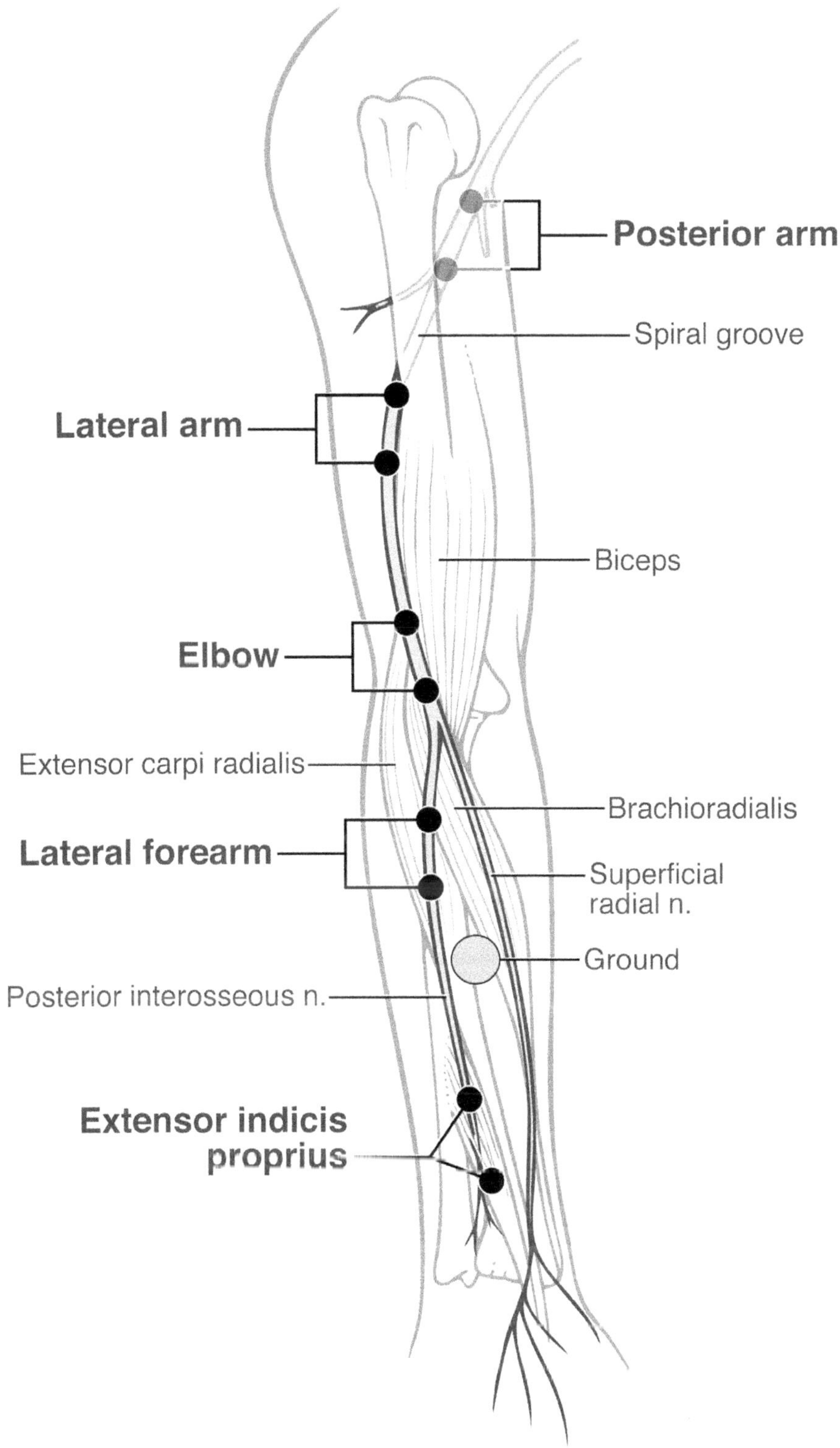

FIGURE 6-6 Radial motor nerve conduction study.

Recording

Active electrode: Position over the belly of the extensor indicis proprius muscle (2 to 3 fingerbreadths proximal to the ulnar styloid, about one-third of the distance between ulna and radius bones). Alternatively, position the active electrode over the distal extensor digitorum communis muscle one-half of the distance between ulna and radius bones.

Reference electrode: Place 3 cm distal to the active electrode or, alternatively, over the ulnar styloid.

Ground electrode: Place on the dorsum of the forearm between stimulating and recording electrodes.

Stimulation

Lateral forearm: Place cathode in the proximal forearm over the dorsolateral aspect of the ulna. The anode is 3 cm proximal to cathode.

Elbow: Place cathode in the groove between the brachioradialis muscle laterally and the biceps medially. The radial nerve is stimulated beneath the brachioradialis muscle. Anode is 3 cm proximal to cathode.

Lateral arm (below spiral groove): Place cathode in the lateral mid-arm between the biceps and triceps muscles. This site lies along the lateral aspect of the humerus bone. Anode is 3 cm proximal to cathode.

Posterior arm (above spiral groove): Place cathode in the upper arm over the posterior aspect of the humerus.

Comment

There are other sites where the radial or posterior interosseous nerve can be stimulated to elicit a CMAP, including at Erb's point and along the course of the nerve in the forearm (Kimura, 1989; Preston and Shapiro, 2005). In addition, short segment stimulation ("inching technique") can be performed across the spiral groove and in the forearm to aid in the localization of a conduction abnormality.

Normal Values

Amplitude (mV) ≥ 2.5

Conduction velocity (m/s) ≥ 50 m/s across all segments

There are no fixed distances in radial motor conduction studies. Normal values differ depending on the distance used and different recording techniques. Radial motor conduction studies should be performed bilaterally because side-to-side comparisons are more useful than normal value tables. An amplitude ≤ 50 % of the unaffected side is evidence of abnormality.

Pitfalls

Technical problems arise from submaximal stimulation in obese or muscular arms. When this occurs with stimulation above the spiral groove, the drop in CMAP amplitude may be misinterpreted as a conduction block.

Imprecise surface measurements over the spiral groove and across the elbow are a source of technical error.

The radial CMAP often has an initial small positive deflection, indicating volume-conduction from coactivation of multiple forearm digital extensors.

Superficial Radial Sensory Nerve Conduction Study

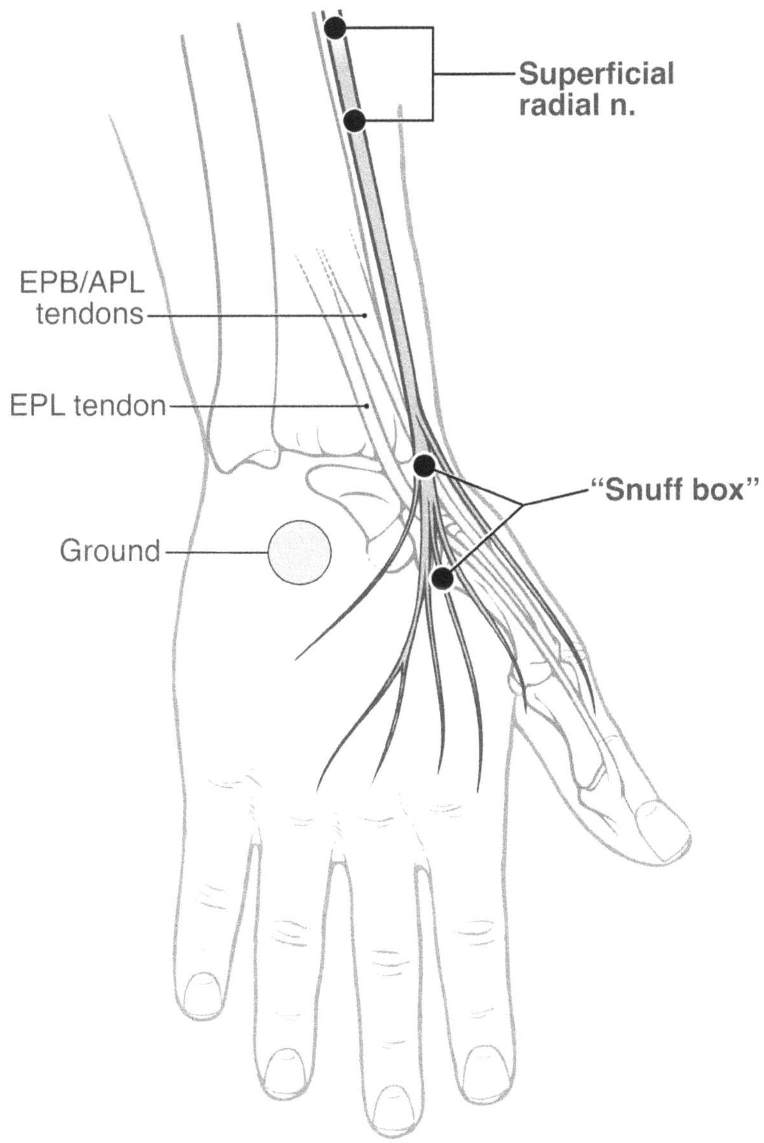

FIGURE 6-7 Superficial radial sensory nerve conduction study (antidromic).

Recording

Active electrode: Position over the anatomical "snuff box," formed by the extensor pollicis brevis (EPB) and abductor pollicis longus (APL) tendons laterally and the extensor pollicis longus (EPL) tendon medially.

Reference electrode: Place 3 cm distal to the active electrode.

Ground electrode: Place on the dorsum of the wrist.

Stimulation

Forearm: Place cathode over the dorsolateral edge of the radius bone, 10 cm from the active recording electrode. The anode is 3 cm proximal to cathode.

Comments

As the name implies, this radial sensory nerve is very superficial and can often be palpated in the region of the anatomical "snuff box."

Normal Values

Latency (ms) ≤ 2.0 (onset latency); ≤ 2.7 (peak latency)
Amplitude (μV) ≥ 20
Conduction velocity (m/s) ≥ 50 m/s

The normal amplitude of the superficial radial SNAP has a large range and standard deviation. Therefore, studies should ideally be performed bilaterally, because side-to-side comparisons are more useful than normal value tables that may not apply to your patient. An amplitude ≤ 50 % of the unaffected side is evidence of abnormality.

REFERENCES

Brown WF, Watson BV. AAEM case report #27: Acute retrohumeral radial neuropathies. *Muscle Nerve* 1993;16:706–711.

Gray's Anatomy. 38th edition, Churchill Livingstone, New York, 1995, pp.1266–1274.

Kimura J. *Electrodiagnosis in Diseases of Nerve and Muscle*. 2nd ed., FA Davis Co., Philadelphia, 1989, pp. 499–500.

Leis AA, Wells KJ. Radial nerve cutaneous innervation to the ulnar dorsum of the hand. *Clin Neurophysiol* 2008;119:662–666.

Preston DC, Shapiro BE. *Electromyography and neuromuscular disorders. Clinical-electrophysiologic correlations.* 2nd ed., Elsevier Butterworth Heinemann, 2005.

Raikin S, Froimson MI. Bilateral brachial plexus compressive neuropathy (crutch palsy). *J Orthop Trauma* 1997;11:136–138.

Sunderland S. *Nerves and Nerve Injuries*. Williams and Wilkins, Baltimore, 1968, pp. 894–938.

Sunderland S. *Nerves and Nerve Injuries*. 2nd ed., Churchill Livingstone, New York, 1978, pp. 820–842.

Extensor Indicis

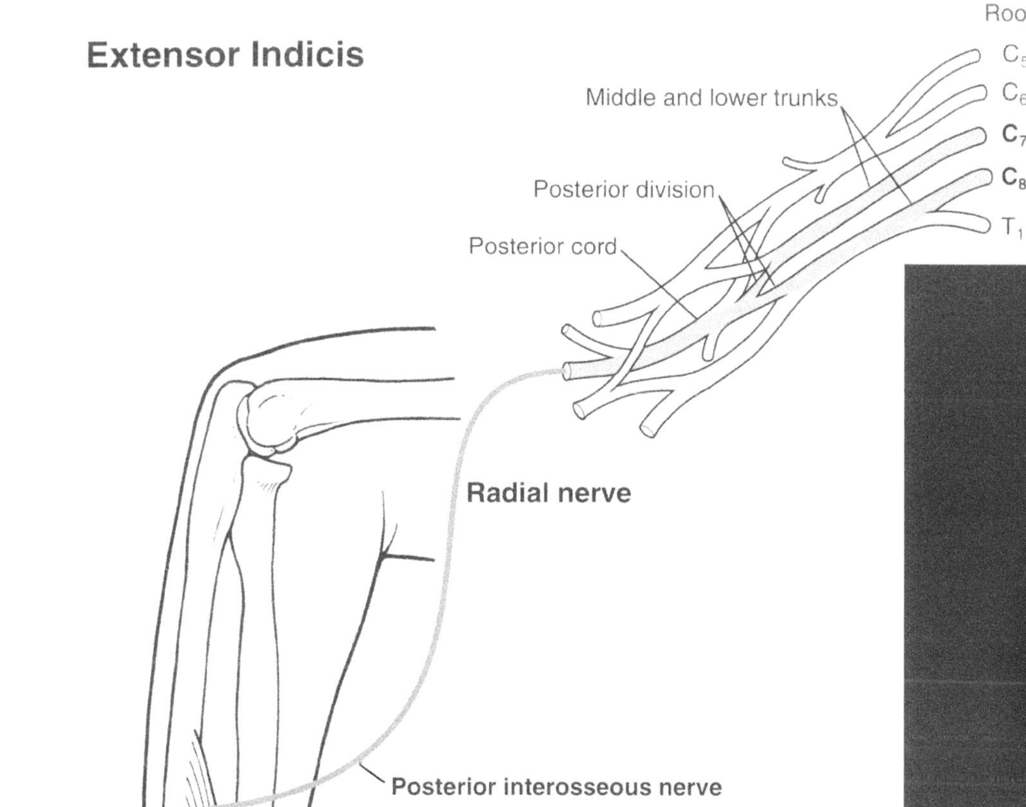

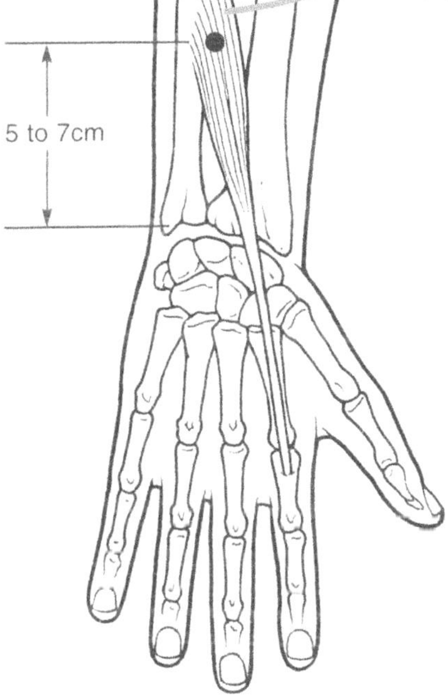

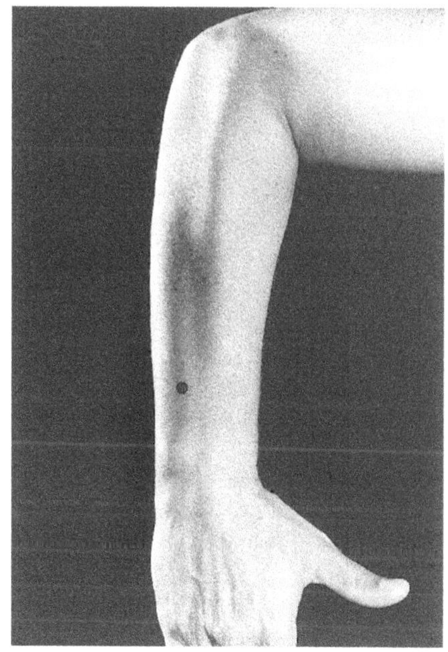

Innervation

Innervation is via the posterior interosseous nerve, radial nerve, posterior cord, middle and lower trunks, and roots C_7, C_8.

Origin

The extensor indicis originates at the posterior surface of the lower half of the shaft of the ulna and adjacent interosseous membrane.

Insertion

The extensor indicis joins the tendon of the extensor digitorum communis to the index finger.

Activation Maneuver

Extension of the index finger activates the muscle.

EMG Needle Insertion

Insert the needle 5–7 cm proximal to the ulnar styloid just radial to the shaft of the ulna. Hint: Follow the tendon proximally to where it intersects the ulna.

Pitfalls

If the needle is inserted too laterally (radially), it may be in the extensor pollicis longus, which also receives innervation from the posterior interosseous nerve.

Clinical Comments

The extensor indicis is usually the most distal muscle innervated by the posterior interosseous branch of the radial nerve.

In a radial nerve lesion at the axilla (crutch neuropathy) or at the arm (Saturday night palsy), needle examination may show neurogenic changes when compression produces axonal loss.

In a posterior interosseous nerve lesion, needle examination may show neurogenic changes when compression at the arcade of Frohse produces axonal loss.

In a C_7, C_8 radiculopathy , needle examination may show neurogenic changes when pathology produces axonal loss.

Extensor Pollicis Brevis

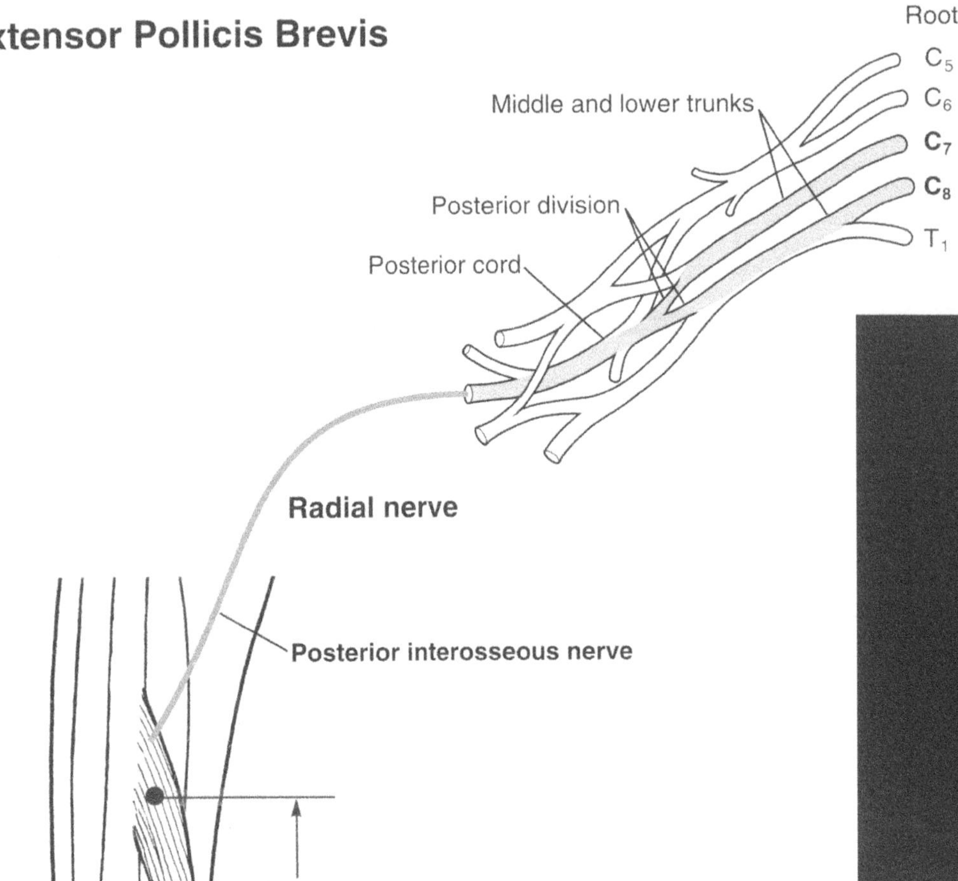

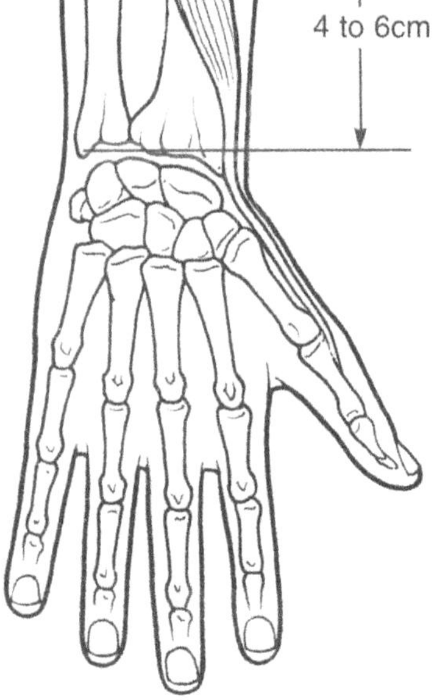

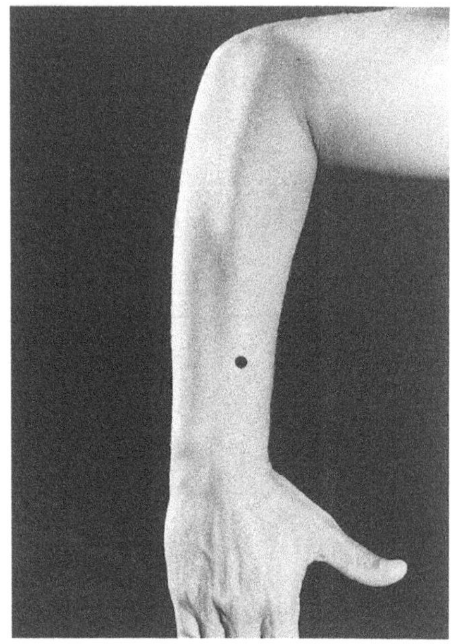

Innervation

Innervation is via the posterior interosseous nerve, radial nerve, posterior cord, middle and lower trunks, and roots C_7, C_8.

Origin

The extensor pollicis brevis originates at the posterior surface of the shaft of the radius, below the origin of the abductor pollicis longus, and adjacent interosseous membrane.

Insertion

Insertion is at the base of the first phalanx of the thumb. (Note: The tendon passes through the same groove as the abductor pollicis longus tendon on the outer side of the styloid process, forming the radial border of the anatomical "snuffbox.")

Activation Maneuver

Extension of the proximal phalanx of the thumb activates the muscle.

EMG Needle Insertion

Insert the needle 4–6 cm proximal co the wrist over the ulnar aspect of the radius.

Pitfalls

If the needle is inserted too proximally, it may be in the abductor pollicis longus, which also receives innervation from the posterior interosseous nerve.

Clinical Comments

In a radial nerve lesion at the axilla (crutch neuropathy) or at the arm (Saturday night palsy), needle examination may show neurogenic changes when compression produces axonal loss.

In a posterior interosseous nerve lesion, needle examination may show neurogenic changes when compression at the arcade of Frohse produces axonal loss.

In C_7, C_8 radiculopathy, needle examination may show neurogenic changes when pathology produces axonal loss.

Extensor Pollicis Longus

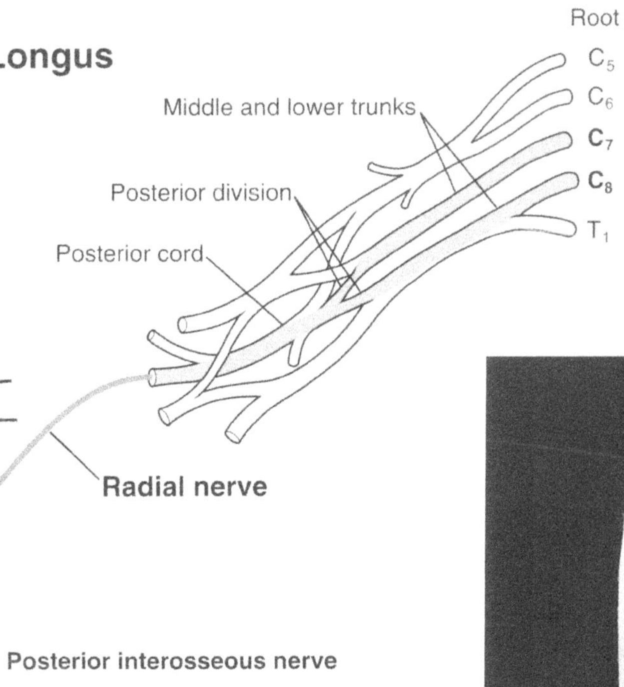

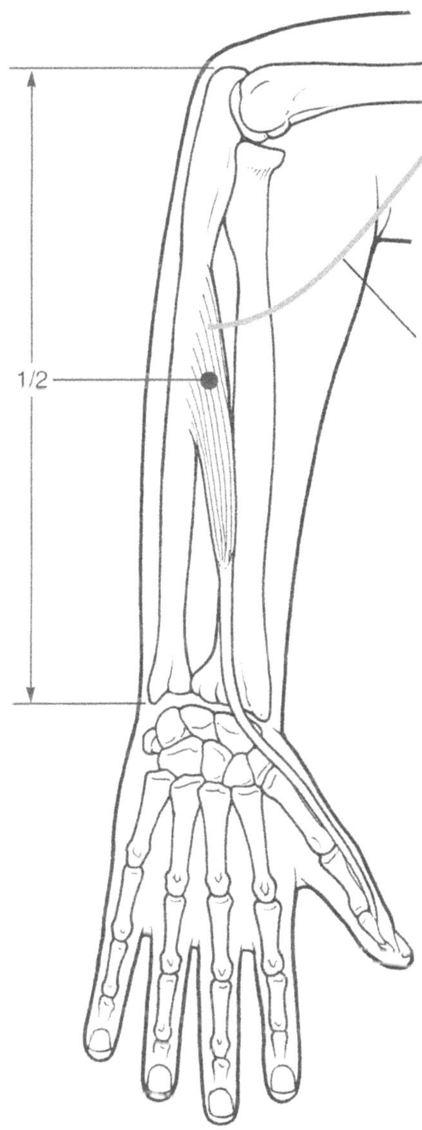

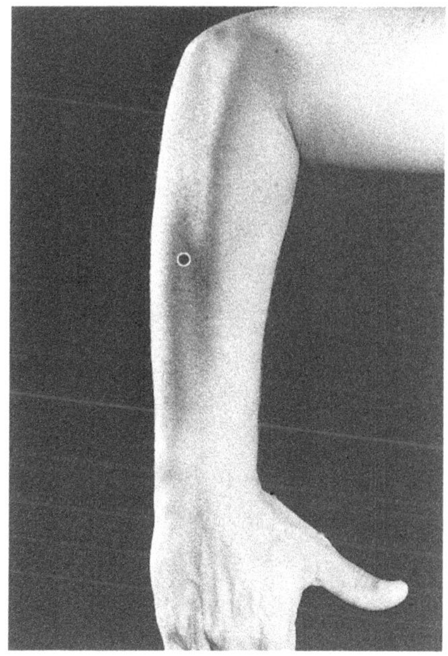

Innervation

Innervation is via the posterior interosseous nerve, radial nerve, posterior cord, middle and lower trunks, and roots C_7, C_8.

Origin

The extensor pollicis longus originates at the posterior surface of the shaft of the ulna, below the origin of the abductor pollicis longus.

Insertion

Insertion is at the base of the terminal phalanx of the thumb. (Note: The tendon forms the ulnar border of the anatomical "snuffbox.")

Activation Maneuver

Extension of the distal phalanx of the thumb activates the muscle.

EMG Needle Insertion

Insert the needle at the mid-forearm along the radial border of the ulna.

Pitfalls

If the needle is inserted too proximally or radially, it may be in the abductor pollicis longus, which also receives innervation from the posterior interosseous nerve.

If the needle is inserted too distally, it may be in the extensor indicts, which is also innervated by the posterior interosseous nerve.

Clinical Comments

In a radial nerve lesion at the axilla (crutch neuropathy) or at the arm (Saturday night palsy), needle examination may show neurogenic changes when compression produces axonal loss.

In a posterior interosseous nerve lesion, needle examination may show neurogenic changes when compression at the arcade of Frohse produces axonal loss.

In C_7, C_8 radiculopathy, needle examination may show neurogenic changes when pathology produces axonal loss.

Abductor Pollicis Longus

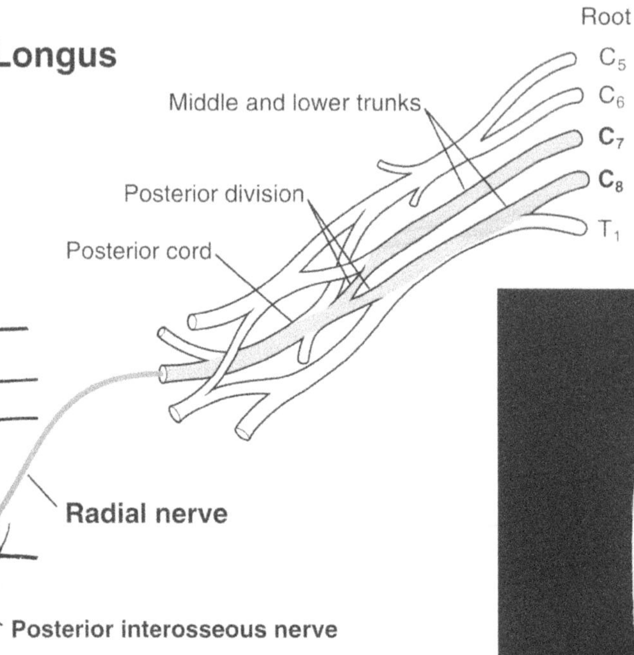

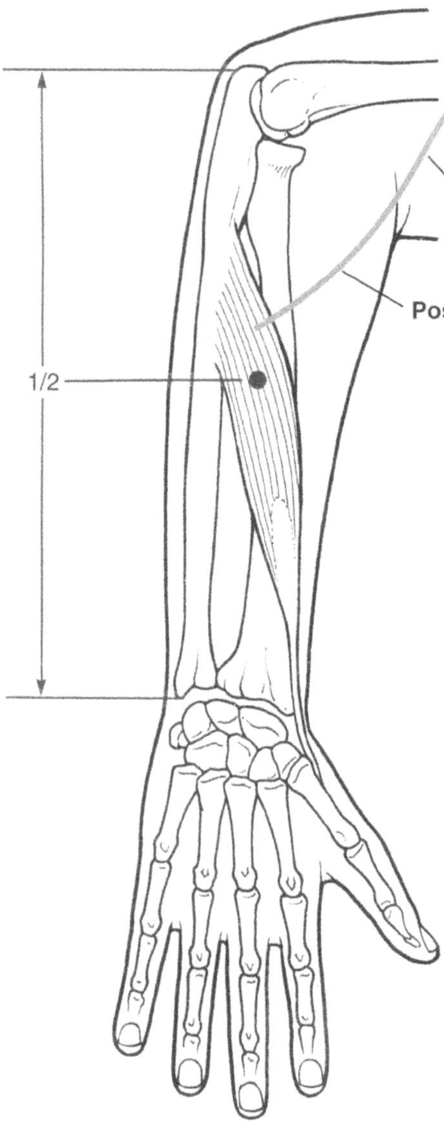

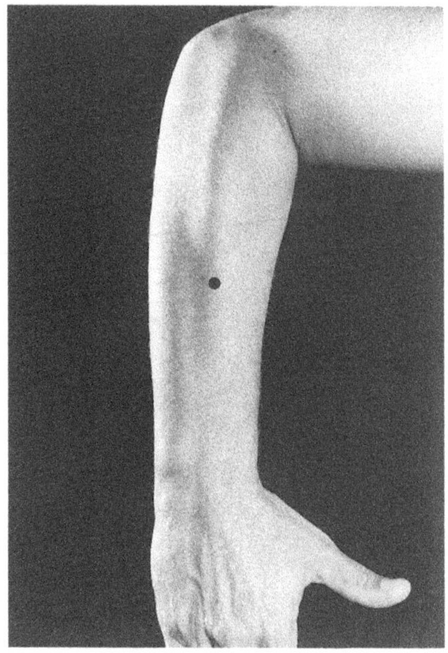

Innervation

Innervation is via the posterior interosseous nerve, radial nerve, posterior cord, middle and lower trunks, and roots C_7, C_8.

Origin

The abductor pollicis longus originates at the posterior surface of the shaft of the ulna, above the origin of the extensor pollicis longus; at the posterior surface of the shaft of the radius, above the origin of the extensor pollicis brevis; and at the adjacent interosseous membrane.

Insertion

Insertion is at the base of the metacarpal bone of the thumb. (Note: The tendon forms the radial border of the anatomical "snuffbox.")

Activation Maneuver

Radial abduction and extension of the thumb activate the muscle.

EMG Needle Insertion

Insert the needle at the mid-forearm along the shaft of the radius.

Pitfalls

If the needle is inserted too distally, it may be in the extensor pollicis brevis, which also receives innervation from the posterior interosseous nerve.

If the needle is inserted too proximally, it may be in the extensor carpi radialis, which is innervated by the radial nerve.

If the needle is inserted too medially (ulnarly), it may be in the extensor digitorum communis, which also receives innervation from the posterior interosseous nerve.

Clinical Comments

In a radial nerve lesion at the axilla (crutch neuropathy) or at the arm (Saturday night palsy), needle examination may show neurogenic changes when compression produces axonal loss.

In a posterior interosseous nerve lesion, needle examination may show neurogenic changes when compression at the arcade of Frohse produces axonal loss.

In C_7, C_8 radiculopathy, needle examination may show neurogenic changes when pathology produces axonal loss.

Extensor Digitorum Communis and Extensor Digiti Minimi

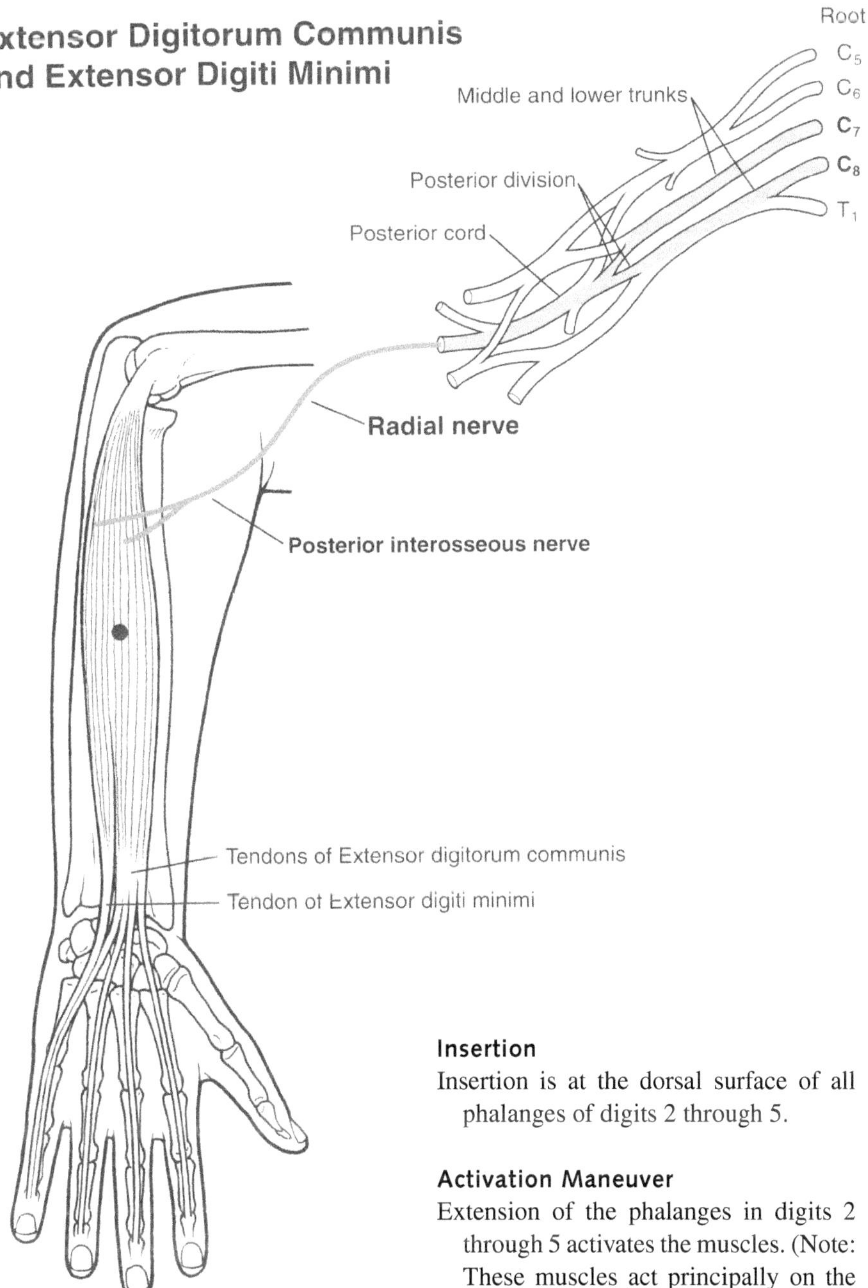

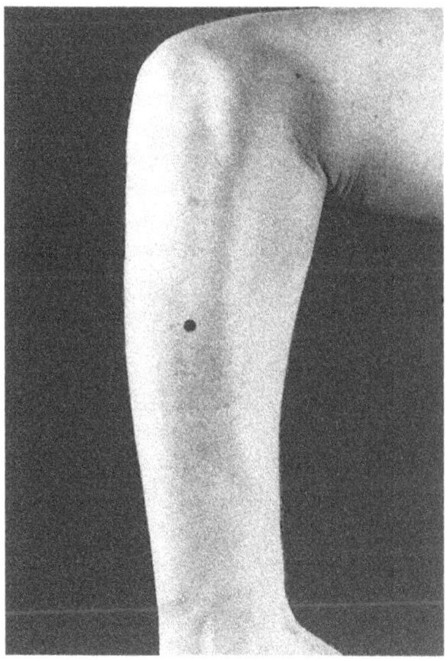

Innervation

Innervation is via the posterior interosseous nerve, radial nerve, posterior cord, middle and lower trunks, and roots C_7, C_8.

Origin

The extensor digitorum communis and extensor digiti minimi originate at the common extensor tendon from the lateral epicondyle of the humerus.

Insertion

Insertion is at the dorsal surface of all phalanges of digits 2 through 5.

Activation Maneuver

Extension of the phalanges in digits 2 through 5 activates the muscles. (Note: These muscles act principally on the proximal phalanges, the middle and distal phalanges being extended by the lumbricals and interossei.)

EMG Needle Insertion

Insert the needle in the mid-forearm midway between the ulna and radius. The extensor digiti minimi is frequently fused with the extensor digitorum communis. The extensor digiti minimi can be found in the mid-forearm on the ulnar border of the extensor digitorum communis.

Pitfalls

If the needle is inserted too laterally (radially), it may be in the extensor carpi radialis, which is innervated by the radial nerve.

If the needle is inserted too medially (ulnarly), it may be in the extensor carpi ulnaris, which also receives innervation from the posterior interosseous nerve.

Clinical Comments

In a radial nerve lesion at the axilla (crutch neuropathy) or at the arm (Saturday night palsy), needle examination may show neurogenic changes when compression produces axonal loss.

In a posterior interosseous nerve lesion, needle examination may show neurogenic changes when compression at the arcade of Frohse produces axonal loss.

In C_7, C_8 radiculopathy, needle examination may show neurogenic changes when pathology produces axonal loss.

Extensor Carpi Ulnaris

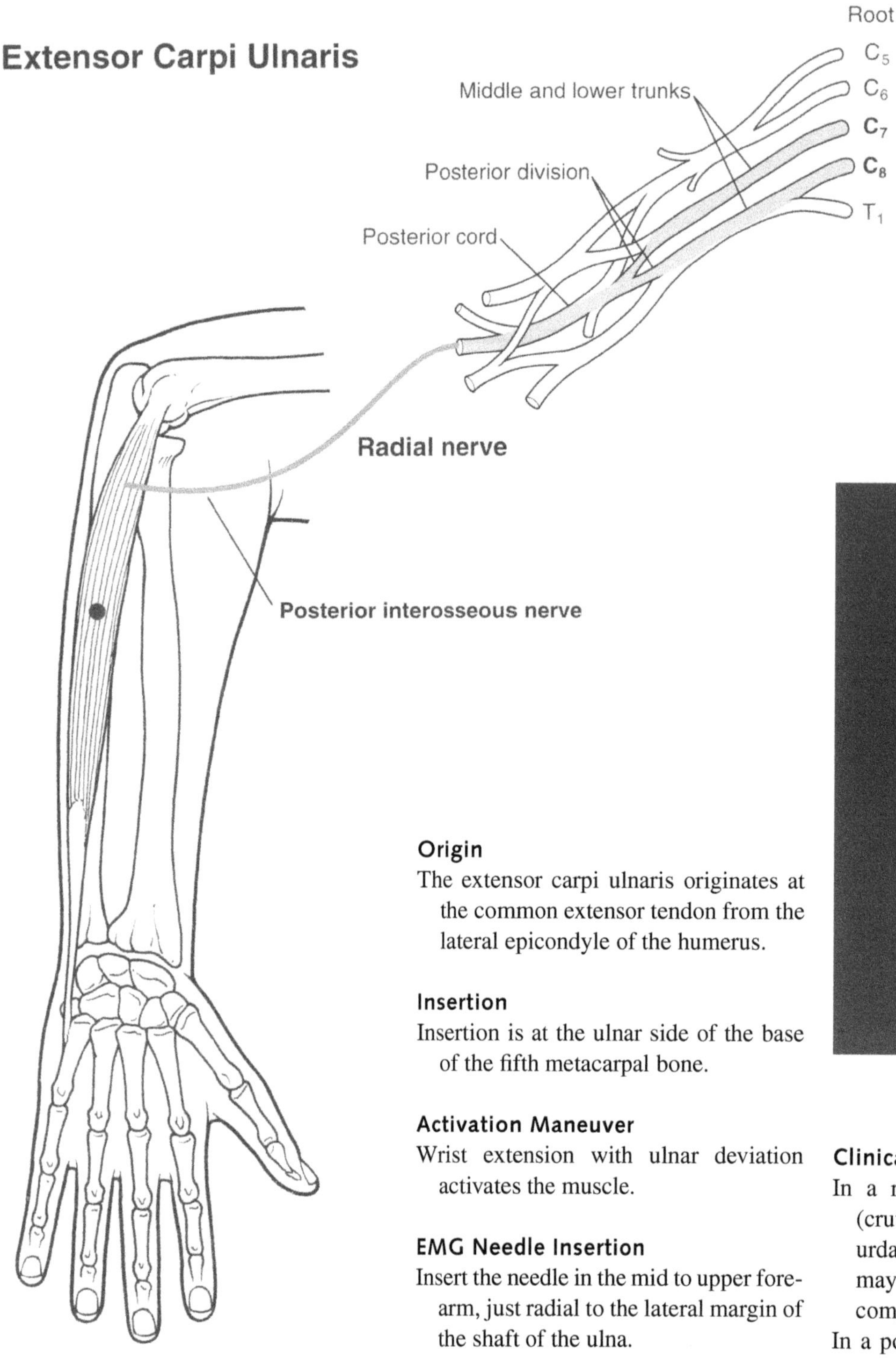

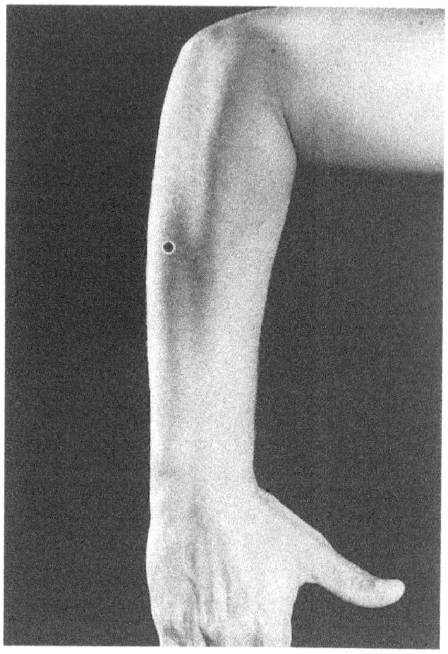

Origin
The extensor carpi ulnaris originates at the common extensor tendon from the lateral epicondyle of the humerus.

Insertion
Insertion is at the ulnar side of the base of the fifth metacarpal bone.

Activation Maneuver
Wrist extension with ulnar deviation activates the muscle.

EMG Needle Insertion
Insert the needle in the mid to upper forearm, just radial to the lateral margin of the shaft of the ulna.

Pitfalls
If the needle is inserted too laterally (radially), it may be in the extensor digiti minimi or extensor digitorum communis; both are innervated by the posterior interosseous nerve.

Innervation
Innervation is via the posterior interosseous nerve, radial nerve, posterior cord, middle and lower trunks, and roots C_7, C_8.

Clinical Comments
In a radial nerve lesion at the axilla (crutch neuropathy) or at the arm (Saturday night palsy), needle examination may show neurogenic changes when compression produces axonal loss.

In a posterior interosseous nerve lesion, needle examination may show neurogenic changes when compression at the arcade of Frohse produces axonal loss.

In C_7, C_8 radiculopathy, needle examination may show neurogenic changes when pathology produces axonal loss.

Supinator

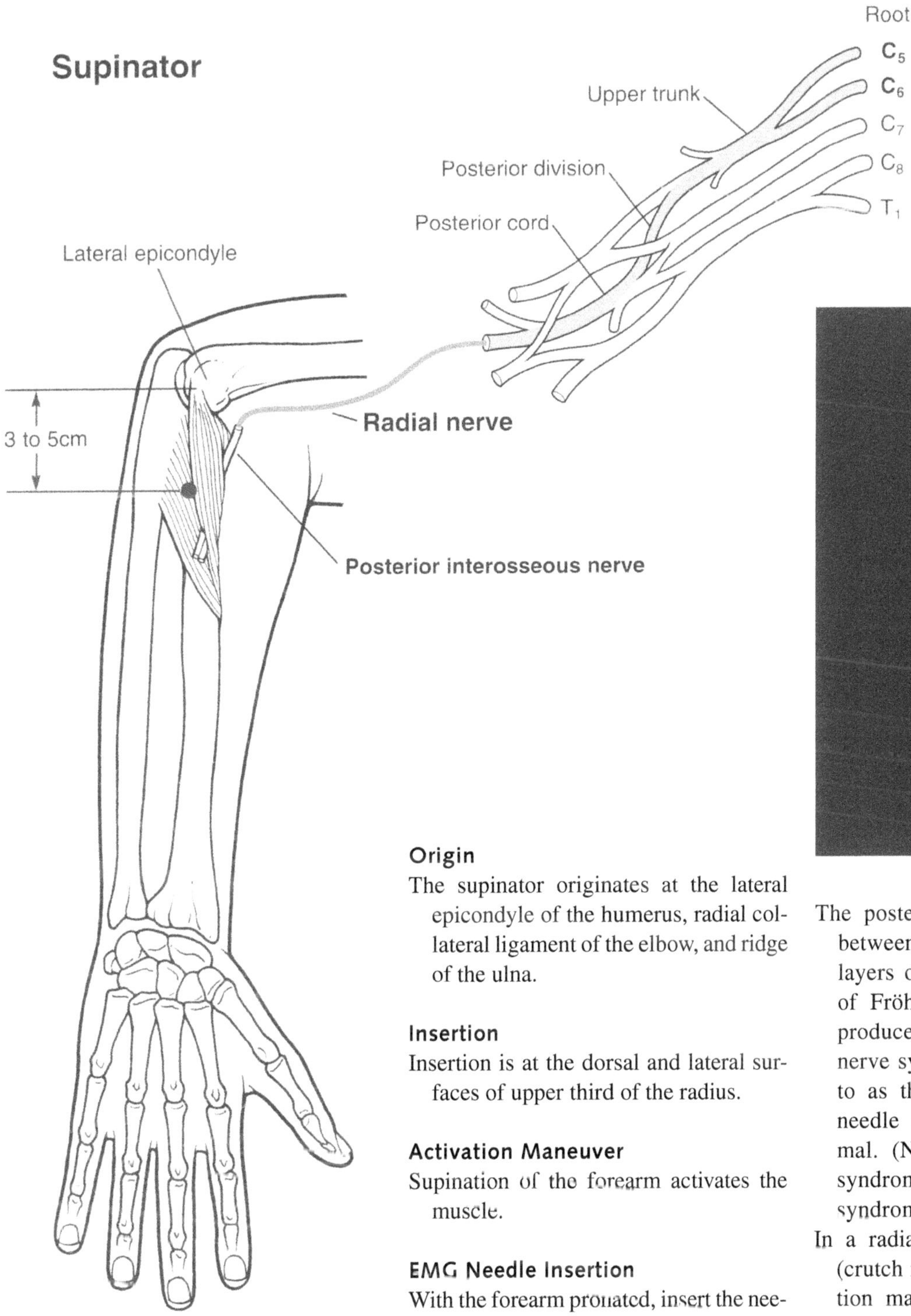

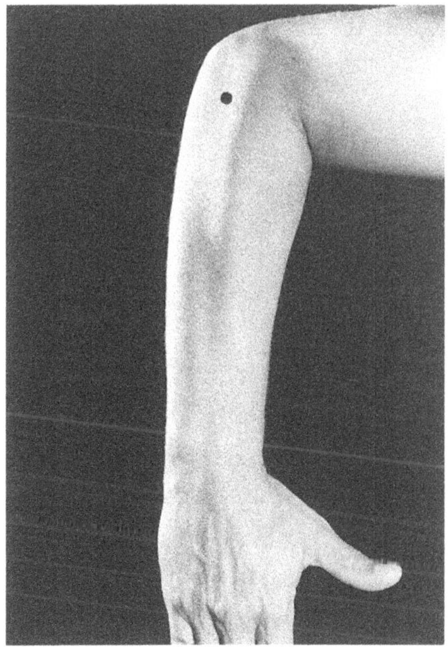

Innervation

Innervation is via the posterior interosseous nerve, radial nerve, posterior cord, upper trunk, and roots C_5, C_6.

Origin

The supinator originates at the lateral epicondyle of the humerus, radial collateral ligament of the elbow, and ridge of the ulna.

Insertion

Insertion is at the dorsal and lateral surfaces of upper third of the radius.

Activation Maneuver

Supination of the forearm activates the muscle.

EMG Needle Insertion

With the forearm pronated, insert the needle 3–5 cm distal to the lateral epicondyle, toward the shaft of the radius.

Pitfalls and Clinical Comments

This muscle lies deep. It is rarely of benefit to test it in a routine EMG evaluation.

The posterior interosseous nerve lies between the superficial and deep layers of this muscle, in the arcade of Fröhse. Entrapment at this site produces the posterior interosseous nerve syndrome, sometimes referred to as the *supinator syndrome*. The needle examination is usually normal. (Note: The muscle naming a syndrome is usually spared in that syndrome.)

In a radial nerve lesion at the axilla (crutch neuropathy), needle examination may show neurogenic changes when compression produces axonal loss.

In a radial nerve lesion at the arm (Saturday night palsy), needle examination may show neurogenic changes when compression at the spiral groove produces axonal loss.

Extensor Carpi Radialis, Longus and Brevis

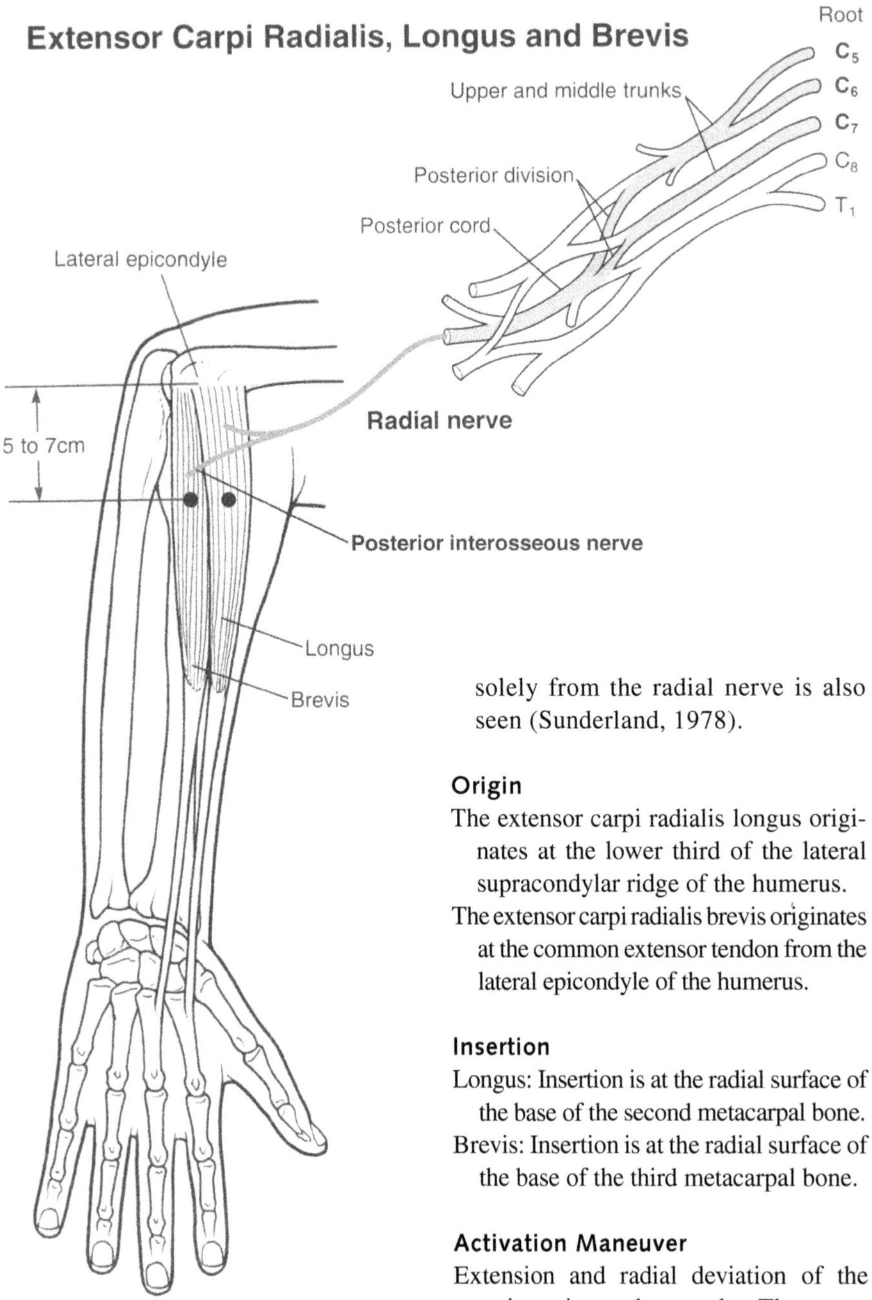

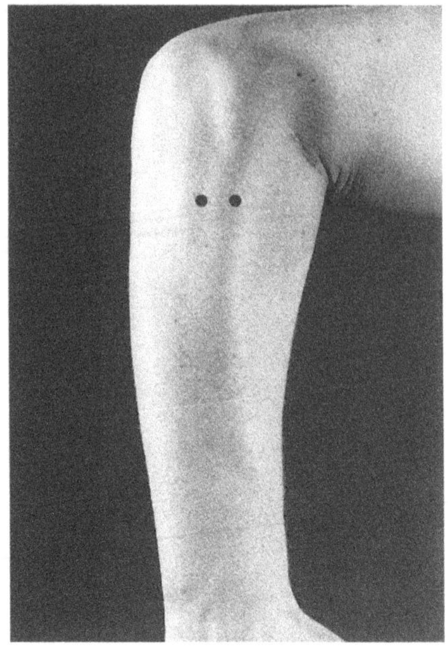

Innervation

Innervation to the extensor carpi radialis longus is via the radial nerve, posterior cord, upper and middle trunks, and roots C_5, C_6, C_7.

Innervation to the extensor carpi radialis brevis is primarily via the posterior interosseous nerve, radial nerve, posterior cord, upper and middle trunks, and roots C_5, C_6, C_7, although supply to this muscle solely from the radial nerve is also seen (Sunderland, 1978).

Origin

The extensor carpi radialis longus originates at the lower third of the lateral supracondylar ridge of the humerus.

The extensor carpi radialis brevis originates at the common extensor tendon from the lateral epicondyle of the humerus.

Insertion

Longus: Insertion is at the radial surface of the base of the second metacarpal bone.

Brevis: Insertion is at the radial surface of the base of the third metacarpal bone.

Activation Maneuver

Extension and radial deviation of the wrist activates the muscles. The extensor carpi radialis longus and brevis are so closely associated that it is impossible to determine whether one or both muscles are contracting. The activation maneuver should be performed while flexing the digits to avoid coactivating the extensor digitorum communis.

EMG Needle Insertion

Longus: Insert the needle in the upper forearm 5–7 cm distal to the lateral epicondyle along a line connecting the epicondyle and second metacarpal bone.

Brevis: Insert the needle in the upper forearm 5–7 cm distal to the lateral epicondyle along a line connecting the epicondyle and third metacarpal bone.

Pitfalls

If the needle is inserted too laterally (radially), it may be in the brachioradialis, which is also innervated by the radial nerve.

If the needle is inserted too medially (ulnarly), it may be in the extensor digitorum communis, which receives innervation from the posterior interosseous nerve.

Clinical Comments

In a radial nerve lesion at the axilla (crutch neuropathy), needle examination may show neurogenic changes when compression produces axonal loss.

In a radial nerve lesion at the upper arm (Saturday night palsy), needle examination may show neurogenic changes when compression at the spiral groove produces axonal loss.

In a posterior interosseous nerve lesion, needle examination of extensor carpi radialis longus will be normal, although needle examination of extensor carpi radialis brevis may show neurogenic changes when pathology produces axonal loss.

Brachioradialis

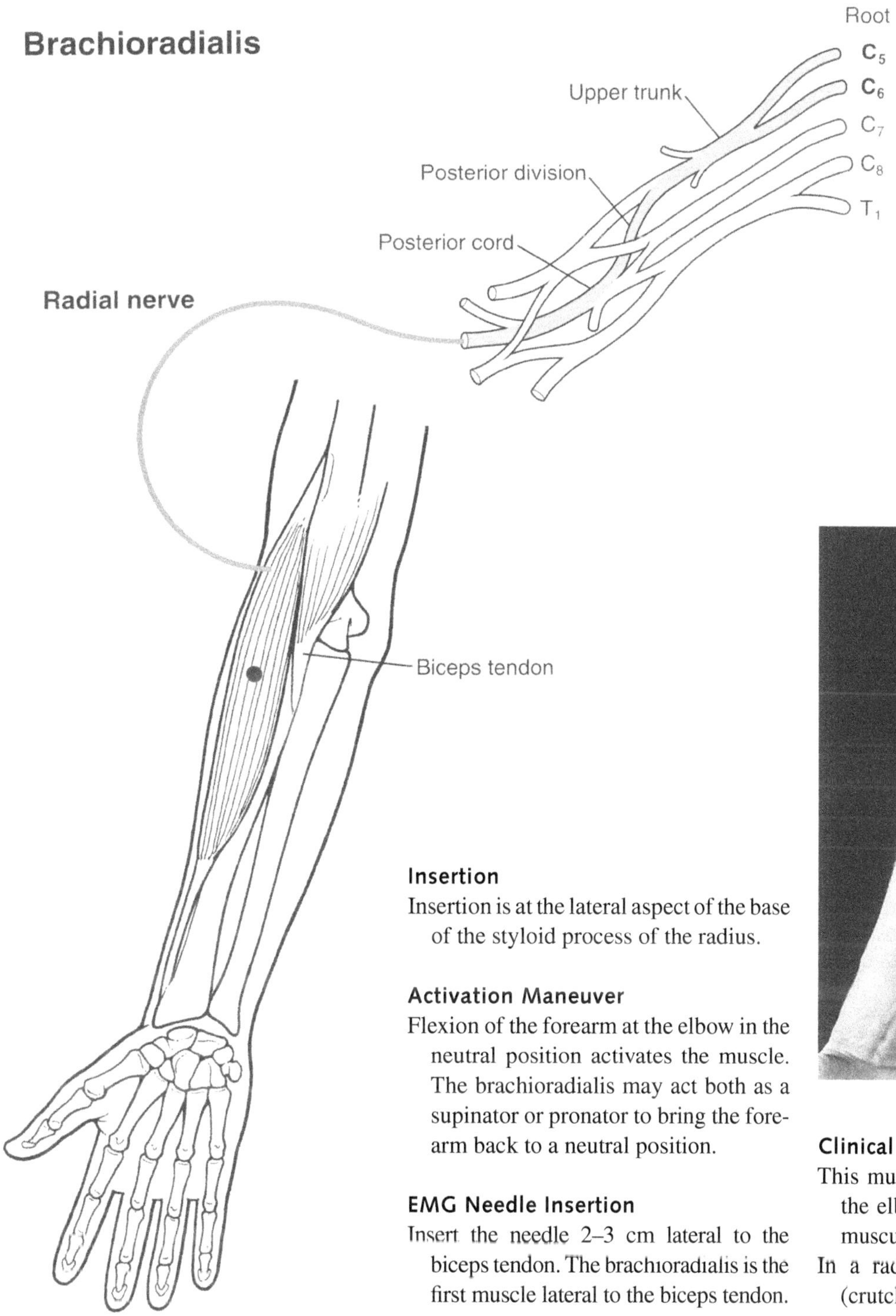

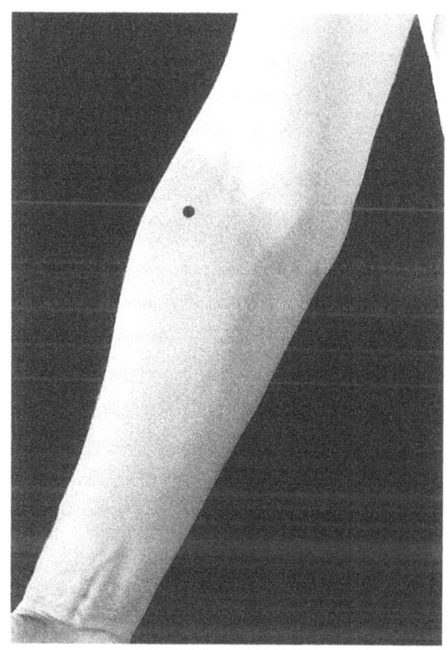

Insertion

Insertion is at the lateral aspect of the base of the styloid process of the radius.

Activation Maneuver

Flexion of the forearm at the elbow in the neutral position activates the muscle. The brachioradialis may act both as a supinator or pronator to bring the forearm back to a neutral position.

EMG Needle Insertion

Insert the needle 2–3 cm lateral to the biceps tendon. The brachioradialis is the first muscle lateral to the biceps tendon.

Innervation

Innervation is via the radial nerve, posterior cord, upper trunk, and roots C_5, C_6.

Origin

The brachioradialis originates at the upper two-thirds of the lateral supracondylar ridge of the humerus.

Pitfalls

If the needle is inserted too laterally (radially), it may be in the extensor carpi radialis, which is also innervated by the radial nerve.

If the needle is inserted too medially (ulnarly) and distally, it may be in the pronator teres, which receives innervation from the median nerve.

Clinical Comments

This muscle is the only major flexor of the elbow joint not innervated by the musculocutaneous nerve.

In a radial nerve lesion at the axilla (crutch neuropathy) or at the spiral groove (Saturday night palsy), needle examination may show neurogenic changes when compression produces axonal loss.

In C_5, C_6 radiculopathy, needle examination may show neurogenic changes when compression produces axonal loss.

In a posterior interosseous nerve lesion, needle examination will be normal.

Anconeus

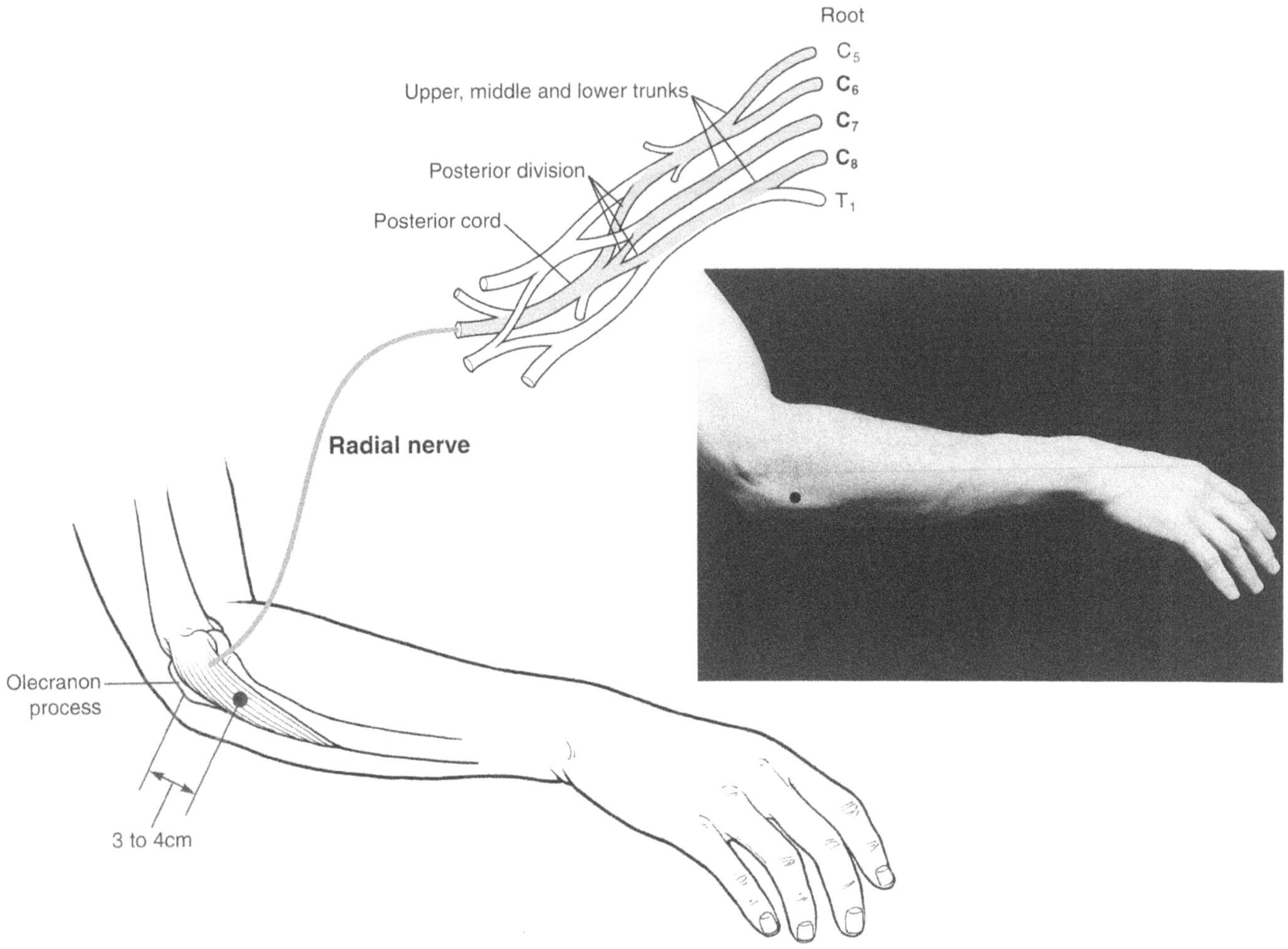

Innervation

Innervation is via the radial nerve, posterior cord, upper, middle, and lower trunks, and roots C_6, C_7, C_8.

Origin

The anconeus originates at the posterior aspect of the lateral epicondyle of the humerus.

Insertion

Insertion is at the lateral aspect of the olecranon process and upper fourth of the posterior surface of the ulna.

Activation Maneuver

Extension of the forearm at the elbow activates the muscle.

EMG Needle Insertion

Insert the needle 3–4 cm distal to the olecranon along the radial border of the ulna.

Pitfalls

If the needle is inserted along the medial (ulnar) border of the ulna, it may be in the flexor digitorum profundus, which is innervated by the ulnar and median nerves.

If the needle is inserted too radially or distally, it may be in the extensor carpi ulnaris, which receives innervation from the posterior interosseous nerve.

If the needle is inserted too deeply, it may be in the supinator, which receives innervation from the posterior interosseous nerve.

Clinical Comments

The anconeus is a continuation of the medial head of the triceps. It is the only forearm muscle innervated by the radial nerve that is spared in lesions at the upper arm (Saturday night palsy).

In a radial nerve lesion at the axilla (crutch neuropathy), needle examination may show neurogenic changes when compression produces axonal loss.

In a posterior interosseous nerve lesion, needle examination will be normal.

Triceps, Lateral Head

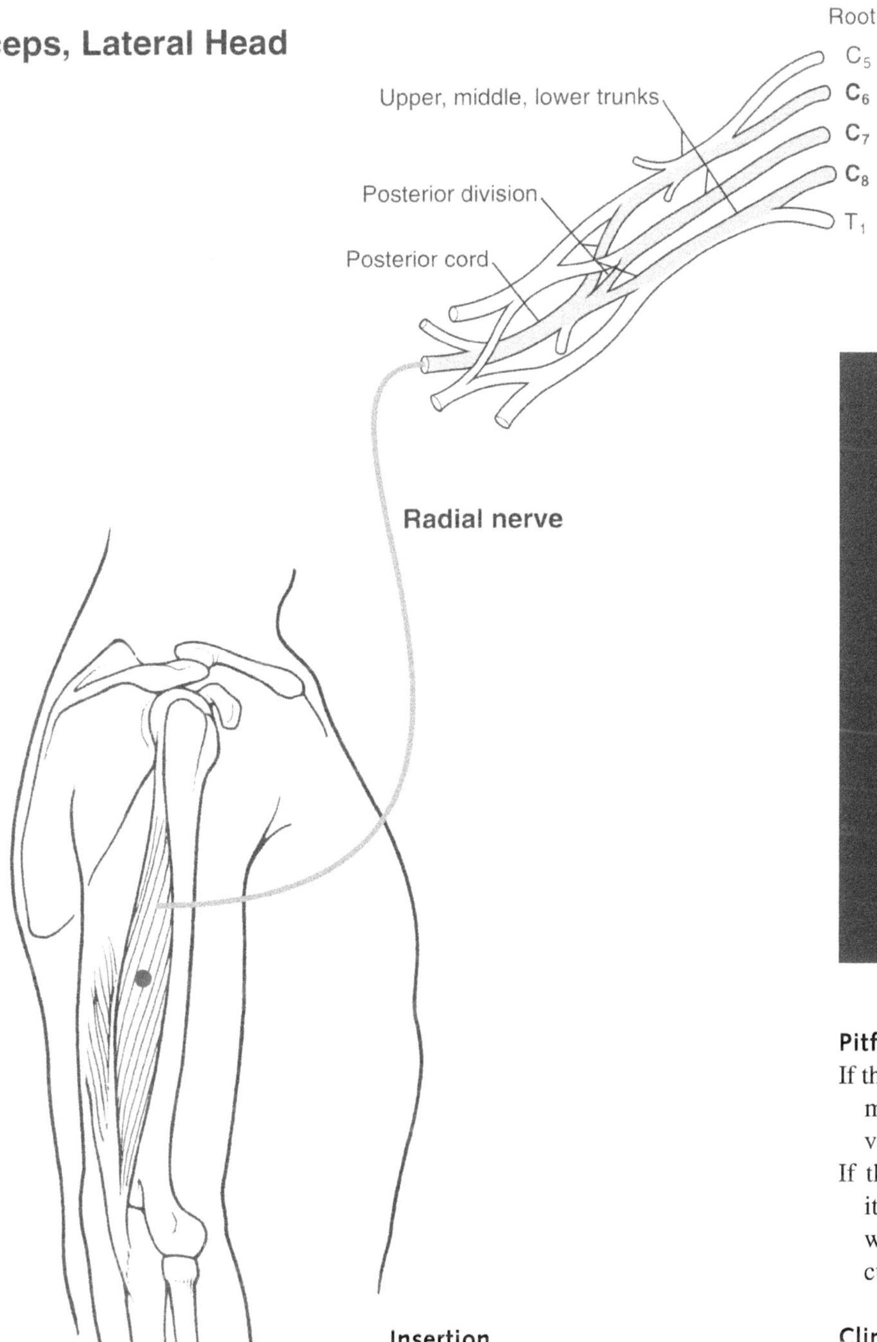

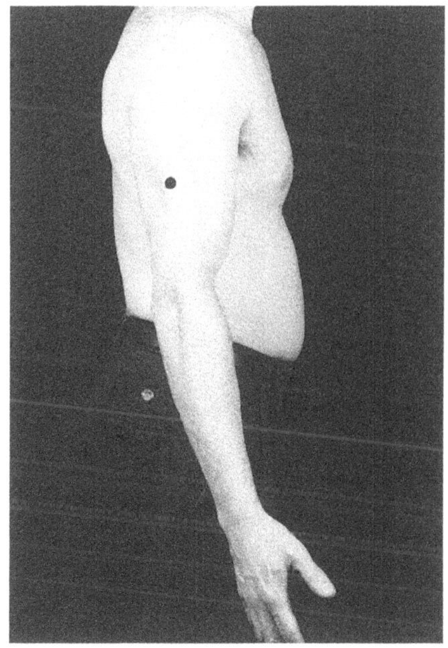

Pitfalls

If the needle is inserted too proximally, it may be in the deltoid, which is innervated by the axillary nerve.

If the needle is inserted too anteriorly, it may be in the lateral or brachialis, which are innervated by the musculocutaneous nerve.

Innervation

Innervation is via the radial nerve, posterior cord, upper, middle, and lower trunks, and roots C_6, C_7, C_8.

Origin

The lateral head of the triceps originates in the posterior aspect of the shaft of the humerus.

Insertion

Insertion is at the posterior aspect of the olecranon process of the ulna.

Activation Maneuver

Extension of the forearm at the elbow joint activates the muscle.

EMG Needle Insertion

Insert the needle at the mid-arm level posterior to the lateral aspect of the shaft of the humerus.

Clinical Comments

In a radial nerve lesion at the spiral groove (Saturday night palsy), needle examination is almost always normal.

In a radial nerve lesion at the axilla (crutch neuropathy) or with C_6-C_8 radiculopathy, needle examination may show neurogenic changes when compression produces axonal loss.

In a posterior interosseous nerve lesion, needle examination will be normal.

Triceps, Long Head

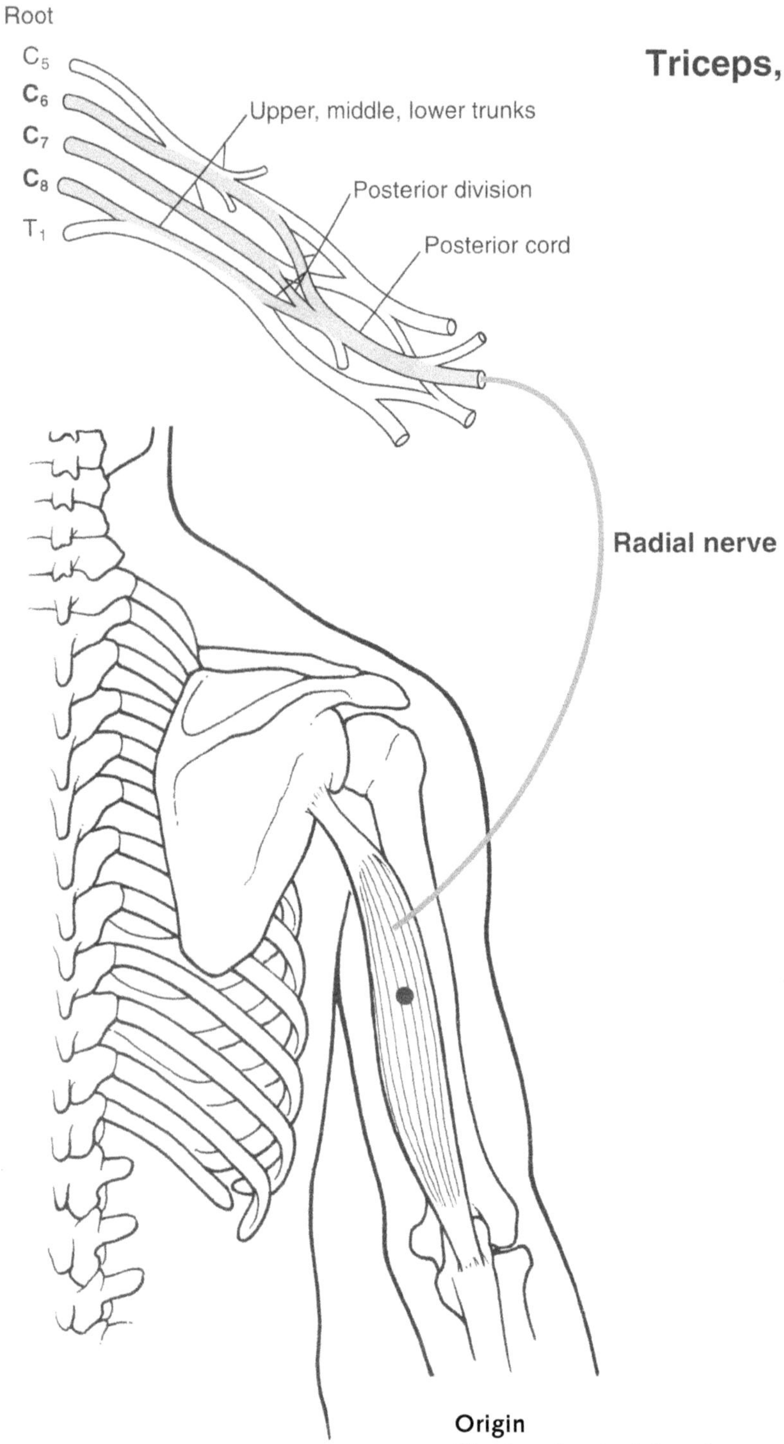

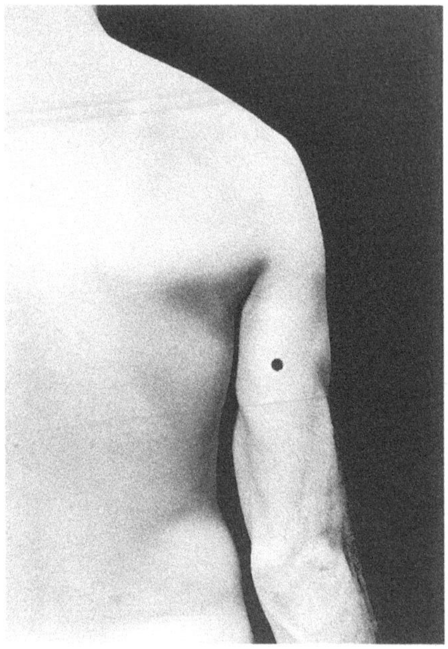

Activation Maneuver

Extension of the forearm at the elbow joint activates the muscle.

EMG Needle Insertion

Insert the needle into the posterior aspect of the arm in the midline, at the junction of the upper and middle thirds of the arm.

Pitfalls

If the needle is inserted too proximally, it may be in the posterior head of the deltoid, which is innervated by the axillary nerve.

Clinical Comments

In a radial nerve lesion at the spiral groove (Saturday night palsy), needle examination is almost always normal.

In a radial nerve lesion at the axilla (crutch neuropathy) or with C_6-C_8 radiculopathy, needle examination may show neurogenic changes when compression produces axonal loss.

In a posterior interosseous nerve lesion, needle examination will be normal.

Origin

The long head of the triceps originates at the scapula, immediately below the glenoid cavity.

Insertion

Insertion is at the posterior aspect of the olecranon process of the ulna.

Innervation

Innervation is via the radial nerve, posterior cord, upper, middle, and lower trunks, and roots C_6, C_7, C_8.

Triceps, Medial Head

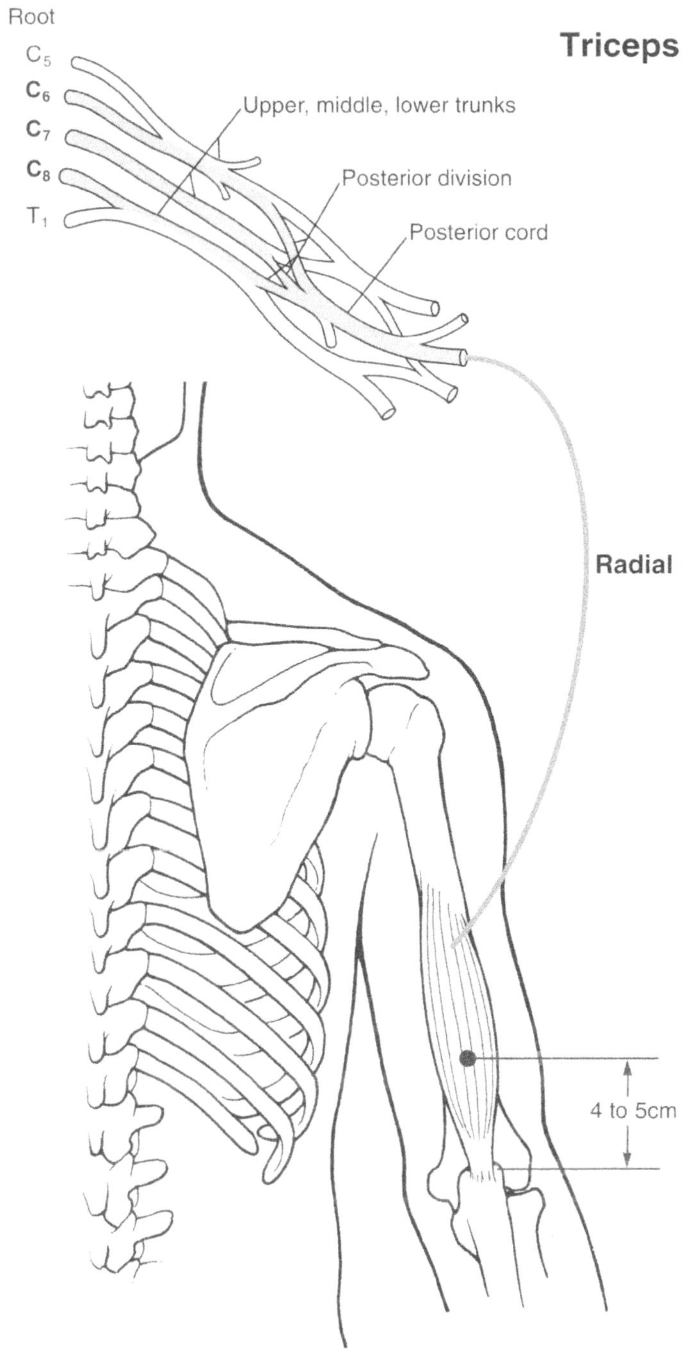

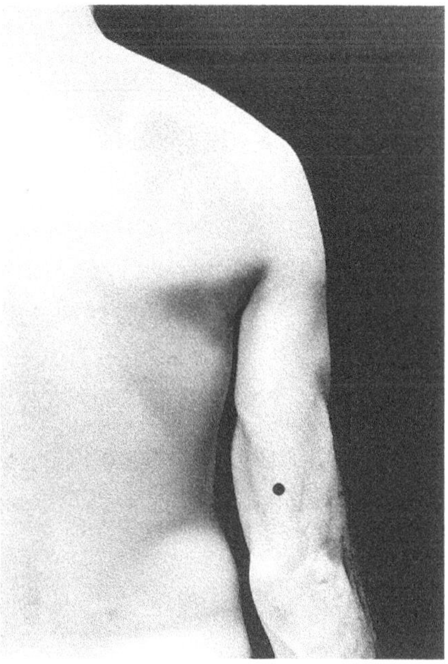

Innervation

Innervation is via the radial nerve, posterior cord, upper, middle, and lower trunks, and roots C_6, C_7, C_8.

Origin

The medial head originates in the posterior surface of the shaft of the humerus, below the spiral groove.

Insertion

Insertion is at the posterior aspect of the olecranon process of the ulna.

Activation Maneuver

Extension of the forearm at the elbow joint activates the muscle.

EMG Needle Insertion

Insert the needle 4–5 cm proximal to the olecranon process just medial to the shaft of the humerus.

Pitfalls

If the needle is inserted too medially, it may be in the medial border of the brachialis or biceps, which are innervated by the musculocutaneous nerve. There is a risk of entering the ulnar or median nerves, or of puncturing the brachial artery.

Clinical Comments

Testing the medial head of the triceps is rarely of benefit in a routine EMG needle evaluation.

In a radial nerve lesion at the spiral groove (Saturday night palsy), needle examination is almost always normal.

In a radial nerve lesion at the axilla (crutch neuropathy) or with C_6-C_8 radiculopathy, needle examination may show neurogenic changes when axonal loss occurs.

In a posterior interosseous nerve lesion, needle examination will be normal.

7

AXILLARY NERVE

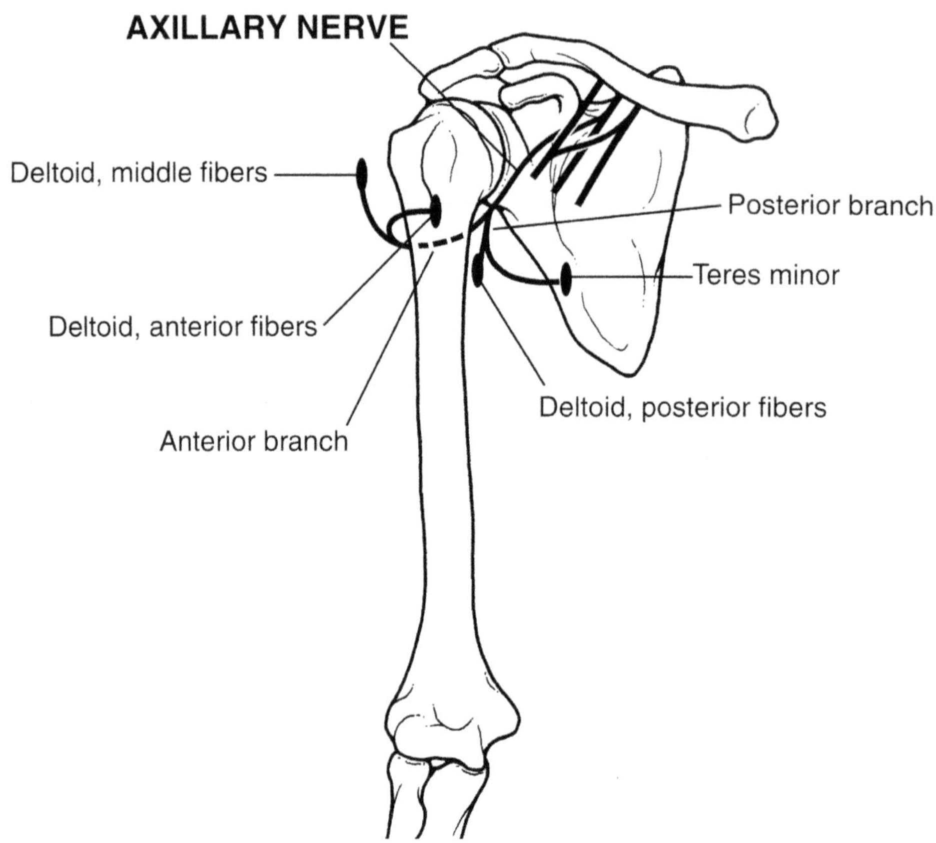

FIGURE 7-1 Diagram of the axillary nerve and the muscles that it supplies.

THE AXILLARY NERVE arises in the axilla as the smaller of the two terminal divisions of the posterior cord. The fibers are derived from the fifth and sixth cervical ventral rami. The nerve descends posterior to the axillary artery and anterior to the subscapularis muscle. At the lower border of the subscapularis, it curves posteriorly through the quadrangular space (quadrilateral space), with the capsule of the shoulder joint above (humeroscapular articular capsule), the surgical neck of the humerus laterally, the long head of the triceps medially, and the teres major below. In this part of its course, it is accompanied by the posterior circumflex artery.

As the nerve emerges from the quadrangular space, it divides into anterior and posterior terminal divisions. The posterior branch deviates medially and supplies the teres minor and the posterior fibers of the deltoid, which take origin from the spine of the scapula. It then gives off a branch, the upper lateral cutaneous nerve of the arm, to reach and ramify over the skin superficial to the deltoid. The anterior branch turns laterally around the surgical neck of the humerus, accompanied by the posterior circumflex artery. It then supplies the middle and anterior fibers of the deltoid, which take origin from the acromion and clavicle, respectively.

AXILLARY NERVE LESION

Etiology

An axillary nerve lesion can occur secondary to inferior dislocation of the humerus at the shoulder joint (the nerve is stretched across the head of the humerus).

An axillary nerve lesion can occur secondary to fractures of the surgical neck of the humerus.

In athletes playing contact sports, a direct blow to anterior or middle deltoid muscle fibers can cause an isolated axillary nerve lesion (Perlmutter et al., 1997).

Deep penetrating wounds and improperly placed injections can injure the axillary nerve.

Upward pressure in the axilla from misused crutches can compress the axillary nerve. Most cases of crutch neuropathy also involve the radial nerve (Sunderland, 1978; Raikin and Froimson, 1997).

The axillary nerve can be entrapped within the quadrangular (quadrilateral) space by fibrous bands, muscle hypertrophy, or repetitive trauma (McClelland and Paxinos, 2008).

Neuralgic amyotrophy (idiopathic brachial plexopathy) can be causative.

General Comments

The most common lesions are those associated with injuries about the shoulder joint.

Clinical Features

Wasting and weakness of the deltoid are present. In the early stages following injury, the arm may hang uselessly by the side. Later, the supplementary actions of other shoulder girdle muscles, including supraspinatus, may result in abduction of the arm even in the absence of deltoid function (Sunderland, 1978).

There is a patch of sensory loss over the outer aspect of the upper arm.

Weakness of the teres minor is not easily demonstrated because other unaffected muscles, such as the infraspinatus, perform the same action.

Most lesions resolve spontaneously. However, if axonal loss injury has occurred, prognosis for recovery of function will be less favorable and will depend on reinnervation and regeneration, which may be slow and incomplete.

Electrodiagnostic Strategy

Demonstrate neurogenic EMG changes limited to the deltoid and teres minor.

EMG of non-axillary innervated C_5, C_6 muscles and cervical paraspinal muscles may be necessary to exclude brachial plexopathy or cervical radiculopathy.

Axillary motor conduction studies may show reduced amplitude on the affected side.

Sensory nerve conduction studies arising from upper trunk of brachial plexus (median sensory response from the thumb, lateral cutaneous nerve of the forearm) and posterior cord (superficial radial sensory response) should be performed to distinguish isolated axillary neuropathy from upper trunk or posterior cord lesion. Abnormal sensory responses suggest brachial plexopathy.

AXILLARY MOTOR NERVE CONDUCTION STUDY

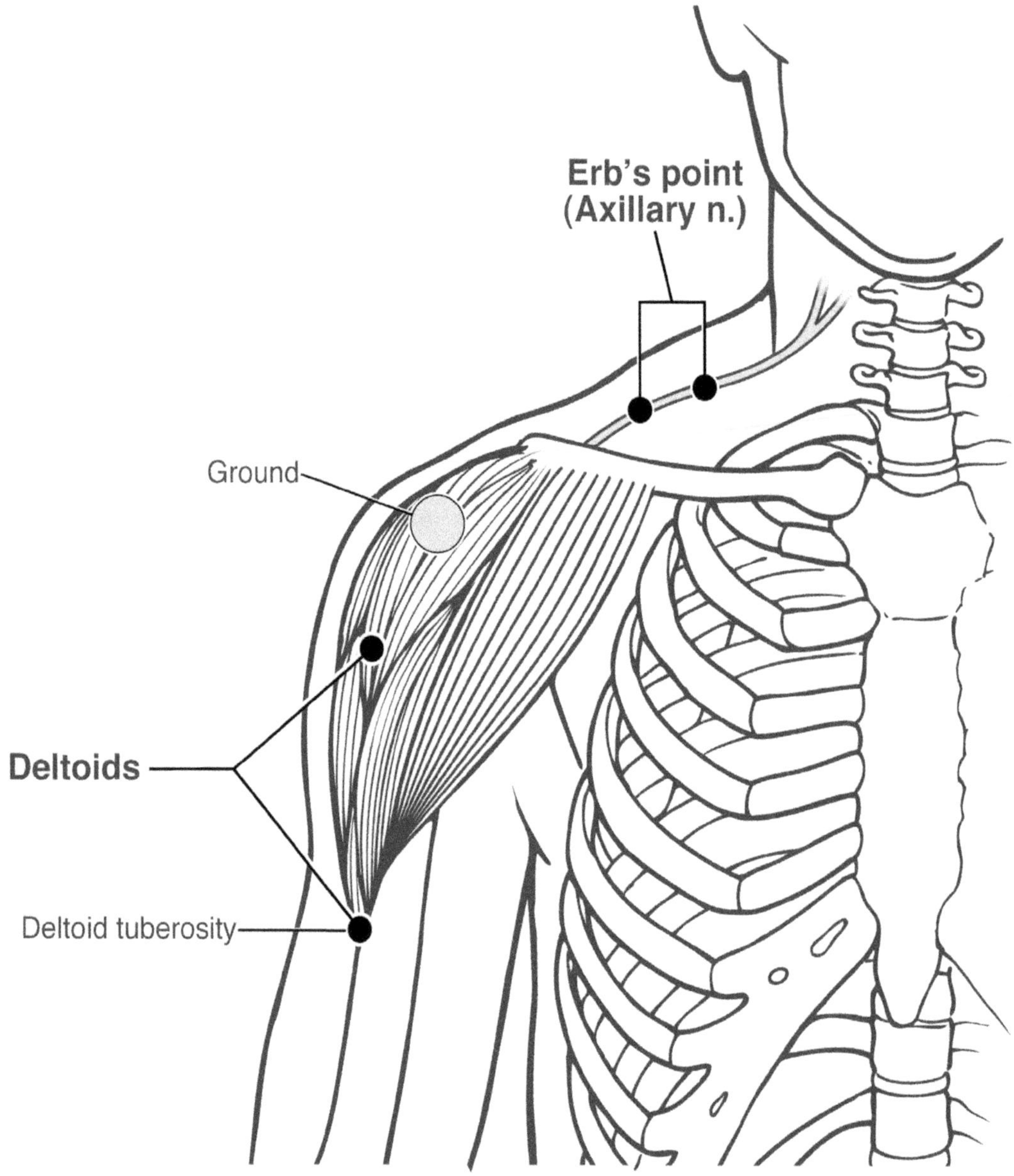

FIGURE 7-2 Axillary motor nerve conduction study.

Recording

Active electrode: Position over the middle fibers of deltoid.

Reference electrode: Place distal to the active electrode over the deltoid tuberosity on the lateral aspect of the humerus mid-shaft.

Ground electrode: Place on the shoulder, between stimulating and recording electrodes.

Stimulation

Erb's point: Place cathode in the supraclavicular region; preferential stimulation of the upper trunk should elicit mechanical abduction and flexion of the arm. Anode is 3 cm proximal to cathode.

Normal Values

Latency (ms) ≤ 5.0
Amplitude (mV) ≥ 3.0

Comments

There is no fixed distance in the axillary motor conduction study. Moreover, surface measurements are often inaccurate at proximal stimulation sites. Accordingly, side-to-side comparisons of latency and amplitude are necessary (Preston and Shapiro, 2005).

A relative latency delay ≥ 1.0 ms or an amplitude ≤ 50 % of the unaffected side is evidence of abnormality.

Pitfalls

Technical problems arise from submaximal stimulation in large or obese individuals. Some patients may not tolerate supramaximal stimulation.

REFERENCES

Gray's Anatomy. 38th edition, Churchill Livingstone, New York, 1995, pp. 1266–1274.

Kimura J. *Electrodiagnosis in Diseases of Nerve and Muscle.* 2nd ed., FA Davis Co., Philadelphia, 1989, p. 499.

McClelland D, Paxinos A. The anatomy of the quadrilateral space with reference to quadrilateral space syndrome. *J Shoulder Elbow Surg* 2008;17:162–164.

Perlmutter GS, Leffert RD, Zarins B. Direct injury to the axillary nerve in athletes playing contact sports. *Am J Sports Med* 1997;25:65–68.

Preston DC, Shapiro BE. *Electromyography and neuromuscular disorders: Clinical-electrophysiologic correlations.* 2nd ed., Philadelphia, Elsevier Butterworth Heinemann, 2005.

Raikin S, Froimson MI. Bilateral brachial plexus compressive neuropathy (crutch palsy). *J Orthop Trauma* 1997;11:136 138.

Sunderland S. *Nerves and Nerve Injuries.* 2nd ed., Churchill Livingstone, New York, 1978, pp. 843–848.

Deltoid, Anterior Fibers

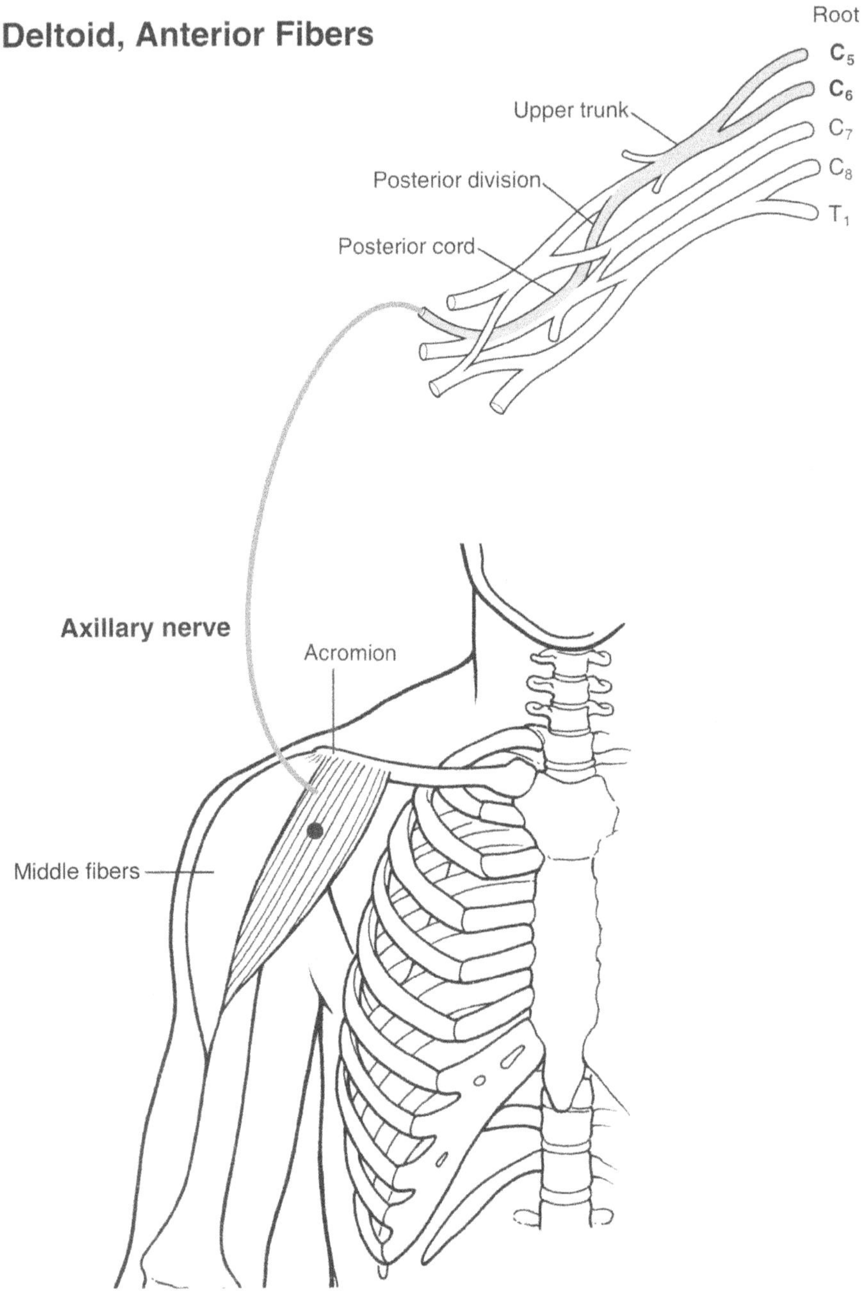

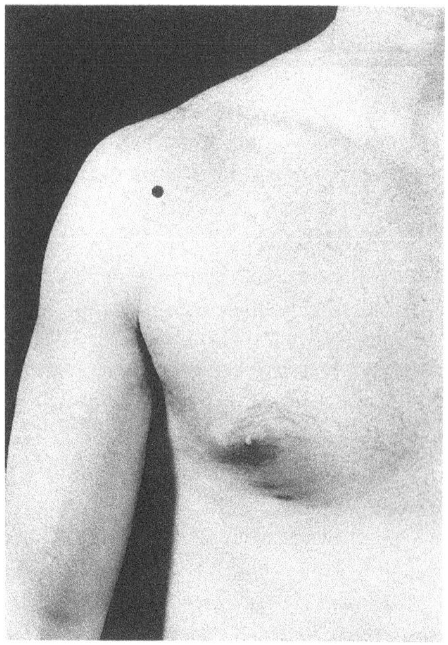

Innervation

Innervation is via the axillary nerve, posterior cord, upper trunk, and roots C_5, C_6.

Origin

The anterior fibers of the deltoid originate at the anterior border and superior surface of the lateral third of the clavicle.

Insertion

Insertion is at the deltoid tuberosity on the lateral aspect of the humerus midshaft.

Activation Maneuver

Forward flexion and medial rotation of the arm activate the anterior fibers of the deltoid (the anterior fibers are assisted by the pectoralis major and coracobrachialis).

EMG Needle Insertion

Insert the needle 3–4 cm directly beneath the anterior margin of the acromion.

Pitfalls

If the needle is inserted too deeply, it may be in the coracobrachialis or tendon of the short head of the biceps. These muscles are supplied by the musculocutaneous nerve.

If the needle is inserted too medially, it may be in the clavicular portion of the pectoralis major, supplied by the medial and lateral pectoral nerves.

Clinical Comments

Needle examination may show neurogenic changes when injury to the axillary nerve produces axonal loss (i.e., blunt trauma, fracture or dislocation of the head of the humerus, brachial plexopathy).

In C_5, C_6 radiculopathy, needle examination may show neurogenic changes when root pathology has resulted in axonal loss (i.e., in moderate to severe radiculopathy).

In Erb's palsy (C_5, C_6 root avulsion), needle examination will show neurogenic changes.

Deltoid, Middle Fibers

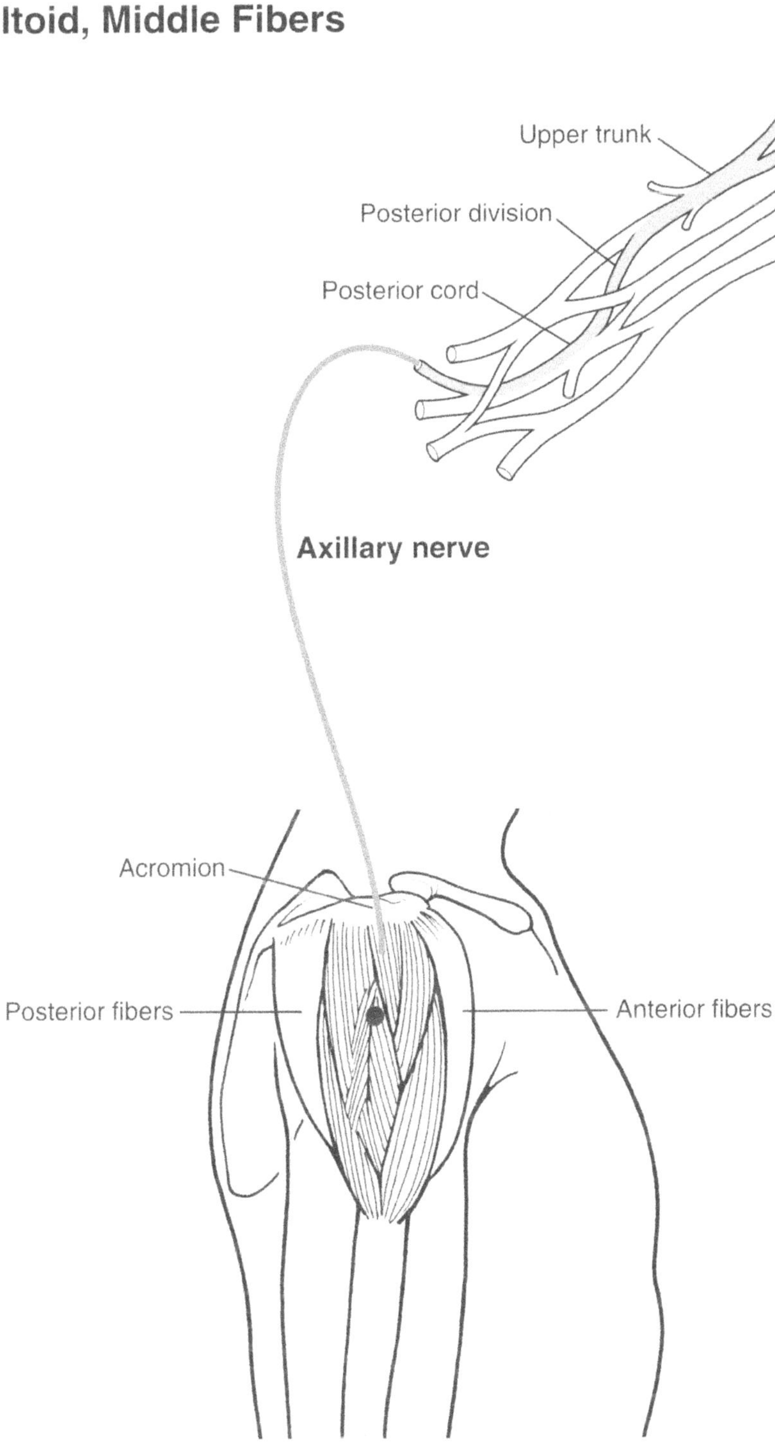

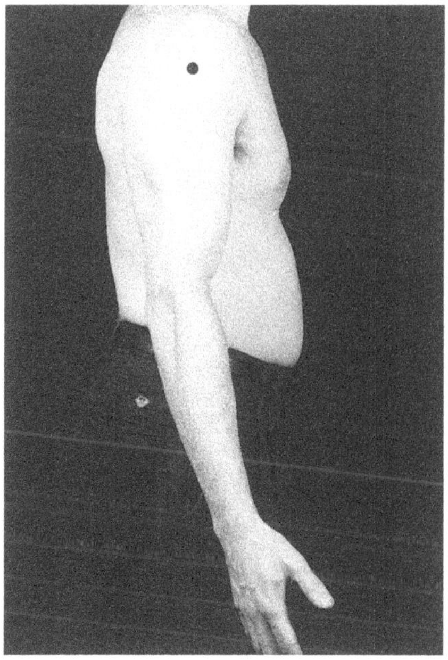

EMG Needle Insertion

Insert the needle 4–5 cm directly beneath the lateral border of the acromion.

Pitfalls

There are no pitfalls.

Clinical Comments

Needle examination may show neurogenic changes when injury to the axillary nerve produces axonal loss (i.e., blunt trauma, fracture or dislocation of the head of the humerus, brachial plexopathy).

A history of multiple intramuscular injections into this muscle may confound needle findings.

In C_5, C_6 radiculopathy, needle examination may show neurogenic changes when root pathology has resulted in axonal loss (i.e., in moderate to severe radiculopathy).

In Erb's palsy (C_5, C_6 root avulsion), needle examination will show neurogenic changes.

Innervation

Innervation is via the axillary nerve, posterior cord, upper trunk, and roots C_5, C_6.

Origin

The middle fibers of the deltoid originate in the lateral margin and superior surface of the acromion.

Insertion

Insertion is at the deltoid tuberosity on the lateral aspect of the humerus midshaft.

Activation Maneuver

Abduction of the arm activates the middle fibers of the deltoid (the middle fibers are assisted by the supraspinatus).

Deltoid, Posterior Fibers

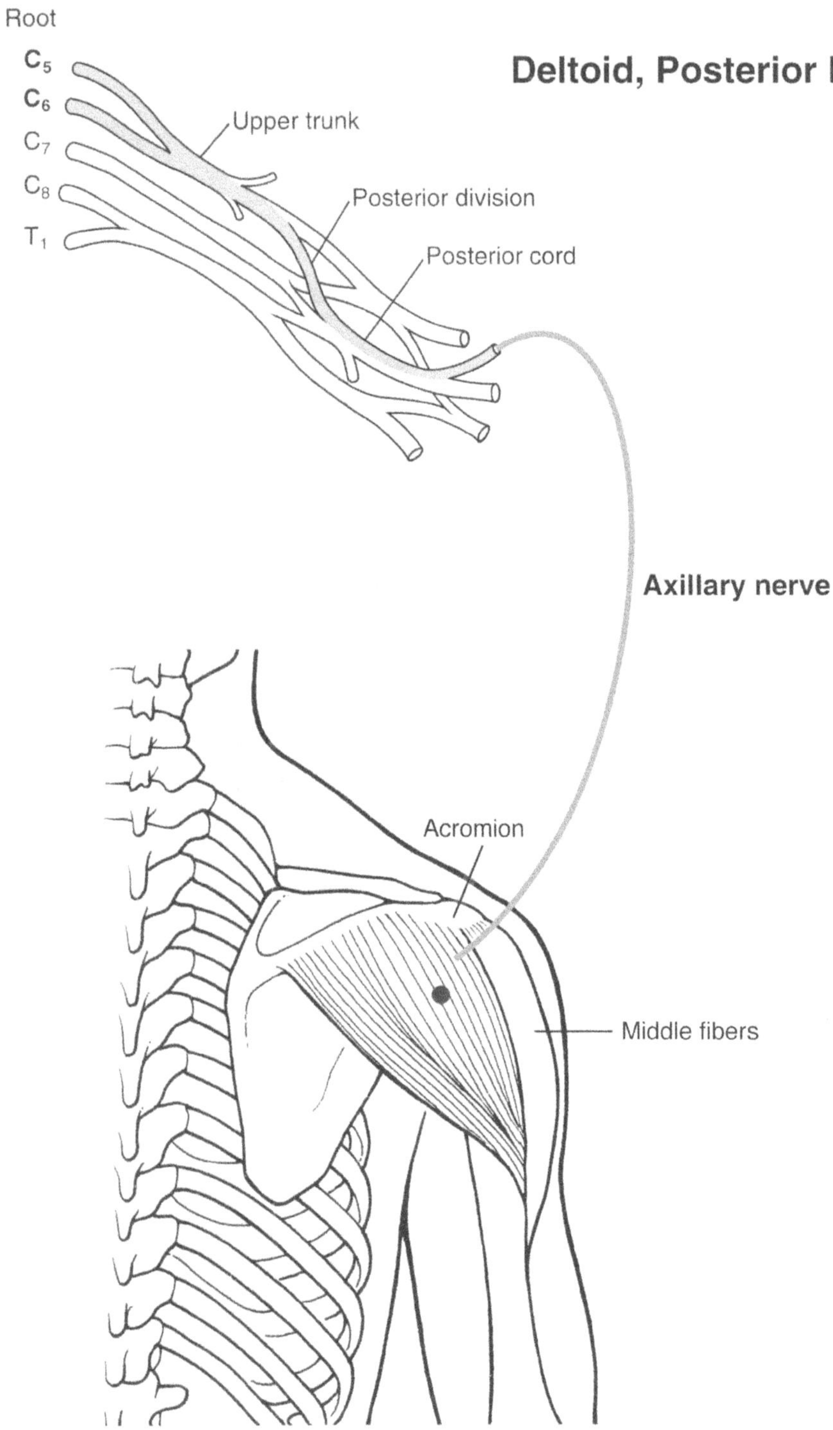

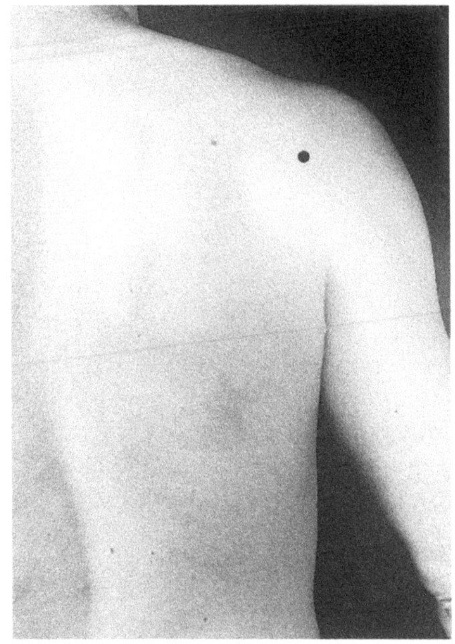

Innervation

Innervation is via the axillary nerve, posterior cord, upper trunk, and roots C_5, C_6.

Origin

The posterior fibers of the deltoid originate at the lower edge of the crest of the spine of the scapula.

Insertion

Insertion is at the deltoid tuberosity of the humerus.

Activation Maneuver

Backward extension and lateral rotation of the arm activate the posterior fibers of the deltoid (the posterior fibers are assisted in backward extension by the latissimus dorsi and teres major).

EMG Needle Insertion

Insert the needle 3–4 cm directly beneath the posterior margin of the acromion.

Pitfalls

If the needle is inserted too deeply, it may be in the teres minor or the long head of the triceps, which are innervated by the axillary and radial nerves, respectively.

If the needle is inserted too medially, it may be in the infraspinatus, which is innervated by the suprascapular nerve.

Clinical Comments

Needle examination may show neurogenic changes when injury to the axillary nerve produces axonal loss, (i.e., blunt trauma, fracture or dislocation of the head of the humerus, brachial plexopathy).

In C_5, C_6 radiculopathy, needle examination may show neurogenic changes when root pathology has resulted in axonal loss (i.e., in moderate to severe radiculopathy).

In Erb's palsy (C_5, C_6 root avulsion), needle examination will show neurogenic changes.

Teres Minor

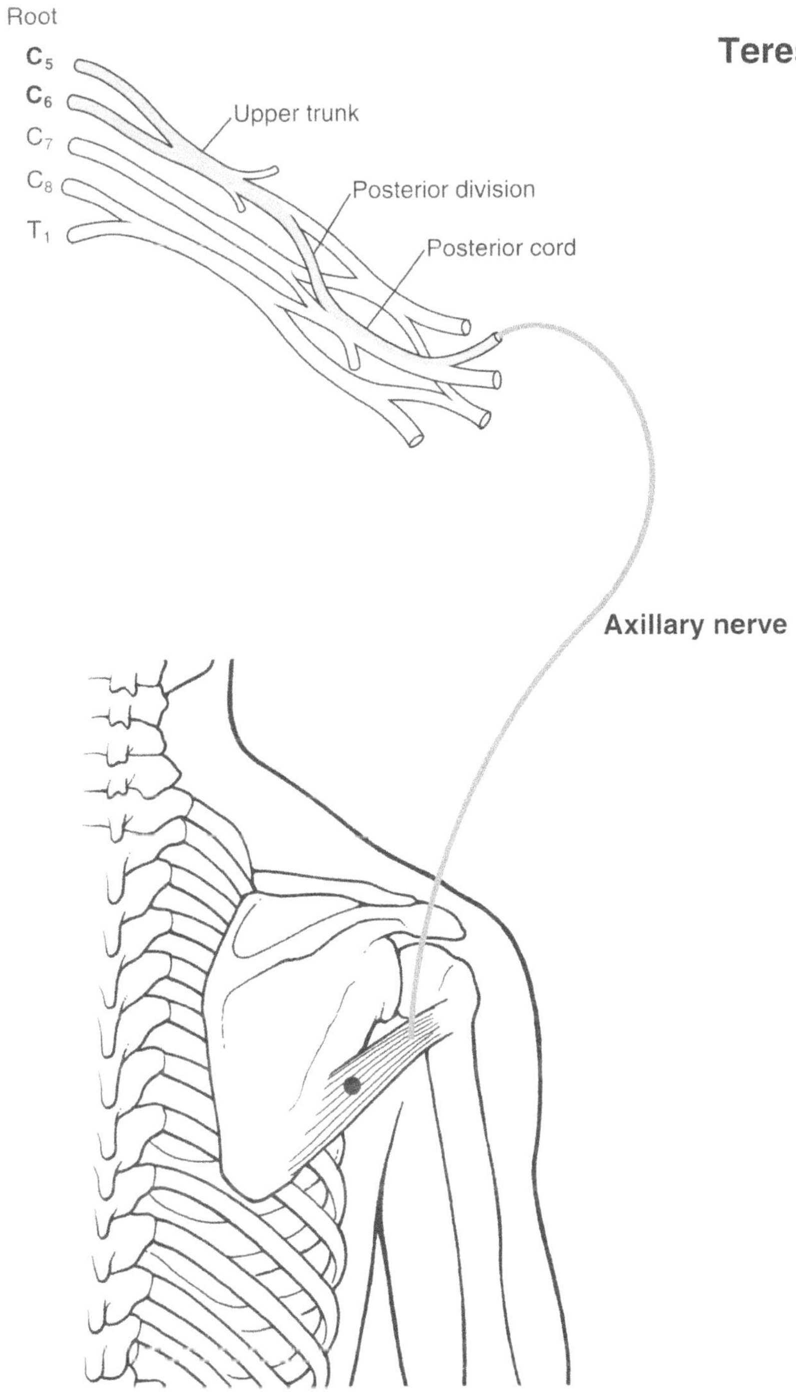

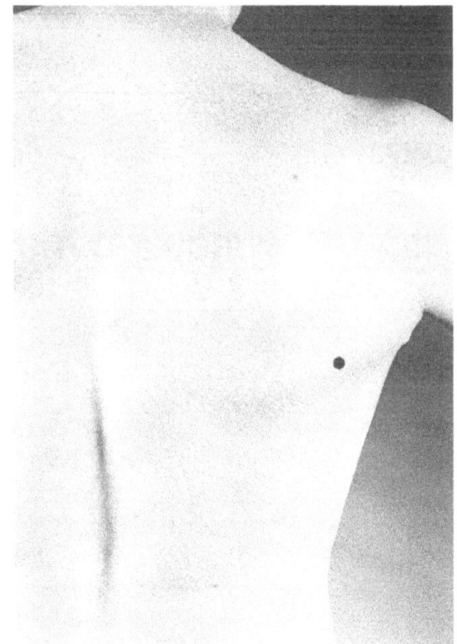

Innervation

Innervation is via the axillary nerve, posterior cord, upper trunk, and roots C_5, C_6.

Origin

The teres minor originates from the middle third of the dorsolateral surface of the scapula.

Insertion

Insertion is at the lowest facet on the greater tubercle of the humerus.

Activation Maneuver

Lateral rotation of the arm (assisted by infraspinatus and posterior fibers of deltoid) activates the muscle.

EMG Needle Insertion

Insert the needle immediately lateral to the middle third of the lateral border of the scapula.

Pitfalls

If the needle is inserted too superficially, it may be in the posterior deltoid, which is also supplied by the axillary nerve.

If the needle is inserted too medially or rostrally, it may be in the infraspinatus, which is innervated by the suprascapular nerve. (Note: The teres minor is sometimes fused with the infraspinatus.)

Clinical Comments

Needle examination may show neurogenic changes when injury to the axillary nerve produces axonal loss (i.e., blunt trauma, fracture or dislocation of the head of the humerus, brachial plexopathy).

In C_5, C_6 radiculopathy, needle examination may show neurogenic changes when root pathology has resulted in axonal loss (i.e., in moderate to severe radiculopathy).

In Erb's palsy (C_5, C_6 root avulsion), needle examination will show neurogenic changes.

8 MUSCULOCUTANEOUS NERVE

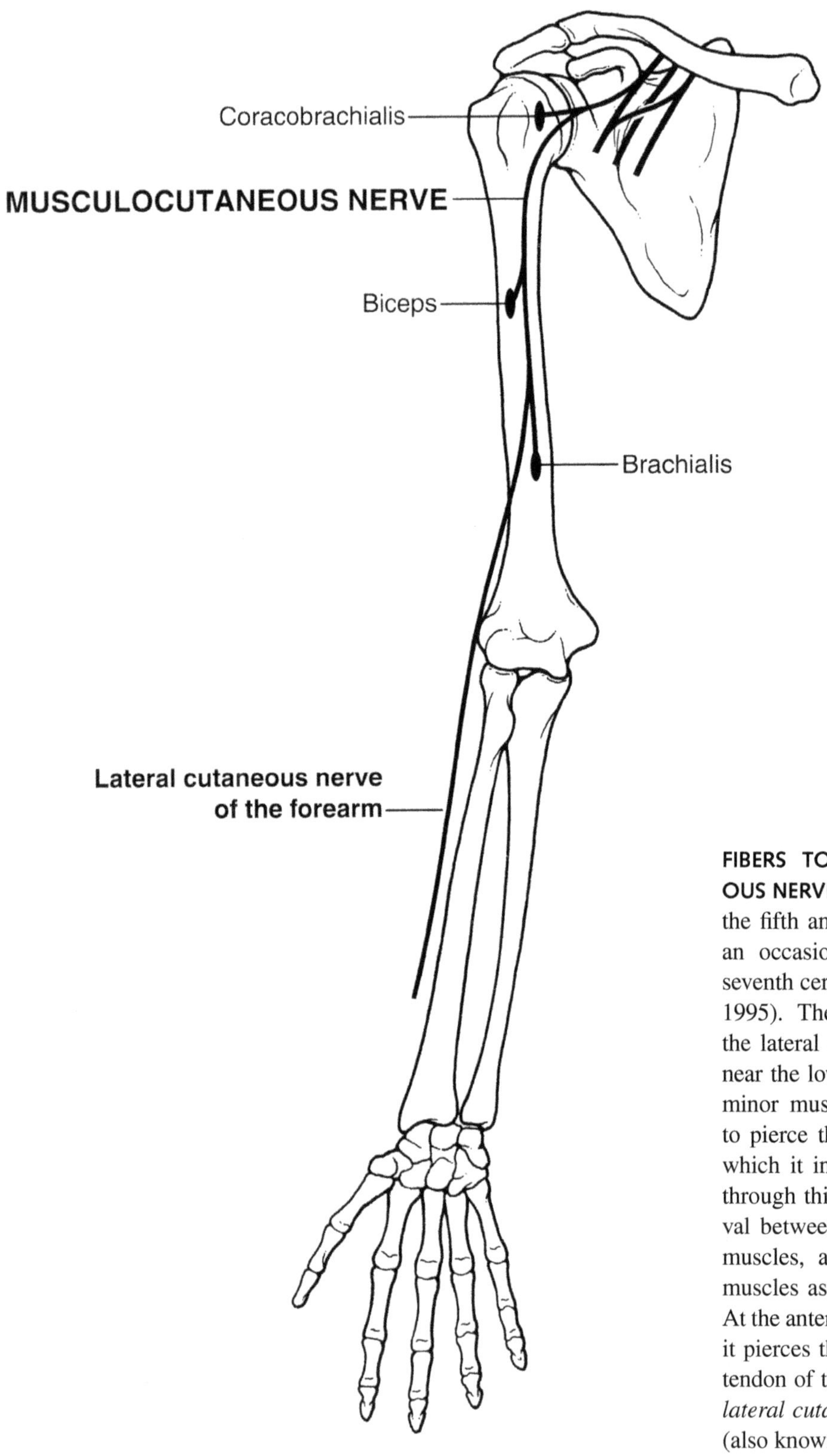

FIGURE 8-1 Diagram of the musculocutaneous nerve and the muscles that it supplies.

FIBERS TO THE MUSCULOCUTANEOUS NERVE are derived primarily from the fifth and sixth cervical roots, with an occasional contribution from the seventh cervical root (*Gray's Anatomy*, 1995). The nerve trunk arises from the lateral cord of the brachial plexus near the lower border of the pectoralis minor muscle. It proceeds downward to pierce the coracobrachialis muscle, which it innervates. The nerve passes through this muscle to reach the interval between the brachialis and biceps muscles, and supplies both of these muscles as it descends between them. At the anterolateral aspect of the elbow, it pierces the deep fascia lateral to the tendon of the biceps, continuing as the *lateral cutaneous nerve of the forearm* (also known as the *lateral antebrachial* *cutaneous nerve*). This pure sensory nerve divides into anterior and posterior branches, which provide cutaneous innervation to the lateral aspect of the forearm, as far as the midline anteriorly and posteriorly, and as distal as the base of the thenar eminence and dorsolateral aspect of the wrist (Sunderland, 1968).

MUSCULOCUTANEOUS NERVE LESION

Etiology

Trauma and deep penetrating wounds can cause a musculocutaneous lesion.

Neuralgic amyotrophy (idiopathic brachial plexopathy) can be causative.

Rarely, vigorous upper extremity exercise can cause entrapment of the musculocutaneous nerve as it passes through the coracobrachialis muscle (Braddom and Wolfe, 1978; Mastaglia, 1986).

Isolated injury to the lateral cutaneous nerve of the forearm can occur. This sensory nerve may be entrapped between the biceps aponeurosis and tendon and brachialis muscle (Bassett and Nunley, 1982). Other causes of isolated injury to the lateral cutaneous nerve of the forearm include hyperextension sports injuries to the elbow and antecubital phlebotomy (Sander et. al., 1998; Stitik et. al., 2001).

General Comments

Trauma almost always results in combined lesions of the musculocutaneous nerve and the lateral cord of the brachial plexus (Sunderland, 1968).

Clinical Features

Wasting and weakness of the coracobrachialis, biceps, and brachialis can occur. In complete lesions of the musculocutaneous nerve, the supinator and brachioradialis muscles hypertrophy and may compensate for the loss of the biceps and brachialis muscles.

Loss of the biceps tendon reflex occurs.

There is sensory loss over the lateral aspect of the forearm.

Electrodiagnostic Strategy

Demonstrate neurogenic EMG changes in the coracobrachialis, biceps, and brachialis.

EMG of other C_5 and C_6 muscles and cervical paraspinal muscles may be necessary to exclude brachial plexopathy or cervical radiculopathy.

Musculocutaneous motor conduction studies may show reduced amplitude or absence on the affected side.

Sensory conduction studies of the lateral cutaneous nerve of the forearm may show reduced amplitude or absence on the affected side.

Sensory nerve conduction studies arising from upper trunk of brachial plexus (median sensory response from the thumb and superficial radial sensory response) should be performed to distinguish isolated musculocutaneous neuropathy from upper trunk lesion. Abnormal sensory responses suggest brachial plexopathy.

Musculocutaneous Motor Nerve Conduction Study

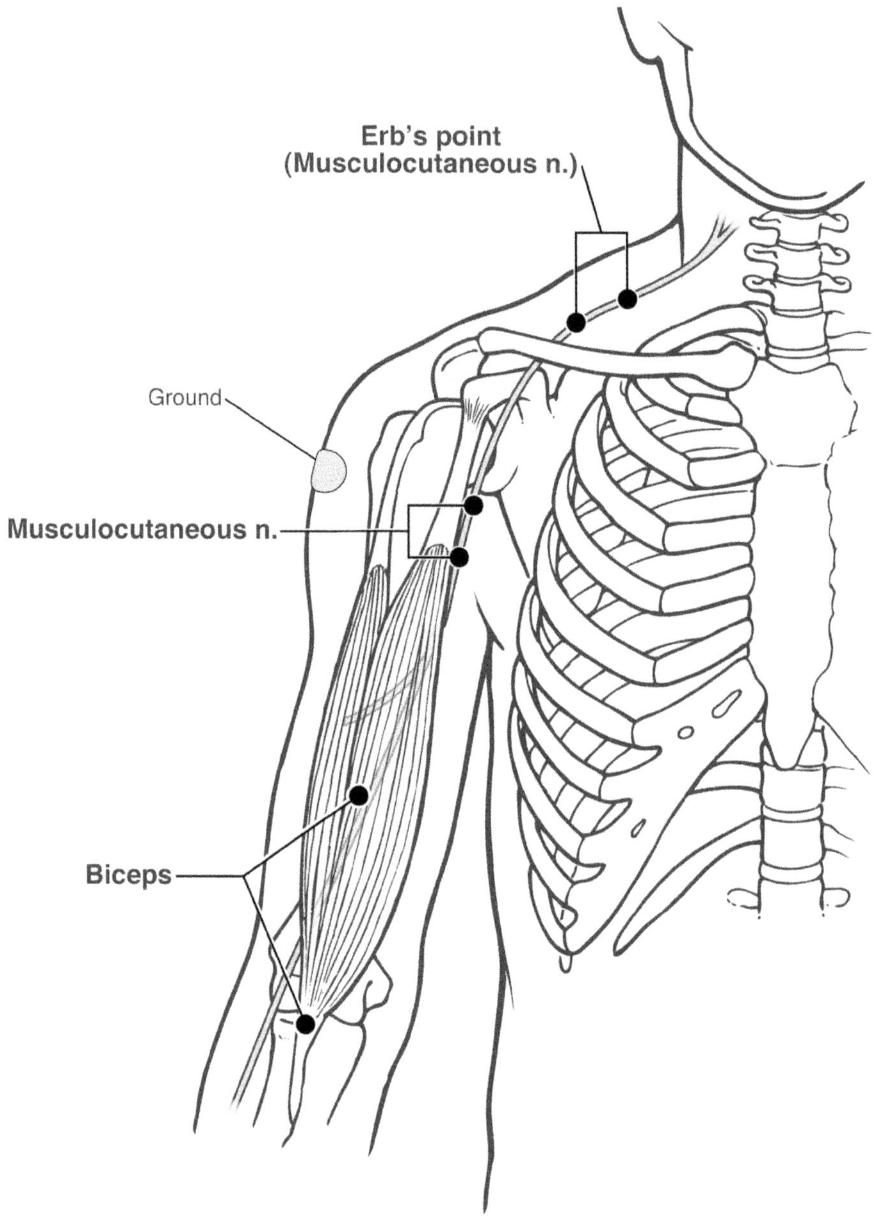

FIGURE 8-2 Musculocutaneous motor nerve conduction study.

Recording

Active electrode: Position over the belly of the biceps.
Reference electrode: Place distal to the active electrode over the biceps tendon.
Ground electrode: Place on the lateral arm.

Stimulation

Axilla: Place cathode just medial to the coracobrachialis muscle and short head of the biceps; stimulation should elicit mechanical flexion of the forearm at the elbow. Anode is 3 cm proximal to cathode.

Erb's point: Place cathode in the supraclavicular region; preferential stimulation of the upper trunk should elicit mechanical abduction and flexion of the arm. Anode is 3 cm proximal to cathode.

Normal Values

Latency (ms) ≤ 5.7 (Erb's point)
Amplitude (mV) ≥ 4.0
Conduction velocity (m/s) ≥ 50 m/s

Comment

There is no fixed distance in the musculocutaneous motor conduction study. Moreover, surface measurements may be inaccurate at proximal stimulation sites. Accordingly, side-to-side comparisons of latency, amplitude, and conduction velocity are necessary (Preston and Shapiro, 2005). A relative latency delay ≥ 1.0 ms or an amplitude ≤ 50 % of the unaffected side is evidence of abnormality.

Pitfalls

Technical problems arise from submaximal stimulation in large or obese individuals.

Lateral Cutaneous Nerve of the Forearm (Lateral Antebrachial Cutaneous) Conduction Study

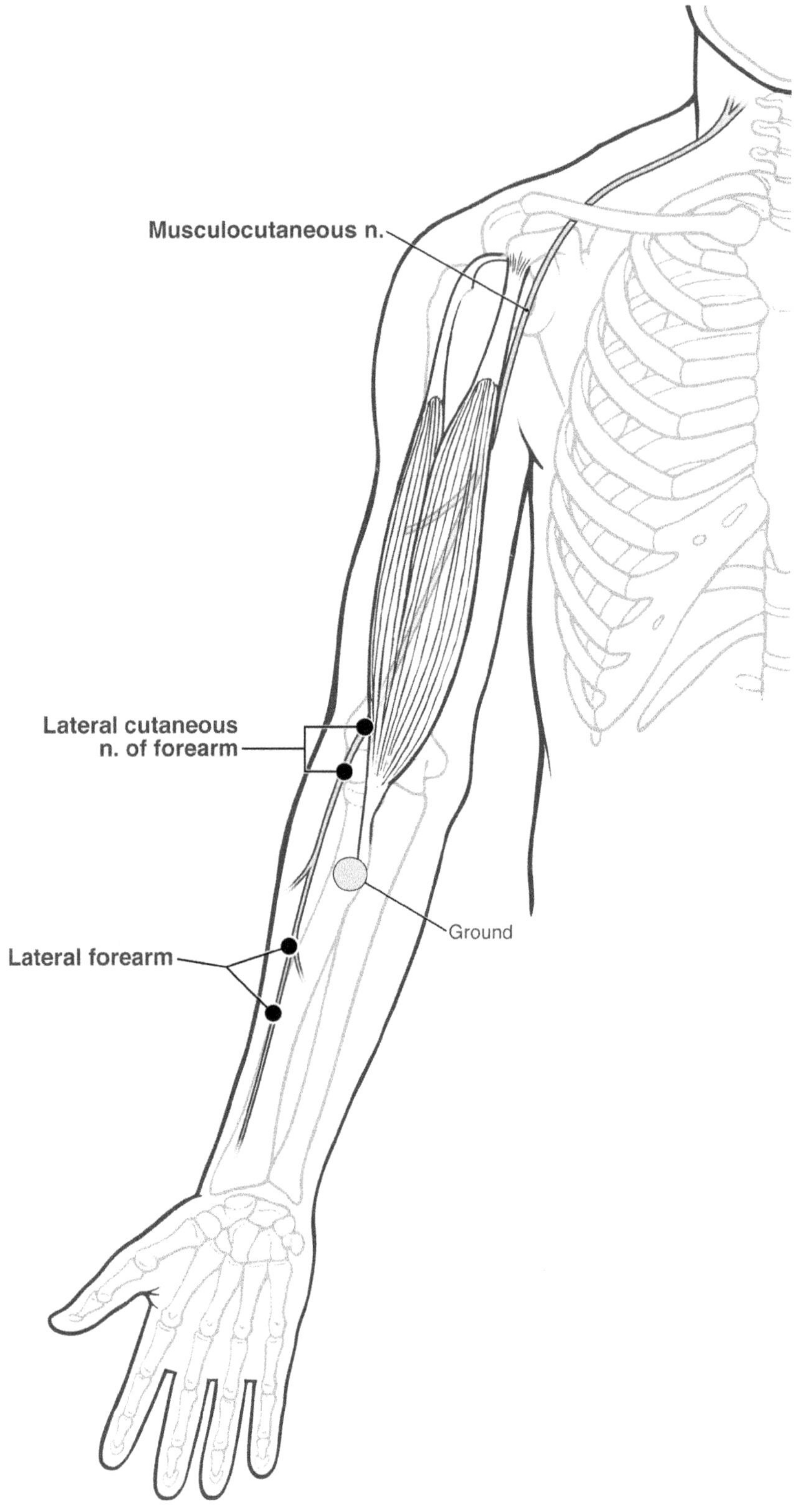

FIGURE 8-3 Lateral cutaneous nerve of the forearm (lateral antebrachial cutaneous) conduction study (antidromic).

Recording

Active electrode: Position over the lateral forearm, 10 cm to 12 cm distal to the cathode, on a line between stimulation site and radial artery pulse at the wrist.

Reference electrode: Place 3 cm distal to the active electrode.

Ground electrode: Place on the anterior forearm between the stimulating and recording electrodes.

Stimulation

Antecubital fossa: Place cathode just lateral to the biceps tendon. The anode is 3 cm proximal to cathode.

Normal Values

Latency (ms) ≤ 2.0 (onset latency at distance 10 cm); ≤ 2.5 (peak latency)

Amplitude (μV) ≥ 15

Conduction velocity (m/s) ≥ 55 m/s

Studies should ideally be performed bilaterally, because side-to-side comparisons are more useful than normal value tables that may not apply to your patient. A relative amplitude ≤ 50 % of the unaffected side is evidence of abnormality.

Comment

In root lesions, the lateral cutaneous nerve of the forearm sensory response will be normal.

In lesions of the lateral cord or upper trunk, the lateral cutaneous nerve of the forearm sensory response will be reduced or absent.

REFERENCES

Bassett FH, Nunley JA. Compression of the musculocutaneous nerve at the elbow. *J Bone Joint Surg* 1982;64:1050–1052.

Braddom RL, Wolfe C. Musculocutaneous nerve injury after heavy exercise. *Arch Phys Med Rehab* 1978;59:290–293.

Gray's Anatomy. 38th edition, Churchill Livingstone, New York, 1995, pp. 1266–1274.

Mastaglia FL. Musculocutaneous neuropathy after strenuous physical activity. *Med J Aust* 1986;145:153–154.

Preston DC, Shapiro BE. *Electromyography and neuromuscular disorders. Clinical-electrophysiologic correlations*. 2nd ed. Philadelphia, Elsevier Butterworth Heinemann, 2005.

Sander HW, Conigliari M, Masdeu JC. Antecubital phlebotomy complicated by lateral antebrachial cutaneous neuropathy. *N Engl J Med*. 1998;339:2024.

Stitik TP, Foye PM, Nadler SF, Brachman GO. Phlebotomy-related lateral antebrachial cutaneous nerve injury. *Am J Phys Med Rehabil* 2001;80:230–234.

Sunderland S. *Nerves and Nerve Injuries*. Williams & Wilkins, Baltimore, 1968, pp. 886–893.

Brachialis

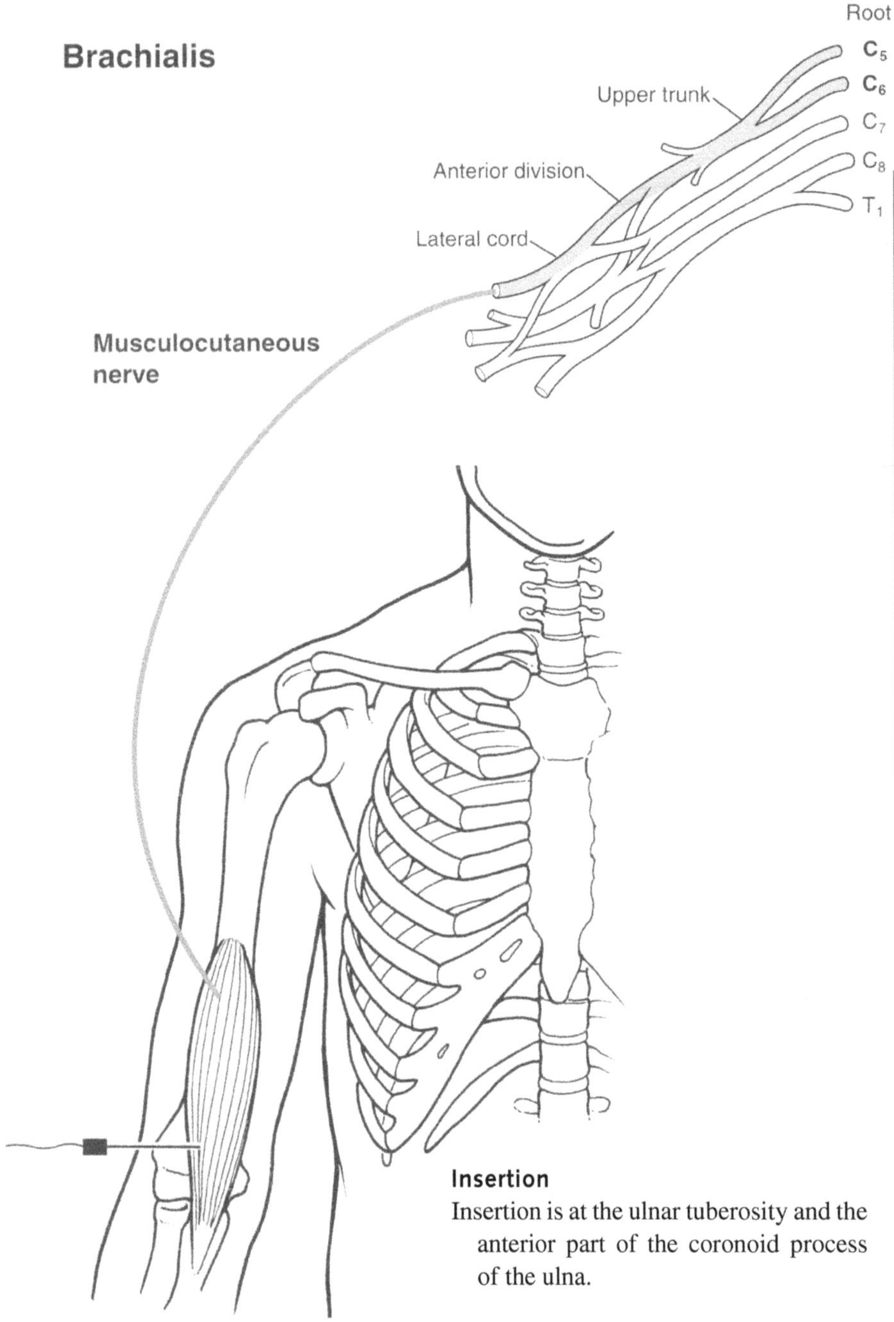

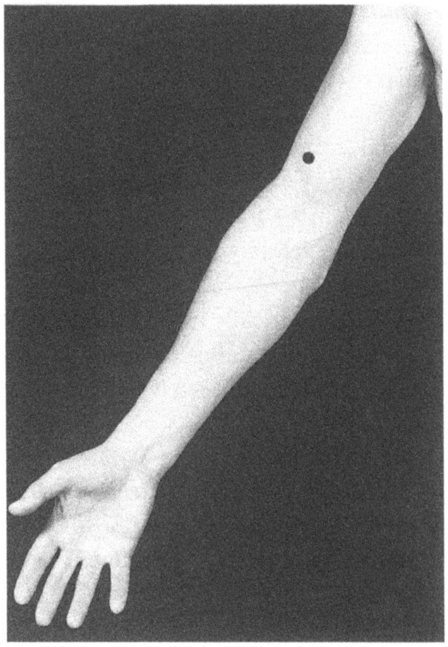

Innervation
Innervation is via the musculocutaneous nerve, lateral cord, upper trunk, and roots C_5, C_6. Note: A small lateral portion of the muscle may receive radial nerve innervation (C_7 root).

Origin
The brachialis originates in the lower half of the anterior surface of the humerus.

Insertion
Insertion is at the ulnar tuberosity and the anterior part of the coronoid process of the ulna.

Activation Maneuver
Flexion of the forearm at the elbow activates the muscle.

EMG Needle Insertion
Lateral approach: Insert the needle 4–5 cm proximal to the elbow crease just lateral to and under the biceps.

Medial approach: This approach is not recommended because it risks injury to the median nerve, brachial artery, and basilic vein.

Pitfalls
If the needle is inserted too distally and posteriorly, it may be in the proximal brachioradialis or extensor carpi radialis longus; these muscles are supplied by the radial nerve.

If the needle is inserted too proximal and posteriorly, it may be in the lateral head of the triceps, which is supplied by the radial nerve.

Clinical Comments
Needle examination may show neurogenic changes when injury to the musculocutaneous nerve produces axonal loss.

In brachial plexopathy, needle examination may show neurogenic changes when lateral cord pathology has resulted in axonal loss.

In C_5, C_6 radiculopathy, needle examination may show neurogenic changes when root pathology has resulted in axonal loss (i.e., in moderate to severe radiculopathy).

In Erb's palsy (C_5, C_6 root avulsion), needle examination will show neurogenic changes.

Biceps Brachii

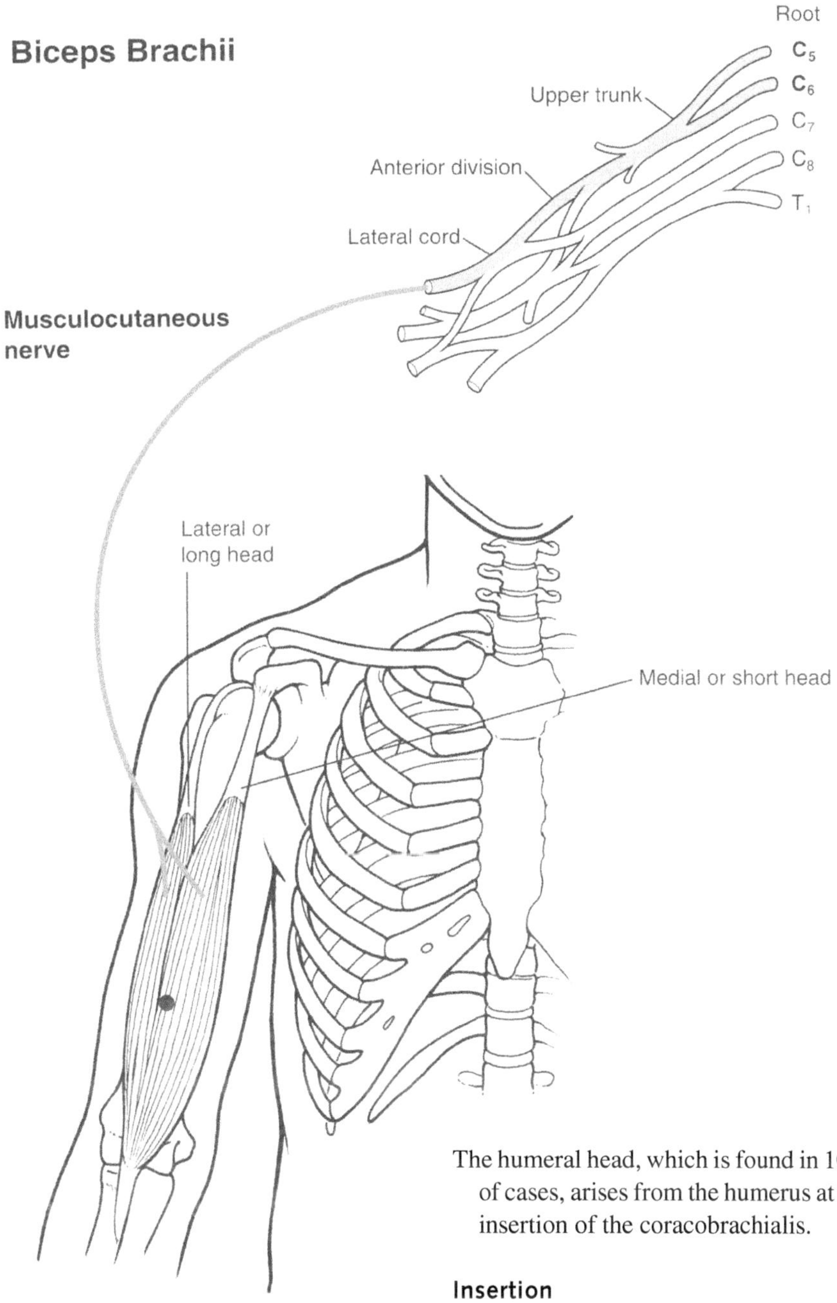

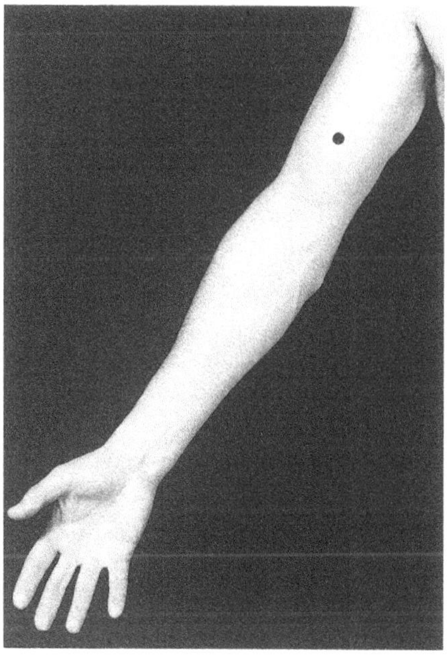

Innervation
Innervation is via the musculocutaneous nerve, lateral cord, upper trunk, and roots C_5, C_6.

Origin
The medial or short head of the biceps brachii originates at the coracoid process of the scapula.

The lateral or long head originates at the supraglenoid tubercle of the scapula.

The humeral head, which is found in 10% of cases, arises from the humerus at the insertion of the coracobrachialis.

Insertion
Insertion is at the posterior aspect of the radial tuberosity (the tuberosity lies distal to the medial part of the neck of the radius).

Activation Maneuver
Flexion and supination of the forearm at the elbow activates the biceps brachii. To a slight extent, the biceps also acts to flex the arm at the shoulder.

EMG Needle Insertion
Insert the needle into the mid-arm anteriorly, into bulk of the muscle.

Pitfalls
If the needle is inserted too proximally, it may be in the anterior deltoid (supplied by the axillary nerve) or the pectoralis major (supplied by the medial and lateral pectoral nerves).

If the needle is inserted too deeply, it may be in the brachialis, which is also supplied by the musculocutaneous nerve.

Clinical Comments
Needle examination may show neurogenic changes when injury to the musculocutaneous nerve produces axonal loss.

In brachial plexopathy, needle examination may show neurogenic changes when lateral cord pathology has resulted in axonal loss.

In C_5, C_6 radiculopathy, needle examination may show neurogenic changes when root pathology has resulted in axonal loss (i.e., in moderate to severe radiculopathy).

In Erb's palsy (C_5, C_6 root avulsion), needle examination will show neurogenic changes.

Coracobrachialis

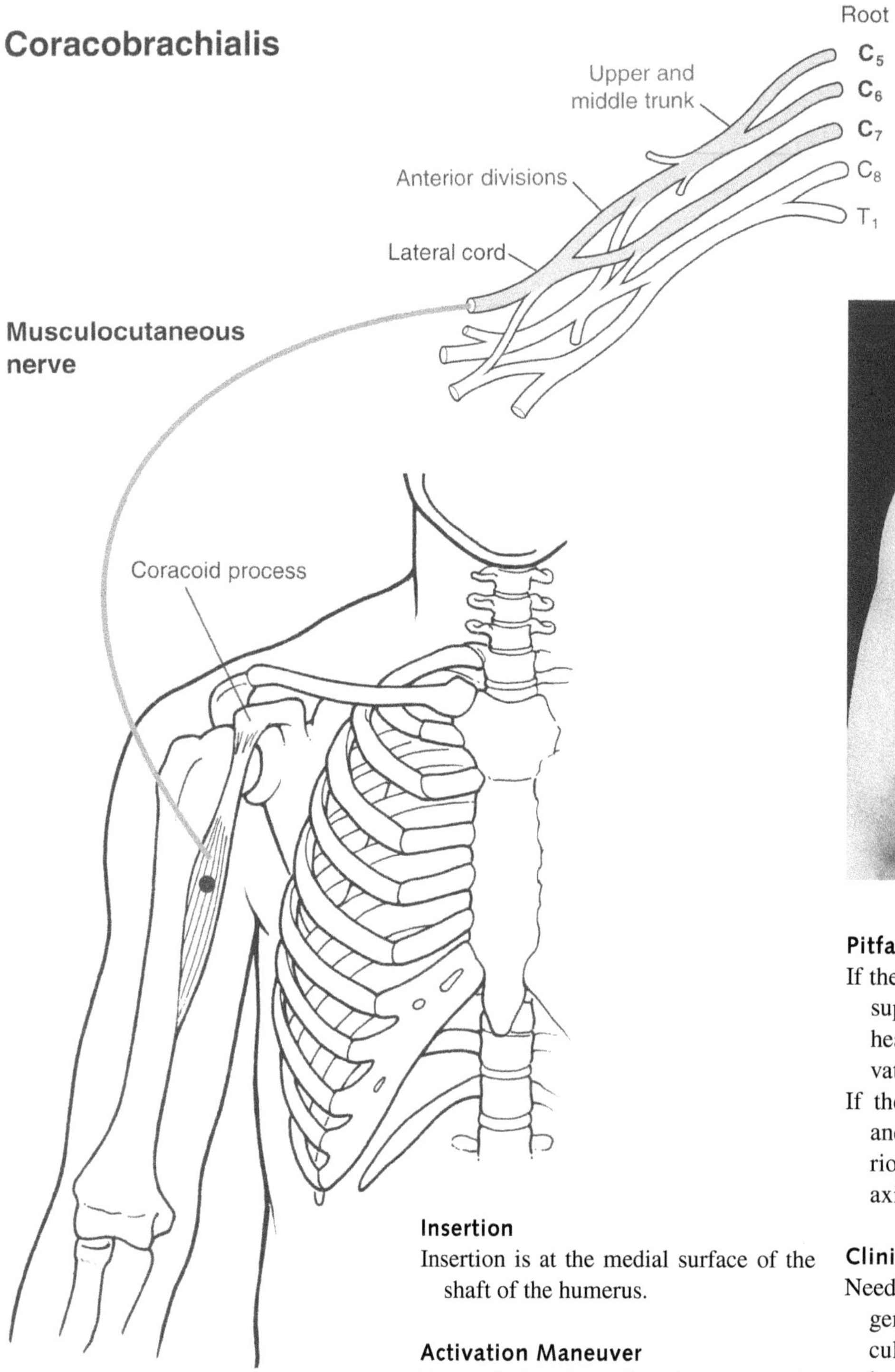

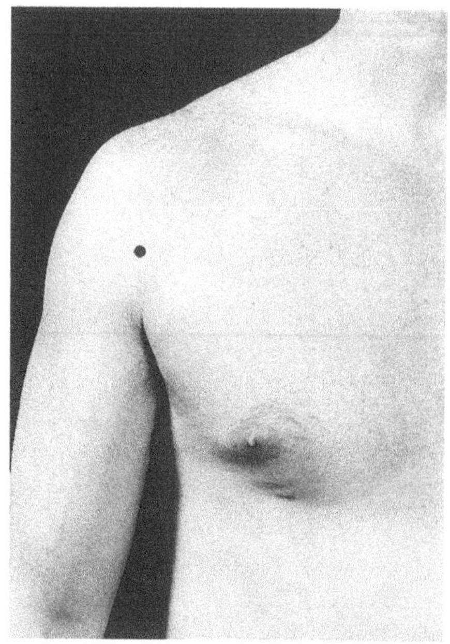

Innervation

Innervation is via the musculocutaneous nerve, lateral cord, upper and middle trunks, and roots C_5, C_6, C_7.

Origin

The coracobrachialis originates at the apex of the coracoid process of the scapula.

Insertion

Insertion is at the medial surface of the shaft of the humerus.

Activation Maneuver

Forward elevation of the humerus activates the muscle. The coracobrachialis stabilizes the head of the humerus in relation to the glenoid fossa of the scapula.

EMG Needle Insertion

Insert the needle 6–8 cm distal to the coracoid process along the volar aspect of the arm.

Pitfalls

If the needle is inserted too laterally and superficially, it may be in the short head of the biceps, which is also innervated by the musculocutaneous nerve.

If the needle is inserted too proximal and superficial, it may be in the anterior deltoid, which is supplied by the axillary nerve.

Clinical Comments

Needle examination may show neurogenic changes when injury to the musculocutaneous nerve produces axonal loss.

In brachial plexopathy, needle examination may show neurogenic changes when lateral cord pathology has resulted in axonal loss.

In C_5, C_6, C_7 radiculopathy, needle examination may show neurogenic changes when root pathology has resulted in axonal loss (i.e., in moderate to severe radiculopathy).

MEDIAL CUTANEOUS NERVE OF THE FOREARM

9

(MEDIAL ANTEBRACHIAL CUTANEOUS NERVE)

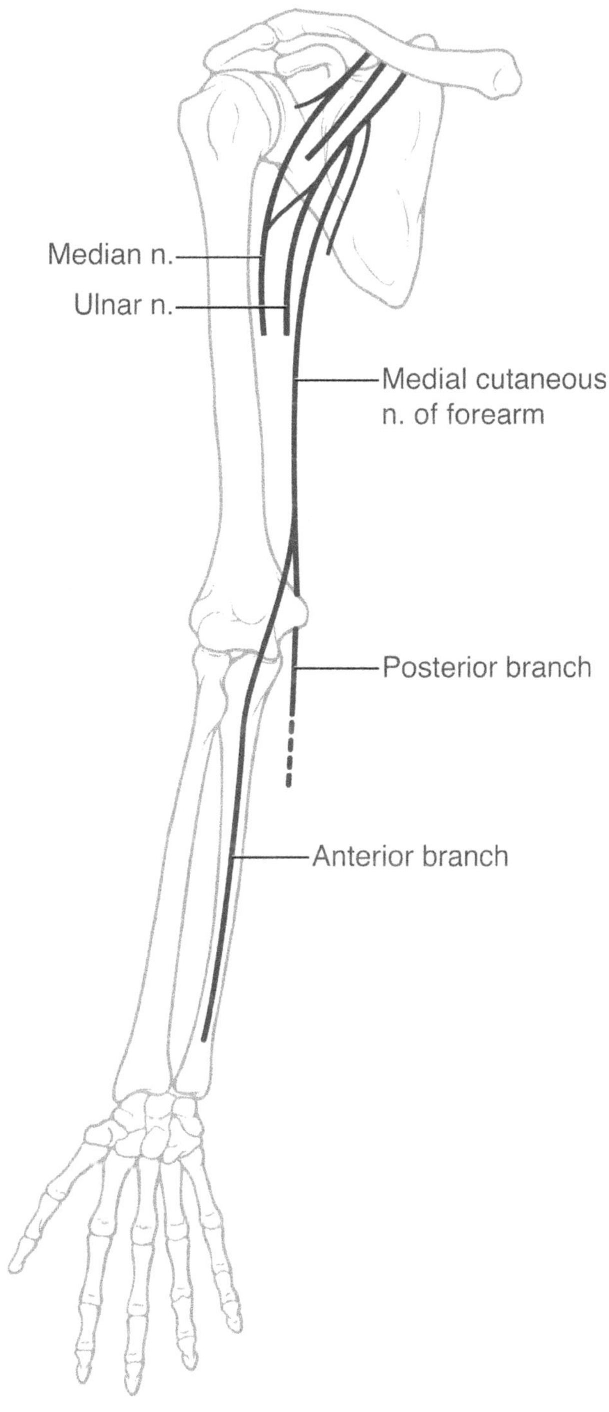

FIGURE 9-1 Medial cutaneous nerve of the forearm.

THE MEDIAL CUTANEOUS NERVE OF THE FOREARM, also known as the *medial antebrachial cutaneous nerve*, arises from the medial cord of the brachial plexus. It derives its fibers from the eighth cervical (C_8) and first thoracic (T_1) roots. It separates from the medial cord proximal to the contribution to the median nerve and the formation of the ulnar nerve. The medial cutaneous nerve of the forearm then descends beneath the deep fascia in the anatomical arm before becoming subcutaneous in the distal third of the arm (Sunderland, 1978). Above the elbow, the nerve divides into anterior and posterior divisions that descend down the anterior and posterior medial forearm, respectively, as far as the wrist. The nerve is purely sensory in function, typically innervating a portion of the medial arm via communications with the medial cutaneous nerve of the arm, and the inner aspect of the forearm from the midline ventrally to the midline dorsally. In some cases, the sensory distribution may extend distally to the hypothenar eminence or ulnar dorsum of hand (Sunderland, 1978).

LESION OF THE MEDIAL CUTANEOUS NERVE OF THE FOREARM

Etiology

Trauma or deep penetrating wounds can cause a medial antebrachial cutaneous nerve lesion.

Iatrogenic nerve injury can occur from invasive medical procedures, including surgical implants (Prahlow and Buschbacher, 2006), surgeries in the medial forearm, and cubital tunnel surgery (Dellon and Mackinnon, 1985).

Antecubital phlebotomy can cause isolated injury to the medial cutaneous nerve of the forearm (Berry and Wallis, 1977).

General Comments

Lesions that affect the lower trunk or medial cord of the brachial plexus will often be associated with injury to the medial cutaneous nerve of the forearm.

Clinical Features

There is sensory loss over the medial aspect of the forearm. However, even after complete section of this nerve, the area of numbness may be limited to a narrow band along the inner forearm, due to extensive overlap of adjacent cutaneous nerves (Sunderland, 1978).

Electrodiagnostic Strategy

Sensory conduction studies of the medial cutaneous nerve of the forearm may show reduced amplitude or absence on the affected side.

Perform additional nerve conduction studies mediated by the medial cord of the brachial plexus (ulnar motor and sensory responses, median motor response) to distinguish isolated medial antebrachial cutaneous neuropathy from medial cord lesion.

EMG of C_8 and T_1 muscles and cervical paraspinal muscles may be necessary to exclude lower trunk brachial plexopathy or cervical radiculopathy.

MEDIAL CUTANEOUS NERVE OF THE FOREARM CONDUCTION STUDY

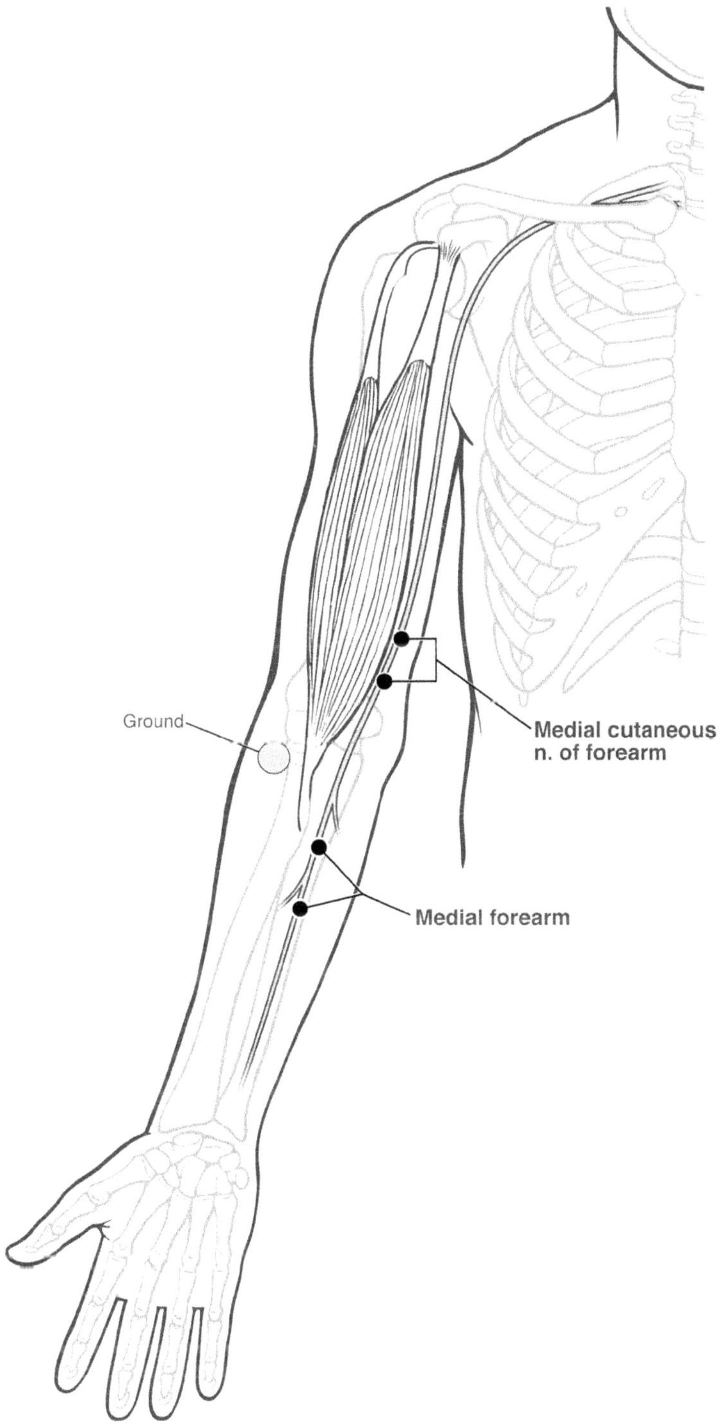

FIGURE 9-2 Medial cutaneous nerve of the forearm conduction study (antidromic).

Recording

Active electrode: Position over the medial forearm, 10 to 12 cm distal to the cathode, on a line between stimulation site and ulnar styloid at the wrist.

Reference electrode: Place 3 cm distal to the active electrode.

Ground electrode: Place on the anterior forearm between the stimulating and recording electrodes.

Stimulation

Medial arm: Place cathode 3 to 4 cm proximal to the midway point between the biceps tendon and the medial epicondyle of the humerus. At this stimulation site, the medial cutaneous nerve lies between the median nerve anteriorly and the ulnar nerve posteriorly. The nerve is superficial, so supramaximal stimulation is achieved at low stimulus intensities (e.g., < 20 mA). Higher stimulus intensities or inappropriate placement of the cathode will coactivate the median or ulnar nerves, causing a mechanical deflection or CMAP that can obscure the desired sensory response. The anode is 3 cm proximal to cathode.

Normal Values

Latency (ms) ≤ 2.0 (onset latency at distance 10 cm); ≤ 2.6 (peak latency)

Amplitude (μV) ≥ 10

Conduction velocity (m/s) ≥ 50 m/s

Studies should be performed bilaterally, because side-to-side comparisons are more useful than normal value tables that may not apply to your patient. A relative amplitude ≤ 50 % of the unaffected side is evidence of abnormality.

Comments

In C_8, T_1 root lesions, the medial cutaneous nerve of the forearm sensory response will be normal.

In lesions of the medial cord or lower trunk, the medial cutaneous nerve of the forearm sensory response will be reduced or absent.

In ulnar neuropathy at the elbow, the medial cutaneous nerve of the forearm sensory response, and sensation in the medial forearm, will be spared.

REFERENCES

Berry PR, Wallis WE. Venepuncture nerve injuries. *Lancet* 1977;1:1236–1237.

Dellon AL, MacKinnon SE. Injury to the medial antebrachial cutaneous nerve during cubital tunnel surgery. *J Hand Surg Br* 1985;10:33–36.

Prahlow ND, Buschbacher RM. An antidromic study of the medial antebrachial cutaneous nerve, with a comparison of the differences between medial and lateral antebrachial cutaneous nerve latencies. *J Long-Term Effects Med Implants* 2006;16:92.

Sunderland S. *Nerves and Nerve Injuries.* 2nd ed., Churchill Livingstone, New York, 1978, p. 620.

SUPRASCAPULAR NERVE

10

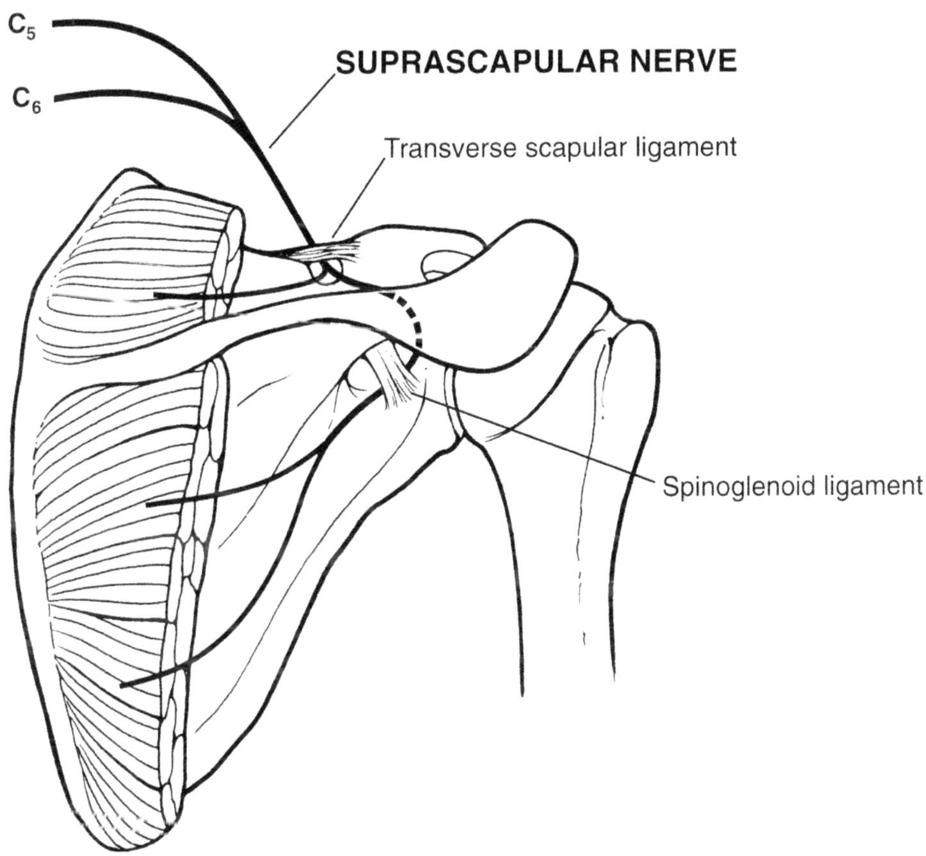

FIGURE 10-1 Diagram of the suprascapular nerve (posterior view) to the supraspinatus and infraspinatus muscles.

FIBERS TO THE SUPRASCAPULAR NERVE are derived from the fifth and sixth cervical roots (*Gray's Anatomy*, 1995). Occasionally, the nerve is derived solely from the fifth, or from the fifth and fourth cervical roots (Sunderland, 1968). The nerve arises from the upper trunk of the brachial plexus and passes obliquely outward beneath the trapezius and omohyoid muscles to reach the suprascapular notch of the scapula. This notch is bridged by the superior transverse scapular ligament to form an osseofibrous foramen through which the suprascapular nerve passes to enter the supraspinous fossa. In the fossa, the nerve lies beneath the supraspinatus muscle, which it innervates.

The nerve then continues around the curved free lateral border of the spine of the scapula to reach the spinoglenoid notch. This notch is covered by the inferior transverse scapular (or spinoglenoid) ligament, which may also form an osseofibrous foramen through which the suprascapular nerve passes to enter the infraspinous fossa. In this fossa, the nerve supplies the infraspinatus muscle. One of the most important uses of the supraspinatus and infraspinatus muscles is the protection they afford to the shoulder joint; the supraspinatus supports it above and prevents displacement of the head of the humerus upward, while the infraspinatus (and teres minor) protect it posteriorly and prevent dislocation backward.

SUPRASCAPULAR NERVE LESION

Etiology

Trauma to the shoulder, fractures of the scapula or humerus, and penetrating wounds can cause direct nerve injury (Hadley et al., 1986).

Mass lesions, such as ganglion cysts or neoplasms, can also cause suprascapular nerve injury (McCluskey et al., 1999).

Entrapment at the suprascapular notch of the scapula, or rarely at the spinoglenoid notch (Aiello et al., 1982; Liveson et al., 1991), can cause a suprascapular nerve lesion.

Neuralgic amyotrophy (idiopathic brachial plexopathy) is causative.

General Comments

Trauma often results in combined lesions of the suprascapular nerve and the upper trunk of the brachial plexus (Sunderland, 1968).

Clinical Features

The shoulder pain is usually described as a deep, dull ache located posterolaterally in the shoulder.

There is wasting of the supraspinatus and infraspinatus muscles.

Initiating of abduction of the arm may be difficult, although the deltoid usually compensates for the loss of the supraspinatus.

Weakness of external rotation of the humerus due to infraspinatus weakness is the major clinical manifestation of a suprascapular nerve lesion. Teres minor only partially compensates for the loss of the infraspinatus.

In a patient with shoulder pain and weakness of external rotation of the arm, a normal EMG of infraspinatus suggests a rotator cuff tear.

There is no sensory loss.

Electrodiagnostic Strategy

Demonstrate neurogenic EMG changes in the supraspinatus and infraspinatus muscles.

EMG of the non-suprascapular innervated C_5, C_6 muscles may be necessary to exclude radiculopathy or coexisting upper trunk lesion.

Perform nerve conduction studies to exclude brachial plexopathy or neuralgic amyotrophy.

Suprascapular motor conduction studies are technically difficult and require a monopolar needle recording in multiple sites for the most accurate assessment (Casazza et. al., 1998).

REFERENCES

Aiello I, Serra G, Traina GC, Tugnoli V. Entrapment of the suprascapular nerve at the spinoglenoid notch. *Ann Neurol* 1982; 12:314–316.

Casazza BA, Young JL, Press JP, Heinemann AW. Suprascapular nerve conduction: A comparative analysis in normal subjects. *Electromyogr Clin Neurophysiol* 1998;38:153–160.

Gray's Anatomy. 38th Edition. Churchill Livingstone, New York, 1995, pp. 1266–1274.

Hadley MN, Sonntag VKH, Pittman HW. Suprascapular nerve entrapment. *J Neurosurg* 1986;64:843–848.

Liveson JA, Bronson MJ, Pollack MA. Suprascapular nerve lesions at the spinoglenoid notch: report of three cases and review of the literature. *J Neurol Neurosurg Psychiatry* 1991;54:241–243.

McCluskey L, Feinberg D, Dolinskas C. Suprascapular neuropathy related to a glenohumeral joint cyst. *Muscle Nerve* 1999;22:772–777.

Reinstein L, Twardzik FG, Mech KF. Pneumothorax: A complication of needle electromyography of the supraspinatus muscle. *Arch Phys Med Rehabil* 1987;68:561–562.

Sunderland S. *Nerves and Nerve Injuries.* Williams & Wilkins, Baltimore, 1968, pp. 1119–1120.

Infraspinatus

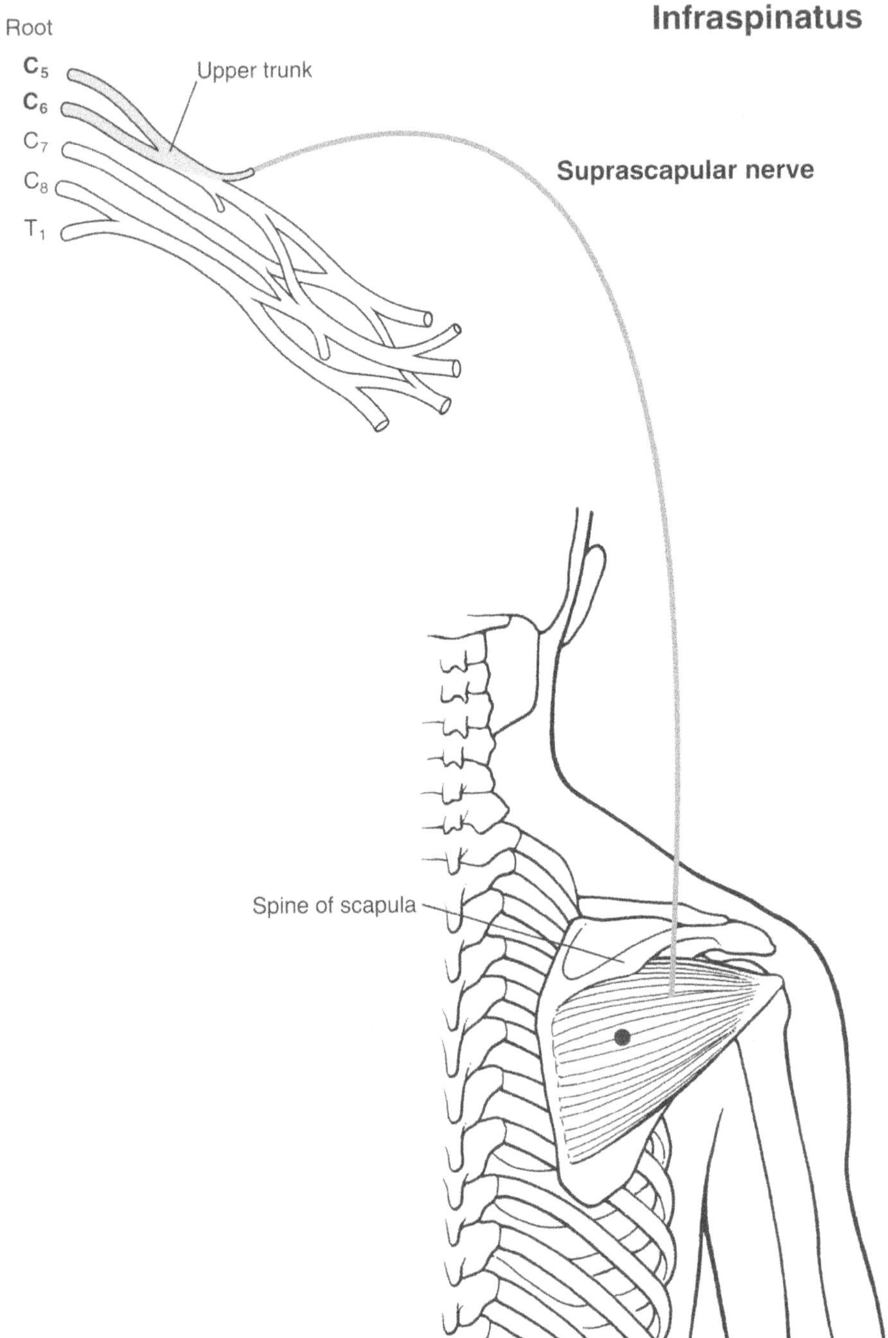

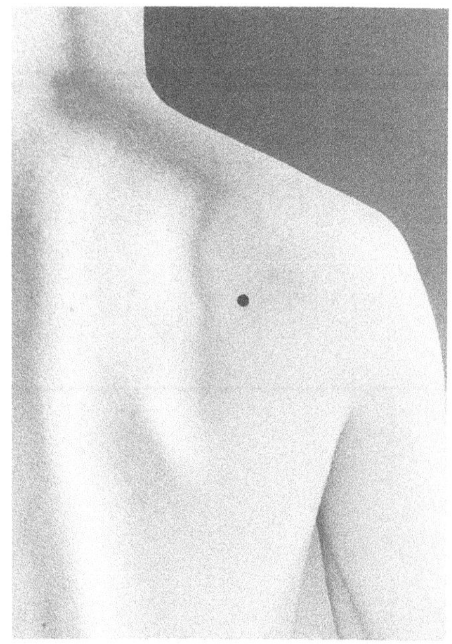

Innervation

Innervation is via the suprascapular nerve, upper trunk, and roots C_5, C_6.

Origin

The infraspinatus originates in the infraspinous fossa of the scapula.

Insertion

Insertion is at the greater tuberosity of the humerus.

Activation Maneuver

External rotation of the humerus activates the muscle.

EMG Needle Insertion

Insert the needle into the infraspinous fossa 2–4 cm below the medial one-third of the spine of the scapula.

Pitfalls

If the needle is inserted too laterally or superficially, it may be in the posterior deltoid, which is supplied by the axillary nerve. Additionally, the trapezius (which is supplied by the spinal accessory nerve) and the latissimus dorsi (supplied by the thoracodorsal nerve) may each lie superficial to the upper and lower margins of the infraspinatus muscle, respectively.

If the needle is placed too caudad, it may be in the teres minor (which is supplied by the axillary nerve) or, rarely, the teres major (supplied by the subscapular nerve).

Clinical Comments

Needle examination may show neurogenic changes when injury to the suprascapular nerve produces axonal loss.

Needle examination may also show neurogenic changes in lesions of the upper trunk and the C_5, C_6 roots, including Erb's palsy.

Supraspinatus

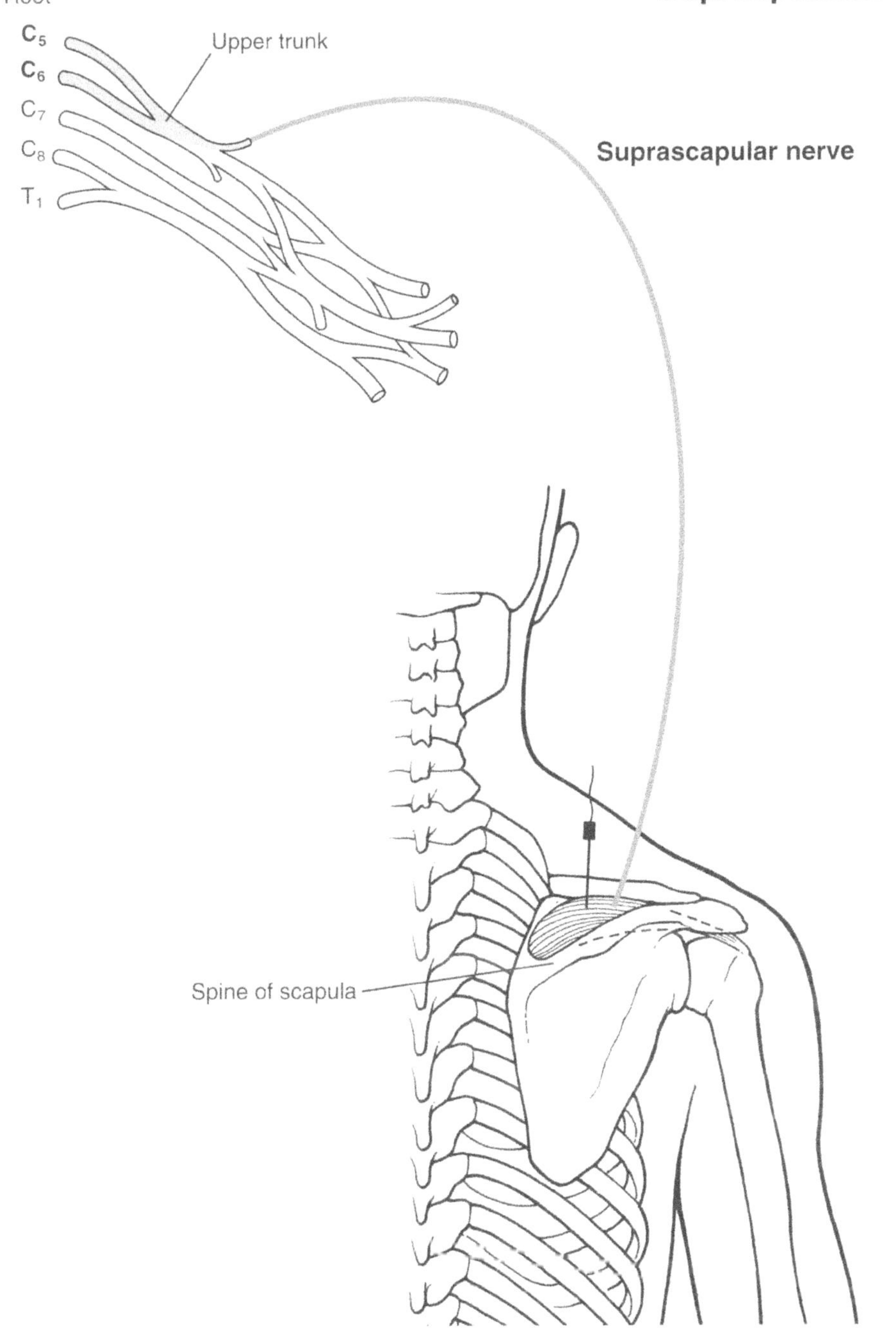

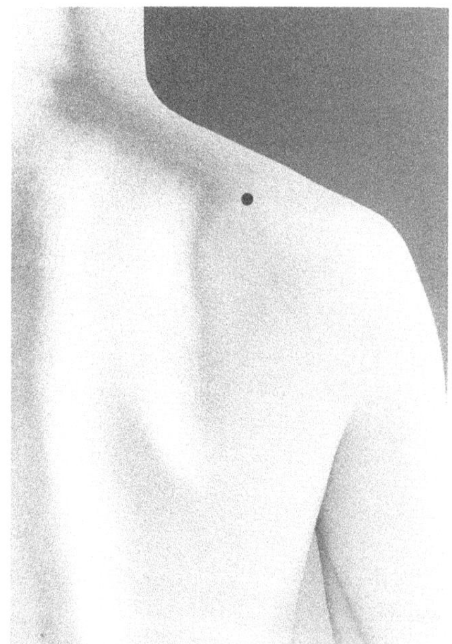

Innervation

Innervation is via the suprascapular nerve, upper trunk, and roots C_5, C_6.

Origin

The supraspinatus originates in the supraspinous fossa of the scapula.

Insertion

Insertion is at the greater tuberosity of the humerus.

Activation Maneuver

Initiation of abduction of the arm activates the muscle.

EMG Needle Insertion

Insert the needle into the supraspinous fossa just above the spine of the scapula (the lateral margin of the spine is usually easier to palpate). Direct the needle to the bone and then retract slightly.

Pitfalls

If the needle is inserted too superficially, it will be in the trapezius muscle, which is supplied by the spinal accessory nerve and C_3 and C_4 spinal nerves.

Pneumothorax following supraspinatus EMG needle examination has been reported in the literature (Reinstein et al., 1987).

Clinical Comments

Needle examination may show neurogenic changes when injury to the suprascapular nerve produces axonal loss.

Needle examination may also show neurogenic changes in lesions of the upper trunk and C_5, C_6 roots, including Erb's palsy.

11 DORSAL SCAPULAR NERVE

THE DORSAL SCAPULAR nerve originates predominantly from the fifth cervical spinal nerve within the substance of the scalenus medius muscle, but it may receive additional fibers from the fourth and sixth spinal nerves (*Gray's Anatomy,* 1995). It may arise in conjunction with the upper root of the long thoracic nerve (Sunderland, 1968). The nerve courses behind the brachial plexus and descends obliquely through the scalenus medius to reach the deep surface of the levator scapulae muscle. It usually sends a twig to this muscle, which receives most of its nerve supply from the third and fourth cervical roots. The nerve continues downward along the medial margin of the scapula to innervate the rhomboideus major and rhomboideus minor muscles (rhomboids).

DORSAL SCAPULAR NERVE LESION

Etiology

Trauma to the back and penetrating wounds can cause direct nerve injury.

Rarely, entrapment due to hypertrophy of the scalenus medius muscle (Kopell and Thompson, 1976) causes a dorsal scapular nerve lesion.

General Comments

Isolated lesions of this nerve are rare.

Clinical Features

Possible shoulder pain is most marked along the medial border of the scapula. Entrapment of the dorsal scapular nerve is a rare but often overlooked cause of shoulder pain.

Wasting of the rhomboid muscles produces slight lateral winging of the scapula, due to the unopposed action of serratus anterior. This manifests as prominence and lateral displacement of the lower medial border and inferior angle of the scapula (Akgun, et al., 2008; Martin and Fish, 2008). Winging is most prominent during lateral abduction of the arm (Washington University).

There is difficulty drawing the scapula directly backward toward the spine.

An isolated nerve lesion may be clinically unrecognized, because the trapezius muscle will partially compensate for paralysis of the rhomboids and levator scapulae (Sunderland, 1968).

Electrodiagnostic Strategy

Demonstrate neurogenic EMG changes in the rhomboids and levator scapulae.

Exclude C_5 radiculopathy by performing EMG in other C_5 muscles. Note: Because isolated lesions of this nerve are rare, neurogenic EMG changes in rhomboids or levator scapulae usually imply C_5 radiculopathy.

Perform nerve conduction studies to exclude an upper trunk lesion.

Dorsal scapular motor conduction studies are not routinely performed.

REFERENCES

Akgun K, Aktas I, Terzi Y. Winged scapula caused by a dorsal scapular nerve lesion: a case report. *Arch Phys Med Rehab* 2008;89:2017–2020.

Gray's Anatomy. 38th Edition. Churchill Livingstone, New York, 1995, pp 835–838.

Kopell HP, Thompson WAL. *Peripheral Entrapment Neuropathies*. 2nd ed. Robert E. Krieger Publishing, New York, 1976, pp. 161–170.

Martin RM, Fish DE. Scapular winging: anatomical review, diagnosis, and treatments. *Curr Rev Musculoskelet Med* 2008;1:1–11.

Miller J. Pneumothorax complication of needle EMG of thoracic wall. *N J Med* 1990;87(8):653.

Sunderland S. *Nerves and Nerve Injuries.* Williams & Wilkins, Baltimore, 1968, p. 1120.

Washington University, St. Louis, Neuromuscular Disease Center. http://neuromuscular.wustl.edu/.

Rhomboideus Major and Minor

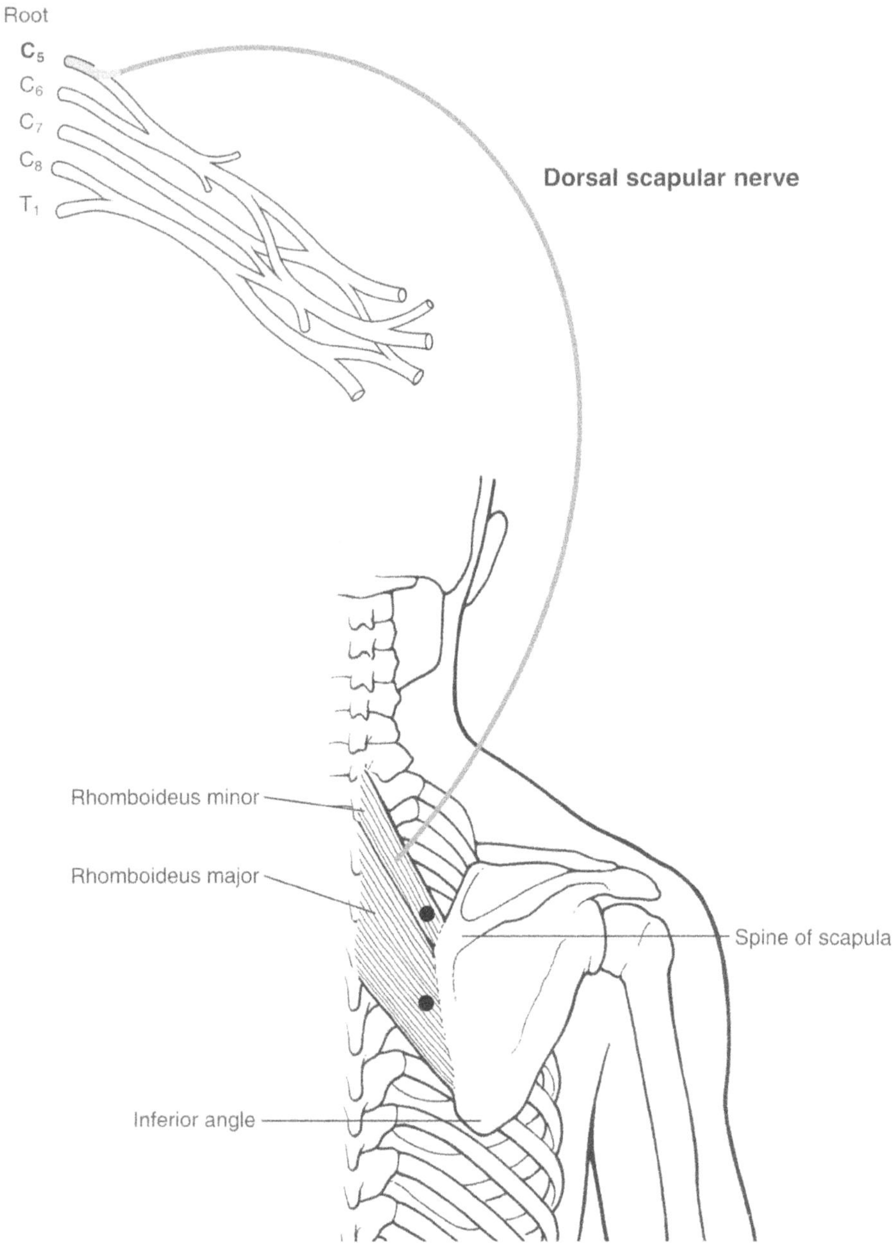

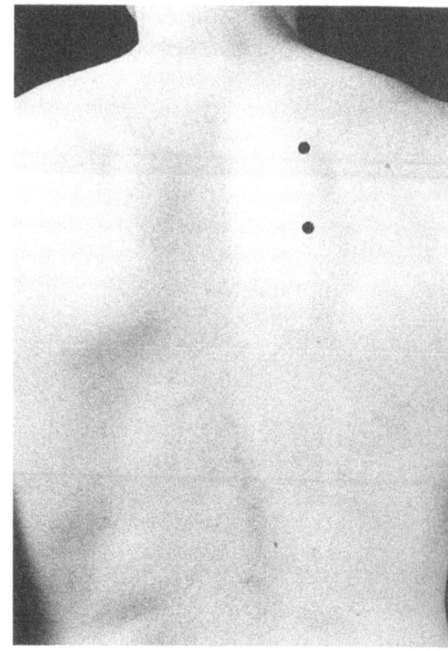

Innervation

Innervation is via the dorsal scapular nerve and root C_5, but may receive additional innervation from the fourth or sixth spinal nerves (*Gray's Anatomy,* 1995).

Origin

The major rhomboideus originates at the spinous processes of the second to fifth thoracic vertebrae.

The minor rhomboideus originates at the spinous processes of the seventh cervical and first thoracic vertebrae.

Insertion

Major: Insertion is at the medial scapular border between the inferior angle and the spine of the scapula.

Minor: Insertion is at the medial scapular border at the base of the spine of the scapula.

Activation Maneuver

Retraction of the scapula (drawing the scapula directly backward toward the vertebral spine) activates the muscles.

EMG Needle Insertion

Major: Insert the needle just medial to the medial margin of the scapula, midway between the scapular spine and the inferior angle.

Minor: Insert the needle just medial to medial border of the scapular spine.

Pitfalls

Major and minor: If the needle is inserted too superficially, it will be in the trapezius muscle, which is supplied by the spinal accessory nerve and C_3 and C_4 spinal roots.

Major only: If the needle is inserted too caudad and superficially, it may be in the latissimus dorsi, which is supplied by the thoracodorsal nerve.

Pneumothorax following needle examination has been reported in the literature (Miller, 1990).

Clinical Comments

Neurogenic changes in the rhomboids on needle examination usually indicate a C_5 radiculopathy.

Look for neurogenic changes in other C_5-innervated muscles.

Levator Scapulae

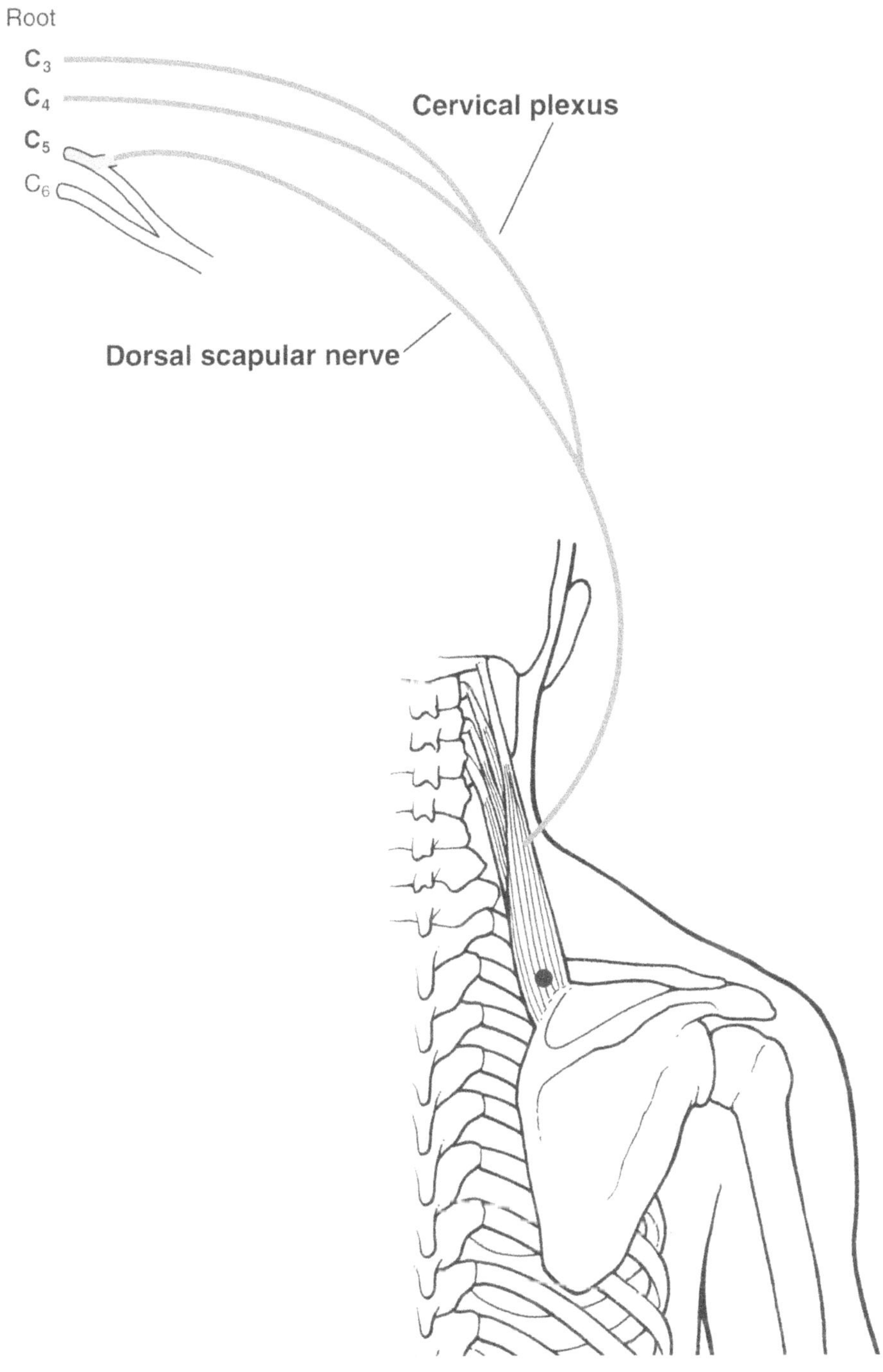

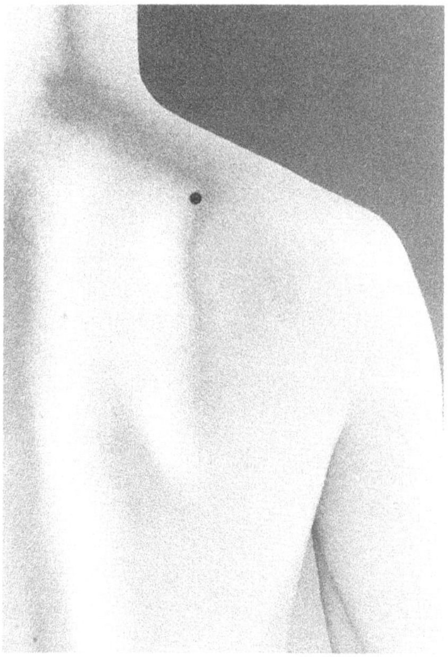

EMG Needle Insertion

Insert the needle along the superomedial margin of the scapula.

Pitfalls

If the needle is inserted too superficially, it will be in the trapezius muscle, which is supplied by C_3 and C_4 spinal nerves and the spinal accessory nerve.

If the needle is inserted too deeply, it may be in the paraspinal muscles, which are supplied by the posterior rami of the spinal nerves.

Innervation

Innervation is via the anterior rami of C_3, C_4, and C_5, the latter branch via the dorsal scapular nerve.

Origin

The levator scapulae originate at the transverse processes of the upper four cervical vertebrae.

Insertion

Insertion is at the posteromedial border of the scapula, between the superior angle and the spine of the scapula.

Activation Maneuver

Elevation of the scapula (which assists the trapezius in shrugging shoulders) activates the levator scapulae.

Clinical Comments

Neurogenic changes in this muscle on needle examination usually indicate a C_3– C_5 radiculopathy.

Look for neurogenic changes in other C_3– C_5 innervated muscles to confirm radiculopathy.

12 LONG THORACIC NERVE

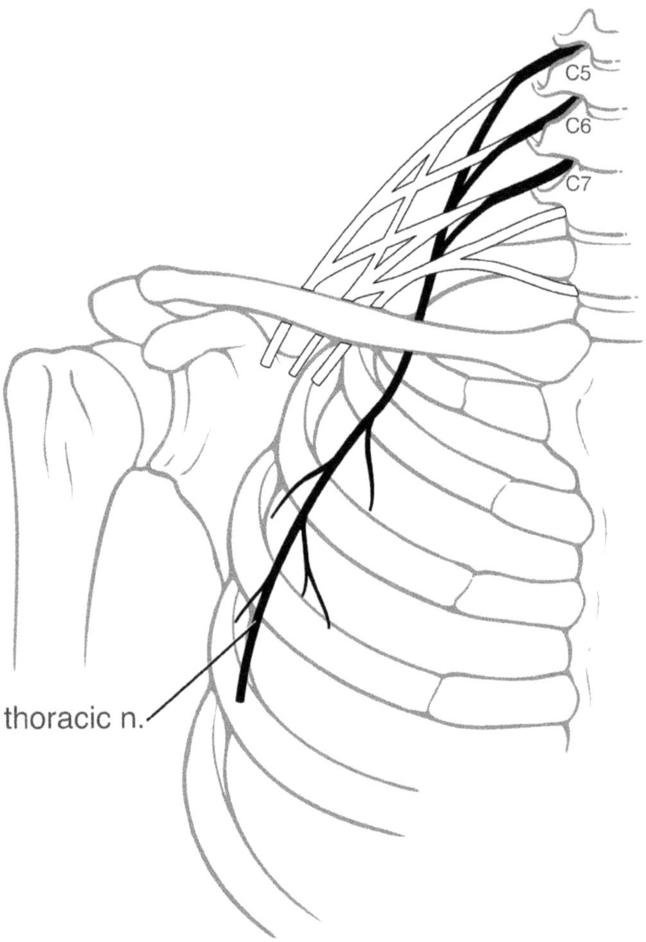

FIGURE 12-1 Diagram of the long thoracic nerve (anterior view) to serratus anterior.

THE LONG THORACIC NERVE is formed by roots from the fifth to the seventh cervical rami (*Gray's Anatomy,* 1995). The upper two roots pierce the scalenus medius obliquely, unite within the muscle, and are then joined by the seventh root, which runs anterior to this muscle. The nerve descends posterior to the brachial plexus, crosses the outer border of the first rib, and descends further along the outer thoracic wall on the surface of the serratus anterior muscle. It supplies this muscle by filaments passing to several digitations of the muscle.

LONG THORACIC NERVE LESION

Etiology

Trauma to the posterior triangle of the neck causes direct nerve injury.

Traction injury occurs when the angle between the neck and the shoulder is forcibly increased (Sunderland, 1968).

Injury may occur in a variety of sports, including archery, ballet, baseball, basketball, body building/weight lifting, bowling, football, golf, gymnastics, hockey, soccer, tennis, and wrestling (Martin and Fish, 2008).

Rarely, entrapment due to hypertrophy of the scalenus medius muscle causes a long thoracic nerve lesion (Kopell and Thompson, 1976).

Neuralgic amyotrophy is causative. Winging of the scapula may be the only manifestation of neuralgic amyotrophy (*Gray's Anatomy*, 1995).

Diseases of muscle (muscular dystrophies, other myopathies) can produce scapular winging.

General Comments

Because the nerve is attached to the scalenus medius above and the serratus anterior below, the nerve is susceptible to stretch injury when the shoulder or chest wall is depressed or the neck is flexed to the opposite side.

Clinical Features

Pain that is dull aching in quality is most marked along the shoulder.

Weakness of serratus anterior produces prominent medial winging of the scapula, due to the unopposed action of trapezius, rhomboids, and other shoulder girdle muscles. This manifests as medial, posterior, and superior displacement of the scapula (inner border protrudes backwards and up off the posterior thoracic wall; Martin and Fish, 2008).

The winging is easily demonstrated by asking the patient to lift the arm forward to 90 degrees at the shoulder, or to push the outstretched arm against a wall.

Electrodiagnostic Strategy

Demonstrate neurogenic EMG changes in the serratus anterior.

Exclude C_5, C_6, or C_7 radiculopathy by performing EMG in other muscles.

Perform nerve conduction studies to exclude a brachial plexus lesion.

EMG in rhomboids and trapezius muscles may be of benefit, since paralysis of trapezius or rhomboids may also cause scapular winging.

Long thoracic nerve motor conduction studies are not routinely performed, although motor conduction studies have been reported to aid in the diagnosis and treatment of long thoracic neuropathy (Depalma et al., 2005; Seror, 2006).

REFERENCES

Depalma MJ, Pease WS, Johnson EW, Kadyan V. A novel technique for recording from the serratus anterior. *Arch Phys Med Rehabil* 2005;86:17–20.

Gray's Anatomy. 38th Edition. Churchill Livingstone, New York, 1995, pp. 835–838.

Johnson EW, Parker WD. Electromyography examination. In Johnson EW, ed. *Practical Electromyography*. Williams & Wilkins, Baltimore, 1980, pp. 1 16.

Kopell HP, Thompson WAL. *Peripheral Entrapment Neuropathies*. 2nd ed., Robert E. Krieger Publishing, New York, 1976, pp 167–168.

Martin RM, Fish DE. Scapular winging: anatomical review, diagnosis, and treatments.

Curr Rev Musculoskelet Med 2008;1:1–11.

Seror P. The long thoracic nerve conduction study revisited in 2006. *Clin Neurophysiol* 2006;117:2446–2450.

Sunderland S. *Nerves and Nerve Injuries*. Williams & Wilkins, Baltimore, 1968, p. 1114–1117.

Serratus Anterior

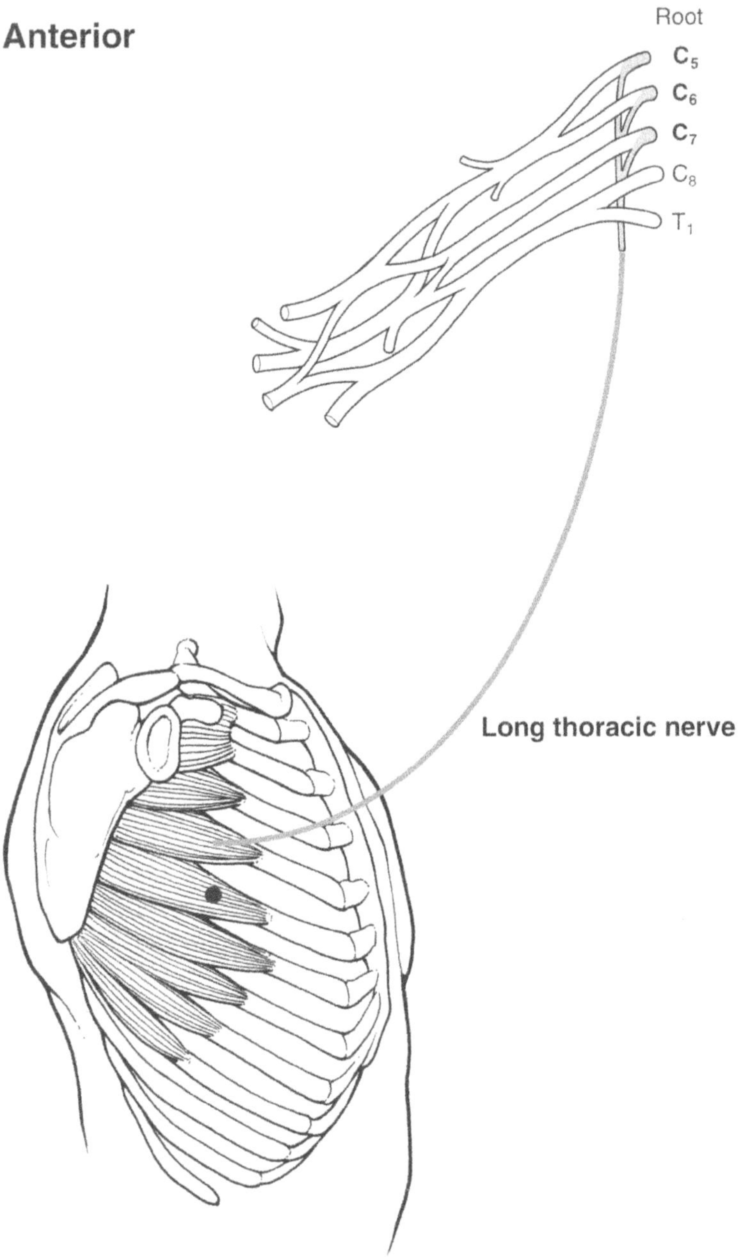

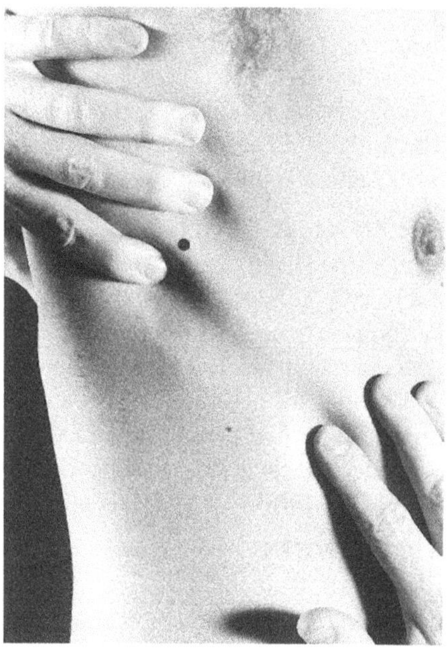

Innervation

Innervation is via the long thoracic nerve and roots C_5, C_6, C_7.

Origin

The serratus anterior originates at the outer surfaces and superior borders of the upper eight or nine ribs.

Insertion

Insertion is at the medial border of the scapula, from the superior angle to the costal surface of the inferior angle.

Activation Maneuver

Forward flexion of the arm and pushing against resistance activate the muscle.

EMG Needle Insertion

Insert the needle along the mid-axillary line directly over the rib, anterior to the bulk of the latissimus dorsi but, in a woman, posterior to breast tissue. Palpating the interspace on either side can isolate a single rib. The serratus anterior is the only muscle between the skin and the rib.

Pitfalls

Pneumothorax following needle examination of the serratus anterior has been reported (Johnson and Parker, 1980).

Clinical Comments

Neurogenic EMG changes limited to the serratus anterior suggest an isolated lesion of the long thoracic nerve.

EMG of other C_5, C_6, or C_7 muscles should be performed to exclude radiculopathy.

SUBSCAPULAR NERVES AND THE THORACODORSAL NERVE

13

THE SUBSCAPULAR NERVES AND THE THORACODORSAL NERVE are all branches of the posterior cord of the brachial plexus. The upper and lower subscapular nerves arise from the fifth and sixth cervical roots, while the thoracodorsal nerve arises from the sixth through eighth cervical roots. The upper and lower subscapular nerves are short and supply the subscapularis and teres major muscles, respectively (Sunderland, 1968).

The subscapularis muscle is of little EMG importance, as it is generally inaccessible to needle examination (it fills the subscapular fossa and terminates in a tendon that inserts on the lesser tuberosity of the humerus). The teres major and latissimus dorsi, however, can be examined during routine EMG evaluation. The nerve to the latissimus dorsi is historically considered to be the middle or long subscapular nerve (Sunderland, 1968; *Gray's Anatomy*, 1977), more recently renamed the *thoracodorsal nerve* (*Gray's Anatomy,* 1995). The thoracodorsal nerve runs a long, exposed course on the posterior wall of the axilla to reach the deep surface of the latissimus dorsi. It is intimately related to lymph nodes along its course, and may be damaged during surgical procedures on the axilla and radical mastectomies. Isolated thoracodorsal nerve injury has been described in bodybuilders (Mondelli et al., 1998). *Paralysis* of the *teres major* muscle may not be clinically noticed, because this muscle acts merely as an aid to the latissimus dorsi.

REFERENCES

Gray's Anatomy. 15th English Edition. Bounty Books/Crown Publishers, New York, 1977, pp. 339–340.

Gray's Anatomy. 38th Edition. Churchill Livingstone, New York, 1995, pp. 835–842.

Mondelli M, Cioni R, Federico A. Rare mononeuropathies of the upper limb in bodybuilders. *Muscle Nerve* 1998;21:809–812.

Sunderland S. *Nerves and Nerve Injuries*. Williams & Wilkins, Baltimore, 1968, p. 1120.

Wu PB, Robinson T, Kingery WS, Date ES. Thoracodorsal nerve conduction study. *Am J Phys Med Rehabil* 1998;77:296–298.

Teres Major

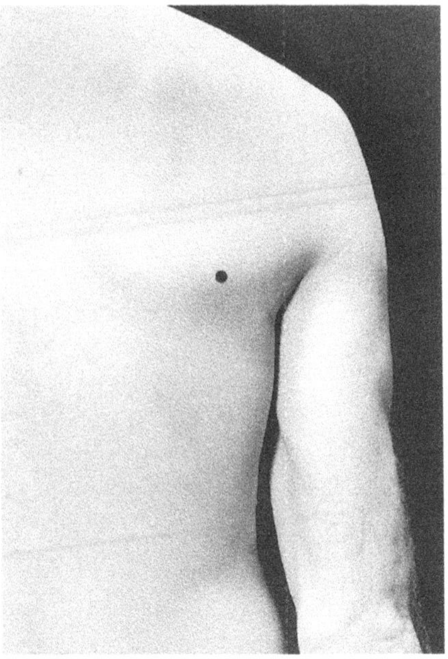

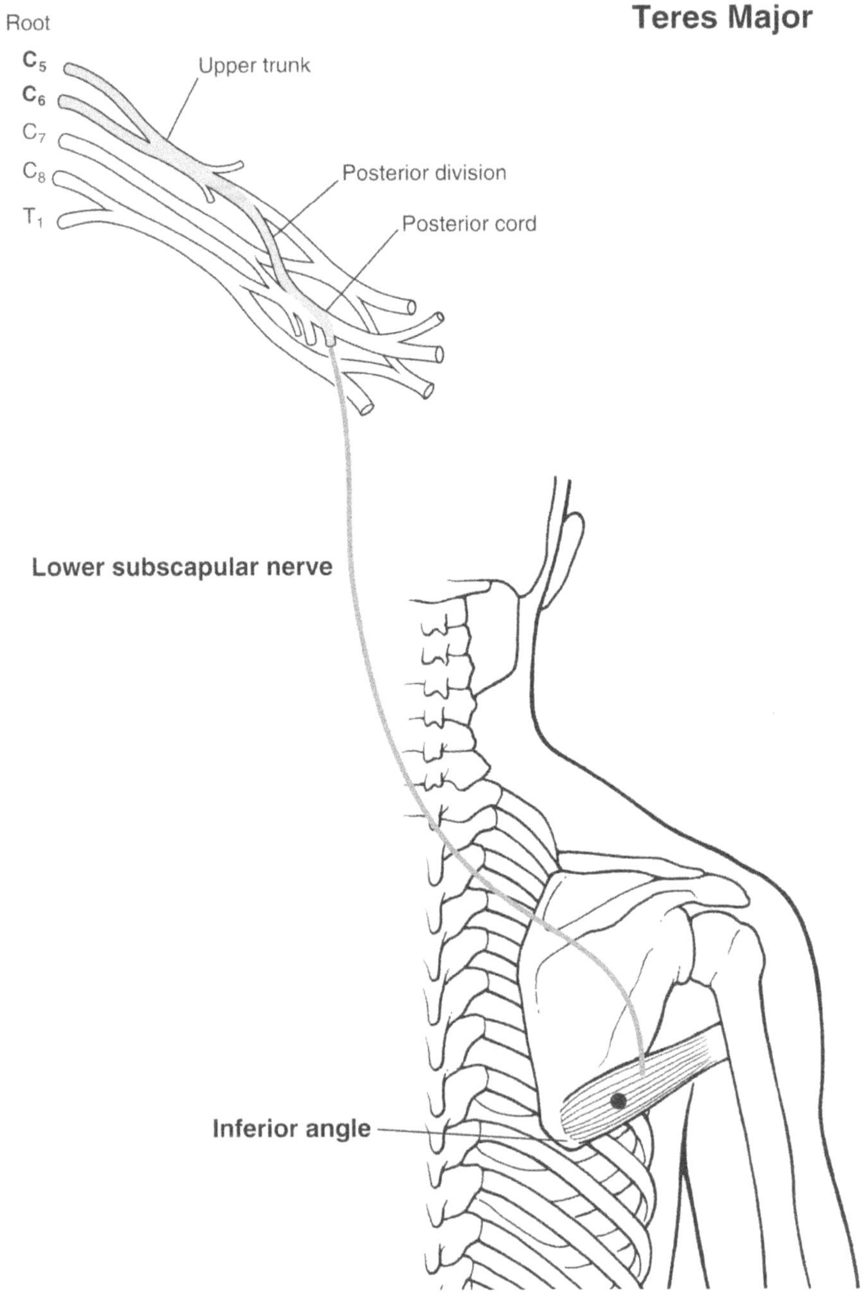

A posterior view of the brachial plexus and the lower subscapular nerve is shown in the drawing and photograph.

Innervation

Innervation is via the lower subscapular nerve, posterior cord, upper trunk, and roots C_5, C_6.

Origin

The teres major originates at the dorsal aspect of the inferior angle of the scapula.

Insertion

Insertion is at the inner bicipital ridge of the humerus.

Activation Maneuver

Internal rotation and adduction of the humerus activates the muscle.

EMG Needle Insertion

Insert the needle along the lateral lower border of the scapula (lateral and rostral to the inferior angle).

Pitfalls

If the needle is inserted too caudally or laterally, it may be in the latissimus dorsi. The latissimus at first covers the origin of the teres major, and then wraps itself obliquely around its lower border so that its tendon ultimately comes to lie in front of that of the teres major.

If the needle is inserted too rostrally (superiorly), it may be in the teres minor, which is supplied by the axillary nerve.

If the needle is inserted too deeply, it may penetrate the serratus anterior, supplied by the long thoracic nerve.

Clinical Comments

An isolated lesion of the lower subscapular nerve is rare. It is unlikely that weakness limited to the teres major would be clinically detectable.

Neurogenic EMG changes in the teres major may be seen with C_5 or C_6 radiculopathy.

A posterior view of the brachial plexus and the thoracodorsal nerve is shown in the drawing and photograph.

Latissimus Dorsi

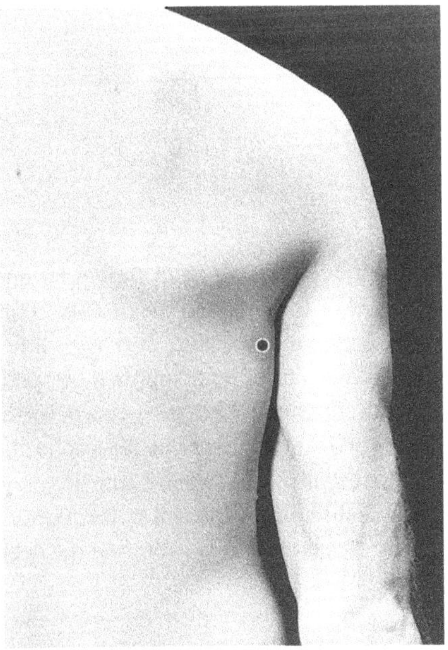

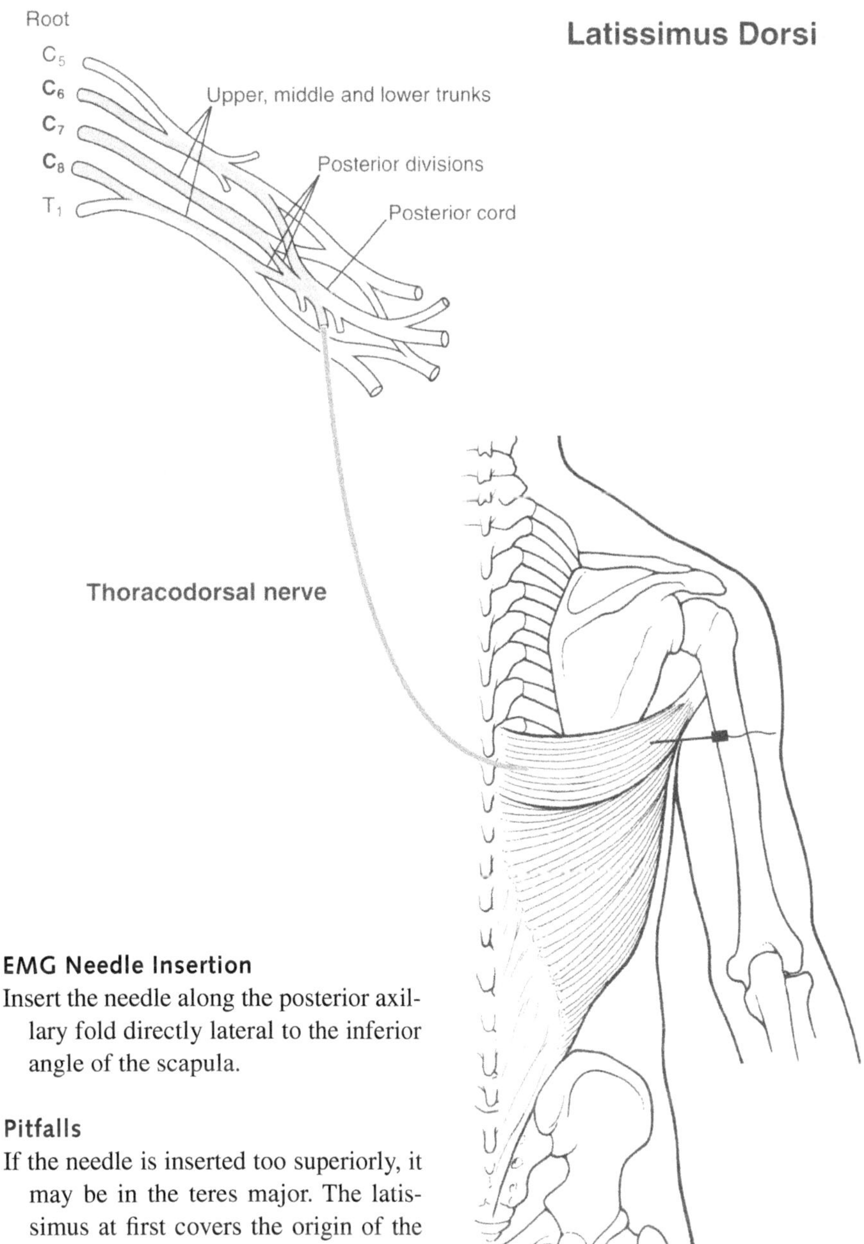

A posterior view of the brachial plexus and the thoracodorsal nerve is shown in the drawing and photograph.

Innervation

Innervation is via the thoracodorsal nerve (formerly the *middle subscapular nerve*), posterior cord, upper, middle, and lower trunks, and roots C_6, C_7, C_8.

Origin

The latissimus dorsi originates at the spinous process of the six inferior thoracic vertebrae, the posterior layer of the lumbar fascia (by which it is attached to the spines of the lumbar and sacral vertebrae), and the crest of the ilium.

Insertion

Insertion is at the bicipital groove of the humerus.

Activation Maneuver

Internal rotation, adduction, and extension (drawing the arm backward) of the humerus activates the muscle.

EMG Needle Insertion

Insert the needle along the posterior axillary fold directly lateral to the inferior angle of the scapula.

Pitfalls

If the needle is inserted too superiorly, it may be in the teres major. The latissimus at first covers the origin of the teres major, and then wraps itself obliquely around its lower border so that its tendon ultimately comes to lie in front of that of the teres major.

Clinical Comments

Atrophy and weakness of the latissimus dorsi is not easily detected, because wasting is not often noticeable and functions (internal rotation, adduction, and extension) can be executed by other muscles (Sunderland, 1968). However, paralysis or paresis of the latissimus dorsi can be exposed by instructing the patient to abduct the arm laterally to 90 degrees at the shoulder, and then to maximally adduct the arm (push down) against the examiner's resistance. The act of maximally bringing the arm down is weakened on the affected side, and atrophy of the muscle can more easily be detected by inspection or palpation.

Neurogenic EMG changes in the latissimus dorsi may be seen with C_6, C_7, or C_8 radiculopathy.

Thoracodorsal nerve motor conduction studies are not routinely performed, although motor conduction studies have been described to evaluate the integrity of the thoracodorsal nerve (Wu et al., 1998).

14 MEDIAL AND LATERAL PECTORAL NERVES

THE LATERAL PECTORAL NERVE is larger than the medial and arises from the upper and middle trunks or by a single branch from the lateral cord of the brachial plexus. Its fibers are derived from the fifth to seventh cervical rami (*Gray's Anatomy,* 1995). It crosses anterior to the axillary artery and vein, pierces the clavipectoral fascia, and supplies the deep surface of the pectoralis major. It sends a small branch to the medial pectoral nerve, forming a loop in front of the first part of the axillary artery, to supply fibers of the pectoralis minor. The medial pectoral nerve is derived from the eighth cervical and first thoracic cervical rami. It arises from the medial cord of the brachial plexus, posterior to the axillary artery. It curves forward to join the branch from the lateral pectoral nerve, entering the deep surface of the pectoralis minor to supply it.

Branches from the medial pectoral nerve emerge from the pectoralis minor to enter and supply portions of the pectoralis major (Macchi et al., 2007). The lateral or medial pectoral nerves may be injured during competitive sports or weight lifting, causing anterior chest wall pain, weakness of arm adduction, and atrophy of pectoralis muscles (Borg-Stein et al., 2006). In addition, medial pectoral neuropathy in body builders may occur because weightlifting and concomitant pectoralis minor hypertrophy produce intramuscular entrapment of the medial pectoral nerve (Rossi et al., 1999). Direct injury to or rupture of the pectoralis muscles may also injure the lateral or medial pectoral nerves.

REFERENCES

Borg-Stein J, Mostoufi SA, Hirschberg R. Chronic pectoral pain following medial pectoral nerve injury: A case report. *J Back Musculoskel* Rehab 2006;19:7–11.

Gray's Anatomy. 38th Edition. Churchill Livingstone, New York, 1995, pp. 838–840, 1269.

Macchi V, Tiengo C, Porzionato A, et al. Medial and lateral pectoral nerves: course and branches. *Clin Anat* 2007;20:157–162.

Pecina MM, Krmpotic-Nemanic J, Markiewitz AD. *Tunnel Syndromes: Peripheral Nerve Compression Syndromes.* 2nd ed., CRC Press, New York, 1997, pp. 36–38.

Rossi F, Triggs WJ, Gonzalez R, Shafer SJ. Bilateral medial pectoral neuropathy in a weight lifter. *Muscle Nerve* 1999;22:1597–1599.

Pectoralis major

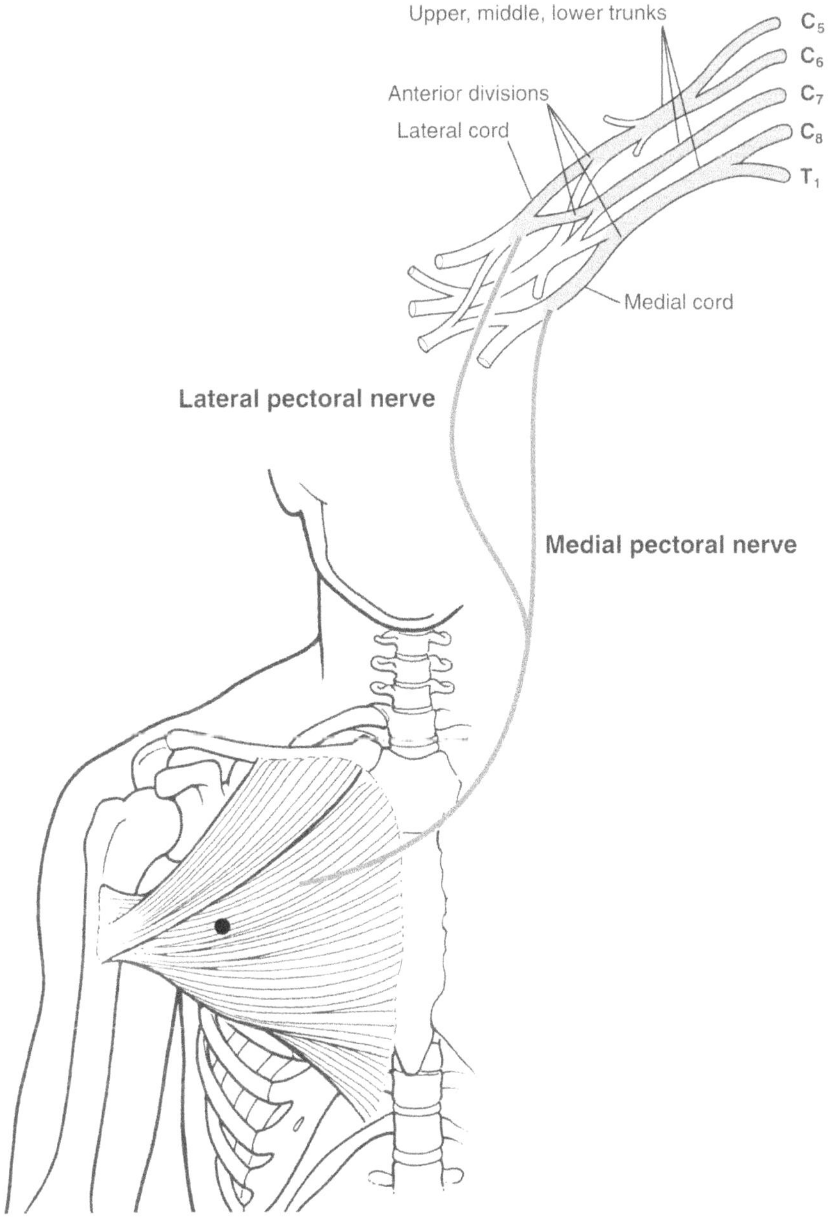

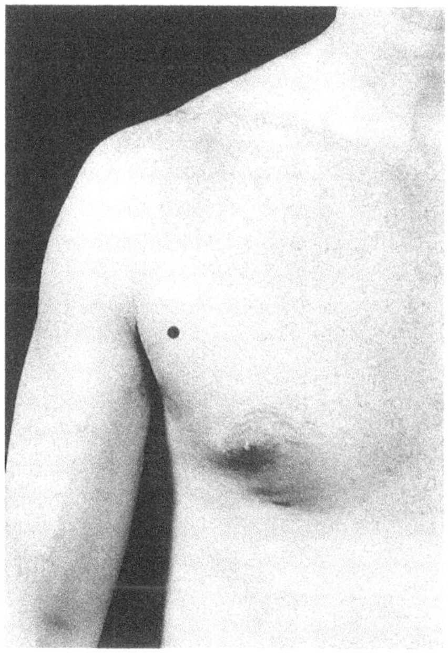

EMG Needle Insertion

Insert the needle just medial to the anterior axillary fold over the bulk of the muscle.

Pitfalls

If the needle is inserted too superiorly, it may be in the anterior fibers of the deltoid, which is supplied by the axillary nerve.

If the needle is inserted too laterally, it may be in the coracobrachialis or the short head of the biceps, which are supplied by the musculocutaneous nerve.

Innervation

Clavicular part: Innervation is via the lateral pectoral nerve, lateral cord, upper trunk, and roots C_5, C_6.

Sternocostal part: Innervation is via the lateral and medial pectoral nerves, lateral and medial cords, middle and lower trunks, and roots C_7, C_8, T_1.

Origin

The clavicular part originates at the sternal half of the clavicle.

The sternocostal part originates at the anterior surface of the sternum, the cartilage of the first six or seven ribs, and the aponeurosis of the external oblique muscle of the abdomen.

Insertion

Insertion is at the lateral lip of the intertubercular sulcus on the shaft of the humerus.

Activation Maneuver

Adduction of the arm activates the muscle.

Clinical Comments

An isolated lesion of the lateral or medial pectoral nerves is rare.

Weakness of the pectoralis major results in limited adduction of the arm.

Neurogenic EMG changes in the pectoralis major may be seen with radiculopathies affecting the C_5–T_1 roots. This muscle is, therefore, of little benefit in localizing a root lesion.

Lateral and medial pectoral nerve conduction studies are not routinely performed.

Pectoralis minor

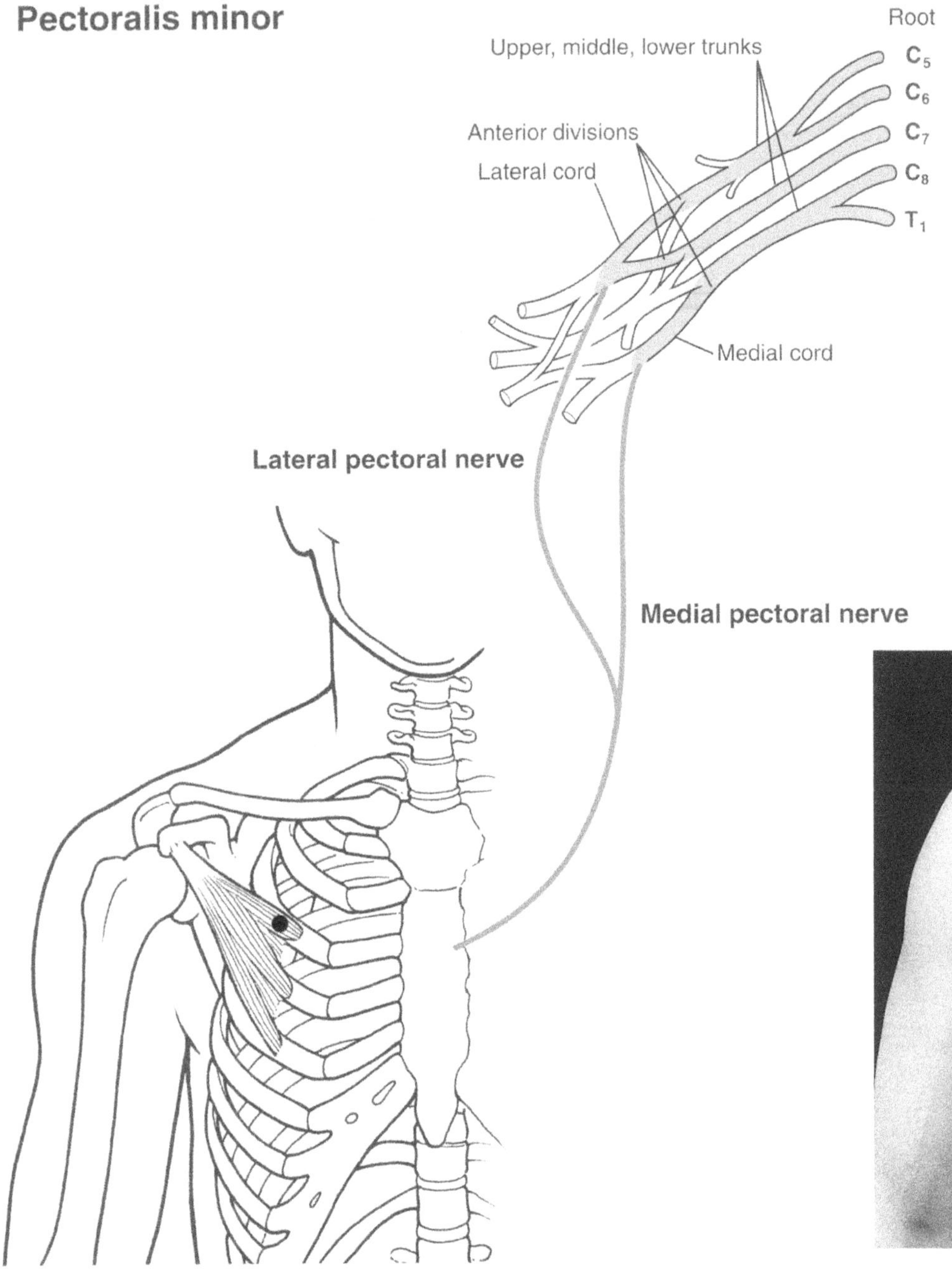

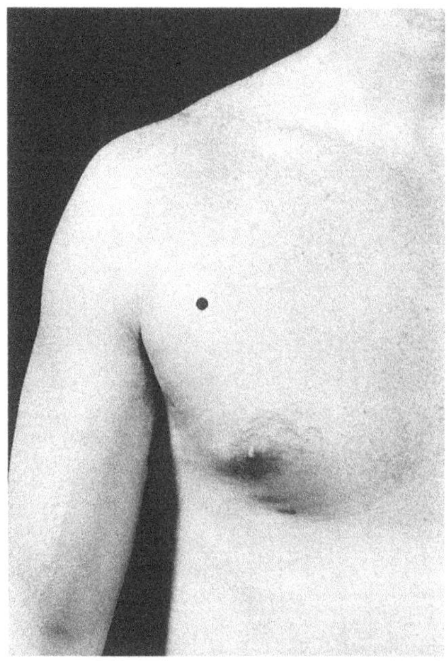

Innervation

Innervation is via the medial and lateral pectoral nerves, medial and lateral cords, upper, middle, and lower trunks, and roots C_5, C_6, C_7, C_8, and T_1.

Origin

The pectoralis minor originates at the outer surfaces of the third to fifth ribs (frequently second to fourth).

Insertion

Insertion is at the coracoid process of the scapula.

Activation Maneuver

Depression of the shoulder activates the muscle.

EMG Needle Insertion

Insert the needle in the midclavicular line overlying the third rib.

Pitfalls

If the needle is inserted too superficially, it will be in the pectoralis major.

Clinical Comments

An isolated lesion of the lateral or medial pectoral nerves is rare.

Weakness of the pectoralis minor is unlikely to be clinically detectable.

Neurogenic EMG changes in the pectoralis minor may be seen with radiculopathies affecting the C_5–T_1 roots. This muscle is, therefore, of little benefit in localizing a root lesion.

In prolonged hyperabduction of the arm, the neurovascular bundle in the axilla can be stretched under the pectoralis minor tendon, resulting in symptoms of neurovascular compression (Pecina et al., 1997).

Lateral and medial pectoral nerve conduction studies are not routinely performed.

CERVICAL PLEXUS

15

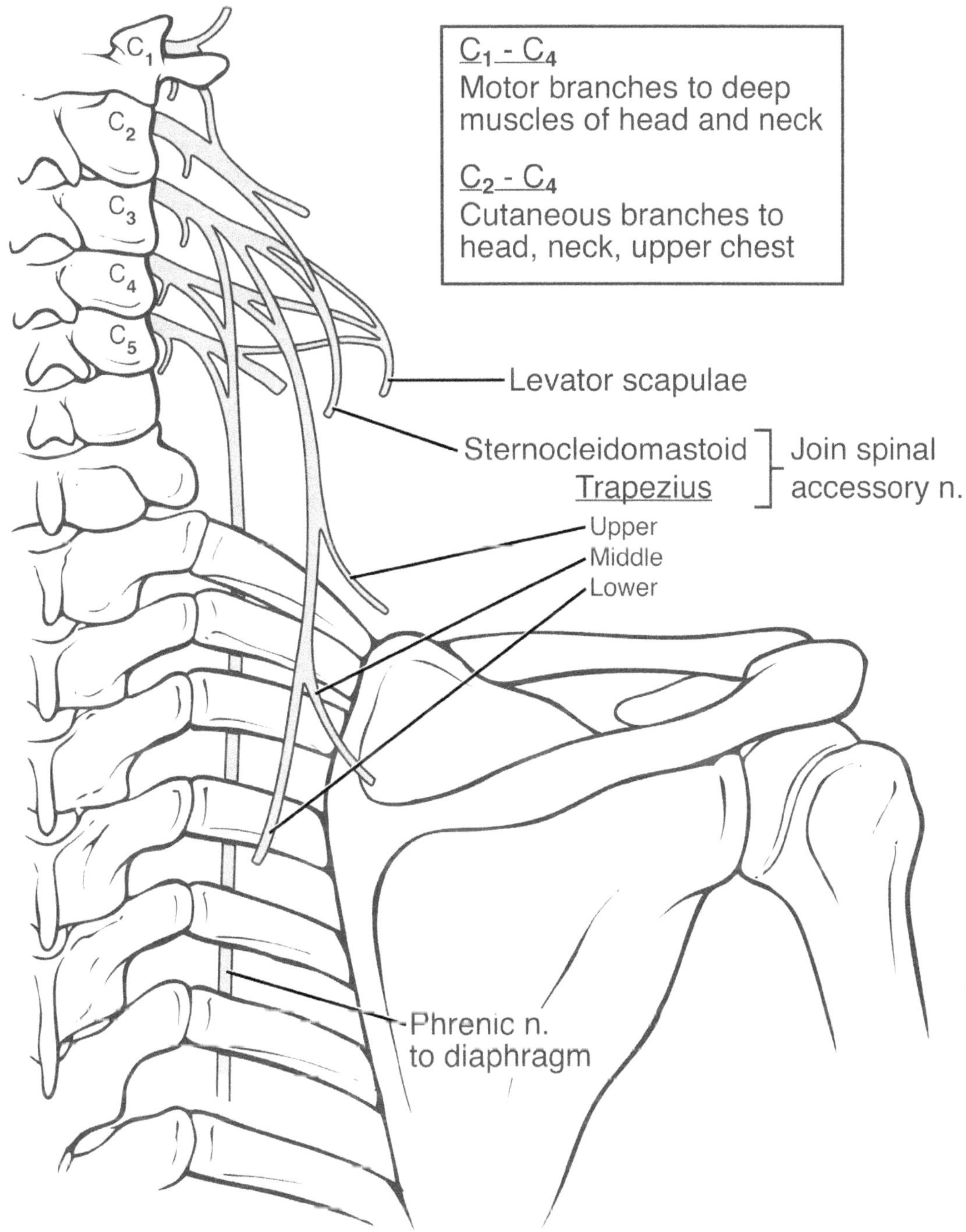

FIGURE 15-1 Diagram of the major muscular branches of the cervical plexus to sternocleidomastoid, trapezius, levator scapulae, and diaphragm (posterior view).

THE CERVICAL PLEXUS is formed by the upper four cervical ventral rami (*Gray's Anatomy*, 1977). It lies deep to the sternocleidomastoid muscle and anterior to the scalenus medius and levator scapulae muscles. Its branches can be divided into two groups, superficial and deep. The superficial branches are primarily sensory branches derived from the second through fourth cervical roots, and provide cutaneous innervation to the head (C_2 dermatome), neck (C_3 dermatome), and chest (C_3 and C_4 dermatomes). These branches include the lesser occipital, great auricular, transverse cervical, and supraclavicular nerves. The deep branches are largely muscular branches derived from the first through fourth cervical roots, and are distributed to deep muscles of the neck, including the anterior recti and rectus capitis lateralis muscles and the scalenus medius. The C_1 through C_3 motor branches also form the *ansa cervicalis*, which is a loop of muscular nerves in the neck that supply infrahyoid muscles, including the sternohyoid, sternothyroid, and omohyoid muscles (Hansen, 2010). Deep muscular branches also supply the sternocleidomastoid, trapezius, levator scapulae, and the diaphragm. From an electromyography perspective, the latter four muscles are the most commonly studied.

The motor branches from the cervical plexus to the trapezius and sternocleidomastoid communicate with the *spinal accessory nerve* (cranial nerve XI, see Chapter 28), which provides most of the innervation to these muscles. Cervical branches to the sternocleidomastoid are derived chiefly from the second and third cervical roots, and occasionally the fourth cervical root, while branches to the trapezius are derived from the third and fourth cervical roots. Branches to the levator scapulae are derived from the third and fourth cervical roots, which are joined by the fifth cervical root via the *dorsal scapular nerve* (see Chapter 11) of the brachial plexus. The diaphragm receives its motor supply from the *phrenic nerve* (see Chapter 16), which arises from the third, fourth, and fifth cervical roots. A useful mnemonic to remember is "C_3, C_4, C_5 keep the diaphragm alive."

REFERENCES

Berry H, MacDonald EA, Mrazek AC. Accessory nerve palsy: A review of 23 cases. *Can J Neurol Sci* 1991;18:337–341.

Donner T, Kline DG. Extracranial spinal accessory nerve injury. *Neurosurgery* 1993;32:907–911.

Gray's Anatomy. 15th English Edition. Bounty Books/Crown Publishers, New York, 1977, pp. 758–764.

Gray's Anatomy. 38th Edition. Churchill Livingstone, New York, 1995, pp 1263–1266.

Hansen JT. *Netter's Clinical Anatomy*. 2nd Edition. Saunders Elsevier, Philadelphia, 2010, pp. 412–415.

Martin RM, Fish DE. Scapular winging: anatomical review, diagnosis, and treatments. *Curr Rev Musculoskelet Med* 2008;1:1–11.

PHRENIC NERVE

16

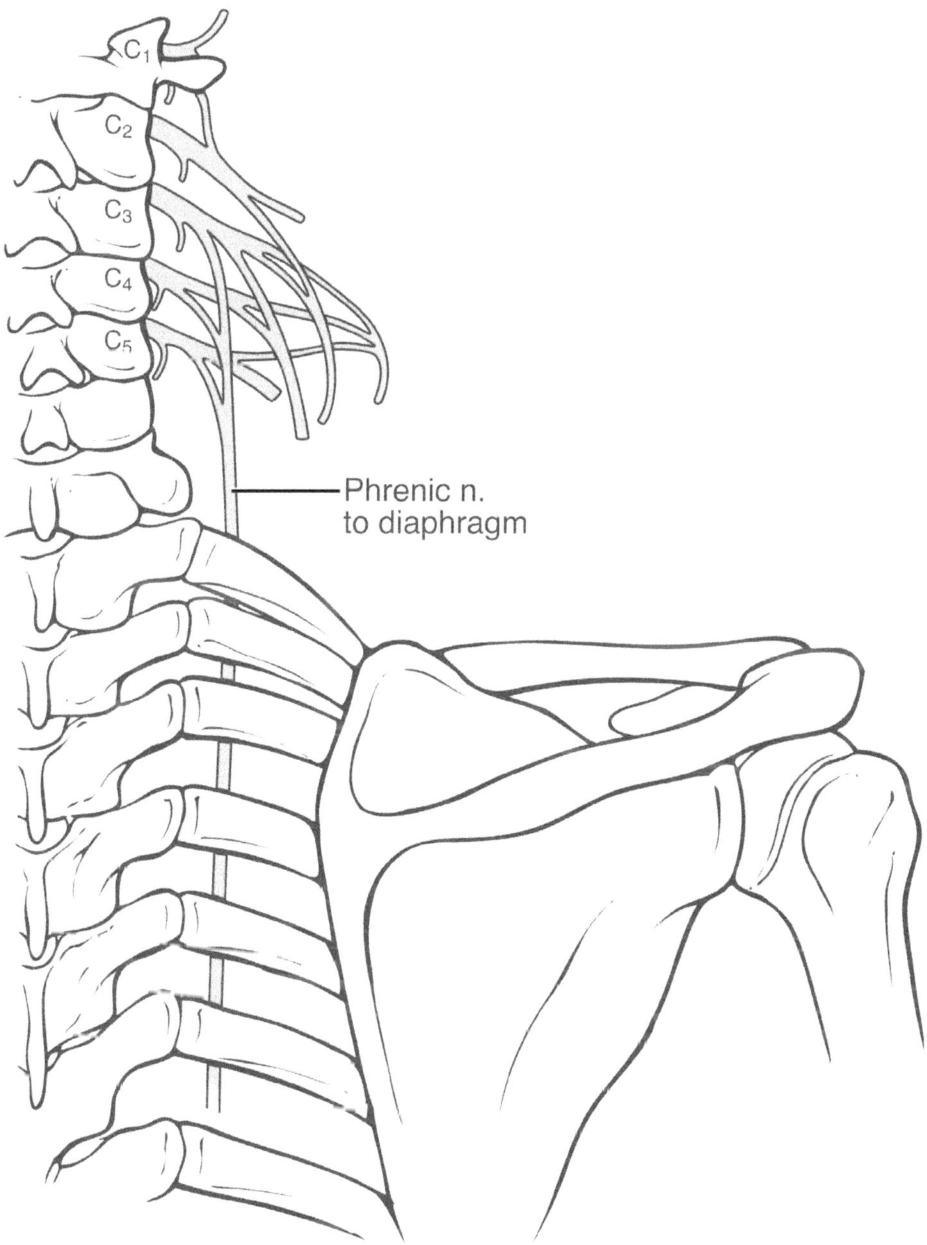

FIGURE 16-1 Diagram of the phrenic nerve to the diaphragm (posterior view).

THE PHRENIC NERVE arises chiefly from the third and fourth cervical nerves, with a communicating branch from the fifth (*Gray's Anatomy,* 1977). It descends to the root of the neck, running obliquely across the anterior surface of the scalenus anterior, and beneath the sternocleidomastoid and the posterior (inferior) belly of the omohyoid muscles. It passes over the first part of the subclavian artery, lying between it and the subclavian vein. Within the chest, the phrenic nerve descends almost vertically in front of the root of the lung and by the side of the pericardium, between it and the mediastinal portion of the pleura. It reaches the diaphragm, where it divides into branches that separately pierce the muscle and are distributed to its undersurface.

The two phrenic nerves differ in their length and in their anatomical relations in the upper thorax. The *right nerve* is shorter, more deeply situated, and more vertical in its descent than the left. It lies on the outer side of the right brachiocephalic vein and superior vena cava. The *left nerve* is longer, due to the inclination of the heart to the left, and from the diaphragm being lower on this side. It enters the thorax behind the left brachiocephalic vein and crosses in front of the vagus nerve, aortic arch, and root of the lung. In the thorax, each phrenic nerve is accompanied by a branch of the internal mammary artery.

PHRENIC NERVE LESION

Etiology

Trauma to the side of the neck causes direct nerve injury.

Iatrogenic causes include cardiac surgery (Tripp and Bolton, 1998), surgery in the neck, compression by retractors or other instruments, and subclavian vein catheterization (Drachler et al., 1976).

Neuralgic amyotrophy is causative.

Malignant neoplasms, including bronchogenic carcinoma and other lesions within the chest, can cause a phrenic nerve lesion.

Abnormalities may occur in spinal cord injury or other pathological conditions affecting the anterior horn cells at the C_3–C_5 segments, including motor neuron disease, poliomyelitis, and syringomyelia.

Radiculopathy involving the C_3–C_5 roots may result in loss of motor axons in the phrenic nerve.

Demyelinating diseases of peripheral nerves, such as Guillain-Barré syndrome or chronic inflammatory demyelinating polyneuropathy (CIDP), can block conduction in the phrenic nerve.

Disorders of the neuromuscular junction, such as myasthenia gravis, can reduce transmission in the phrenic nerves.

Diseases of muscle (critical illness myopathy, inflammatory myopathies) can weaken the diaphragm.

General Comments

The phrenic nerve has a relatively long course before reaching its final destination. Lower motor neuron damage may occur anywhere from the anterior horn cells at the C_3–C_5 segments to the terminal innervation of the diaphragm (Bolton, 1993).

The diaphragm is the major muscle of respiration. Respiratory compromise always occurs when excursion of the diaphragm bilaterally is moderately diminished or absent. However, unilateral diaphragm dysfunction may go undiagnosed.

Clinical Features

Dyspnea (shortness of breath) occurs with bilateral phrenic nerve lesions, associated with orthopnea (shortness of breath when lying flat) and tachypnea (rapid, shallow breathing). For example, in incomplete high cervical spinal cord injury, respiratory movements will be weak and breathing will be rapid and shallow.

Weakness of the diaphragm typically causes paradoxic respiration, in which all or part of the affected lung is deflated during inhalation and inflated during exhalation, the opposite of normal chest motion. Paradoxic abdominal wall motion also occurs, with retraction or inward movement of the abdominal wall during inspiration and outward movement during expiration.

Weakness of the diaphragm also results in decreased breath sounds on the affected side, and dullness upon percussion of the lower chest on the involved side.

Electrodiagnostic Strategy

Perform phrenic nerve conduction studies (Bolton, 1993). In axonal loss lesions affecting the phrenic nerve, compound muscle action potentials from the diaphragm will be reduced or absent. In demyelinating lesions, phrenic nerve conduction latencies may be markedly prolonged.

Demonstrate neurogenic EMG changes in the diaphragm.

Evaluate for C_3, C_4, or C_5 radiculopathy by performing EMG in other muscles that have C_3–C_5 innervation (cervical paraspinals, sternocleidomastoid, trapezius, levator scapulae, and rhomboids).

Perform nerve conduction studies to assess for cervical or brachial plexus lesions.

In cases of respiratory dysfunction of undetermined etiology, assess for acquired myopathies (inflammatory, critical illness), axonal or demyelinating polyneuropathies, and disorders of neuromuscular transmission.

PHRENIC NERVE CONDUCTION STUDY

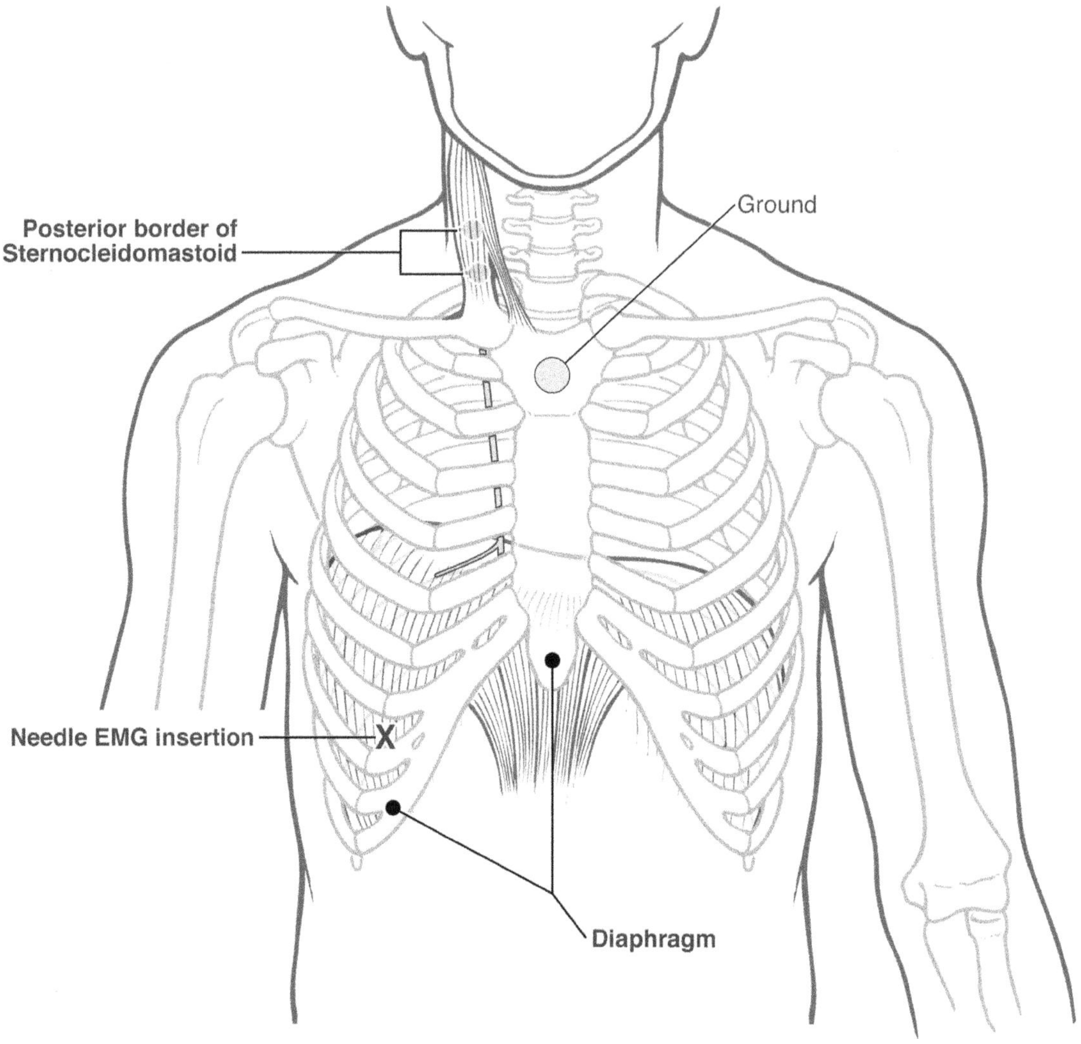

FIGURE 16-2 Phrenic nerve conduction study.

Recording (Bolton, 1993)

Active electrode: Position over the xiphoid process, which marks the inferior extent of the sternum and the anterior attachment point of the diaphragm (Hansen, 2010).

Reference electrode: Place 16 cm inferior and lateral to the active electrode, over the cartilaginous lower costal margin.

Ground electrode: Place on the sternum, between stimulating and recording electrodes.

Stimulation

Neck: Place cathode at the posterior border of the sternocleidomastoid muscle, about 3 cm above the clavicle. The anode is 3 cm superior to the cathode.

Comments

Small adjustments in the electrode position and stimulus intensity may be necessary to ensure a supramaximal diaphragm CMAP, particularly in patients with large necks.

Normal Values (Bolton, 1993)
Latency (ms) 6.3 ± 0.8
Amplitude (μV) 600 ± 140

Note that the amplitude of the diaphragm CMAP is relatively small compared with other motor responses. Phrenic nerve conduction studies should be performed bilaterally. An amplitude ≤ 50% of the unaffected side is evidence of abnormality.

Pitfalls

Technical problems arise when the brachial plexus is inadvertently coactivated by the electrical stimulation. This results in a CMAP that is volume-conducted from chest wall muscles (e.g., pectoralis major and minor, serratus anterior), and is characterized by an initial positive deflection and a shorter latency. When this occurs, repositioning the cathode so that the phrenic nerve is preferentially stimulated should eliminate the problem.

The electrocardiogram will produce a discharge that will interfere with the desired diaphragm CMAP. However, this artifact is obvious because it is time-locked to the heart rate. Stimulation to the phrenic nerve can be repeated to avoid this artifact.

The diaphragm CMAP amplitude varies with respiration, and is usually greater during inspiration using the current technique. Accordingly, phrenic nerve stimulation should be performed during quiet respirations.

Additional Comments

Fluoroscopic examination of the diaphragm is useful in assessing diaphragmatic function. The fluoroscopic "sniff test," in which paradoxical elevation of the paralyzed hemidiaphragm is observed with rapid inspiration, can confirm chest radiographic findings of unilateral diaphragmatic paralysis.

Fluoroscopy may also be employed at the time of phrenic nerve conduction studies to confirm diaphragmatic movement, particularly in patients with high spinal cord injury. Rapid repetitive stimulation (e.g., 20 stimuli at 20 Hz) may be necessary to better visualize diaphragmatic movement.

REFERENCES

Bolton CF. AAEM minimonograph #40: Clinical neurophysiology of the respiratory system. *Muscle Nerve* 1993;16:809–818.

Bolton CF. Grand'Maison F, Parkes A, Shkrum M. Needle electromyography of the diaphragm. *Muscle Nerve* 1992;15:678–681.

Drachler DH, Koepke GH, Weg JG. Phrenic nerve injury from subclavian vein catheterization: Diagnosis by electromyography. *JAMA* 1976;236:2880–2881.

Gray's Anatomy. 15th English Edition. Bounty Books/Crown Publishers, New York, 1977, pp. 758–764.

Hansen JT. *Netter's Clinical Anatomy*. 2nd Edition. Saunders Elsevier, Philadelphia, 2010, pp. 73–78.

Koepke GH, Smith EM, Murphy AJ, Dickinson DG. Sequence of action of the diaphragm and intercostal muscles during respiration: I. Inspiration. *Arch Phys Med Rehabil* 1958;39:426–430.

Preston DC, Shapiro BE. *Electromyography and neuromuscular disorders. Clinical-electrophysiologic correlations*. 2nd ed. Philadelphia, Elsevier Butterworth Heinemann, 2005, p. 655.

Tripp HF, Bolton JWR. Phrenic nerve injury following cardiac surgery: a review. *J Cardiac Surg* 1998;13:218–223.

Diaphragm

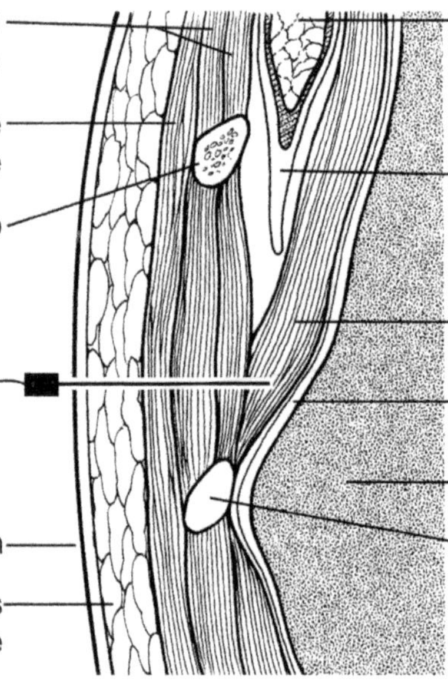

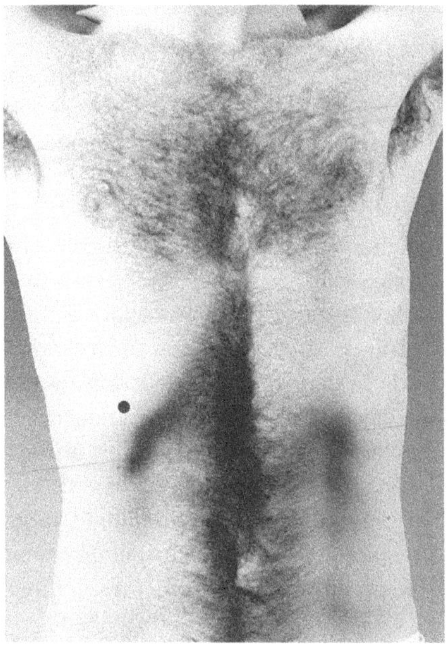

The technique of needle EMG of the diaphragm (adopted from Koepke et al., 1958 and Bolton, 1993). EMG is recorded with the needle inserted at right angles to the chest wall in any one of several interspaces between the anterior axillary and medial clavicular lines (see Figure 16-2; in this example the needle is inserted between the seventh and eighth rib interspace). There is at least 1.5 cm between the pleura above and the lower costal margin below, upon which the diaphragm inserts. Bursts of motor unit potentials characteristically occur with each inspiration when the needle is in the diaphragm. The various structures that the needle traverses in reaching the diaphragm are shown. The distance between the cartilaginous lower costal margin and the pleural reflection is about 1.5 cm. In quiet respiration, the lung is well removed from the path of the needle. Entry of the needle into the peritoneum is associated with pain and loss of muscle insertional activity.

Innervation

Innervation is via the anterior rami of C_3, C_4, and C_5 ("C_3, C_4, C_5 keep the diaphragm alive").

Origin

The diaphragm originates at the circumference of the thoracic cavity. The diaphragm separates the thorax from the abdomen.

Insertion

Anteriorly and laterally: Insertion is to the inner surface of the xiphoid cartilage and cartilages and bony portions of the six or seven inferior ribs.

Posteriorly: Insertion is to the aponeurotic arches and crura that attach to the lumbar vertebrae.

Activation Maneuver

There is activation of the diaphragm with each inspiration. Motor unit potentials (MUPs) in the diaphragm are of shorter duration and smaller amplitude, but are more numerous than MUPs from chest wall muscles (the needle will first pass through the external oblique or rectus abdominis muscles and the external and internal intercostal muscles before entering the diaphragm). With quiet respiration, the chest wall muscles do not fire or only recruit a few MUPs (Bolton, 1993).

EMG Needle Insertion

Introduce the needle at a right angle to the chest wall in any one of several interspaces (usually the seventh, eighth, or ninth rib interspace) between the anterior axillary and midclavicular lines. *The needle should be inserted just above the costal margin*, where there is an approximately 1.5 cm distance between the pleural reflection and the lower costal cartilage upon which the diaphragm inserts (see illustrations and Figure 16-2). Thus, the needle does not traverse either the pleural space or the lung.

Pitfalls

If the needle is inserted too deeply, it will enter the peritoneum. Entry of the needle into the peritoneum produces pain and loss of muscle insertional activity.

If the needle is inserted below the costal margin or at a more proximal interspace, it may penetrate the neurovascular bundle (intercostal nerve, artery, and vein) and continue into the pleura and lung.

Clinical Comments

The technique is reported to be safe, causes little discomfort, and provides good recordings of diaphragm activity (Bolton et al., 1992; Bolton, 1993).

Pneumothorax is a rare complication of this technique, particularly in patients with chronic obstructive pulmonary disease. Some investigators believe that the risk-to-benefit ratio of sampling this muscle is too high to justify its assessment in routine electromyography (Preston and Shapiro, 2005).

Neurogenic changes, including abnormal spontaneous activity, can be recorded from chest wall muscles and diaphragm (Bolton, 1993).

If there is total denervation of the diaphragm, MUPs will not fire with attempted inspiration. Hence, an important sign that the needle is in the diaphragm will be lost.

The phrenic nerve may be unilaterally damaged, as in radiculopathy, tumor, trauma, or surgery.

In high cervical spinal cord injury, denervation will usually be present in one or both diaphragms; MUPs will recruit in a neurogenic pattern or not at all if denervation is complete.

Look for neurogenic changes in other C_3–C_5 innervated muscles to support the diagnosis of radiculopathy or high cervical spinal cord injury. Muscles to be examined include cervical paraspinals, trapezius, levator scapulae, and rhomboids.

17 SACRAL PLEXUS

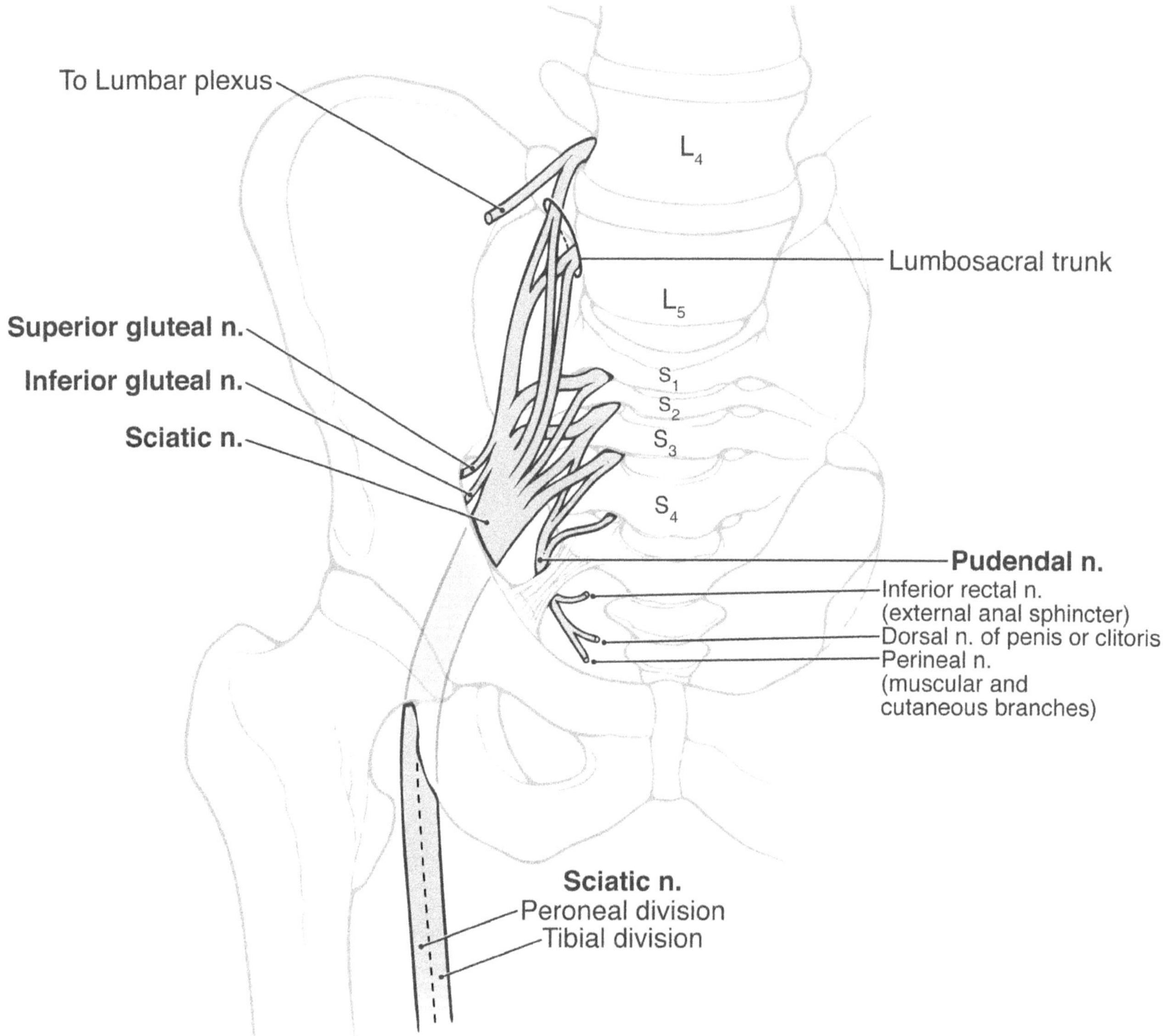

FIGURE 17-1 Diagram of the sacral plexus (anterior view) and its branches.

THE SACRAL PLEXUS is formed by the lumbosacral trunk (a small branch of the fourth lumbar ventral ramus that joins the fifth lumbar ventral ramus), the first through the third sacral ventral rami, and part of the fourth sacral ventral ramus (*Gray's Anatomy,* 1995). It adjoins the posterior pelvic wall anterior to the piriformis muscle and posterior to the internal iliac vessels, ureter, sigmoid colon, and terminal ileum. Pelvic fascia separates the sacral plexus from the viscera of the pelvis. The upper rami proceed obliquely downward and outward, while the lower rami proceed nearly horizontally. All rami converge toward the greater sciatic foramen and unite to form two cords, an upper, larger one and a lower, smaller cord. The upper, larger cord is formed by the lumbosacral trunk (L_4, L_5) and the first (S_1), second (S_2), and part of the third (S_3) sacral ventral rami. This cord becomes the *sciatic nerve*, which supplies the hamstring muscles (semitendinosus, semimembranosus, biceps femoris long and short heads) and the medial part of the adductor magnus, before splitting into tibial and common peroneal nerves. The lower, smaller cord is formed by portions of the second (S_2), third (S_3), and fourth (S_4) sacral ventral rami. This becomes the *pudendal nerve*, which provides muscular and cutaneous innervation to the perineum and pelvic floor. The sacral plexus also gives rise to the *superior gluteal nerve* (L_4, L_5, S_1), which supplies the gluteus medius, gluteus minimus, and tensor fasciae latae; the *inferior gluteal nerve* (L_5, S_1, S_2) to the gluteus maximus; the posterior cutaneous nerve of the thigh (S_1, S_2, S_3); and the perforating cutaneous nerve (S_2, S_3). In addition, muscular branches of the sacral plexus innervate short muscles around the hip joint, including quadratus femoris and gemellus inferior (L_4, L_5, S_1), obturator internus and gemellus superior (L_5, S_1, S_2), and piriformis (S_1, S_2). These muscles are largely inaccessible to direct observation and, because of their intimate relationship to important neurovascular structures, they are usually avoided in the routine needle EMG examination. The sacral plexus can also be divided into anterior and posterior divisions, with the tibial portion of the sciatic nerve formed by the anterior division and the peroneal portion formed by the posterior division.

A lesion of the sacral plexus produces a clinical picture similar to that seen with a sciatic nerve lesion, but with additional involvement of the gluteal muscles, tensor fasciae latae, and, occasionally, the anal sphincter.

SACRAL PLEXUS LESION

Etiology

Tumors and metastatic lesions can cause a sacral plexus lesion. Malignant infiltration is the most common cause of involvement of the lumbosacral plexus, usually due to spread of carcinoma of the cervix, uterus, prostate, or rectum (*Gray's Anatomy,* 1995).

Neuralgic amyotrophy (also known as *idiopathic lumbosacral plexopathy, acute idiopathic mononeuropathy*, or *lumbosacral plexus neuropathy*; Kimura, 1989) is causative.

Trauma, including pelvic fractures, stab wounds, or gunshot wounds, can cause a sacral plexus lesion.

Traction injury during orthopedic or other surgical manipulation (common during hip joint replacement) can cause a sacral plexus lesion.

Radiation plexopathy is causative.

Compression plexopathy occurs due to retroperitoneal hematomas, usually in hemophiliacs, in those with coagulopathies, or during anticoagulation therapy.

Compression lesions against the bony pelvis also occur, and affect the common peroneal fibers maximally or exclusively. The greater vulnerability of the peroneal fibers is due, in part, to the more direct relationship of the posterior division, which comprises peroneal fibers, with the bony pelvis (Sunderland, 1968).

General Comments

Malignant infiltration usually gives rise to *painful* and slowly progressive paralysis unilaterally (Kimura, 1989).

Radiation plexopathy causes very slowly progressive, *painless* leg weakness, often bilateral.

Neuralgic amyotrophy is characterized by acute pain in one or both legs that precedes the onset of weakness and areflexia.

Clinical Features

The distribution of weakness is similar to that seen with a sciatic nerve lesion.

There can be additional weakness of the gluteal muscles, tensor fasciae latae, or anal sphincter.

Wasting of lower limb muscles occurs.

Numbness occurs over the posterior thigh, lateral half of the leg, and entire foot.

There is an absent or reduced Achilles stretch reflex.

Electrodiagnostic Strategy

Use nerve conduction studies to confirm a lesion involving the sacral plexus (absent or low amplitude sensory responses from sural and superficial peroneal nerves, absent or low amplitude motor responses from tibial and peroneal nerves, absent or delayed H-reflex responses). Sensory responses are usually normal in radiculopathies because the lesion is proximal to the dorsal root ganglion (preganglionic lesion) and the cell bodies in the ganglion maintain viability of peripheral sensory fibers.

Demonstrate neurogenic EMG needle examination (i.e., spontaneous activity, abnormal motor unit potentials, and abnormal recruitment) in muscles supplied by the sacral plexus.

Use needle EMG to exclude lumbosacral radiculopathies. Radiculopathies produce neurogenic findings in paraspinal muscles as well as in limb muscles; plexopathies never do so because the plexus is formed by *ventral rami*, whereas paraspinal muscles are innervated by *posterior rami* (Wilbourn, 1985).

REFERENCES

Gray's Anatomy. 38th Edition. Churchill Livingstone, New York, 1995, pp. 1282–1288.

Kimura J. *Electrodiagnosis in Diseases of Nerve and Muscle.* 2nd Edition. FA Davis, Philadelphia, 1989, pp. 456–457.

Sunderland S. *Nerves and Nerve Injuries.* Williams & Wilkins, Baltimore, 1968, pp. 1069–1095.

Wilbourn AJ. Electrodiagnosis of plexopathies. *Neurol Clin* 1985;3:511–529.

SCIATIC NERVE

18

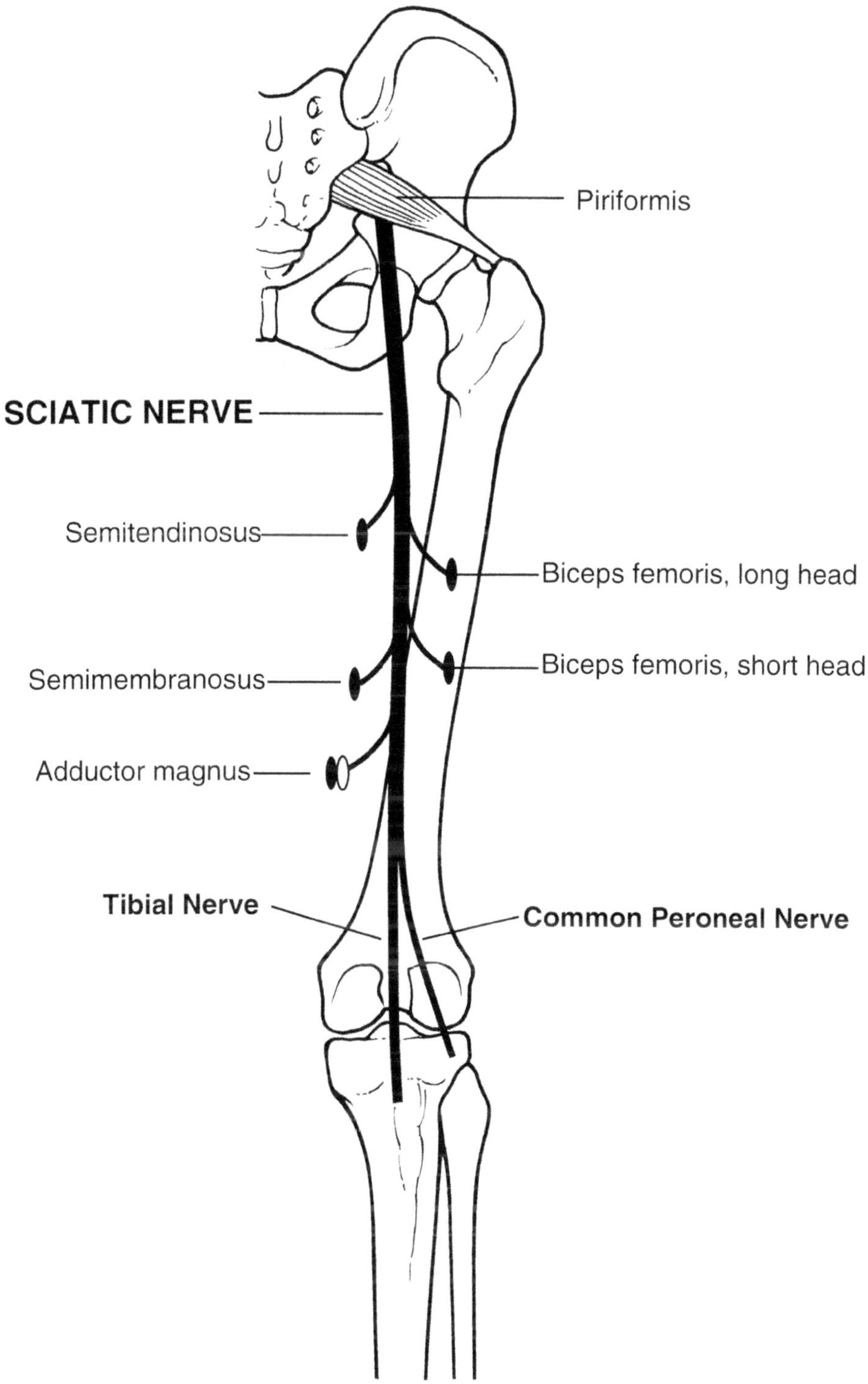

FIGURE 18-1 Diagram of the sciatic nerve (posterior view) and its branches. Note: The white oval signifies that a muscle receives part of its innervation from another peripheral nerve.

THE SCIATIC NERVE is a continuation of the upper, larger cord of the sacral plexus, and is formed by the lumbosacral trunk (L_4, L_5) and the first, second, and part of the third sacral ventral rami (*Gray's Anatomy,* 1995). It is the broadest nerve of the human body (2 cm at its origin) and is composed of independent tibial and common peroneal divisions that are usually united as far as the lower part of the thigh, although simple dissection reveals the double structure. In about 10% of cases, the two divisions remain distinct from the outset. The sciatic nerve leaves the pelvis via the greater sciatic foramen below the lower margin of the *piriformis* muscle and descends between the greater trochanter of the femur and ischial tuberosity along the back of the thigh. Just above the popliteal fossa it separates into its two terminal divisions.

In the gluteal region (after emerging below the piriformis), the nerve is deep to the gluteus maximus. On leaving the gluteal region, the nerve continues down the midline of the thigh closely related to the shaft of the femur. Muscular branches are given to the biceps femoris (the short head is supplied by peroneal division and the long head by tibial division), semitendinosus, semimembranosus, and the ischiocondylar part of the adductor magnus. Articular branches supply the hip joint.

Although the sciatic nerve, or its branches, may be involved by penetrating injuries at any level, there are regions where the nerve is prone to certain types of injury. Anatomical features of particular clinical significance are found in the pelvis (see Chapter 17), the gluteal region, and the thigh (Sunderland, 1968). On leaving the pelvis, the nerve may rarely be entrapped by the piriformis muscle (piriformis syndrome). In the gluteal region, the sciatic nerve is at risk because the buttock is a common site for therapeutic injections. The nerve is also intimately related to the hip joint and may be involved with injuries to that joint. Damage may also occur during operations on the hip joint or femur. In the thigh, the nerve may be injured during fractures of the femur or when compressed against the firm edge of a seat.

SCIATIC NERVE LESION

Etiology

Tumors and metastatic lesions can cause a sciatic nerve lesion.

Trauma, including hip fracture or dislocation, or more distal fractures of the femur can cause a sciatic nerve lesion.

A traction injury can occur during orthopedic or other surgical manipulation (common during hip joint replacement).

Radiation therapy (usually related to radiation plexopathy) is causative.

Compression injury can occur in the gluteal region. As the nerve appears from beneath the gluteus maximus, it is relatively superficial and may be compressed when seated on a firm surface. Common peroneal fibers are maximally or exclusively affected (Sunderland, 1968).

Entrapment by the piriformis muscle (piriformis syndrome) is an uncommon cause of sciatic pain or "sciatica" that involves the buttock and leg. However, this syndrome is controversial and there is some doubt as to whether such an entrapment exists (Halpin and Ganju, 2009; Tiel, 2008).

Intramuscular injections can cause a sciatic nerve lesion. The nerve may be damaged by the needle, by sclerosing or toxic agents, or later by scarring that follows the tissue reaction (Sunderland, 1968).

General Comments

Malignant infiltration usually involves the nerve roots contributing to the formation of the sciatic nerve in the pelvis. It gives rise to *painful* and slowly progressive paralysis unilaterally (Kimura, 1989).

Radiation injury causes very slowly progressive *painless* leg weakness.

There is a greater vulnerability of the common peroneal fibers to most injuries of the sciatic nerve. This may be related to various factors, including the more exposed position of the peroneal division in the thigh, and to the poorer blood supply (less nutrient arteries). In addition, the size, number, and disposition of the funiculi may predispose the peroneal division to injury because it is composed of fewer and larger bundles with less connective tissue than the tibial division. Peroneal fibers are also securely fixed at both the sciatic notch and the neck of the fibula, and therefore subjected to greater stretch (Sunderland, 1968).

Clinical Features

Weakness or wasting involves the hamstring muscles as well as the muscles supplied by the common peroneal and tibial nerves.

Numbness occurs over the lateral half of the leg and the entire foot.

The Achilles stretch reflex is absent or reduced.

Electrodiagnostic Strategy

Use nerve conduction studies to confirm a lesion involving the tibial and common peroneal fibers (absent or low amplitude sensory responses from sural and superficial peroneal nerves, absent or low amplitude motor responses from tibial and peroneal nerves, absent or delayed H-reflex response).

Demonstrate neurogenic EMG needle examination (i.e., spontaneous activity, abnormal motor unit potentials, abnormal recruitment) in muscles supplied by the sciatic nerve (hamstrings) and muscles supplied by the common peroneal and tibial nerves.

Use needle EMG to exclude lumbosacral radiculopathies. Radiculopathies produce neurogenic findings in paraspinal muscles as well as in limb muscles; peripheral nerve injury never does so because the peripheral nerve is formed by the *ventral rami,* whereas the paraspinal muscles are innervated by the *posterior rami* (Wilbourn, 1985).

REFERENCES

Gray's Anatomy. 38th Edition. Churchill Livingstone, New York, 1995, pp. 1282–1288.

Halpin RJ, Ganju A. Piriformis syndrome: a real pain in the buttock? *Neurosurgery* 2009;65(4 Suppl):A197–202.

Kimura J. *Electrodiagnosis in Diseases of Nerve and Muscle.* 2nd Edition. FA Davis, Philadelphia, 1989, pp 456–457.

Sunderland S. *Nerves and Nerve Injuries.* Williams & Wilkins, Baltimore, 1968, pp. 1069–1095.

Tiel RL. Piriformis and related entrapment syndromes: myth & fallacy. *Neurosurg Clin N Am* 2008;19:623–627.

Wilbourn AJ. Electrodiagnosis of plexopathies. *Neurol Clin* 1985;3:511–529.

Wilbourn AJ. AAEE case report #12: Common peroneal mononeuropathy at the fibular head. *Muscle Nerve* 1986;9:825–836.

Semitendinosus

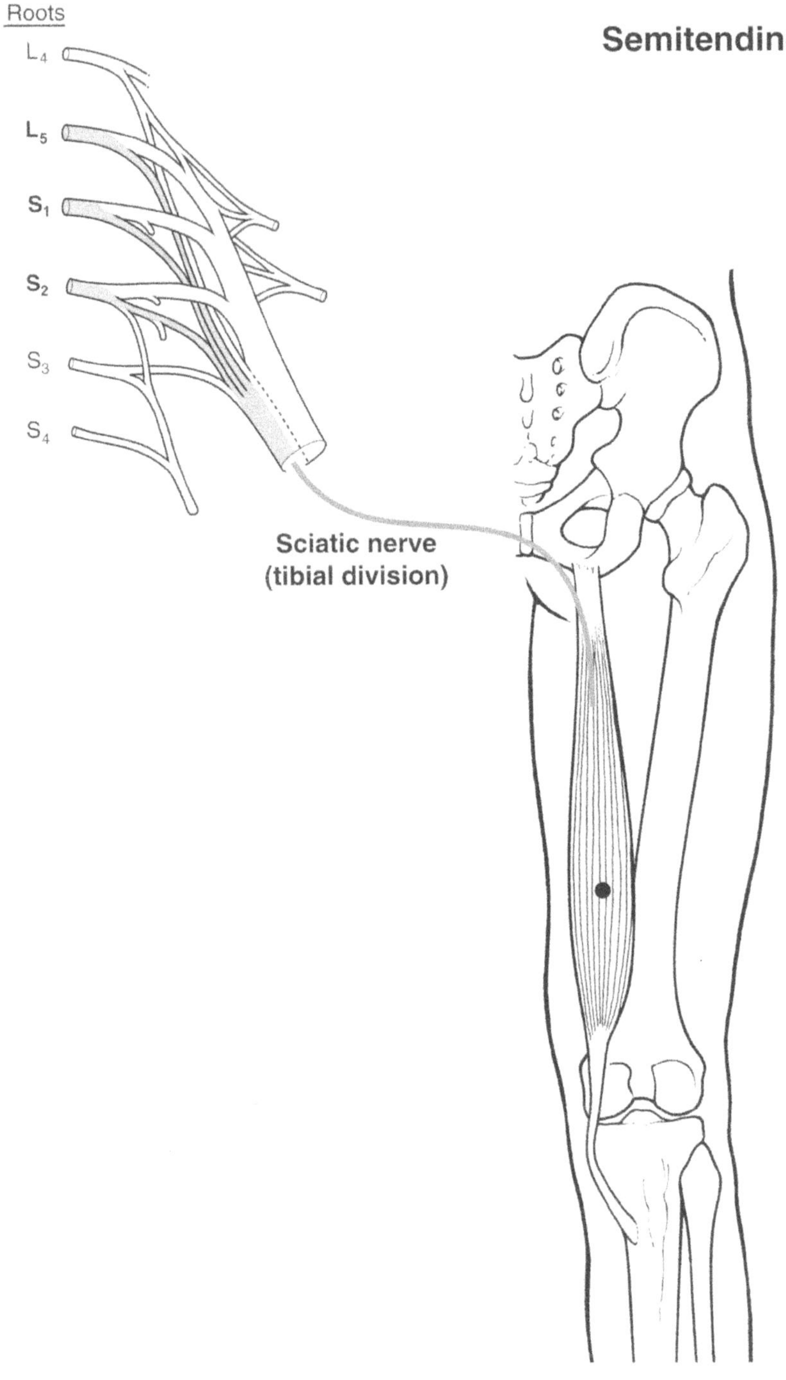

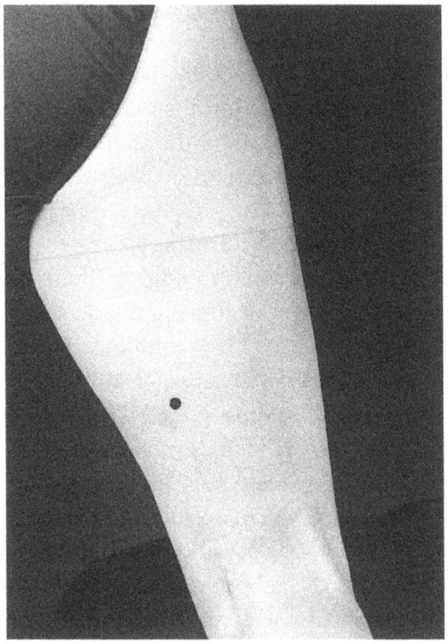

Innervation

Innervation is via the sciatic nerve (tibial division), sacral plexus, and roots L_5, S_1, S_2.

Origin

The semitendinosus originates at the ischial tuberosity.

Insertion

Insertion is at the upper part of the medial surface of the shaft of the tibia.

Activation Maneuver

Flexion of the knee activates the muscle. Note: The "hamstrings" cross both hip and knee joints, integrating extension at the hip with flexion of the knee. In addition, the semitendinosus can act as a medial rotator of the leg.

EMG Needle Insertion

Insert the needle one-third to midway along a line connecting the semitendinosus tendon (easily palpable as it forms the proximal medial margin of the popliteal fossa) with the ischial tuberosity.

Pitfalls

There are no pitfalls. If the needle is inserted too laterally, it may be in the biceps femoris long head, which is also supplied by the tibial division of sciatic nerve and roots L_5, S_1, and S_2. If the needle is inserted too medially, it may be in the semimembranosus (also the tibial division of the sciatic nerve and roots L_5, S_1, S_2).

Clinical Comments

Neurogenic changes on needle examination may be seen with lesions of the tibial division of the sciatic nerve, sacral plexus, and roots L_5, S_1, or S_2.

Semimembranosus

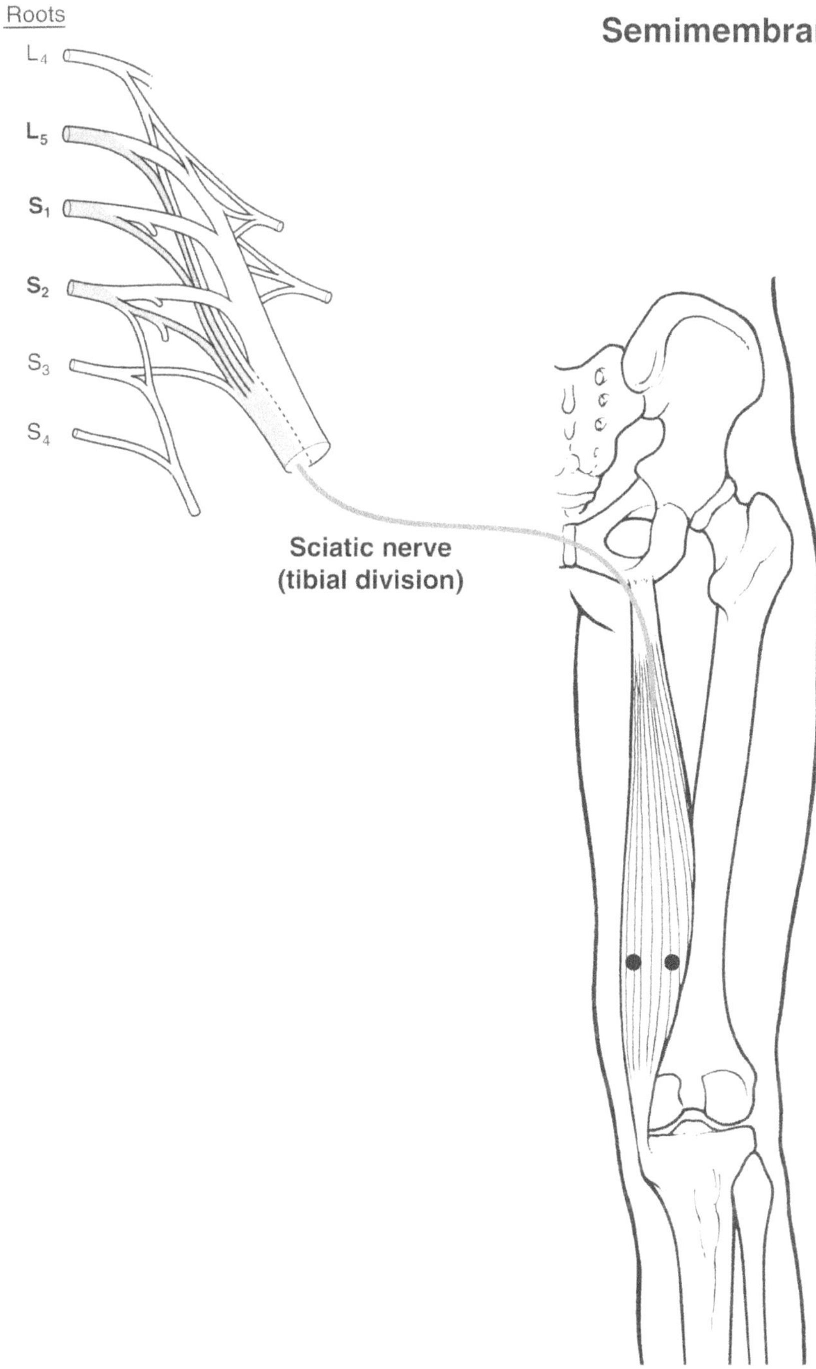

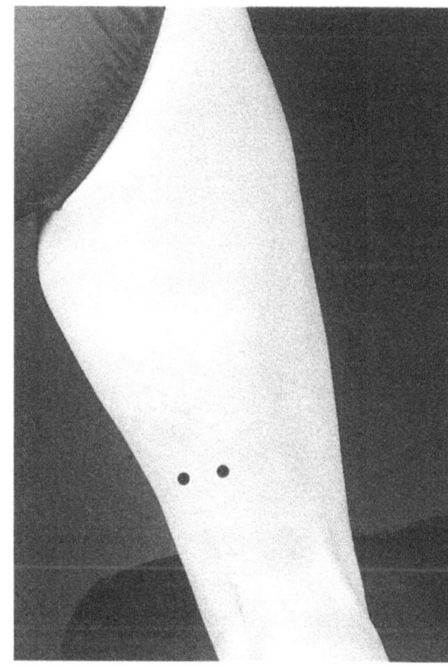

Innervation

Innervation is via the sciatic nerve (tibial division), sacral plexus, and roots L_5, S_1, S_2.

Origin

The semimembranosus originates at the ischial tuberosity.

Insertion

Insertion is at the medial condyle of the tibia (major insertion); it also inserts on the medial shaft of the tibia and the fascia over the popliteus and contributes to an expansion that inserts on the lateral femoral condyle.

Activation Maneuver

Flexion of the knee activates the muscle. Note: The "hamstrings" cross both hip and knee joints, integrating extension at the hip with flexion of the knee. In addition, the semimembranosus can act as a medial rotator of the leg.

EMG Needle Insertion

Palpate the semitendinosus tendon in the proximal popliteal fossa. Insert the needle on either side of the semitendinosus tendon.

Pitfalls

If the needle is inserted too laterally, it may be in the biceps femoris short head, which is supplied by the peroneal division of the sciatic nerve and roots L_5, S_1, S_2.

If the needle is inserted too medially and proximally, it may be in the adductor magnus or gracilis. The adductor magnus is supplied by the obturator nerve (L_2–L_4 roots) and the tibial division of the sciatic nerve (L_4 root), while the gracilis receives innervation from the obturator nerve (L_2–L_4 roots).

Clinical Comments

Neurogenic changes on needle examination may be seen with lesions of the tibial division of the sciatic nerve, sacral plexus, and roots L_5, S_1 or S_2.

Biceps Femoris (Long Head)

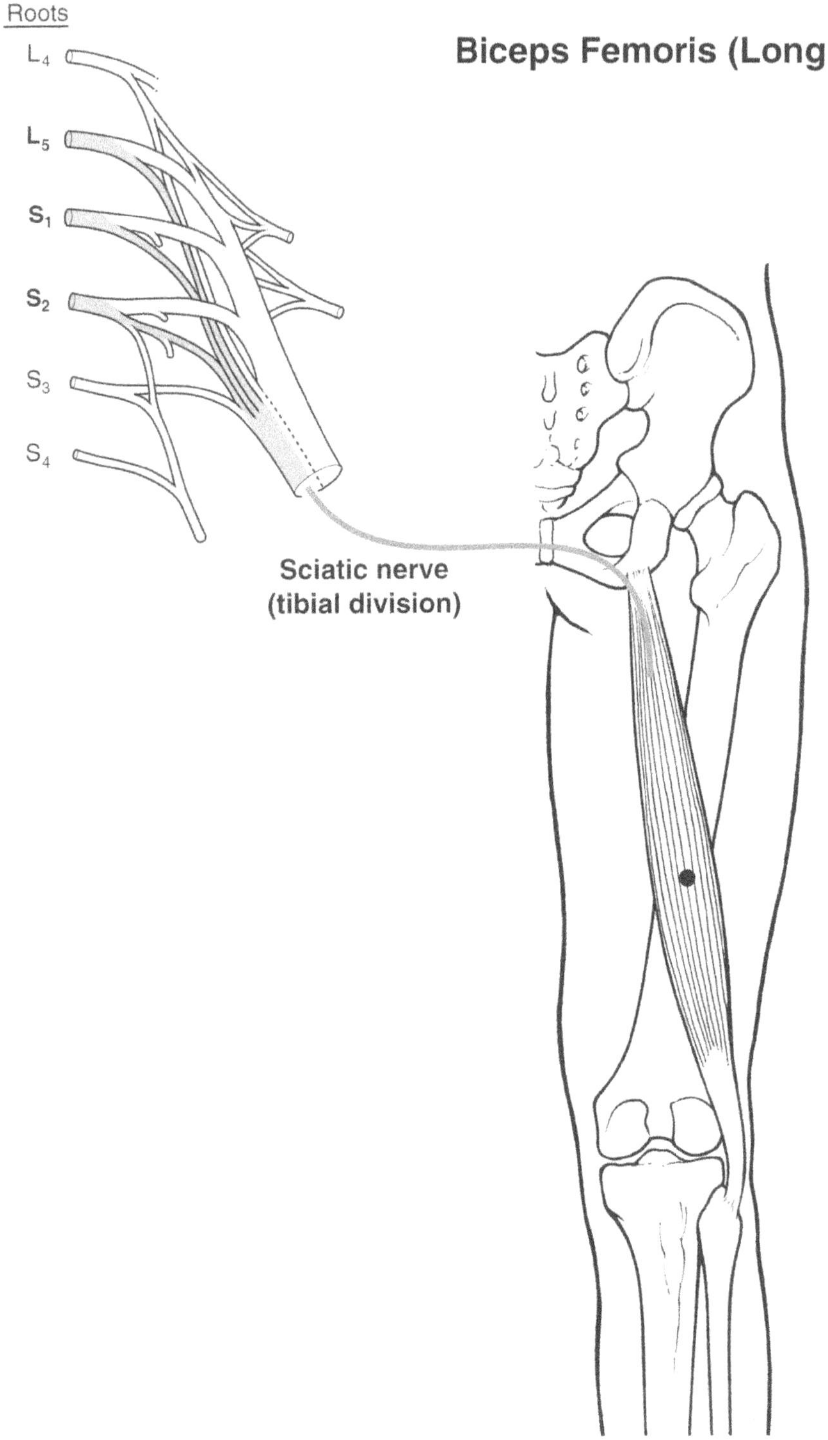

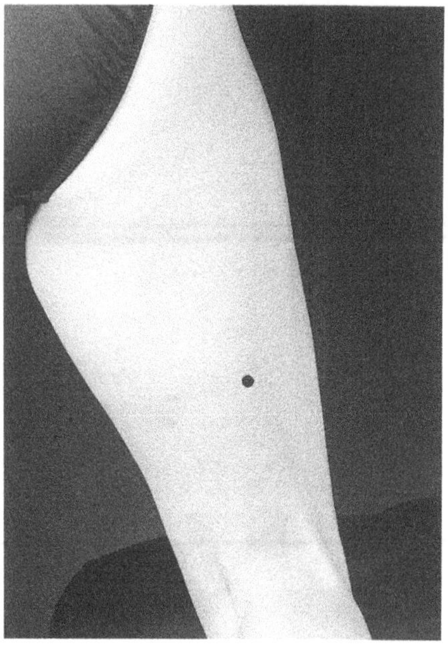

Innervation

Innervation is via the sciatic nerve (tibial division), sacral plexus, and roots L_5, S_1, S_2.

Origin

The long head of the biceps femoris originates at the ischial tuberosity.

Insertion

Insertion is at the head of the fibula.

Activation Maneuver

Flexion of the knee activates the muscle. Note: The "hamstrings" cross both hip and knee joints, integrating extension at the hip with flexion of the knee. In addition, the biceps femoris can act as a lateral rotator of the leg.

EMG Needle Insertion

Insert the needle one-third to midway along a line connecting the fibular head with the ischial tuberosity.

Pitfalls

If the needle is inserted too distally, it may be in the short head of the biceps femoris, which is supplied by the peroneal division of the sciatic nerve and roots L_5, S_1, S_2 (at the mid-thigh, the fibers of the short head are narrow and deep).

If the needle is inserted too laterally, it may be in the vastus lateralis, which is supplied by the femoral nerve (L_2–L_4 roots).

If the needle is inserted too medially, it may be in the semitendinosus, which is also supplied by the tibial division of the sciatic nerve (L_5–S_2 roots).

Clinical Comments

Neurogenic changes on needle examination may be seen with lesions of the tibial division of the sciatic nerve, sacral plexus, and roots L_5, S_1, or S_2.

Biceps Femoris (Short Head)

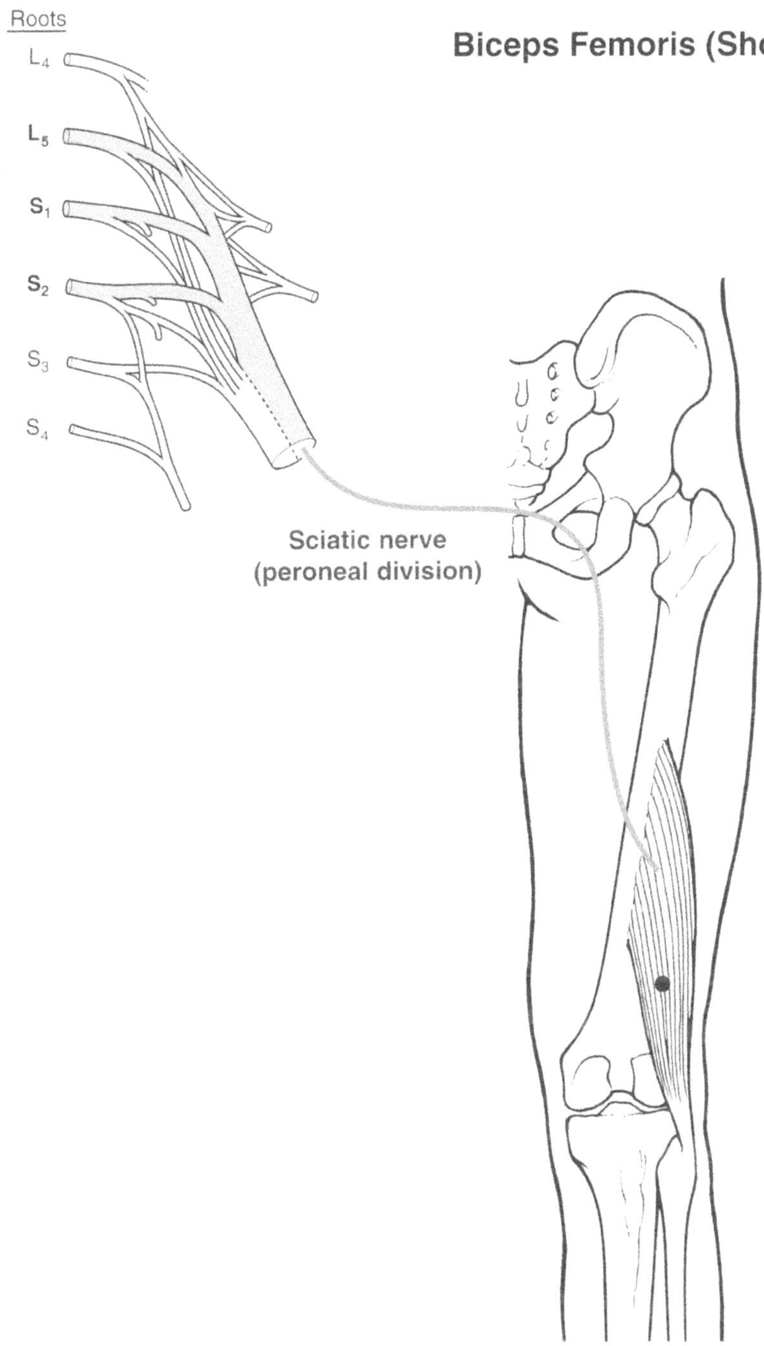

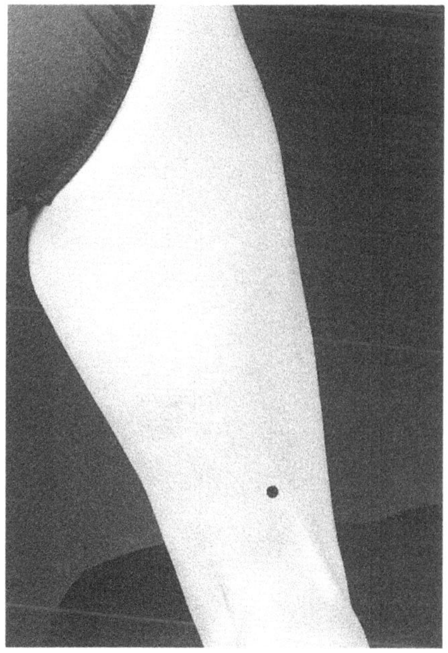

Insert the needle just medial to the tendon.

Pitfalls

If the needle is inserted too laterally it may penetrate the long head of the biceps femoris, which is supplied by the tibial division of the sciatic nerve (roots L_5, S_1, S_2).

If the needle is inserted too medially, it may be in the semimembranosus, which is supplied by the tibial division of the sciatic nerve (roots L_5, S_1, S_2).

Innervation

Innervation is via the sciatic nerve (peroneal division), sacral plexus, and roots L_5, S_1, S_2.

Origin

The short head of the biceps femoris originates at the lateral lip of the linea aspera on the posterolateral surface of the shaft of the femur, and from the lateral intermuscular septum.

Insertion

Insertion is at the head of the fibula.

Activation Maneuver

Flexion of the knee activates the muscle. The short head of the biceps femoris does not cross the hip joint; it cannot contribute to hip extension, but it can act as a lateral rotator of the leg.

EMG Needle Insertion

Palpate the tendon of the long head of the biceps femoris in the popliteal fossa.

Clinical Comments

Neurogenic changes on needle examination may be seen with lesions of the peroneal division of the sciatic nerve, sacral plexus, and L_5, S_1, or S_2 roots.

This is the only muscle in the thigh innervated by the peroneal division of the sciatic nerve.

This muscle is of great importance in the electrodiagnostic evaluation of peroneal nerve lesions because it is crucial in defining the proximal extent of the lesion. If neurogenic EMG changes are present in this muscle, the lesion must be at or proximal to the mid-thigh (Wilbourn, 1986).

19 TIBIAL NERVE

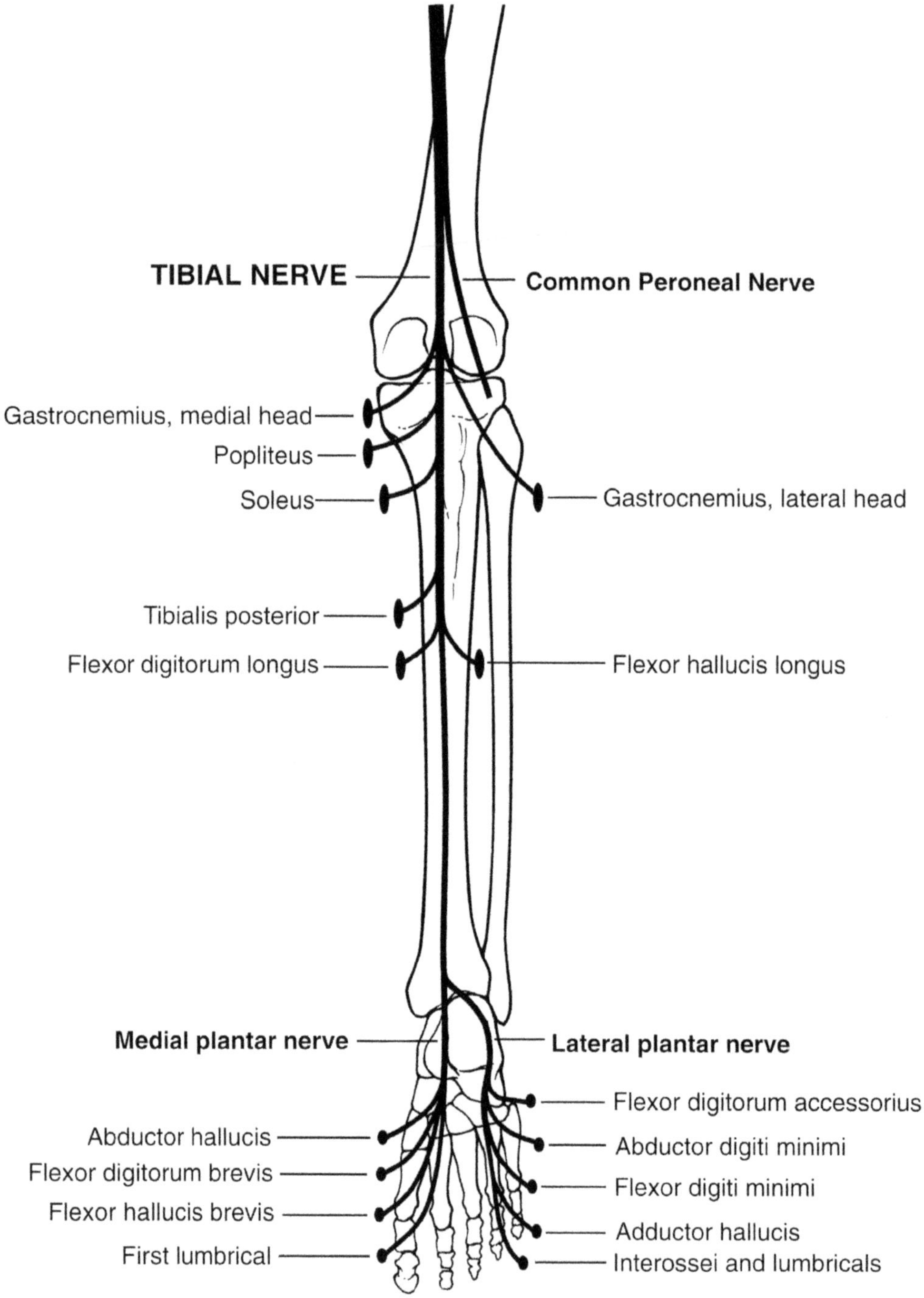

FIGURE 19-1 Diagram of the tibial nerve (posterior view) and its branches.

THE TIBIAL NERVE (also known as the *posterior tibial nerve*) is the larger sciatic division and is formed by the fourth and fifth lumbar and the first to third sacral ventral rami (Gray's Anatomy, 1995). It descends along the back of the thigh and the popliteal fossa to the distal border of the popliteus muscle, passing anterior to the aponeurotic arch of the soleus with the popliteal artery and vein to enter the leg. In the distal thigh, it is overlapped by the hamstring muscles, but becomes more superficial in the popliteal fossa where it is lateral to the popliteal vessels, becoming superficial to them at the knee and crossing to the medial side of the vessels as it enters the leg. In the distal fossa, it is overlapped by the junction of the two heads of the gastrocnemius muscles.

In the leg, the tibial nerve descends with the posterior tibial artery and vein, crossing lateral to the vessels. Proximally, the nerve is deep to the soleus and gastrocnemius, but in the distal one-third of the leg it is covered only by skin and fascia, sometimes overlapped by the flexor hallucis longus. It reaches the medial malleolus, ending under the flexor retinaculum, where it divides into medial and lateral plantar nerves.

The tibial nerve gives off articular branches to the knee joint. Just before it divides it also supplies the ankle joint. Most of the articular branches are nociceptive in nature. Muscular branches supply the two heads of the gastrocnemius, plantaris (a small, almost vestigial muscle that is the lower limb equivalent of the palmaris longus), soleus, popliteus, tibialis posterior, flexor digitorum longus, and flexor hallucis longus. Cutaneous branches include the sural and medial calcaneal nerves. The *sural nerve* is joined by a sural communicating branch of the common peroneal nerve and descends along the calf and lateral border of the Achilles tendon to the region between the lateral malleolus and the calcaneus. It supplies the posterior and lateral skin of the distal third of the leg, the skin overlying the lateral malleolus, and the lateral aspect of the foot and little toe (Sunderland, 1968). The medial calcaneal branch supplies the skin of the heel and the medial side of the sole.

The *medial plantar nerve* also gives off articular, cutaneous, and muscular branches. The cutaneous branches supply the skin of the sole of the foot, including the digital branches to the hallux, the second, third, and half of the fourth toe (the digital branches of the medial plantar nerve are like those of the median nerve). Muscular branches supply the abductor hallucis, flexor digitorum brevis, flexor hallucis brevis, and the first lumbrical (the muscular branches of the medial plantar nerve also correspond closely with those of the median nerve).

The *lateral plantar nerve* supplies the skin of the fifth toe, the lateral half of the fourth toe, and the lateral part of the sole of the foot (like the ulnar nerve in the hand). Muscular branches supply most deep muscles of the foot, including the flexor digitorum accessorius, abductor digiti minimi (quinti), flexor digiti minimi brevis, interossei, second to fourth lumbricals, and adductor hallucis.

The tibial nerve, or its branches, may be involved by penetrating injuries at any level. Of the two terminal divisions of the sciatic nerve, however, the tibial is the more deeply situated and better protected (Sunderland, 1968). At the ankle, the tibial nerve may rarely be subjected to compression beneath the flexor retinaculum (tarsal tunnel). This may result in the *tarsal tunnel syndrome*.

TARSAL TUNNEL SYNDROME

Etiology

Tarsal tunnel syndrome is caused by compression of the tibial nerve or its branches in the tarsal tunnel (Figure 19-2).

General Comments

Tarsal tunnel syndrome is a rare entrapment neuropathy.

Symptoms usually involve one foot (Dawson et al., 1990), although they may be bilateral.

Predisposing conditions include trauma, such as fracture or dislocation at the ankle, deformity or hypermobility at the ankle, peripheral neuropathy, rheumatoid arthritis, or

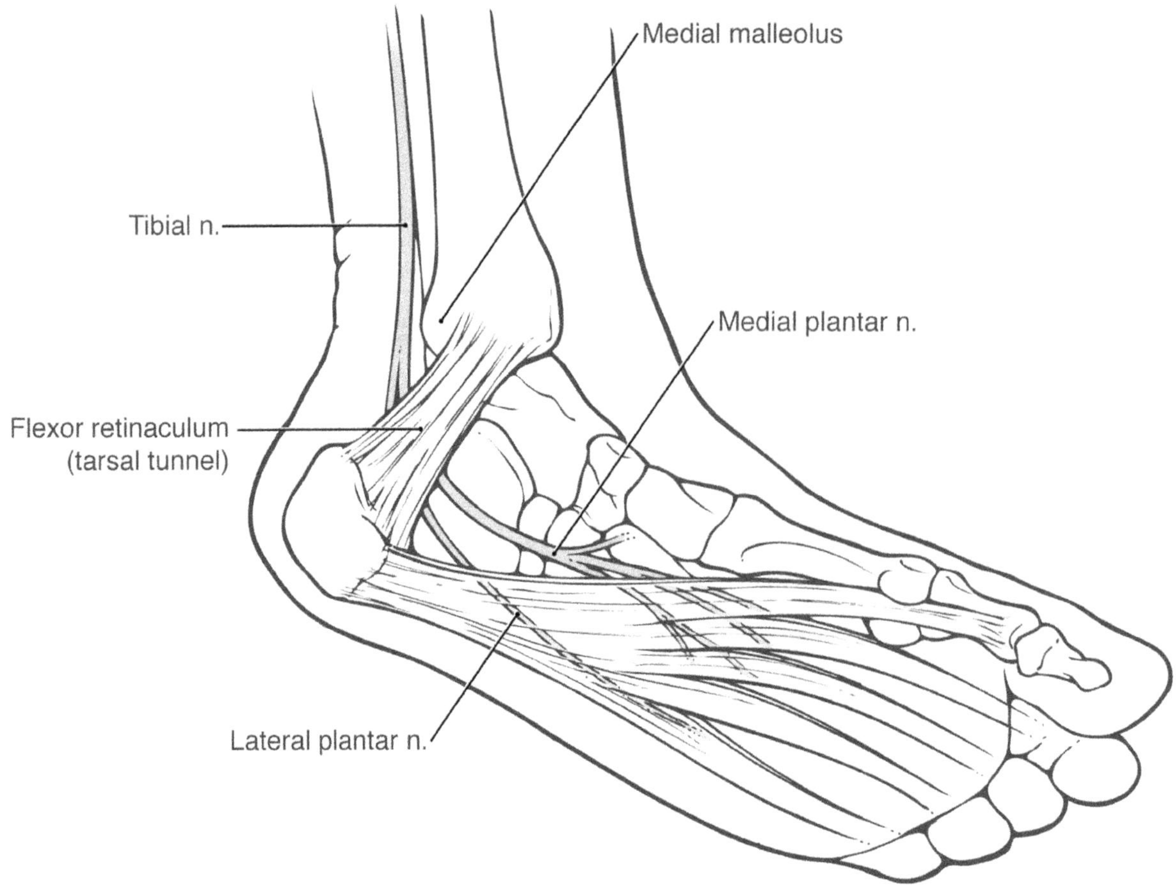

FIGURE 19-2 Anatomy of the tarsal tunnel.

other conditions associated with focal inflammation, and masses in the tunnel such as lipomas, ganglion cysts, or neoplasms.

Radiologic studies of the ankle may reveal evidence of degenerative arthritis, old fractures, bone spicules or accessory ossicles (DeLisa and Saeed, 1983).

Differential diagnoses include early polyneuropathy and orthopedic conditions such as plantar fasciitis and tendonitis.

Pes planus (flat feet) may predispose to lateral and medial plantar neuropathies due to chronic compression. This type of compression occurs in the sole of the foot rather than at the tarsal tunnel and typically manifests in obese individuals (Leis, personal observation).

Clinical Features

Pain, reportedly burning in quality, occurs in the sole of the foot.

Patients may awaken at night with symptoms (nocturnal paresthesias).

Numbness may involve the medial plantar or lateral plantar areas and occasionally the whole surface of the foot, including the medial calcaneal distribution (Dawson et al., 1990).

Tinel's sign over the tarsal tunnel may be present (Oh et al., 1979).

Weakness and atrophy of the intrinsic foot muscles are difficult to detect clinically.

Electrodiagnostic Strategy

Use nerve conduction studies to confirm a focal lesion of the tibial sensory or motor fibers in the tarsal tunnel. Techniques have been developed for identifying conduction abnormalities within the tarsal tunnel (Oh et al., 1979; DeLisa and Saeed, 1983).

Perform EMG needle examination in the foot muscles innervated by both the medial and lateral plantar nerves. In tarsal tunnel syndrome associated with loss of motor fibers,

EMG may show neurogenic changes (i.e., spontaneous activity, abnormal motor unit potentials, and abnormal recruitment).

If EMG examination of the foot muscles is abnormal, study the proximal tibial-innervated muscles to exclude a tibial nerve lesion above the ankle. Compare with the findings in the other foot, because tarsal tunnel syndrome is often unilateral. Also, study the S_1 and S_2 muscles innervated by other nerves to exclude radiculopathy.

TIBIAL NERVE CONDUCTION STUDIES

Tibial Motor Nerve Conduction Studies

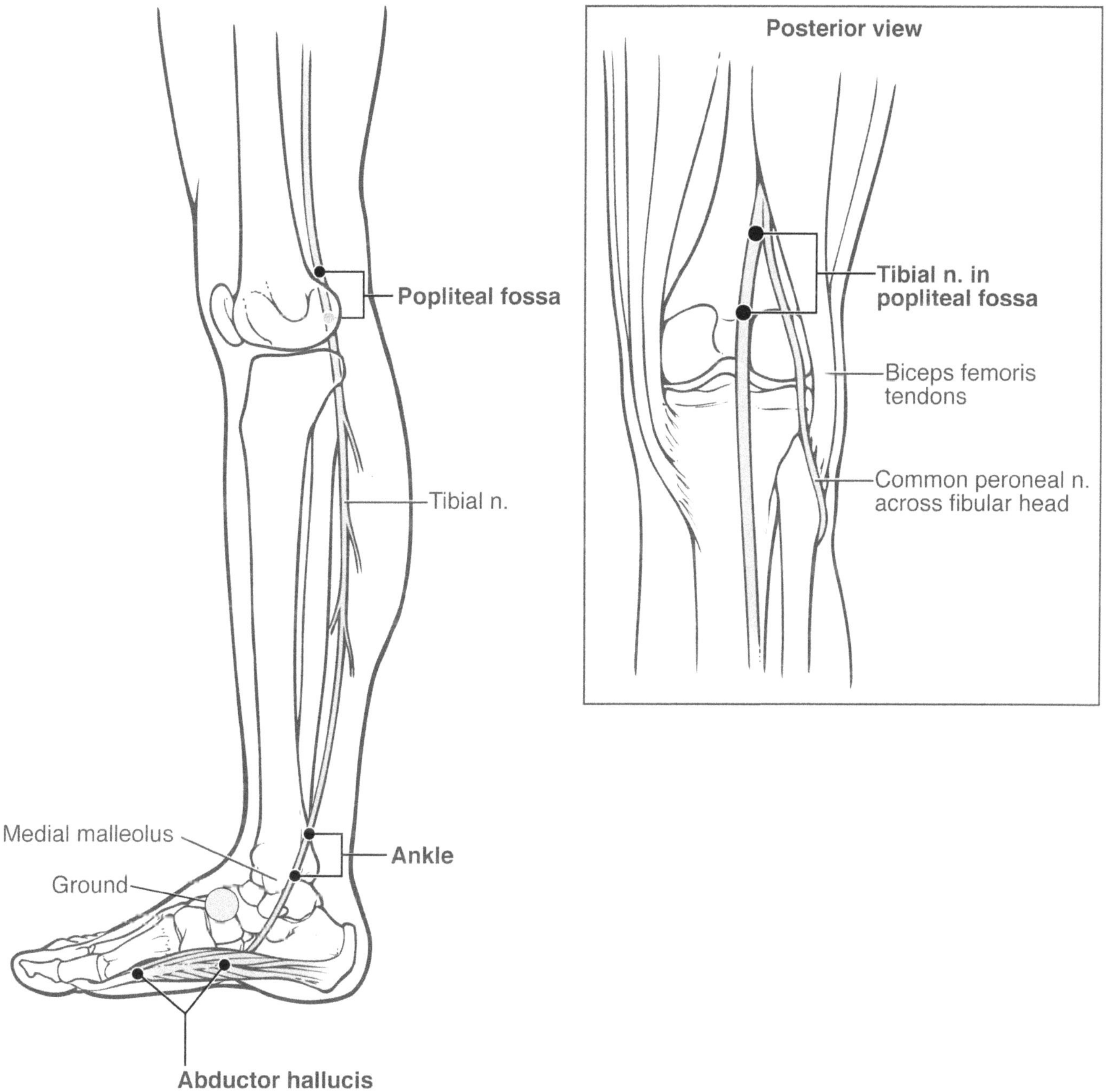

FIGURE 19-3 Tibial motor nerve conduction study.

Recording (Figure 19-3)

Active electrode: Position over the belly of the abductor hallucis muscle on the medial aspect of the foot directly beneath the navicular bone.

Reference electrode: Place distal to the active electrode over the tendon of the abductor hallucis muscle ("belly tendon" recording).

Ground electrode: Place on the dorsum of the foot, between stimulating and recording electrodes.

Stimulation

Ankle: Place cathode posterior to the medial malleolus. The anode is 3 cm proximal to cathode.

Popliteal fossa: Place cathode 1 to 2 finger breadths medial to the biceps femoris tendons. The anode is 3 cm proximal to cathode.

Comment

The tibial motor conduction study recording from abductor hallucis is performed routinely in most electrodiagnostic laboratories.

The tibial CMAP can also be recorded from the abductor digiti minimi quinti muscle (Preston and Shapiro, 2005). This provides additional conduction data about fascicles in the lateral plantar nerve.

Normal Values

Distal latency (ms) ≤ 6.0
Amplitude (mV) ≥ 3.5
Conduction velocity (m/s) ≥ 40 m/s

Normal values differ depending on the distance used. Tibial motor conduction studies should be performed bilaterally, because side-to-side comparisons are more useful than normal value tables. An amplitude ≤ 50 % of the unaffected side is evidence of abnormality.

Pitfalls

The tibial nerve lies relatively deep in the popliteal fossa and technical problems arise from submaximal stimulation, particularly in obese subjects. Greater pressure on the cathode and increased stimulus intensity and duration may be required to evoke the motor response. Accordingly, a drop in CMAP amplitude with popliteal fossa stimulation compared with ankle stimulation should not be misinterpreted as a conduction block.

Tibial F-waves

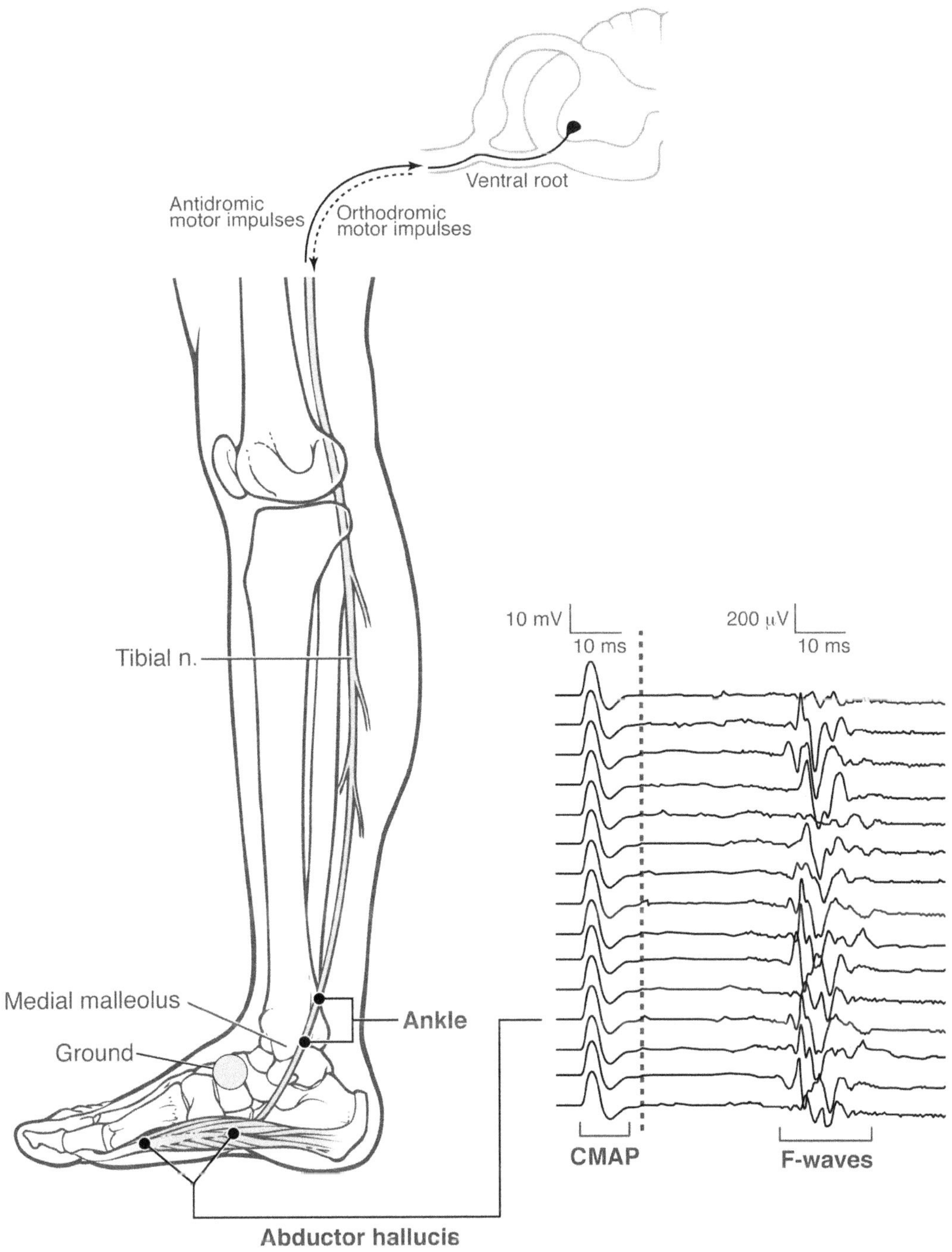

FIGURE 19-4 Tibial F-waves.

Recording F-waves (Figure 19-4)

Identical recording technique to that utilized to elicit the CMAP from abductor hallucis, except that the gain is set from 200 to 500 μV and sweep speed 10 ms/division to visualize this late response. At least 10 to 20 stimuli are delivered to elicit the F-wave responses.

Stimulation

Identical stimulation technique to that utilized for distal stimulation at the ankle (place cathode in the same site and deliver supramaximal stimuli). By convention, the anode is rotated 180 degrees from its original position to avoid the theoretical possibility of nerve hyperpolarization under the anode (anodal conduction block). However, in routine clinical practice, anodal block is not observed (Wee et al., 2000).

F-wave Measurements and Normal Values

Minimum F-wave latency is the most commonly obtained measurement. In leg muscles, upper limits of minimum F-wave latency are 44 ms for height 4'11" (150 cm), 53 ms for height 5'7" (170 cm) and 62 ms for height 6'3" (190 cm). A right–left asymmetry of minimal F-wave latency >3.5 ms in leg muscles is considered abnormal (Kimura, 1989; Fisher, 1992; Puksa et al. 2003).

Mean F-wave latency is calculated by adding all individual F-wave latencies and dividing this sum by the number of F-waves recorded (Fisher, 1992). The upper limits of normal for this value will be approximately 2 ms longer than minimum F-wave latency for the corresponding heights (Nobrega, et al. 2004).

Maximum F-wave latency is the longest onset latency of all recorded F-waves. The upper limits of this value will be about 4 ms longer than minimum F-wave latency for the corresponding heights (Nobrega et al., 2004).

F-wave dispersion (or chronodispersion) provides a measure of the range of conductions and is calculated as the difference between minimum and maximum F-wave latencies. In leg muscles, a typical upper limit of normal F-wave dispersion is <8 ms (Puksa et al., 2003). Excessive chronodispersion suggests temporal dispersion and demyelination.

F-wave amplitude usually measures <5% of the maximal CMAP or M-wave amplitude (F/M amplitude ratio). This is a measure of the proportion of the motor neuron pool activated by antidromic stimulation. F-wave amplitude may be increased in upper motor neuron dysfunction, especially when spasticity is present.

F-wave persistence is the percentage of F-waves obtained following a series of stimulations (i.e., the number of measureable F-waves divided by the number of stimuli). This reflects the antidromic excitability of a particular motor neuron pool (Fisher, 1992). F-wave persistence in median, ulnar, and tibial nerves is normally >50%, although in the peroneal nerve it can be <25%. F-wave persistence is often decreased in lower motor neuron dysfunction and increased in upper motor neuron dysfunction, particularly when spasticity is present.

Comments

In radiculopathy, F-waves are of limited value and less sensitive than needle EMG examination in assessing motor fiber involvement.

F-waves are commonly abnormal in a variety of axonal and demyelinating polyneuropathies. In Guillain-Barré syndrome, F-waves may be absent or delayed during the acute stages when other nerve conduction studies are normal. Increased F-wave dispersion suggests temporal dispersion and demyelination.

F-waves provide a means of assessing motor neuron excitability (Fisher, 1992). F-waves are typically absent or decreased in spinal shock (Leis et al., 1996) and early after acute stroke, compatible with a decreased central excitability state. In contrast, F-waves are typically increased in patients with established spasticity.

Sural Sensory Nerve Conduction Study

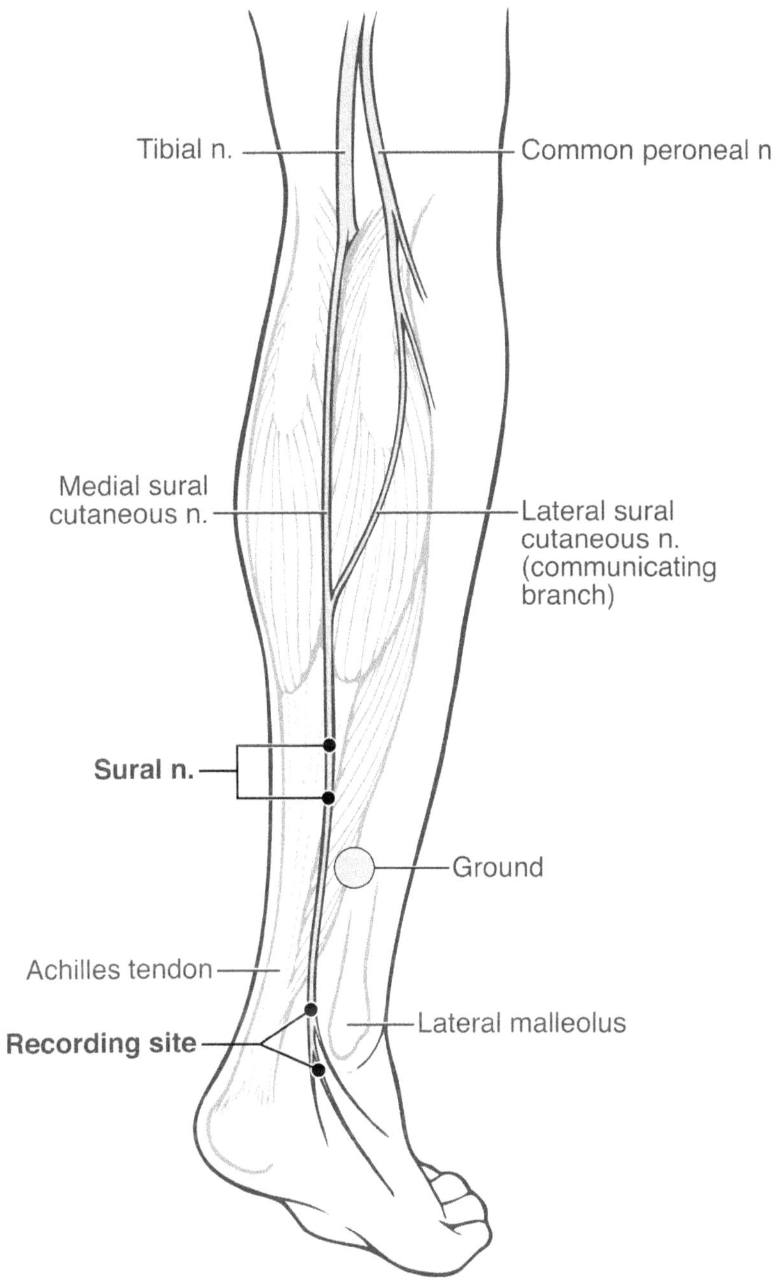

FIGURE 19-5 Sural sensory nerve conduction study (antidromic).

Recording (Figure 19-5)

Active electrode: Place between the lateral malleolus and the Achilles tendon.

Reference electrode: Place 3 cm distal to the active electrode.

Ground electrode: Place on the distal lateral leg, between stimulating and recording electrodes.

Stimulation

Leg: Place cathode over the distal posterolateral leg (slightly lateral to the midline of the posterior leg), 10 cm to 16 cm above the active recording electrode (most laboratories use 14 cm). The stimulator may need to be moved slightly laterally or medially to elicit a maximal sensory response. The anode is 3 cm proximal to cathode.

Normal Values

Latency (ms) ≤ 2.8 (onset latency); ≤ 3.5 (peak latency)
Amplitude (μV) ≥ 8
Conduction velocity (m/s) ≥ 40 m/s

Comments

The normal amplitude of the sural SNAP has a large range and standard deviation. Therefore, studies should ideally be performed bilaterally because side-to-side comparisons are more useful than normal value tables that may not apply to your patient. An amplitude ≤ 50 % of the unaffected side is evidence of abnormality.

Temperature has a profound effect on nerve conduction studies. Low temperature is common in feet, and will prolong distal latencies, slow conduction velocity, and increase action potential amplitudes (see Chapter 1).

Pedal edema will reduce the amplitude of foot sensory responses.

The sural nerve conduction study offers one of the most sensitive means of detecting abnormalities in various types of peripheral neuropathies (Kimura, 1989).

Although the sural nerve is joined by a communicating branch from the common peroneal nerve, this conduction technique only evaluates the tibial component. Hence, the sural sensory response is characteristically reduced or absent in axonal loss lesions involving the tibial nerve and spared in peroneal nerve lesions.

H-reflex

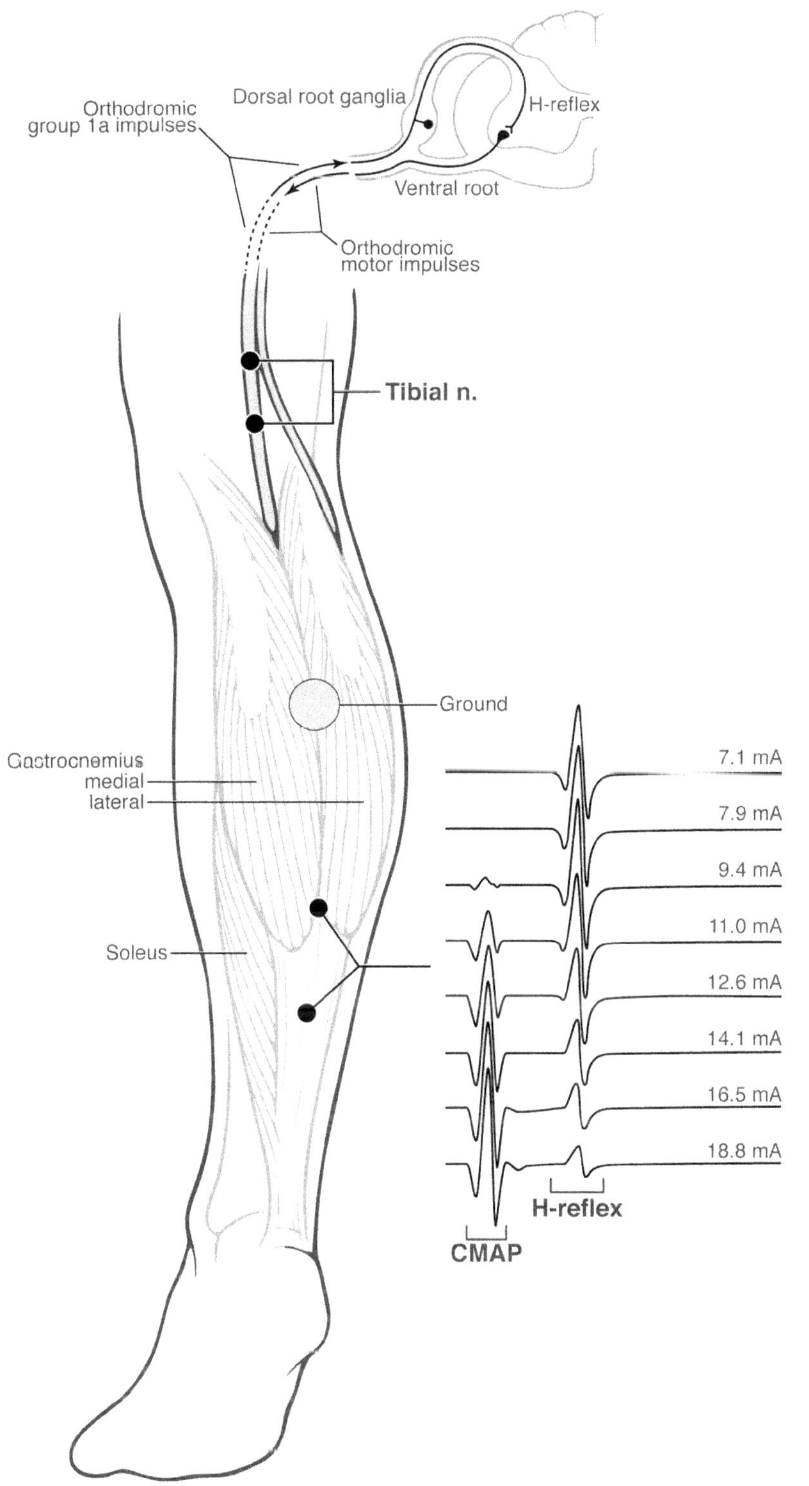

FIGURE 19-6 H-reflex.

The H-reflex is a monosynaptic reflex evoked by direct electrical stimulation of large group Ia afferent fibers in the mixed nerve. The afferent limb of the reflex arc transmits orthodromic sensory (Ia) impulses while the efferent limb of the reflex conveys orthodromic motor impulses.

Recording the H-reflex (Figure 19-6)

Active electrode: Place distal to the lower border of the gastrocnemius muscles, approximately at the junction of the middle and lower thirds of the leg. Alternatively, the recording electrode can be placed at the junction of the soleus and medial gastrocnemius muscles.

Reference electrode: Place over the Achilles tendon, distal to the active electrode.

Ground electrode: Place on the posterior leg between stimulating and recording electrodes.

The gain is set at 1 mV with a sweep speed of 10 ms/division to allow visualization of this late response. If an H-reflex is difficult to elicit, a sensitivity of 200 to 500 μV/division should be used before concluding that the response is absent. Multiple H-reflex responses are recorded following consecutive single stimuli of increasing stimulus intensity.

The latency of the H-reflex responses is rather constant compared with that of the F-wave responses.

Stimulation

Popliteal fossa: Place cathode 1 to 2 finger breadths medial to the biceps femoris tendons. By convention, the cathode is placed proximal to the anode to avoid the possibility of anodal conduction block. However, in routine clinical practice, anodal block is not observed (Wee et al., 2000).

The stimulator may need to be moved slightly laterally or medially to elicit a maximal H-reflex response.

To elicit the H-reflex, stimulus pulses of long duration (usually 1 ms) are used to preferentially activate the large group Ia fibers.

The H-reflex is initially evoked by a low intensity stimulus that is subthreshold for the direct motor response. This can occur because there is central amplification of the motor response due to reflex activation of motor neurons (Fisher, 1992). With increases in stimulus intensity, the amplitude of the direct motor response progressively increases, whereas the H-reflex amplitude progressively decreases (see Figure 19-6 waveforms).

H-reflex Normal Values

H-reflex onset latency is the most commonly obtained measurement. The upper limit of normal latency is directly related to height and leg length. For a height of 4'11" (150 cm) the upper limit of normal is 29 ms; for a height of 5'7" (170 cm) it is 32 ms, and for height 6'3" (190 cm) it is 35 ms. A right–left latency asymmetry of >1.5 ms is considered abnormal (Fisher, 1992).

The ratio of the peak-to-peak maximum H-reflex to maximum direct motor response (H/M ratio) provides a measure of motor neuron pool activation. The H/M ratio for calf H-reflexes is normally <0.7 (Fisher, 1992).

H-reflex amplitude is not usually interpreted, although a fourfold amplitude difference between sides suggests abnormality.

Clinical Application

The H-reflex is most often used to evaluate a possible S_1 radiculopathy. In the proper clinical setting, a unilaterally delayed or absent H-reflex suggests an S_1 radiculopathy.

H-reflexes are commonly abnormal in a variety of axonal and demyelinating polyneuropathies. In Guillain-Barré syndrome, H-reflexes (and F-waves) may be absent or delayed during the acute stages when other nerve conduction studies are normal.

H-reflexes provide a means of assessing motor neuron excitability (Fisher, 1992). H-reflexes are absent or decreased immediately after spinal cord injury (Leis et al., 1996A; Leis et al., 1996B), compatible with a decreased central excitability state. In contrast, H-reflexes may be abnormally widespread and H/M ratio may be increased in patients with chronic CNS lesions, consistent with increased excitability of the spinal motor neuron pool.

The presence of the H and Achilles reflexes are highly correlated (Fisher, 1992).

Limitations of H-reflexes

In neonates, H-reflex responses are widely distributed. Beyond infancy, the H-reflex is routinely recorded from only calf muscles (gastrocnemii and soleus). Less commonly, an H-reflex can also be recorded from flexor carpi radialis muscle. In routine electrophysiology, only the S_1 root is usually evaluated.

An abnormal H-reflex is not synonymous with an S_1 radiculopathy, because the H-reflex pathway includes conduction in tibial nerve, sciatic nerve, sacral plexus, spinal cord, and S_1 sensory and motor roots. Lesions at any of these levels can produce identical H-reflex abnormalities.

Once the H-reflex is lost because of S_1 root compromise, it may remain absent indefinitely. Accordingly, evaluation of patients with previous lumbosacral radiculopathies or low back surgery may be of limited value.

H-reflex responses are often absent bilaterally in patients with polyneuropathy and in subjects over age 60.

Medial and Lateral Plantar Nerve Conduction Studies

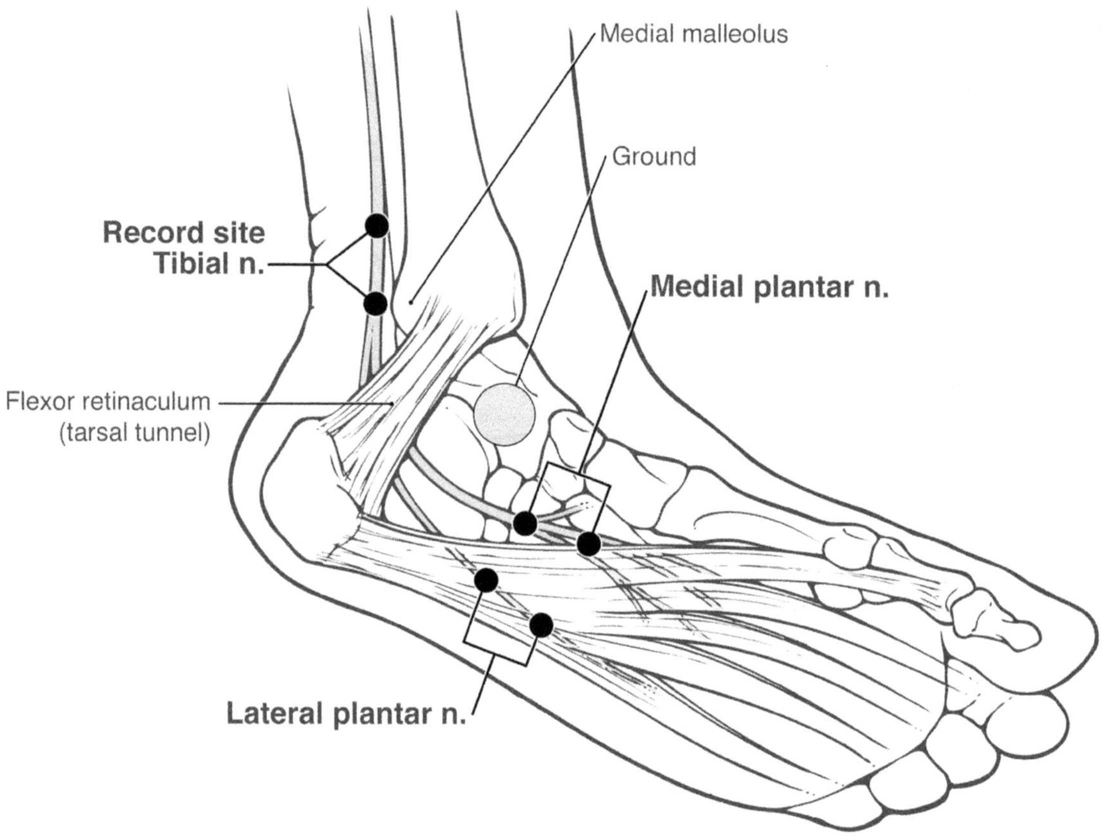

FIGURE 19-7 Medial and lateral plantar nerve conduction studies (mixed nerve technique).

Recording

Active electrode: Position over the tibial nerve just posterior to the medial malleolus.

Reference electrode: Place 3 cm proximal to the active electrode.

Ground electrode: Place on the medial aspect of the foot, between stimulating and recording electrodes.

Note: The potentials may be small and difficult to record. In some cases, electronic averaging of responses may be required.

Stimulation

Medial plantar nerve: Place cathode over the medial aspect of the plantar surface of the foot. The anode is 3 cm distal to the cathode.

Lateral plantar nerve: Place cathode over the lateral aspect of the plantar surface of the foot. The anode is 3 cm distal to the cathode.

Normal Values

Distal latency (ms) onset ≤ 3.5; peak ≤ 4.2
Amplitude (μV) ≥ 4.0
Conduction velocity (m/s) ≥ 40 m/s

Normal values are the same for medial and lateral plantar nerves. Stimulation is ideally performed at a set distance (often 14 cm) from the recording electrode.

Pitfalls

This is a technically difficult study. Stimulus artifact may obscure the recording, particularly in persons with thickened skin on the soles of the feet.

The lateral plantar nerve response is usually smaller and more difficult to elicit than the medial. Averaging may be required.

In some normal subjects, particularly those over age 50, plantar nerve responses may be very small or even absent. Accordingly, before interpreting a low or absent potential as abnormal, side-to-side comparison is necessary. An amplitude ≤ 50% of the unaffected side is evidence of abnormality.

In obese individuals with pes planus (flat feet), chronic compression may result in lateral and medial plantar neuropathies. This type of compression occurs in the sole of the foot rather than at the tarsal tunnel (Leis, personal observation).

Medial and lateral plantar nerve responses are often absent bilaterally in patients with polyneuropathy and in the elderly.

REFERENCES

Dawson DM, Hallett M, Millender LH. *Entrapment Neuropathies.* 2nd Edition. Little, Brown, Boston, 1990, pp. 291–299.

DeLisa JA, Saeed MA: AAEE case report #8: The tarsal tunnel syndrome. *Muscle Nerve* 1983;6:664–670.

Fisher MA. AAEM Minimonograph#13: H reflexes and F waves: physiology and clinical indications. *Muscle Nerve* 1992;15(11):1223–1233. Review.

Gray's Anatomy. 38th Edition. Churchill Livingstone, New York, 1995, pp. 1282–1288.

Kimura J. *Electrodiagnosis in Diseases of Nerve and Muscle.* 2nd ed., FA Davis Co., Philadelphia, 1989.

Leis AA, Kronenberg MF, Stetkarova I, Paske WC, Stokic DS. Spinal motoneuron excitability following acute spinal cord injury in man. *Neurology* 1996;47:231–237.

Leis AA, Zhou HH, Mehta M, Harkey HL, Paske WC. Behavior of the H-reflex in humans following mechanical perturbation or injury to rostral spinal cord. *Muscle Nerve* 1996;19:1373–1382.

Nobrega JAM, Pinhiero DS, Manzano GM, Kimura J. Various aspects of F-wave values in a healthy population. *Clin Neurophysiol* 2004;115:2336–2342.

Oh SJ, Sarala PK, Kuba T, Elmore RS. Tarsal tunnel syndrome: electrophysiologic study. *Ann Neurol* 1979;5:327–330.

Preston DC, Shapiro BE. Electromyography and neuromuscular disorders. Clinical-electrophysiologic correlations. 2nd ed. Philadelphia, Elsevier Butterworth Heinemann, 2005.

Puksa L, Stalberg E, Falck B. Reference values of F wave parameters in healthy subjects. *Clin Neurophysiol* 2003;114:1079–1090.

Sunderland S. *Nerves and Nerve Injuries.* Williams & Wilkins, Baltimore, 1968, pp. 1069–1095.

Wee AS, Leis AA, Kuhn AR, Gilbert RW. Anodal block: can this occur during routine nerve conduction studies? *Electromyogr Clin Neurophysiol* 2000;40:387–391.

Gastrocnemius, Medial Head

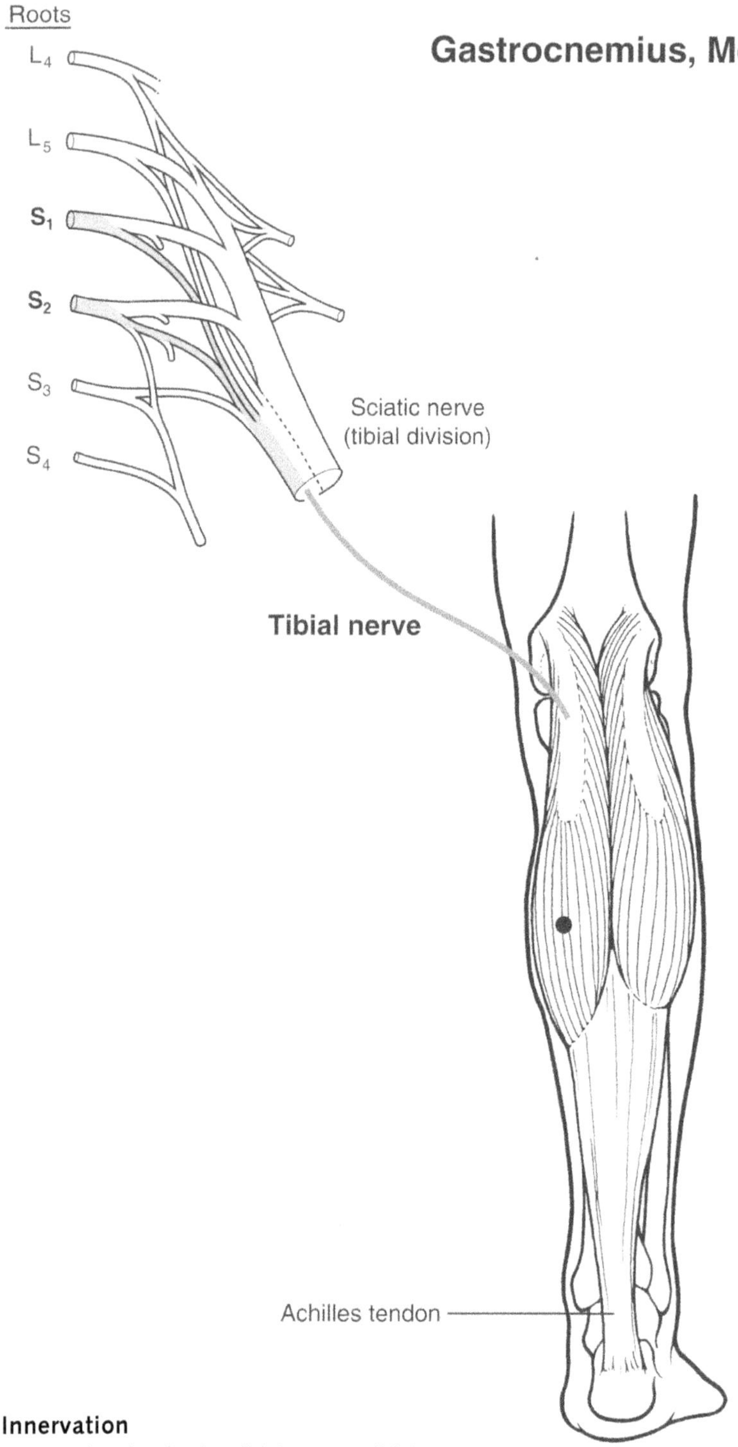

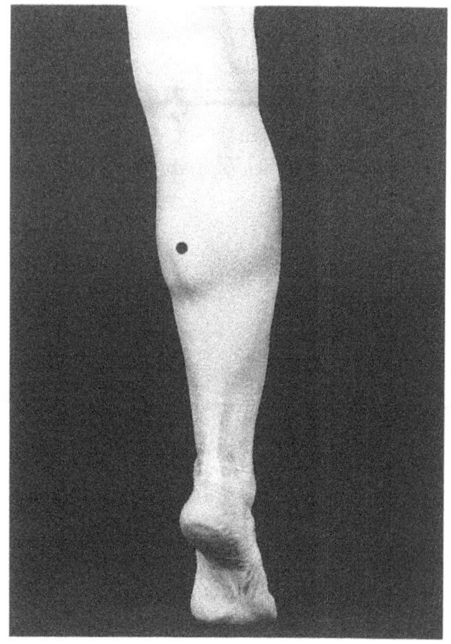

Innervation

Innervation is via the tibial nerve, tibial division of the sciatic nerve, sacral plexus, and roots S_1, S_2.

Origin

The medial head of the gastrocnemius originates at the medial condyle of the femur.

Insertion

Insertion is at the calcaneus via the Achilles tendon.

Activation Maneuver

Plantar flexion of the foot against resistance activates the muscle.

EMG Needle Insertion

Insert the needle into the medial mass of the calf.

Pitfalls

If the needle is inserted too deeply, it may be in the soleus, which is also supplied by the tibial nerve and S_1, S_2.

If the needle is inserted still deeper, it may be in the flexor digitorum longus or tibialis posterior (both muscles supplied by the tibial nerve and L_5, S_1). These muscles may show neurogenic changes on needle examination in an L_5 radiculopathy.

Clinical Comments

Neurogenic changes in the medial gastrocnemius on needle examination may be seen with lesions of the tibial nerve, sciatic nerve, sacral plexus, and S_1 or S_2 roots.

Gastrocnemius, Lateral Head

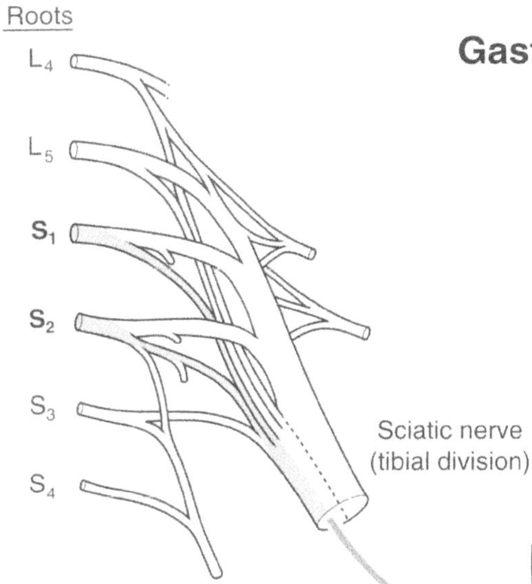

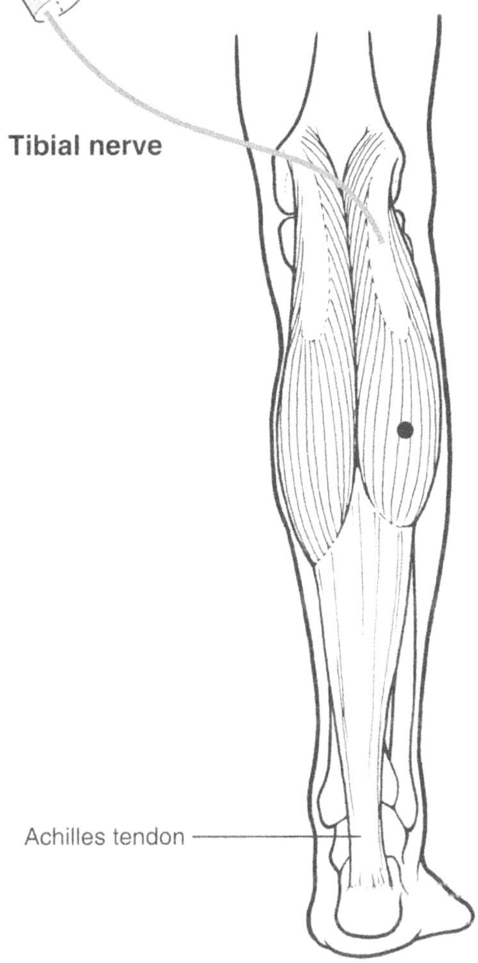

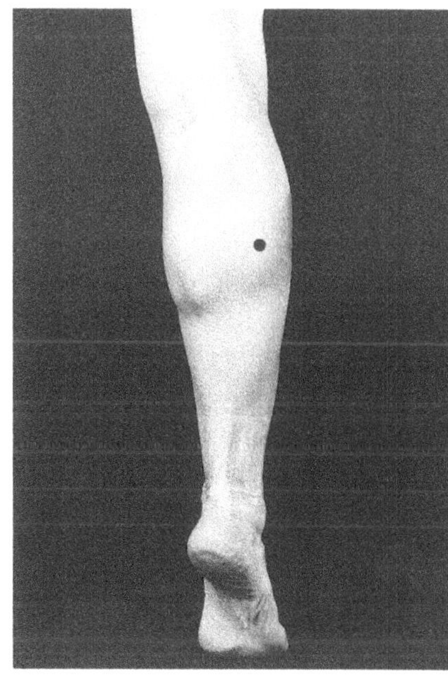

Innervation
Innervation is via the tibial nerve, tibial division of the sciatic nerve, sacral plexus, and roots S_1, S_2.

Origin
The lateral head of the gastrocnemius originates at the lateral condyle of the femur.

Insertion
Insertion is at the calcaneus via the Achilles tendon.

Activation Maneuver
Plantar flexion of the foot against resistance activates the muscle.

EMG Needle Insertion
Insert the needle into the lateral mass of the calf.

Pitfalls
If the needle is inserted too deeply, it may be in the soleus, which is also supplied by the tibial nerve and S_1, S_2.

If the needle is inserted too laterally and anteriorly, it may be in the peroneus longus or brevis, which are supplied by the superficial peroneal nerve. The outer border of the lateral gastrocnemius contacts the peronei muscles.

Clinical Comments
Neurogenic changes in this muscle on needle examination may be seen with lesions of the tibial nerve, sciatic nerve, sacral plexus, and S_1 or S_2 roots.

Soleus

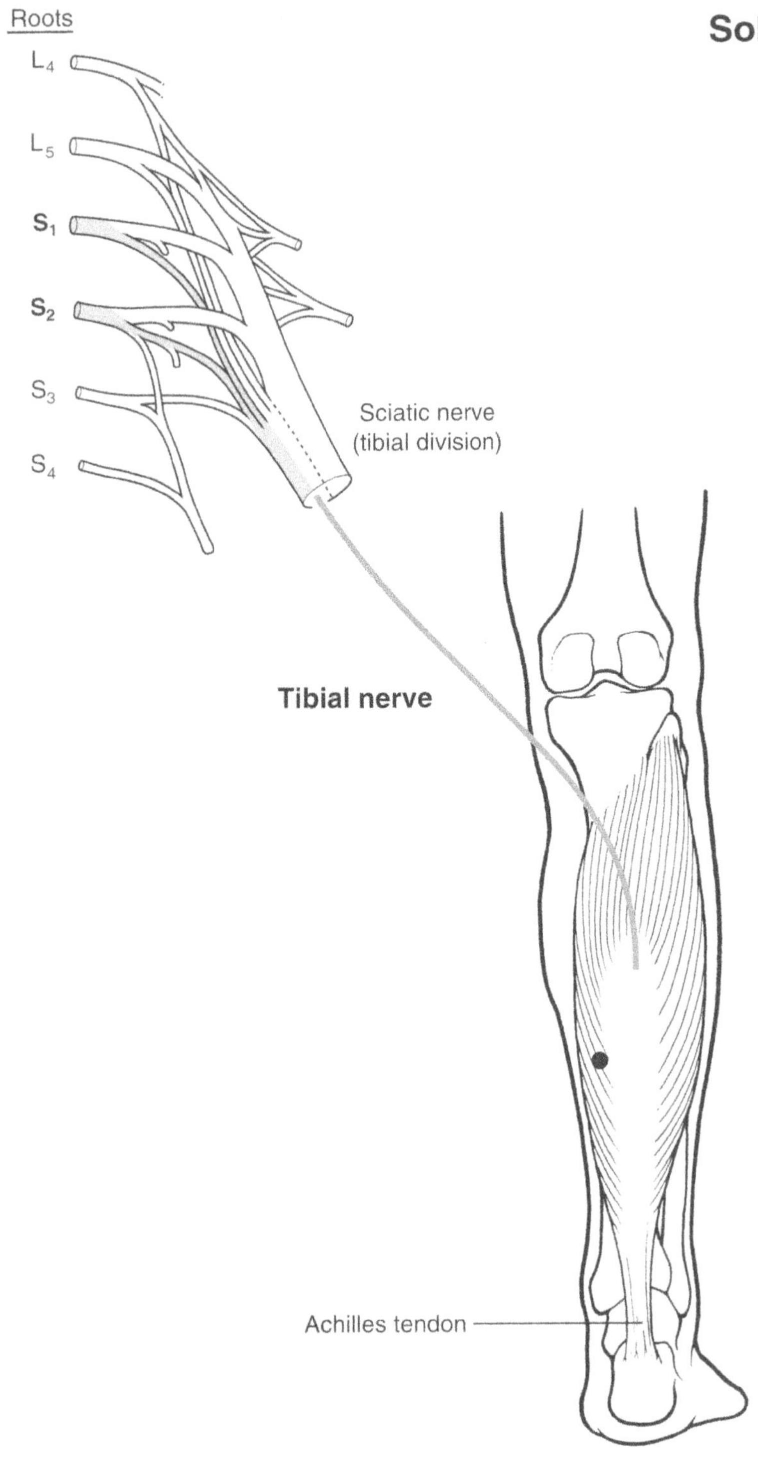

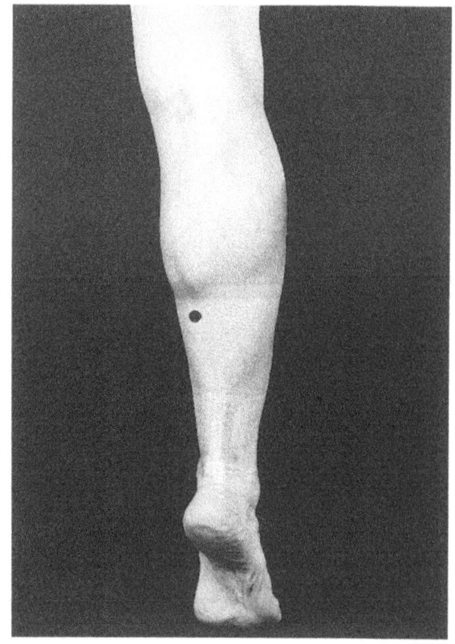

Innervation
Innervation is via the tibial nerve, tibial division of the sciatic nerve, sacral plexus, and roots S_1, S_2 (may also receive an L_5 contribution from the internal popliteal branch).

Origin
The soleus originates at the head of the fibula and the upper third of the posterior surface of its shaft and from the oblique line of the tibia and middle third of the medial surface of its shaft.

Insertion
Insertion is at the calcaneus via the Achilles tendon. Note: The Achilles tendon is the common tendon of the medial and lateral gastrocnemius and soleus muscles. These three muscles are sometimes referred to as the *triceps surae*.

Activation Maneuver
Plantar flexion of the foot against resistance activates the muscle.

EMG Needle Insertion
Insert the needle just distal to the belly of the medial gastrocnemius, medial to the Achilles tendon.

Pitfalls
If the needle is inserted too deeply, it may be in the flexor digitorum longus or tibialis posterior, which are supplied by the tibial nerve and L_5, S_1. These muscles may show neurogenic changes on needle examination in an L_5 radiculopathy.

Clinical Comments
Neurogenic changes in the soleus on needle examination may be seen with lesions of the tibial nerve, sciatic nerve, sacral plexus, and S_1 or S_2 roots. The soleus usually does not show neurogenic changes in an L_5 radiculopathy.

Tibialis Posterior

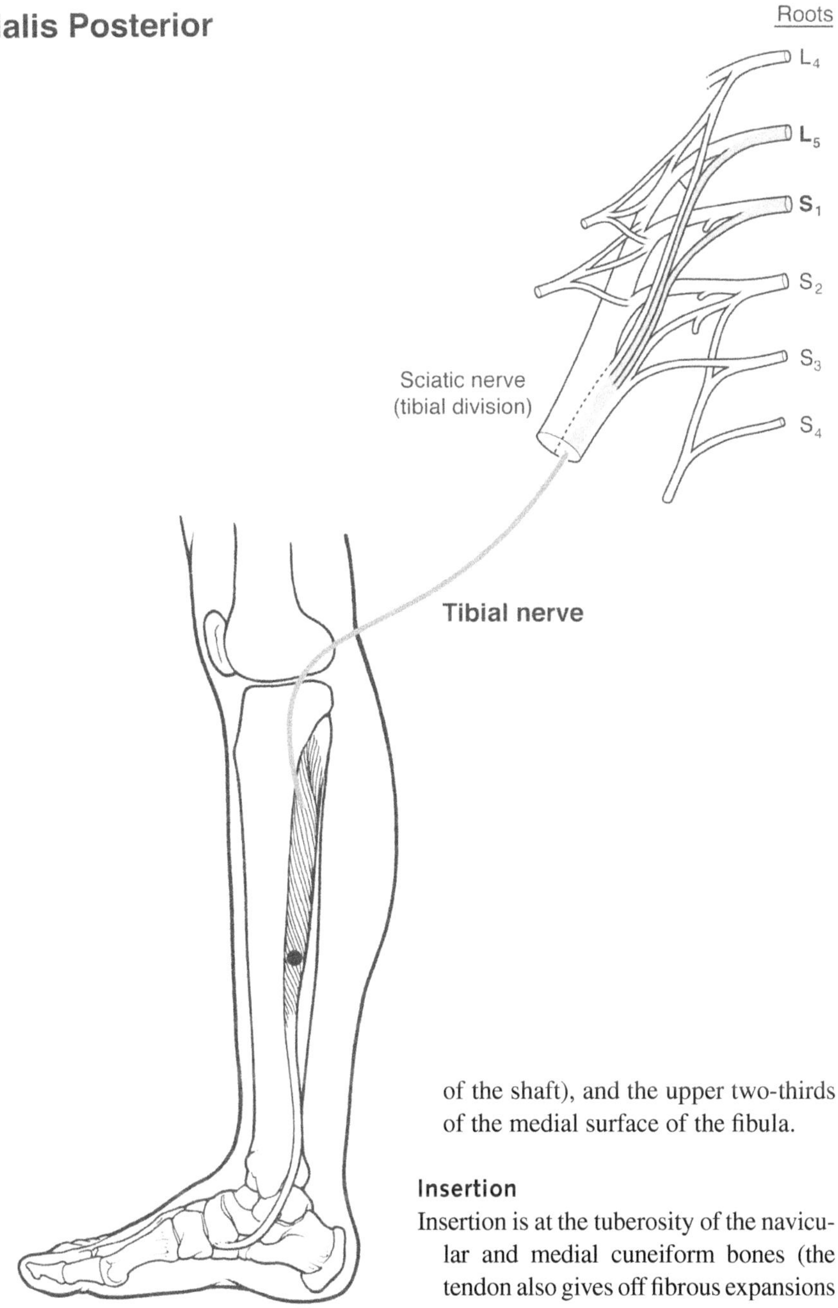

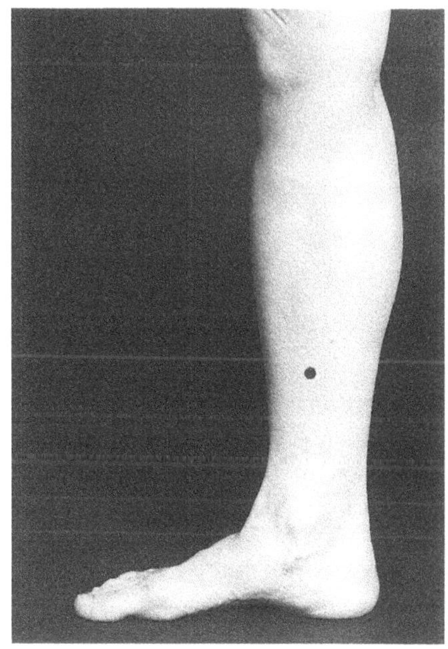

Innervation

Innervation is via the tibial nerve, tibial division of the sciatic nerve, sacral plexus, and roots L_5, S_1.

Origin

The tibialis posterior originates at the posterior surface of the interosseous membrane throughout the entire length except at the lowest part, the posterior surface of the shaft of the tibia (between the oblique line and the junction of the middle and lower thirds of the shaft), and the upper two-thirds of the medial surface of the fibula.

Insertion

Insertion is at the tuberosity of the navicular and medial cuneiform bones (the tendon also gives off fibrous expansions to the sustentaculum tali of the calcaneus, middle and lateral cuneiform and cuboid bones, and bases of the second through fourth metatarsal bones).

Activation Maneuver

Inversion of the foot activates the muscle.

EMG Needle Insertion

Insert the needle 1–2 cm medial to the margin of the tibia at the junction of the upper two-thirds with the lower third of the shaft. Direct the needle obliquely (underneath the shaft) through the soleus and flexor digitorum muscles.

Pitfalls

If the needle is inserted too superficially, it will be in the flexor digitorum longus (also supplied by the tibial nerve and L_5, S_1) or soleus (supplied by the tibial nerve and S_1, S_2).

Clinical Comments

Neurogenic changes on needle examination may be seen with lesions of the tibial nerve, sciatic nerve, sacral plexus, and L_5, S_1 roots.

The tibialis posterior and flexor digitorum longus are usually abnormal in severe "foot drop" due to L_5 radiculopathy. Conversely, these muscles are normal in foot drop due to peroneal mononeuropathy.

Flexor Digitorum Longus

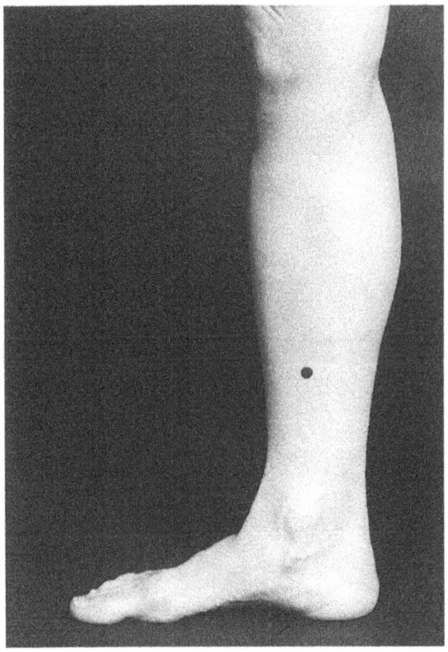

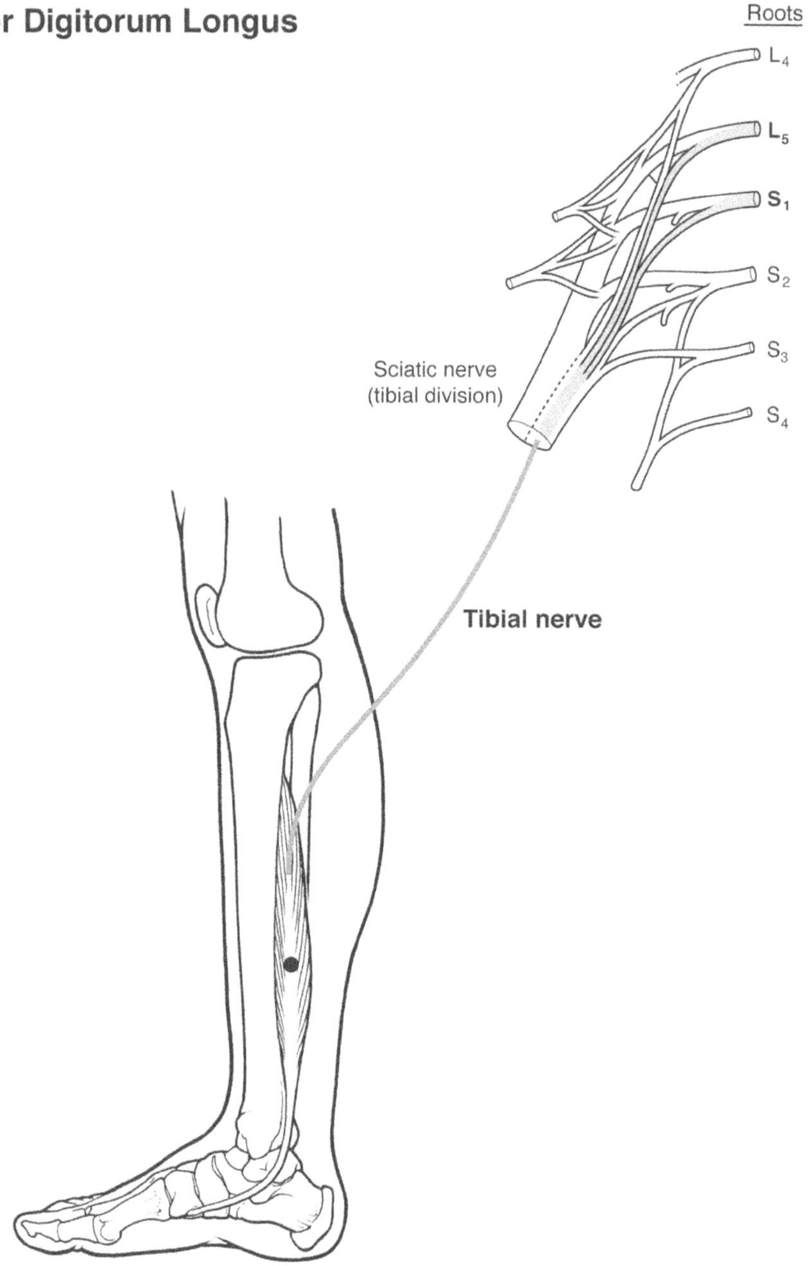

Innervation

Innervation is via the tibial nerve, tibial division of the sciatic nerve, sacral plexus, and roots L_5, S_1.

Origin

The flexor digitorum longus originates at the posterior surface of the midshaft of the tibia immediately below the oblique line.

Insertion

Insertion is at the bases of the distal phalanges of the four lesser toes.

Activation Maneuver

Flexion of the four lesser toes without plantar flexion or inversion the foot (i.e., do not coactivate the soleus or tibialis posterior muscles) activates the muscle.

EMG Needle Insertion

Insert the needle 1–2 cm medial to the margin of the tibia at the junction of the upper two-thirds with the lower third of the shaft. Direct the needle obliquely (underneath the shaft) through the soleus muscle.

Pitfalls

If the needle is inserted too superficially, it will be in the soleus muscle (supplied by the tibial nerve and S_1, S_2).

If the needle is inserted too deeply, it will be in the tibialis posterior (also supplied by the tibial nerve and L_5, S_1).

Clinical Comments

Neurogenic changes on needle examination may be seen with lesions of the tibial nerve, sciatic nerve, sacral plexus, and L_5, S_1 roots.

The tibialis posterior and flexor digitorum longus are usually abnormal in severe "foot drop" due to L_5 radiculopathy. Conversely, these muscles are normal in foot drop due to peroneal mononeuropathy.

Flexor Hallucis Longus

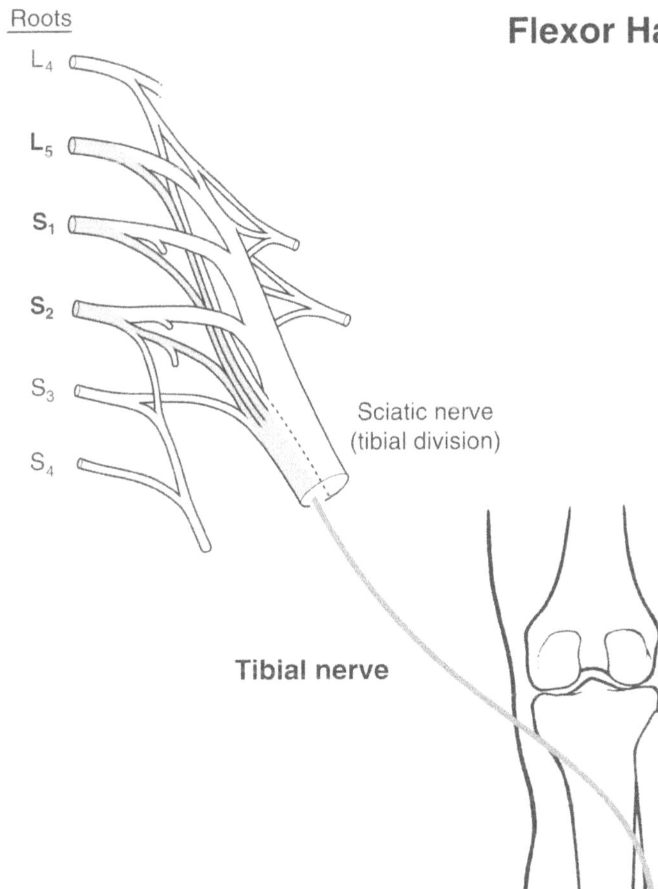

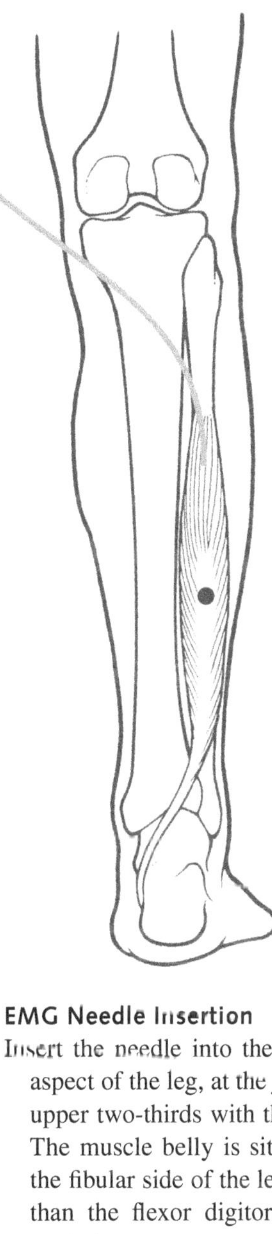

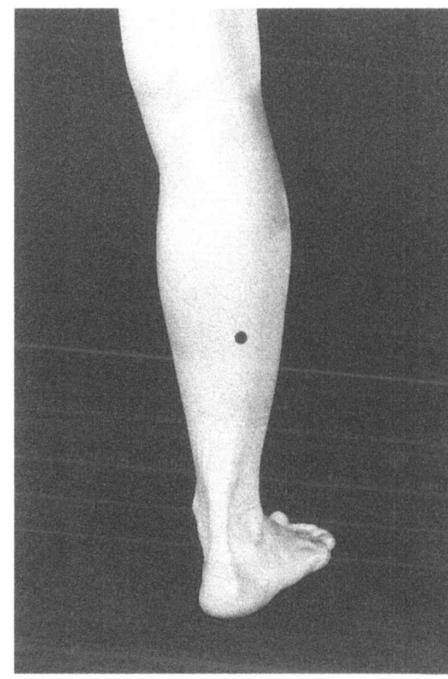

Innervation

Innervation is via the tibial nerve, tibial division of the sciatic nerve, sacral plexus, and roots L_5, S_1, S_2.

Origin

The flexor hallucis longus originates at the posterior surface of the distal two-thirds of the shaft of the fibula and the interosseous membrane.

Insertion

Insertion is at the base of the distal phalanx of the great toe.

Activation Maneuver

Flexion of the great toe without coactivation of other muscles activates the flexor hallucis longus.

EMG Needle Insertion

Insert the needle into the posterolateral aspect of the leg, at the junction of the upper two-thirds with the lower third. The muscle belly is situated deep on the fibular side of the leg and is larger than the flexor digitorum or tibialis posterior.

Pitfalls

If the needle is inserted too superficially, it will be in the soleus muscle (supplied by the tibial nerve and S_1, S_2).

If the needle is inserted too medially and deeply, it will be in the tibialis posterior (also supplied by the tibial nerve and L_5, S_1).

If the needle is inserted too laterally, it will be in the peroneus longus or brevis (supplied by the superficial peroneal nerve and L_5, S_1). The outer border of the flexor hallucis longus abuts the peronei muscles.

Clinical Comments

Neurogenic changes on needle examination may be seen with lesions of the tibial nerve, sciatic nerve, sacral plexus, and L_5, S_1, or S_2 roots.

Popliteus

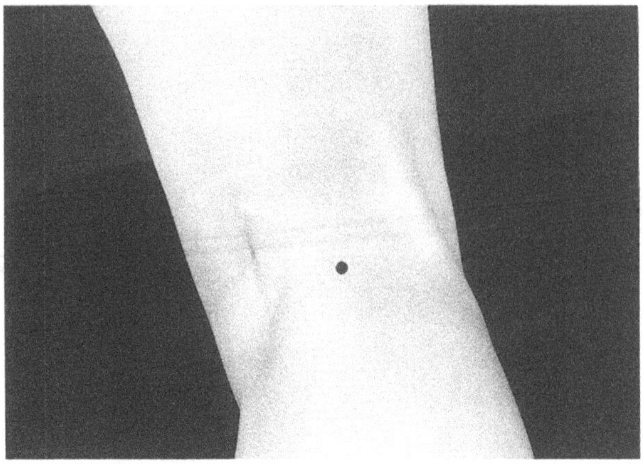

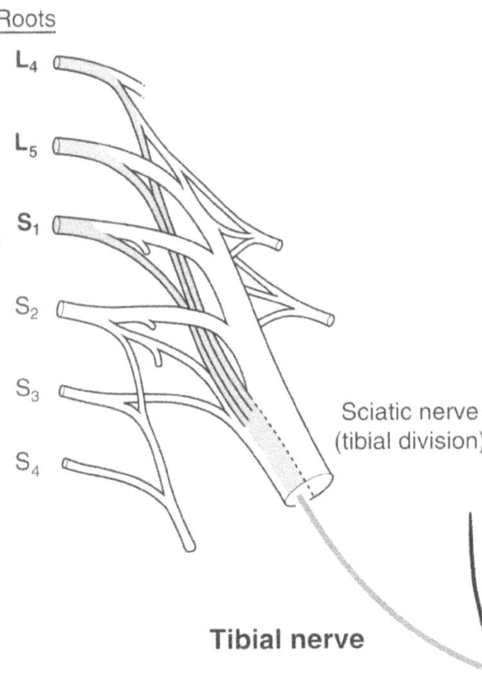

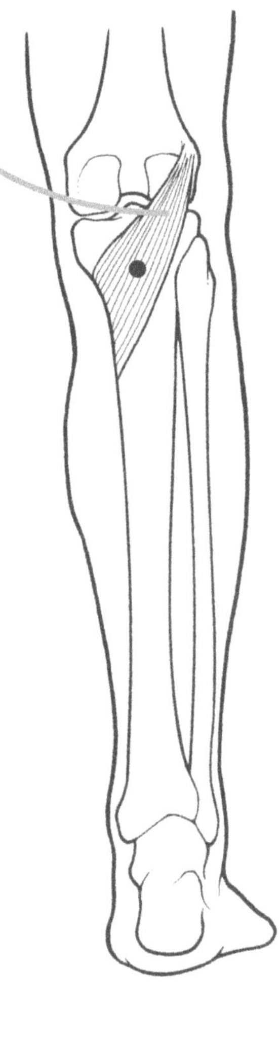

Innervation

Innervation is via the tibial nerve, tibial division of the sciatic nerve, the sacral plexus, and roots L_4, L_5, S_1.

Origin

The popliteus originates at the lateral condyle of the femur and the posterior ligament of the knee joint.

Insertion

Insertion is at the posterior surface of the shaft of the tibia above the oblique line.

Activation Maneuver

Flexion of the knee joint activates the muscle. (The popliteus produces a slight inward rotation of the tibia, which is essential during the early stages of bending the knee.)

EMG Needle Insertion

Insert the needle into the floor of the popliteal fossa in the proximal leg midway between the insertions of the outer and inner hamstring tendons.

Pitfalls

Testing of the popliteus is rarely useful in routine electromyography due to the muscle's thinness and proximity to the popliteal vessels.

If the needle is inserted too superficially, it will be in the gastrocnemius muscles (supplied by the tibial nerve and S_1, S_2).

Clinical Comments

Neurogenic changes on needle examination may be seen with lesions of the tibial nerve, sciatic nerve, sacral plexus, and roots L_4, L_5, or S_1.

Abductor Hallucis

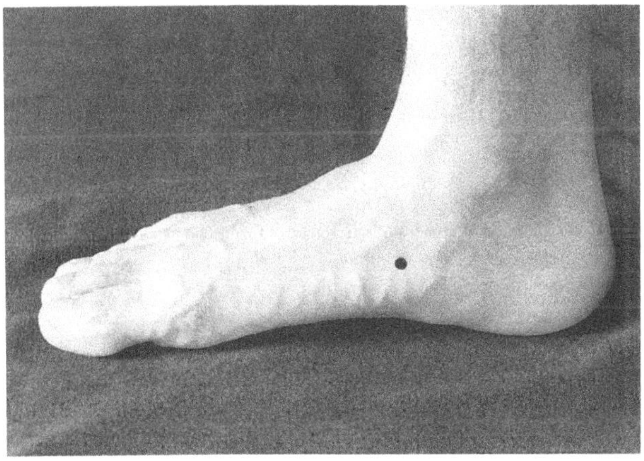

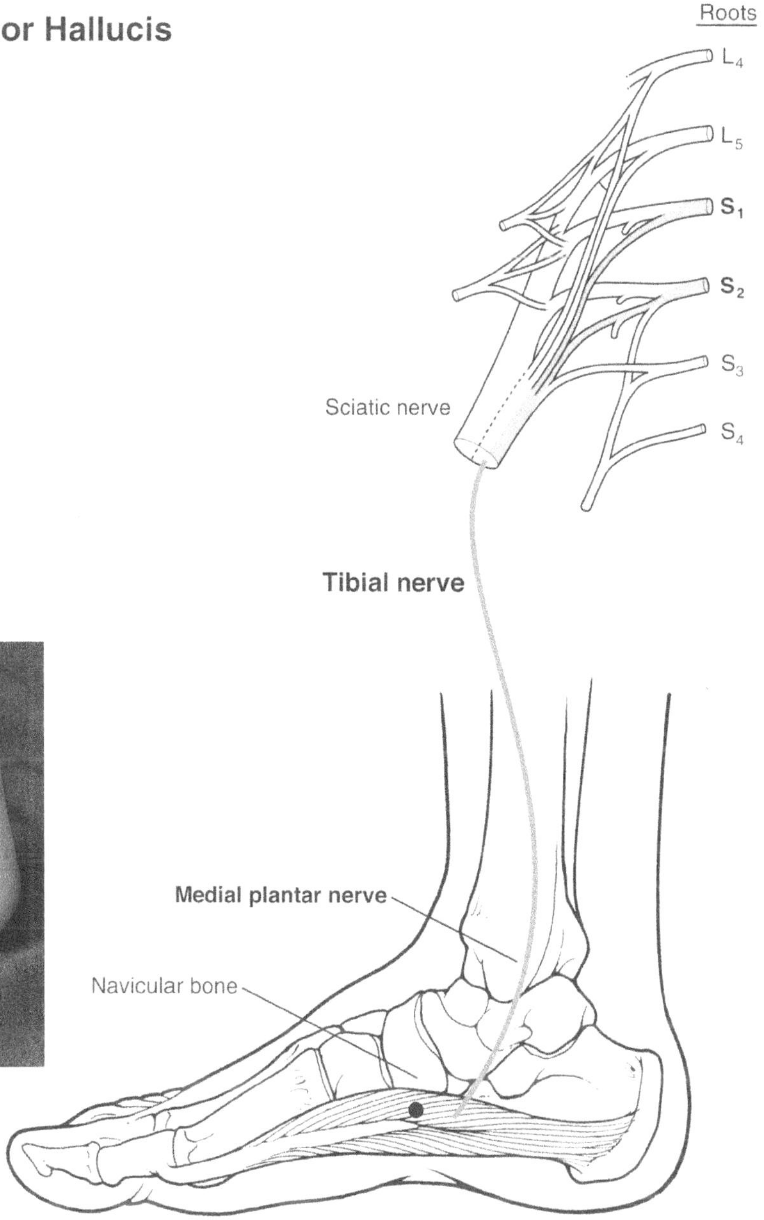

Innervation
Innervation is via the medial plantar nerve, tibial nerve, tibial division of the sciatic nerve, sacral plexus, and roots S_1, S_2.

Origin
The abductor hallucis originates at the medial process of the calcaneus (heel bone).

Insertion
Insertion is at the base of the first phalanx of the great toe.

Activation Maneuver
Abduction of the great toe activates the muscle.

EMG Needle Insertion
Insert the needle into the muscle belly directly beneath the navicular bone.

Pitfalls
Some subjects may not be able to voluntarily activate this muscle.

If the needle is inserted too deeply, it may be in the flexor hallucis brevis muscle (also supplied by the medial plantar nerve and S_1, S_2).

Clinical Comments
Neurogenic changes on needle examination may be seen with lesions of the medial plantar nerve, tibial nerve, sciatic nerve, sacral plexus, and S_1 or S_2 root.

The abductor hallucis is involved in the tarsal tunnel syndrome.

The abductor hallucis is also involved early in length-dependent peripheral neuropathies.

Flexor Digitorum Brevis

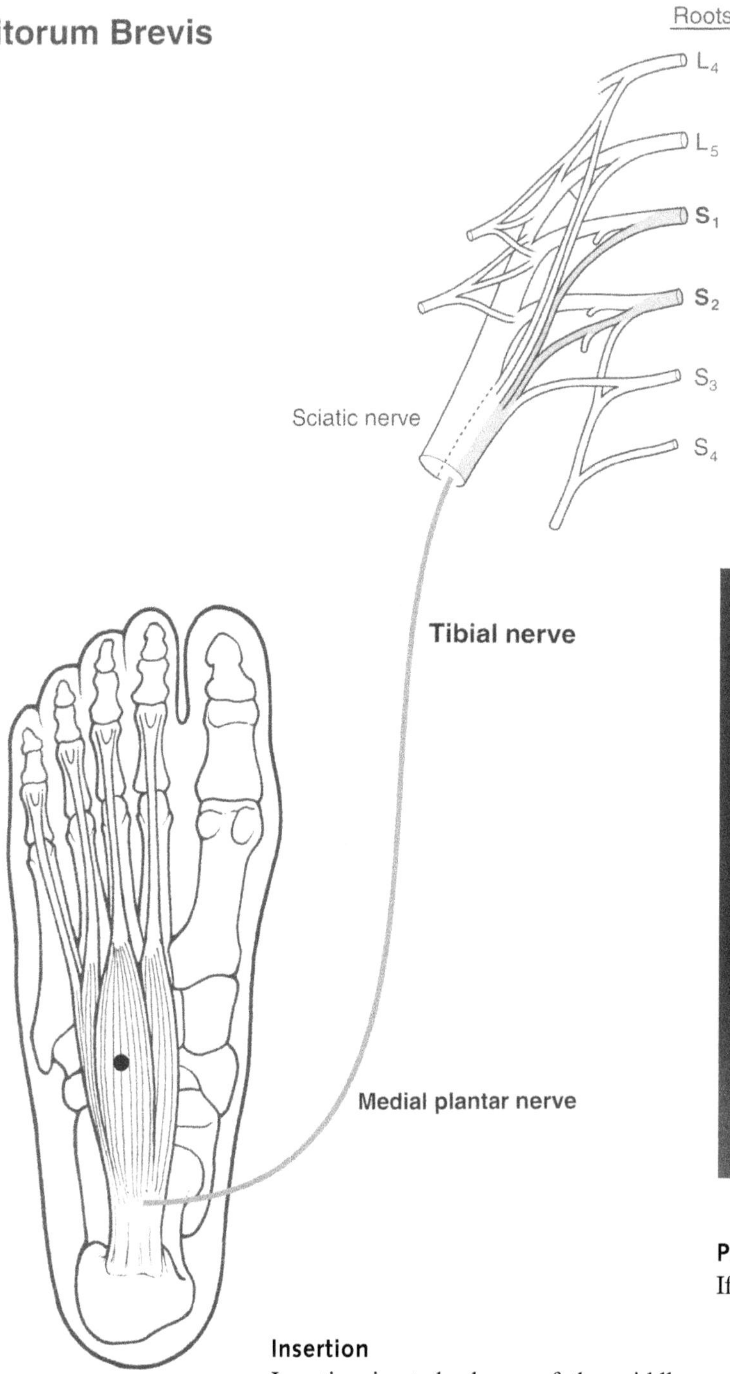

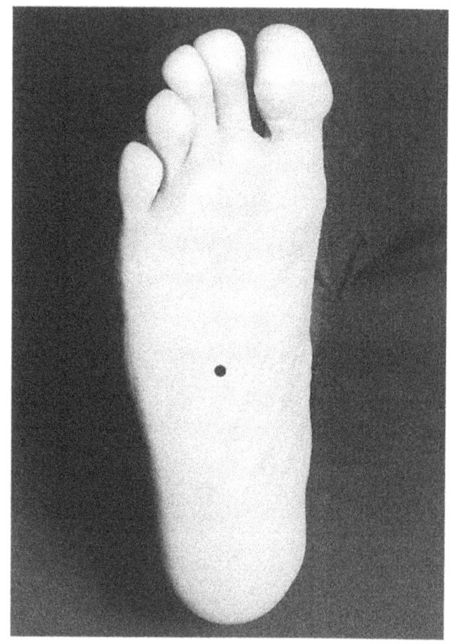

Innervation
Innervation is via the medial plantar nerve, tibial nerve, tibial division of the sciatic nerve, sacral plexus, and roots S_1, S_2.

Origin
The flexor digitorum brevis originates at the medial process of the calcaneus (heel bone) and the central part of the plantar aponeurosis.

Insertion
Insertion is at the bases of the middle phalanges of the second, third, fourth, and fifth toes.

Activation Maneuver
Flexion of the four lesser toes activates the muscle.

EMG Needle Insertion
Insert the needle midway between the third metatarsal head and the calcaneus. The muscle is superficial.

Pitfalls
If the needle is inserted too laterally, it may be in the abductor digiti minimi (quinti) or other muscles innervated by the lateral plantar nerve.

Clinical Comments
Neurogenic changes on needle examination may be seen with lesions of the medial plantar nerve, tibial nerve, sciatic nerve, sacral plexus, and S_1 or S_2 root.

The flexor digitorum brevis is involved in tarsal tunnel syndrome.

The flexor digitorum brevis is also involved early in length-dependent peripheral neuropathies.

Flexor Hallucis Brevis

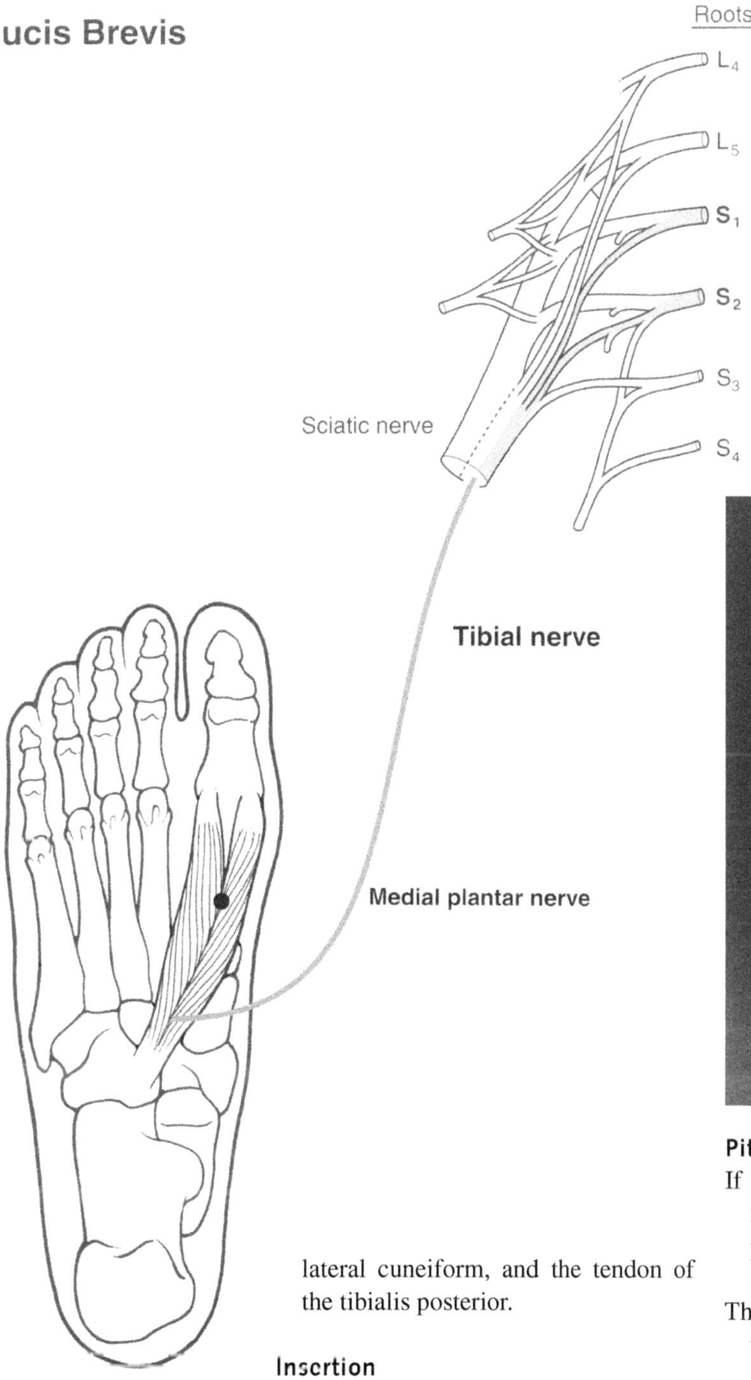

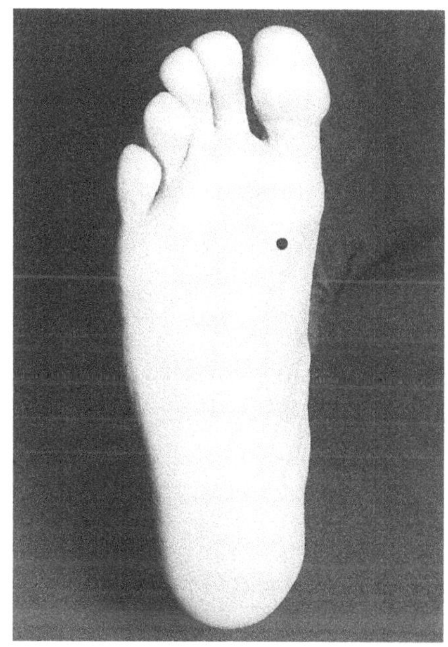

Innervation

Innervation is via the medial plantar nerve, tibial nerve, tibial division of the sciatic nerve, sacral plexus, and roots S_1, S_2.

Origin

The flexor hallucis brevis originates at the plantar surface of the cuboid, the lateral cuneiform, and the tendon of the tibialis posterior.

Insertion

Twin tendons attach to the base of the first phalanx of the great toe.

Activation Maneuver

Flexion of the great toe at the metatarsophalangeal joint activates the muscle.

EMG Needle Insertion

Insert the needle into the plantar surface of the foot 2 cm proximal to the first metatarsal head.

Pitfalls

If the needle is inserted too laterally, it may be in the adductor hallucis (supplied by the lateral plantar nerve and S_1, S_2, S_3).

The abductor hallucis is superficial to the flexor hallucis brevis, but it is also innervated by the medial plantar nerve and S_1, S_2.

Clinical Comments

Neurogenic changes on needle examination may be seen with lesions of the medial plantar nerve, tibial nerve, sciatic nerve, sacral plexus, and S_1 or S_2 root.

The flexor hallucis brevis is involved in the tarsal tunnel syndrome.

The flexor hallucis brevis is also involved early in length-dependent peripheral neuropathies.

Abductor Digiti Minimi (Quinti)

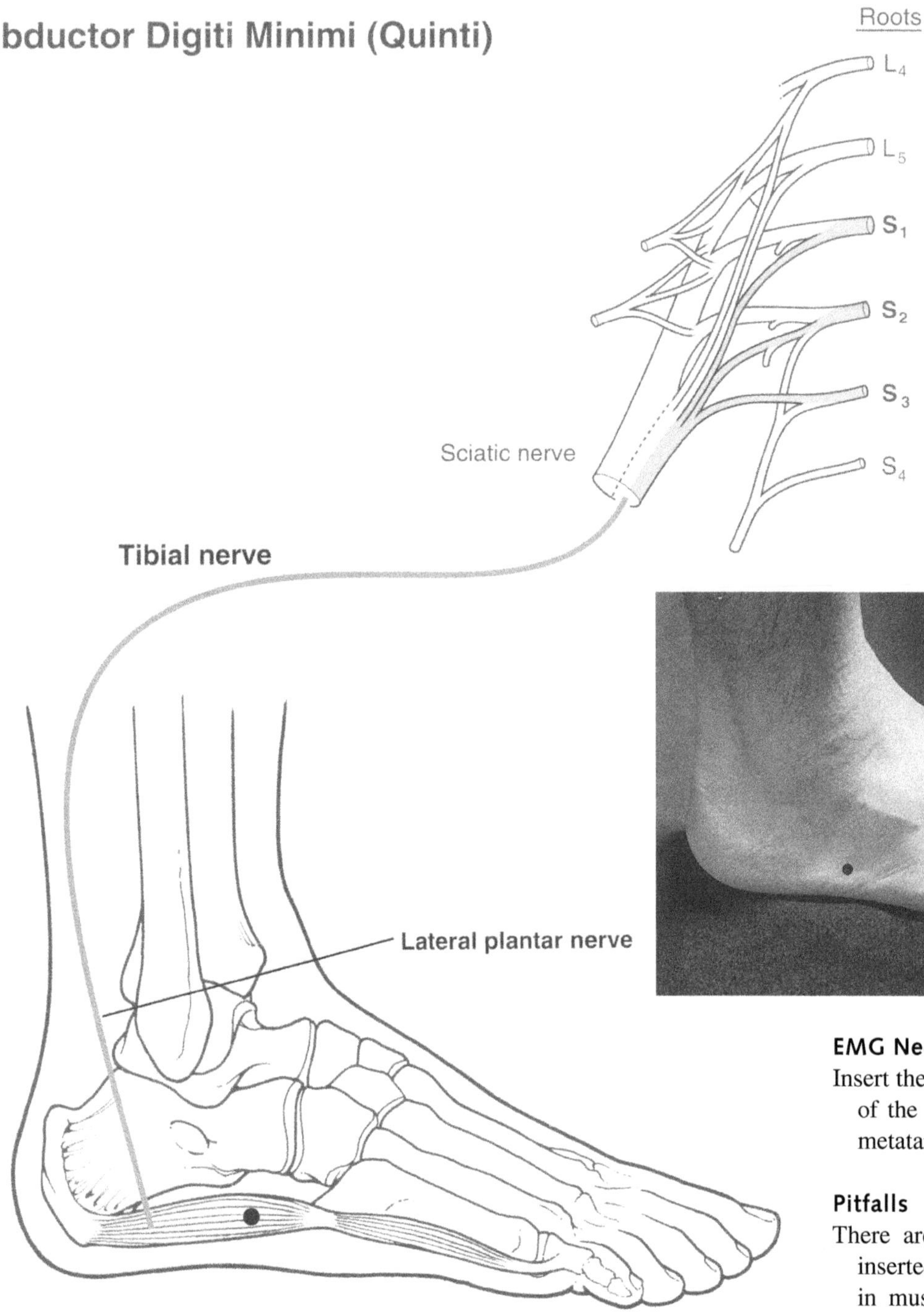

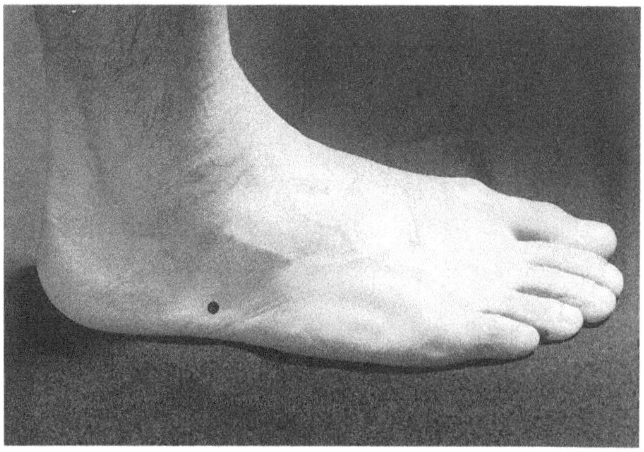

Innervation

Innervation is via the lateral plantar nerve, tibial nerve, tibial division of the sciatic nerve, sacral plexus, and roots S_1, S_2, S_3.

Origin

The abductor digiti minimi (quinti) originates at the medial and lateral processes of the calcaneus (heel bone) and the plantar aponeurosis. This muscle lies superficially along the lateral border of the foot.

Insertion

Insertion is at the lateral side of the base of the proximal phalanx of the fifth toe.

Activation Maneuver

Abduction or flexion of the fifth toe activates the muscle.

EMG Needle Insertion

Insert the needle along the lateral border of the foot midway between the fifth metatarsal head and the calcaneus.

Pitfalls

There are no pitfalls. If the needle is inserted too deeply, it will still be in muscles innervated by the lateral plantar nerve.

Clinical Comments

Neurogenic changes on needle examination may be seen with lesions of the lateral plantar nerve, tibial nerve, sciatic nerve, sacral plexus, and roots S_1, S_2, or S_3.

The abductor digiti minimi (quinti) is involved in the tarsal tunnel syndrome.

The abductor digiti minimi (quinti) is also involved early in length-dependent peripheral neuropathies.

Adductor Hallucis

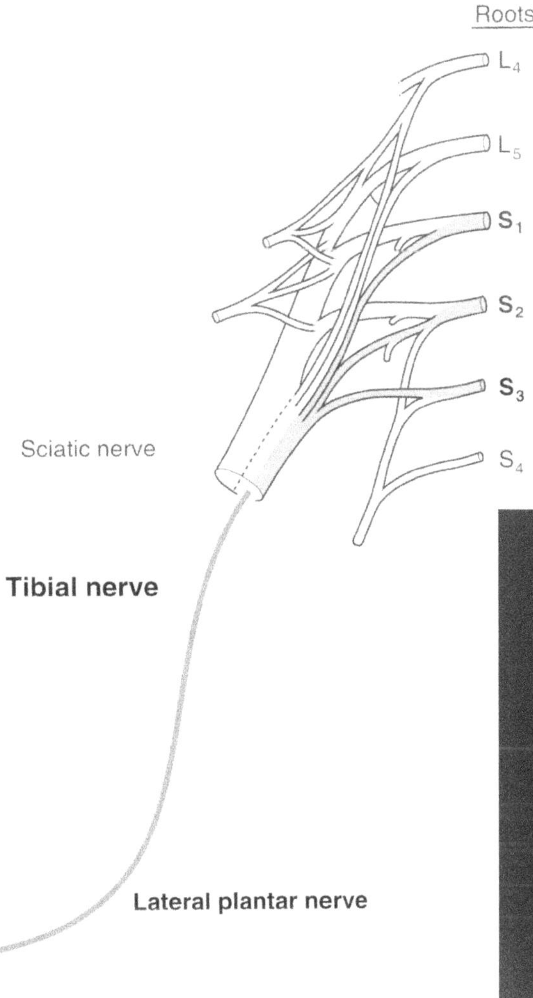

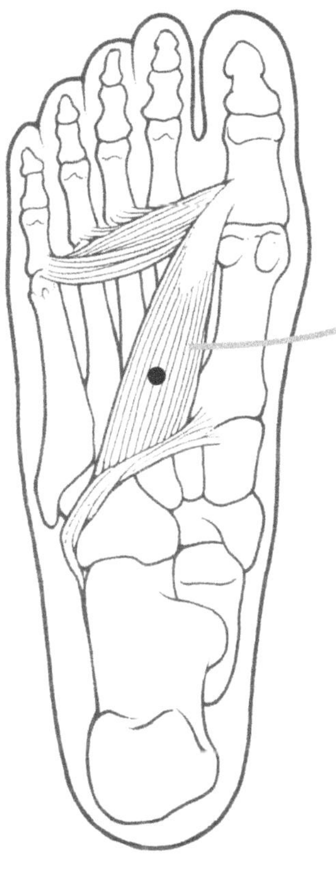

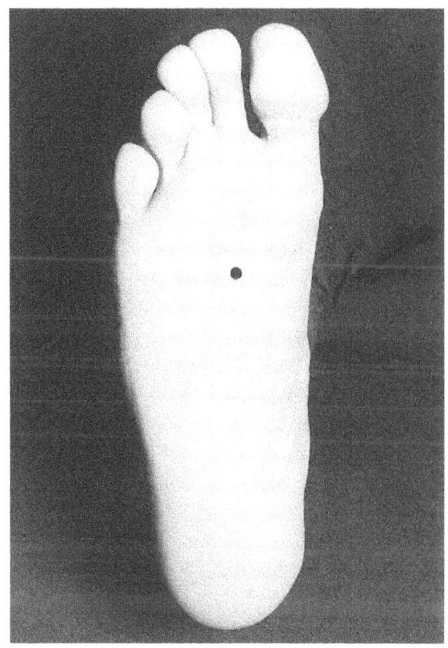

Innervation

Innervation is via the lateral plantar nerve, tibial nerve, tibial division of the sciatic nerve, sacral plexus, and roots S_1, S_2, S_3.

Origin

The oblique head originates from the bases of the second, third, and fourth metatarsal bones and from the fibrous sheath of the tendon of the peroneus longus.

The transverse head originates from the plantar metatarsophalangeal ligaments of the third, fourth, and fifth toes.

Insertion

Insertion is at the medial side of the base of the proximal phalanx of the great toe and the lateral sesamoid bone of the great toe.

Activation Maneuver

Adduction of the great toe activates the muscle.

EMG Needle Insertion

Insert the needle 4–5 cm proximal to the second or third metatarsal head to a depth of 2 cm or more (the muscle lies deep). This will access the thick, fleshy oblique head.

Pitfalls

If the needle is inserted too medially, it may be in the flexor hallucis brevis, which is innervated by the medial planter nerve.

If the needle is inserted too superficially, it may be in the first lumbrical, which is innervated by the medial plantar nerve.

Clinical Comments

Neurogenic changes on needle examination may be seen with lesions of the lateral plantar nerve, tibial nerve, sciatic nerve, sacral plexus, and roots S_1, S_2, or S_3.

The adductor hallucis is involved in the tarsal tunnel syndrome.

The adductor hallucis is also involved early in length-dependent peripheral neuropathies.

20 COMMON PERONEAL NERVE

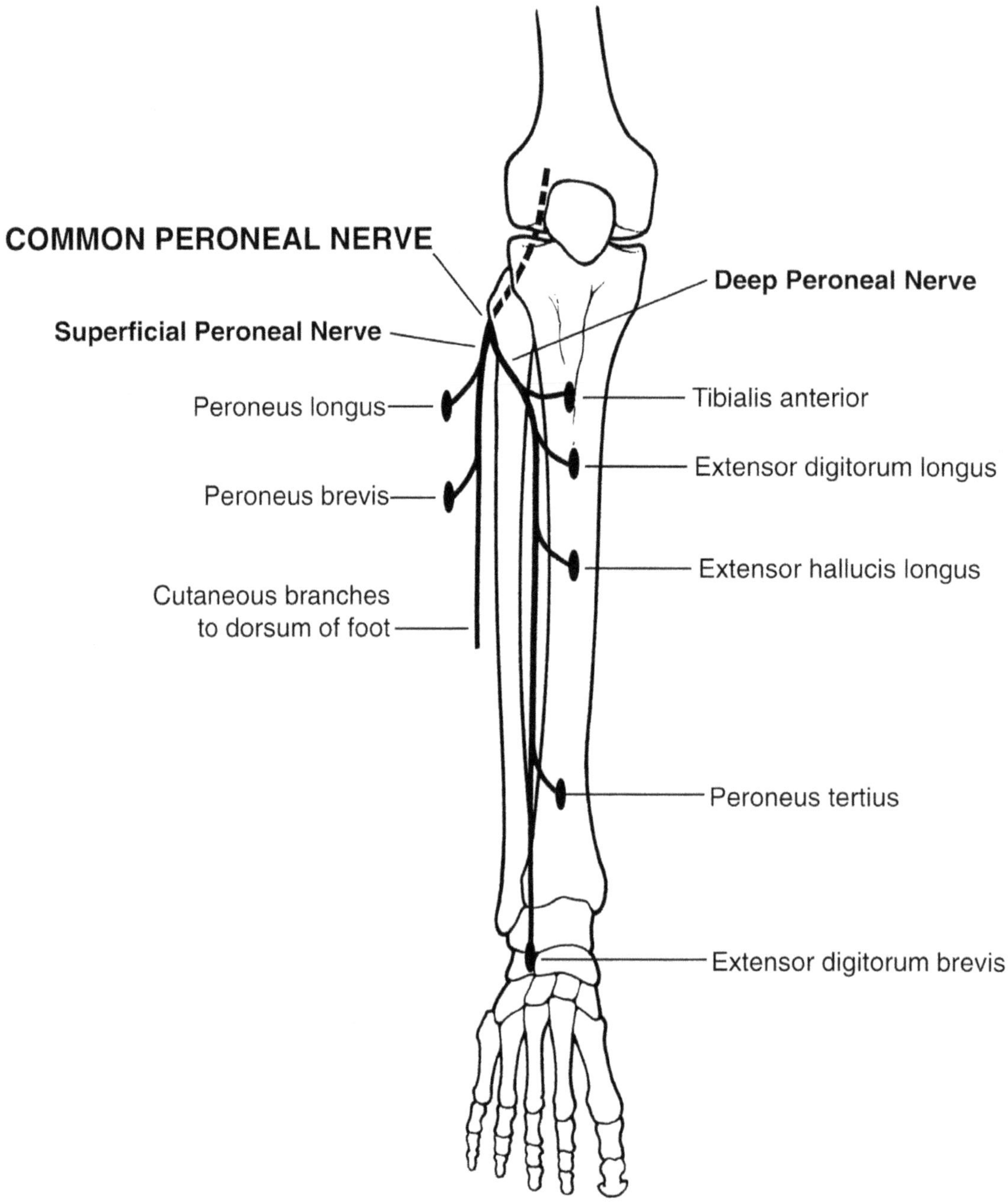

Figure 20-1 Diagram of the common peroneal nerve (anterior view) and its branches.

THE COMMON PERONEAL NERVE is derived from the fourth and fifth lumbar and first sacral ventral rami, with occasional contribution from the second sacral ventral ramus (*Gray's Anatomy,* 1995). It descends obliquely along the lateral side of the popliteal fossa, medial to the tendon of the biceps femoris as far as the attachment of the latter to the head of the fibula.

It gives off two cutaneous branches, the lateral sural nerve (lateral cutaneous nerve of the calf) and the sural communicating nerve. The former supplies the skin of the anterior, lateral, and posterior aspects of the leg; the latter descends medially to join the sural nerve in the furrow between the two gastrocnemius muscles. Articular branches in the fossa supply the knee joint. The nerve then curves laterally around the neck of the fibula, passing through a fibro-osseous opening in the peroneus longus muscle. This opening can be quite tough, and can result in the nerve angulating through it at an acute angle. In addition, considerable fibrous connective tissue secures the nerve to this proximal portion of the fibula, potentially compromising the nerve. The nerve then divides into its two terminal branches: the *superficial peroneal* and the *deep peroneal* nerves. At the neck of the fibula, the nerve is flattened and superficial and can be easily rolled against the bone (Sunderland, 1968).

The deep peroneal nerve (also known as the *anterior tibial nerve*) passes medially deep to the extensor digitorum longus and in front of the interosseous membrane. It descends on the interosseous membrane to the ankle, dividing there into lateral and medial terminal branches. Muscular branches in the leg supply the tibialis anterior, extensor digitorum longus, extensor hallucis longus, and peroneus tertius. The lateral terminal branch runs laterally on the dorsum of the foot to supply the extensor digitorum brevis. It also gives off interosseous branches to the tarsal and metatarsophalangeal joints, and to the second dorsal interosseous muscle. The medial terminal branch runs distally on the dorsum of the foot and terminates in the first interspace, where it provides cutaneous innervation to the skin on the contiguous sides of the great and second toes. It also gives off branches to the tarsal and metatarsophalangeal joints and the first dorsal interosseous muscle.

The superficial peroneal nerve turns downward between the peroneus longus and the extensor digitorum longus and emerges from between them at the mid to lower third of the leg, where it divides into lateral and medial terminal branches. In its course, it supplies the peroneus longus and the peroneus brevis. The two terminal branches are cutaneous. The medial supplies the medial aspect of the dorsum of the foot, medial side of the great toe, and the contiguous sides of the second and third toes. The lateral supplies the lateral aspect of the dorsum of the foot and adjoining sides of the third and fourth, and the fourth and fifth toes.

While the common peroneal nerve, or its branches, may be involved by penetrating injuries at any level, there are regions where the nerve is prone to certain types of injury. In the popliteal fossa, the nerve is intimately related to the knee joint as it curves laterally to reach the head of the fibula. In this position the nerve may be stretched or torn in dislocations of the knee joint (Sunderland, 1968). At the head and neck of the fibula, the nerve is superficial and may be damaged by fractures of the fibula, blows to the lateral side of the knee, superficial lacerations, pressure from improperly applied casts, compression or ischemia resulting from habitual leg crossing, or compression against any hard surface. Emaciation and weight loss are also conditions that predispose the nerve to injury.

COMMON PERONEAL MONONEUROPATHY AT THE KNEE

Etiology

Injury to the common peroneal nerve or its branches as the nerve winds around the head and neck of the fibula can cause common peroneal mononeuropathy at the knee.

The condition is usually traumatic in origin due to blunt trauma to the lateral knee, compression (tight casts, high boots, high-pressure support stockings, sedation, intoxication, prolonged anesthesia), traction (repetitive stretch from squatting or other causes of sustained hyperflexion at the knee, habitual leg crossing), or laceration.

Mass lesions (ganglia, tumors, cysts) can cause common peroneal mononeuropathy at the knee (Preston and Shapiro, 2005).

General Comments

Mononeuropathy is common. Most peroneal nerve injuries occur at the region of the fibular head.

People who are extremely thin or emaciated may develop common peroneal nerve injury. This condition is known as *slimmer's paralysis* (Sotaniemi, 1985).

Individuals who spend long hours in a squatting position can develop peroneal nerve compression. This condition is known as *strawberry pickers' palsy* (Koller and Blank, 1980).

Compression can cause nerve dysfunction by both a single episode (e.g., compression during coma) and by repeated episodes (e.g., habitual leg crossing).

Preexisting medical conditions, such as diabetic or alcoholic polyneuropathy, can predispose to common peroneal nerve injury.

Unilateral symptoms are more common, but bilateral asymmetrical involvement is often seen in patients with greater risk factors or underlying peripheral neuropathy (Wilbourn, 1986).

Clinical Features

There is weakness of foot dorsiflexion ("foot drop") associated with "slapping" or high-steppage gait. This is the chief complaint in almost all patients.

Weakness occurs during extension of the toes ("toe drop").

Weakness of foot eversion commonly occurs, due to involvement of the superficial peroneal fibers that supply the peroneus longus and brevis.

Loss of sensation or numbness commonly occurs over the anterolateral part of the leg and the dorsum of the foot.

Electrodiagnostic Strategy

Use nerve conduction studies to confirm a focal lesion of common peroneal motor and sensory fibers at the fibular head. Routine techniques are available that can identify conduction abnormalities across the fibular head (Katirji and Wilbourn, 1984; Wilbourn, 1986).

Perform EMG needle examination in muscles innervated by both the deep peroneal nerve and the superficial peroneal nerve. In common peroneal mononeuropathy associated with loss of motor fibers, EMG will show neurogenic changes (i.e., spontaneous activity, abnormal motor unit potentials, and abnormal recruitment).

If EMG is abnormal in muscles innervated by the common peroneal nerve, study the biceps femoris (short head) to define the proximal extent of the lesion (i.e., neurogenic changes in this muscle suggest a sciatic mononeuropathy with disproportionate involvement of common peroneal fibers).

Exclude L_5 radiculopathy as the etiology of foot drop. Perform a needle examination in the flexor digitorum longus, tibialis posterior, tensor fasciae latae, gluteus medius, and lumbosacral paraspinal muscles. These muscles are usually abnormal in foot drop due to L_5 radiculopathy. Conversely, these muscles are normal in foot drop due to common peroneal neuropathy.

Common Peroneal Motor Nerve Conduction Study from Extensor Digitorum Brevis

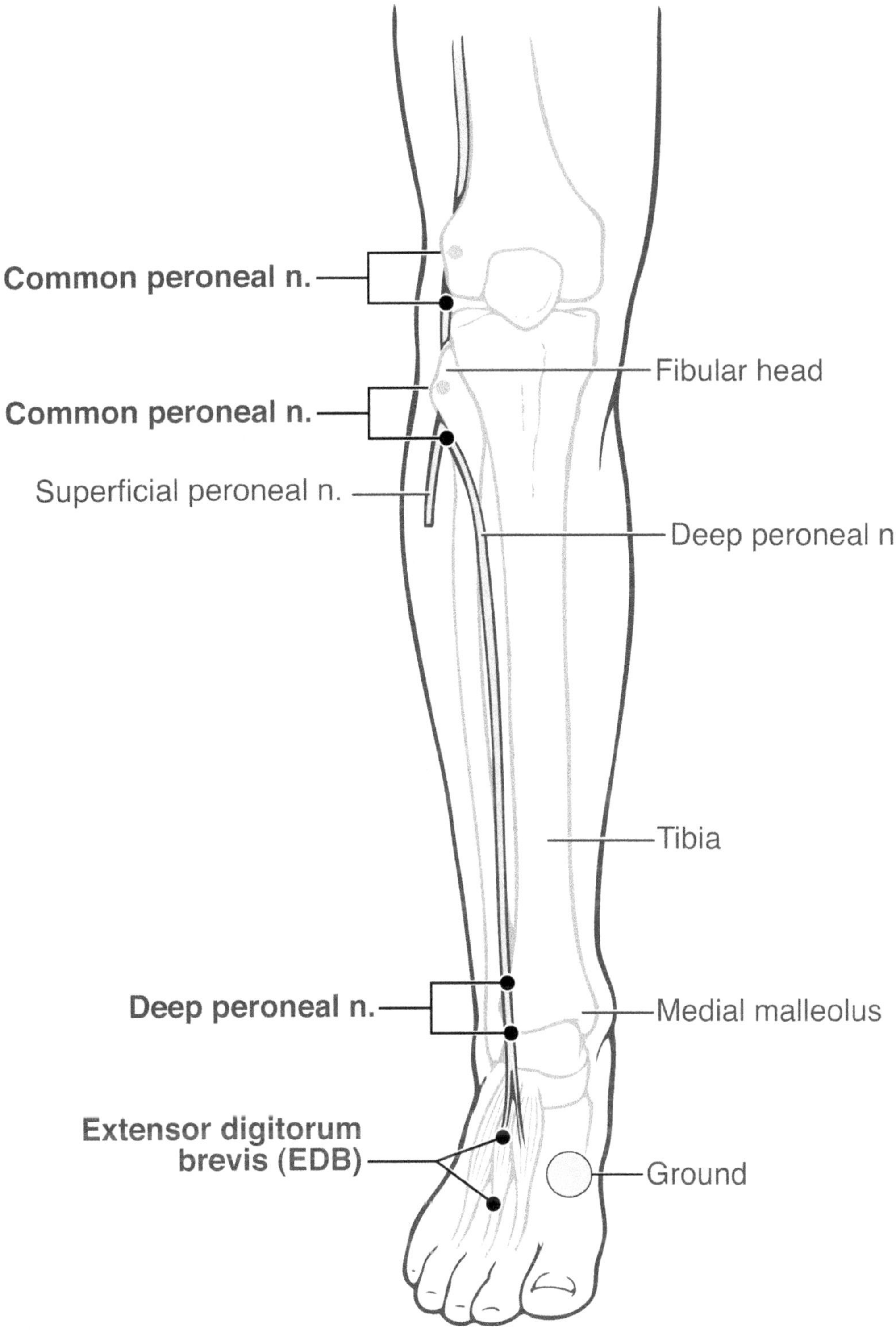

FIGURE 20-2 Common peroneal motor nerve conduction study from Extensor Digitorum Brevis.

Recording (Figure 20-2)

Active electrode: Position over the belly of the extensor digitorum brevis (EDB) muscle on the dorsal aspect of the foot.

Reference electrode: Place distal to the active electrode over the tendon of the EDB ("belly tendon" recording).

Ground electrode: Place on the dorsum of the foot between stimulating and recording electrodes.

Stimulation

Ankle: Place cathode over the anterior ankle. The anode is 3 cm proximal to cathode.

Below the knee: Place cathode just below the head of the fibula. The anode is 3 cm proximal to cathode.

Above the knee: Place cathode above the head of the fibula in the lateral popliteal fossa. The distance between the below and above knee stimulation sites is usually about 8 to 10 cm. The anode is 3 cm proximal to cathode.

Normal Values

Distal latency (ms) ≤ 6.0

Amplitude (mV) ≥ 2.0

Conduction velocity (m/s) ≥ 40 m/s in the ankle to below-knee segment and across the fibular head.

Pitfalls

Coactivation of the tibial nerve may occur with stimulating in the popliteal fossa. Therefore, observation of the mechanical movement of the foot is important to avoid recording a volume-conducted response (obvious foot dorsiflexion occurs with correct stimulation of the peroneal nerve in the popliteal fossa, whereas coactivation of the tibial nerve produces a muted deflection or plantar flexion of the foot).

Failure to recognize the anomalous accessory deep peroneal nerve to EDB muscle (see Figure 20-4) may cause confusion when evaluating lesions of the common peroneal nerve (Gutmann, 1993). This anomaly is common, affecting about 1 in 5 persons.

In patients with foot drop, recording the peroneal motor response from the tibialis anterior is required, because weakness in this muscle accounts for the clinical deficit. In some cases of foot drop, conduction abnormalities may be seen only when recording from the tibialis anterior (Preston and Shapiro, 2005).

Peroneal F-waves

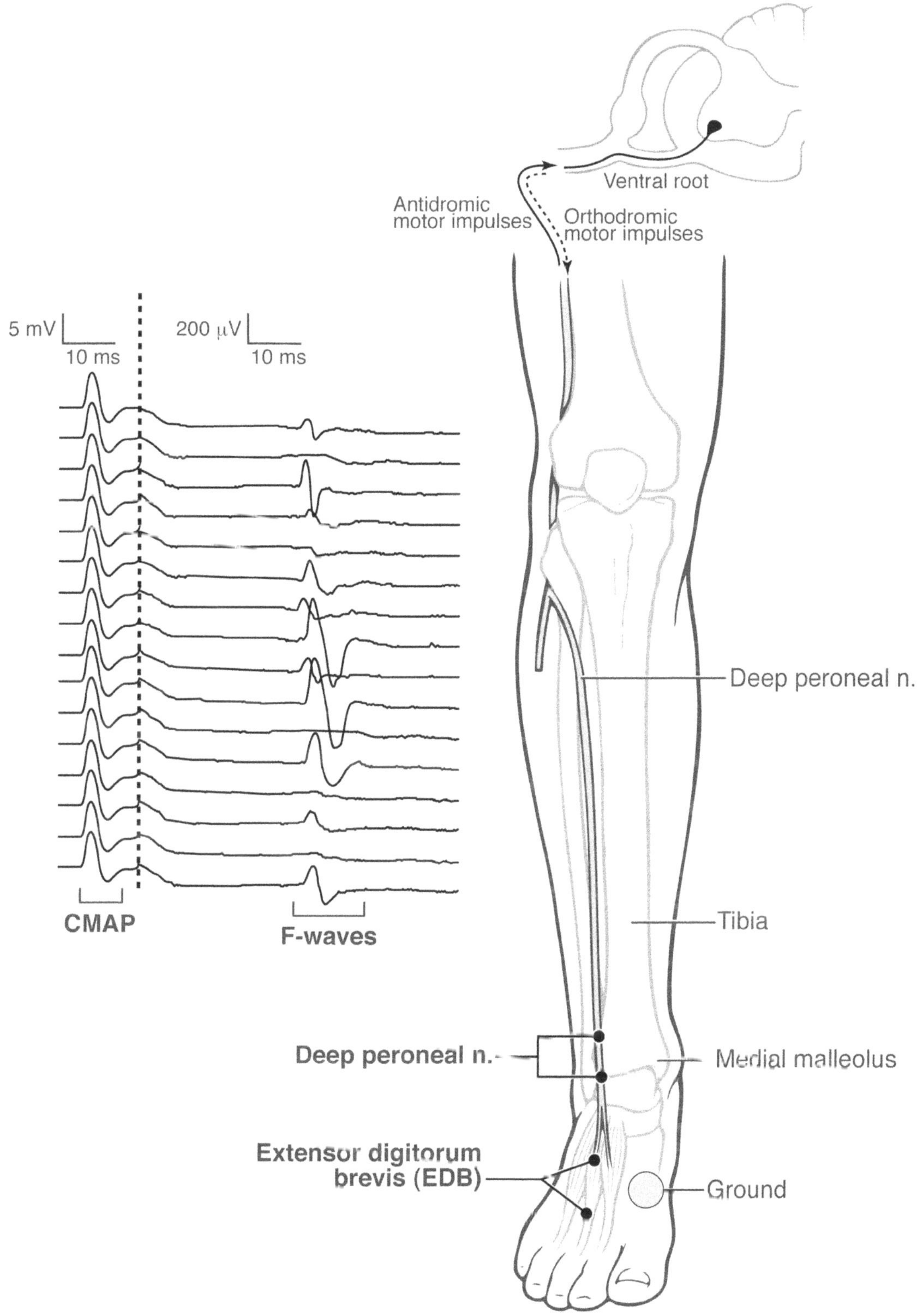

FIGURE 20-3 Peroneal F-waves.

Recording F-waves

Identical recording technique to that utilized to elicit the CMAP from EDB, except that the gain is set from 200 μV to 500 μV and sweep speed 10 ms/division to allow visualization of this late response. At least 10 to 20 stimulation trials are recorded.

Stimulation

Identical stimulation technique to that utilized for distal stimulation at the ankle (place cathode in the same site and deliver supramaximal stimuli). By convention, the anode is rotated 180 degrees from its original position to avoid the theoretical possibility of anodal conduction block. However, in routine clinical practice, anodal block is not observed (Wee et al., 2000).

F-wave Measurements and Normal Values

Minimum F-wave latency is the most commonly obtained measurement. In leg muscles, upper limits of minimum F-wave latency are 44 ms for height 4'11" (150 cm), 53 ms for height 5'7" (170 cm) and 62 ms for height 6'3" (190 cm). A right–left asymmetry of minimal F-wave latency >3.5 ms in leg muscles is considered abnormal (Fisher, 1992; Puksa et al., 2003).

Mean F-wave latency is calculated by adding all individual F-wave latencies and dividing this sum by the number of F-waves recorded (Fisher, 1992). The upper limits of normal for this value will be approximately 2 ms longer than minimum F-wave latency for the corresponding heights (Nobrega et al., 2004).

Maximum F-wave latency is the longest onset latency of all recorded F-waves. The upper limits of this value will be about 4 ms longer than minimum F-wave latency for the corresponding heights (Nobrega et al., 2004).

F-wave dispersion (or chronodispersion) provides a measure of the range of conductions and is calculated as the difference between minimum and maximum F-wave latencies. In leg muscles, a typical upper limit of normal F-wave dispersion is <8 ms (Puksa et al., 2003). Excessive chronodispersion suggests temporal dispersion and demyelination.

F-wave amplitude usually measures <5% of the maximal CMAP or M-wave amplitude (F/M amplitude ratio). This is a measure of the proportion of the motor neuron pool activated by antidromic stimulation. F-wave amplitude may be increased in upper motor neuron dysfunction, especially when spasticity is present.

F-wave persistence is the percentage of F-waves obtained following a series of stimulations (i.e., the number of measureable F-waves divided by the number of stimuli). This reflects the antidromic excitability of a particular motor neuron pool (Fisher, 1992). F-wave persistence in median, ulnar, and tibial nerves is normally >50%, although in the peroneal nerve it can be <25%. Hence, *absence of F-waves in the peroneal nerve cannot be regarded as evidence of abnormality.* F-wave persistence is often decreased in lower motor neuron dysfunction and increased in upper motor neuron dysfunction, particularly when spasticity is present.

Comments

In radiculopathy, F-waves are of limited value and less sensitive than needle EMG examination in assessing motor fiber involvement.

F-waves are commonly abnormal in a variety of axonal and demyelinating polyneuropathies. In Guillain-Barré syndrome, F-waves may be absent or delayed during the acute stages when other nerve conduction studies are normal. Increased F-wave dispersion suggests temporal dispersion and demyelination.

F-waves provide a means of assessing motor neuron excitability (Fisher, 1992). F-waves are typically absent or decreased in spinal shock (Leis et al., 1996) and early after acute stroke, compatible with a decreased central excitability state. In contrast, F-waves are typically increased in patients with established spasticity.

Accessory Deep Peroneal Nerve

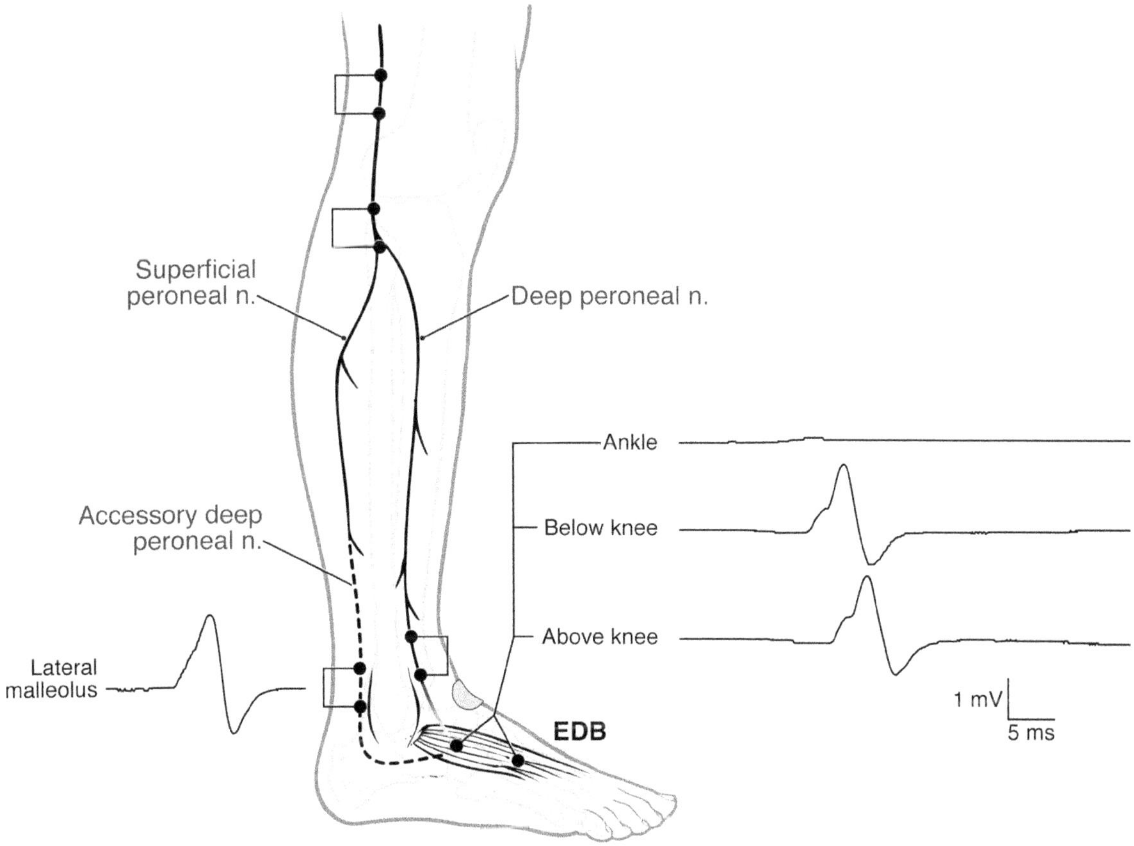

FIGURE 20-4 Accessory deep peroneal nerve.

The accessory deep peroneal nerve (Figure 20-4) is a common anomaly in which motor fibers from the superficial peroneal nerve provide partial innervation to the extensor digitorum brevis (EDB) muscle (Gutmann, 1993). The accessory deep peroneal fibers descend behind the lateral malleolus to supply the lateral portion of the EDB, although occasionally the entire muscle can be innervated by this anomalous branch.

When performing routine peroneal nerve conduction studies, the presence of an accessory deep peroneal nerve can be recognized by a CMAP that is larger with stimulation of the peroneal nerve at proximal sites than at the ankle. This occurs because the accessory deep peroneal nerve, situated behind the lateral malleolus, provides abundant innervation to the EDB. In such cases, an accessory deep peroneal nerve can be confirmed by stimulating posterior to the lateral malleolus. This will elicit the "missing" CMAP from the EDB.

Although this anomaly is not clinically relevant, failure to recognize it can confound the electrodiagnostic interpretation. For example, in a patient with a dominant accessory deep peroneal nerve and peroneal neuropathy at the fibular head due to conduction block, routine stimulation of the peroneal nerve at the ankle and above the knee may fail to elicit a CMAP, whereas peroneal nerve stimulation below the knee may elicit the only recordable motor response. This produces a confusing picture if the electromyographer is unaware of the existence of an accessory deep peroneal nerve.

Common Peroneal Motor Nerve Conduction Study from Tibialis Anterior

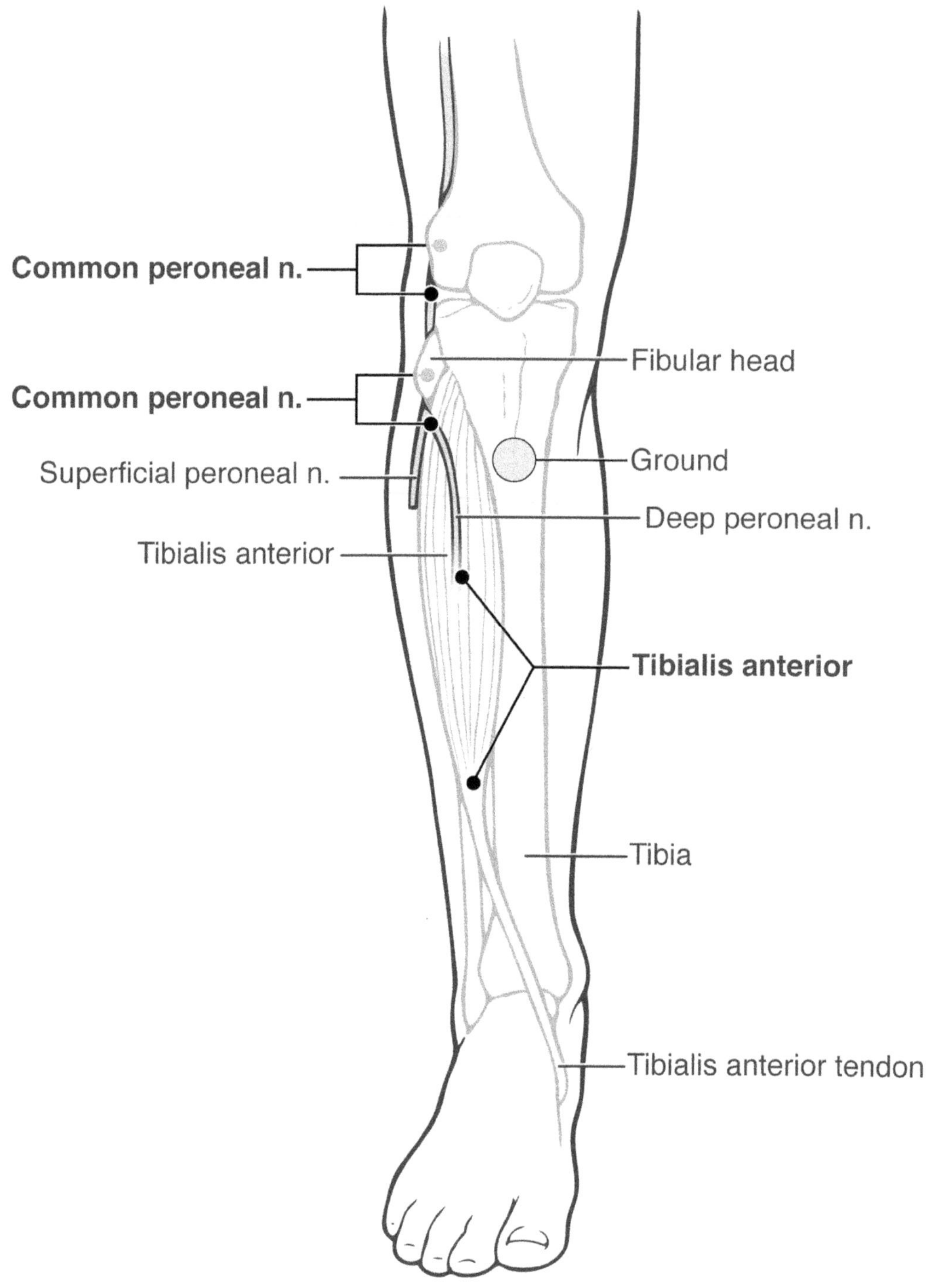

FIGURE 20-5 Common peroneal motor nerve conduction study from tibialis anterior.

Recording (Figure 20-5)

Active electrode: Position over the belly of the tibialis anterior muscle on the lateral aspect of the leg.

Reference electrode: Place distal to the active electrode over the tendon of the tibialis anterior ("belly tendon" recording).

Ground electrode: Place on the anterior surface of the leg between stimulating and recording electrodes.

Stimulation

Below the knee: Place cathode just below the head of the fibula. The anode is 3 cm proximal to cathode.

Above the knee: Place cathode above the head of the fibula in the lateral popliteal fossa. The distance between the below-knee and above-knee stimulation sites is usually about 8 to 10 cm. The anode is 3 cm proximal to cathode.

Normal Values

Amplitude (mV) ≥ 3.0

Conduction velocity (m/s) ≥ 40 m/s in the segment across the fibular head.

There is no fixed distance in the peroneal nerve tibialis anterior motor conduction study. Accordingly, side-to-side comparisons using identical recording and stimulating techniques are necessary. A relative latency delay ≥ 1.0 ms or an amplitude ≤ 50 % of the unaffected side is evidence of abnormality.

Comments

In patients with foot drop, recording the motor response from the tibialis anterior is mandatory, because weakness in this muscle accounts for the clinical deficit. In some cases, conduction abnormalities localized to the fibular head may be seen only when recording from the tibialis anterior, but not the EDB muscle (Preston and Shapiro, 2005).

In patients with chronic diffuse polyneuropathy, the EDB muscle may be atrophied. Hence, recording the peroneal motor response from the tibialis anterior can provide information about the length-dependent nature of the polyneuropathy, and whether there is slowing of conduction velocity at a physiologic compression site.

Short segment stimulation across the fibular head ("inching technique") may be very helpful in precisely localizing a peroneal palsy (Figure 20-6).

Short Segment Stimulation across the Fibular Head ("Inching Technique")

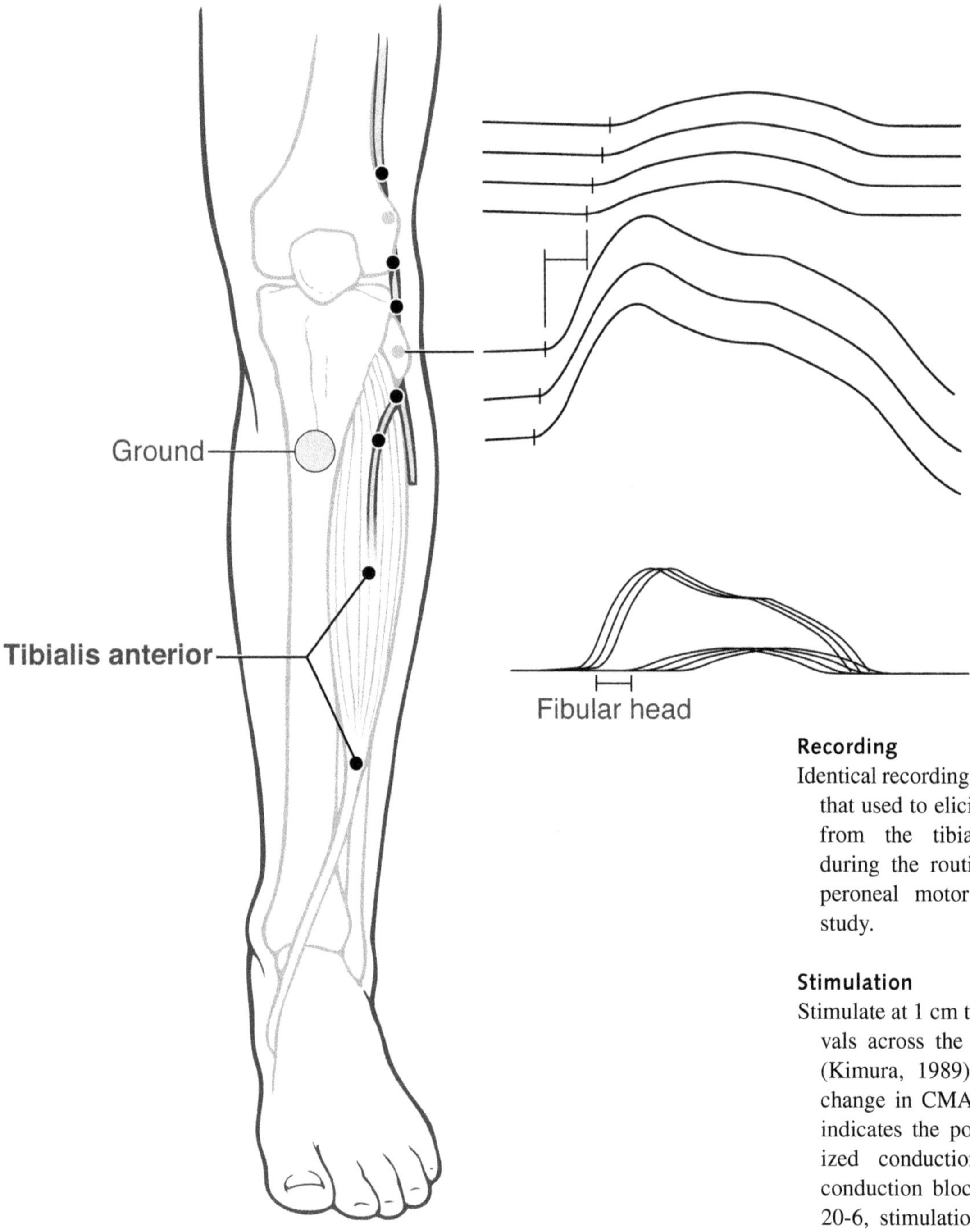

FIGURE 20-6 Short segment stimulation across the fibular head ("inching technique").

Recording

Identical recording technique to that used to elicit the CMAP from the tibialis anterior during the routine common peroneal motor conduction study.

Stimulation

Stimulate at 1 cm to 2 cm intervals across the fibular head (Kimura, 1989). An abrupt change in CMAP waveform indicates the point of localized conduction delay or conduction block. In Figure 20-6, stimulation at 1.5 cm increments results in a motor conduction velocity of <10 m/s localized to just above the fibular head, associated with a marked conduction block (focal demyelination).

Superficial Peroneal Sensory Nerve Conduction Study

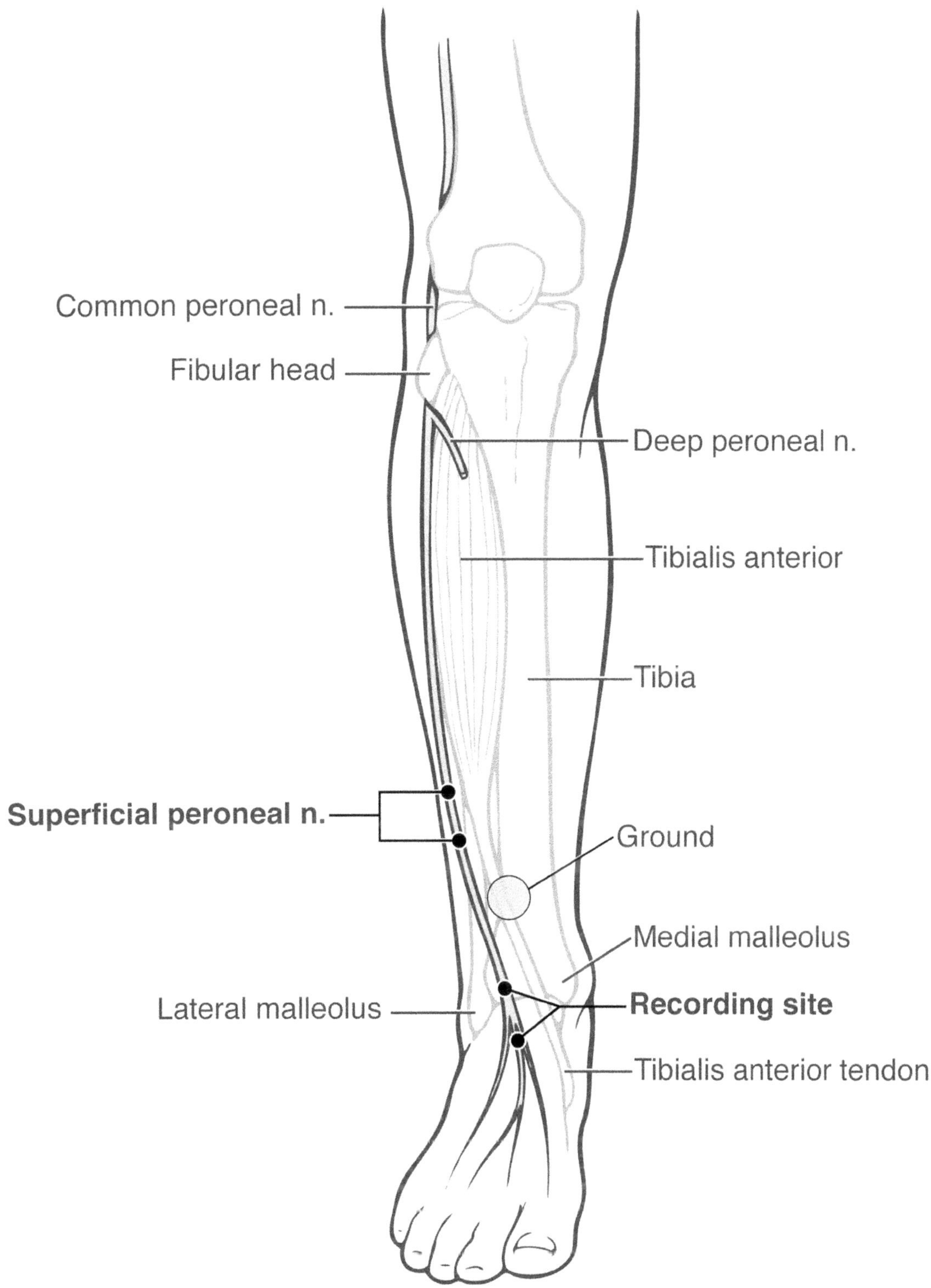

FIGURE 20-7 Superficial peroneal sensory nerve conduction study (antidromic).

Recording

Active electrode: Place over the dorsum of the foot at the level of the malleoli slightly lateral to the midline.

Reference electrode: Place 3 cm distal to the active electrode.

Ground electrode: Place on the distal leg, between stimulating and recording electrodes.

Stimulation

Leg: Place cathode over the distal anterolateral leg about 10 cm to 14 cm proximal to the lateral malleolus. The stimulator may need to be moved slightly laterally or medially to elicit a maximal sensory response. The anode is 3 cm proximal to cathode.

Normal Values

Latency (ms) ≤ 3.0 (onset latency); ≤ 3.5 (peak latency)
Amplitude (μV) ≥ 4
Conduction velocity (m/s) ≥ 40 m/s

Comments

The superficial peroneal sensory response is very useful in evaluating a common peroneal neuropathy at the fibular head associated with focal demyelination (conduction block). In a purely demyelinating lesion, the sensory response will be normal because the axons are spared, and both the stimulating and recording sites are distal to the lesion site. In contrast, the sensory response will be reduced in amplitude or absent in lesions causing axonal loss.

The normal amplitude of the superficial peroneal SNAP has a large range and standard deviation. Therefore, studies should ideally be performed bilaterally, because side-to-side comparisons are more useful than normal value tables that may not apply to your patient. An amplitude ≤ 50 % of the unaffected side is evidence of abnormality.

Temperature has a profound effect on nerve conduction studies. Low temperature is common in feet, and will prolong distal latencies, slow conduction velocity, and increase action potential amplitudes.

Pedal edema will reduce the amplitude of foot sensory responses.

The fibers underlying the stimulating and recording electrodes are derived primarily or exclusively from the L_5 root.

REFERENCES

Dawson DM, Hallett M, Millender LH. *Entrapment Neuropathies.* 2nd edition. Little, Brown, Boston, 1990, pp. 295–299.

Fisher MA. AAEM Minimonograph#13. H reflexes and F waves: physiology and clinical indications. *Muscle Nerve* 1992;15(11):1223–1233. Review.

Gray's Anatomy. 38th Edition. Churchill Livingstone, New York, 1995, pp. 1282–1288.

Gutmann L. AAEM Minimonograph #2. Important anomalous innervations of the extremities. *Muscle Nerve* 1993;16:339–347.

Katirji MB, Wilbourn AJ. Common peroneal mononeuropathy: A clinical electrophysiological study of 100 cases. *Neurology* 1984:34:142.

Kimura J. *Electrodiagnosis in Diseases of Nerve and Muscle.* 2nd ed., FA Davis Co., Philadelphia, 1989.

Koller RL, Blank NK. Strawberry pickers' palsy. *Arch Neurol* 1980;37:320.

Leis AA, Kronenberg MF, Stetkarova I, Paske WC, Stokic DS. Spinal motoneuron excit-ability following acute spinal cord injury in man. *Neurology* 1996;47:231–237.

Nobrega JAM, Pinhiero DS, Manzano GM, Kimura J. Various aspects of F-wave values in a healthy population. *Clin Neurophysiol* 2004;115:2336–2342.

Preston DC, Shapiro BE. Electromyography and neuromuscular disorders. Clinical-electrophysiologic correlations. 2nd ed. Philadelphia, Elsevier Butterworth Heinemann, 2005.

Puksa L, Stalberg E, Falck B. Reference values of F wave parameters in healthy subjects. *Clin Neurophysiol* 2003;114:1079–1090.

Sotaniemi KA. Slimmer's paralysis—peroneal neuropathy during weight reduction. *J Neurol Neurosurg Psychiatry.* 1984;47:564–566.

Sunderland S. *Nerves and Nerve Injuries.* Williams & Wilkins, Baltimore, 1968, pp. 1069–1095.

Wilbourn AJ. AAEE case report #12: Common peroneal mononeuropathy at the fibular head. *Muscle Nerve* 1986;9:825–836.

Tibialis Anterior

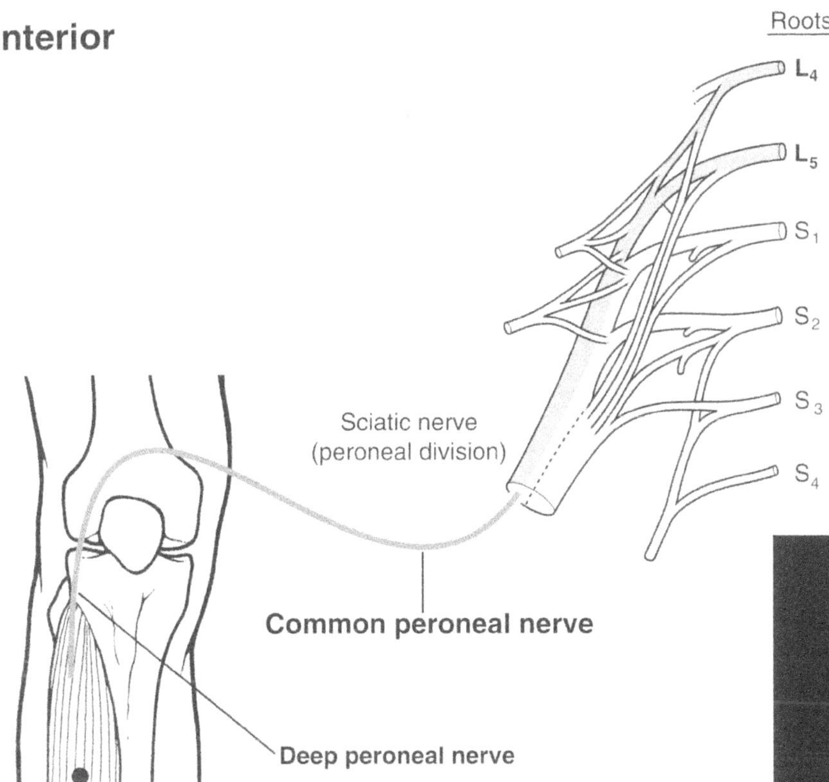

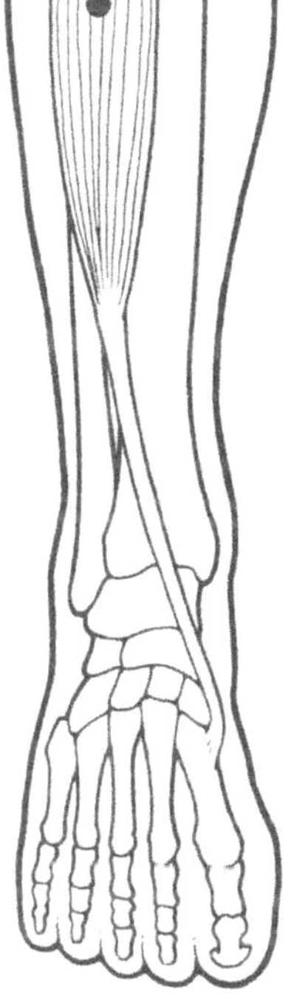

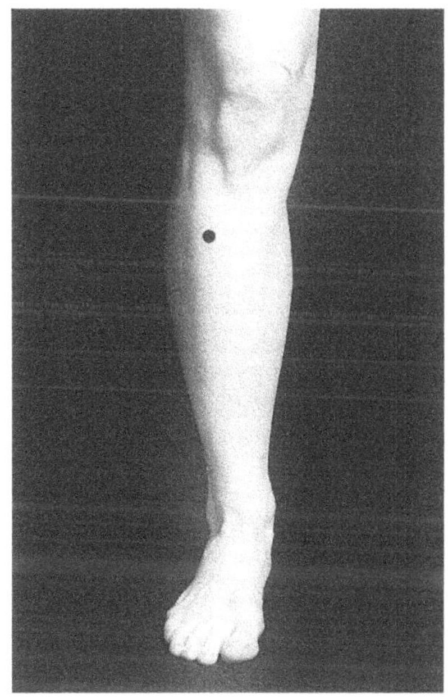

Innervation
Innervation is via the deep peroneal nerve, common peroneal nerve, peroneal division of the sciatic nerve, sacral plexus, and roots L_4, L_5.

Origin
The tibialis anterior originates from the lateral condyle of the tibia and the proximal half of the lateral surface of the shaft of the tibia.

Insertion
Insertion is at the medial cuneiform bone and adjoining part of the base of the first metatarsal bone.

Activation Maneuver
Dorsiflexion of the foot activates the muscle.

EMG Needle Insertion
Insert the needle just lateral to the proximal half of the shaft of the tibia (the muscle is superficial and readily palpable lateral to the tibia).

Pitfalls
There are no pitfalls. If the needle is inserted too laterally or deeply, it will be in the extensor digitorum longus, which is also innervated by the deep peroneal nerve.

Clinical Comments
Neurogenic changes on needle examination may be seen with lesions of the deep peroneal nerve, common peroneal nerve, peroneal division of the sciatic nerve, sacral plexus, or L_4, L_5 roots.

In the evaluation of severe "foot drop," always examine L_5 muscles that are not supplied by the common peroneal nerve (i.e., tibialis posterior, flexor digitorum longus, tensor fasciae latae, gluteus medius, or paraspinals) to exclude an L_5 radiculopathy. Conversely, these muscles are normal in foot drop due solely to peroneal mononeuropathy.

The tibialis anterior may also contribute to *inversion* of the foot because its tendon inserts on the medial aspect of the foot.

Extensor Digitorum Longus

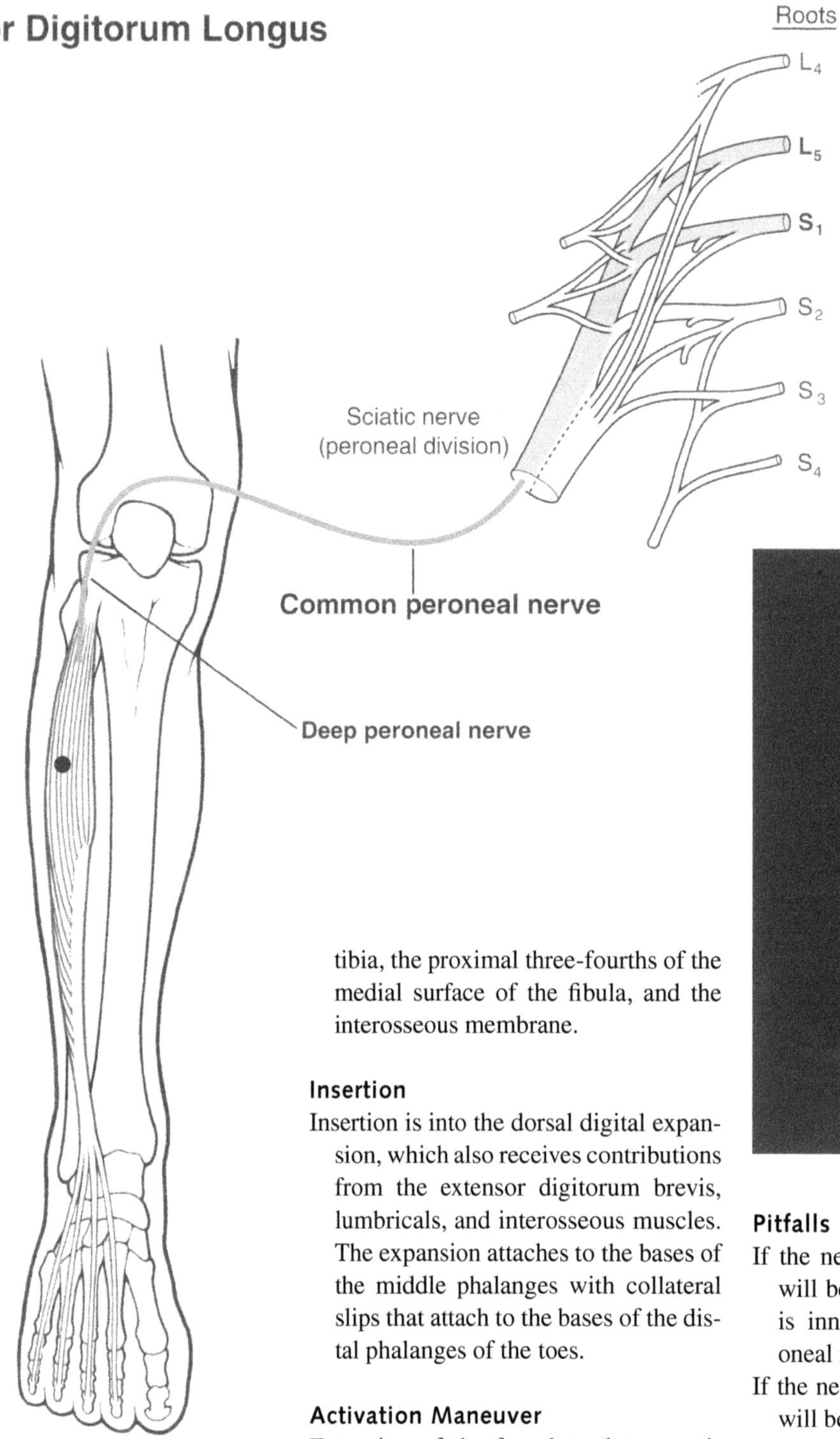

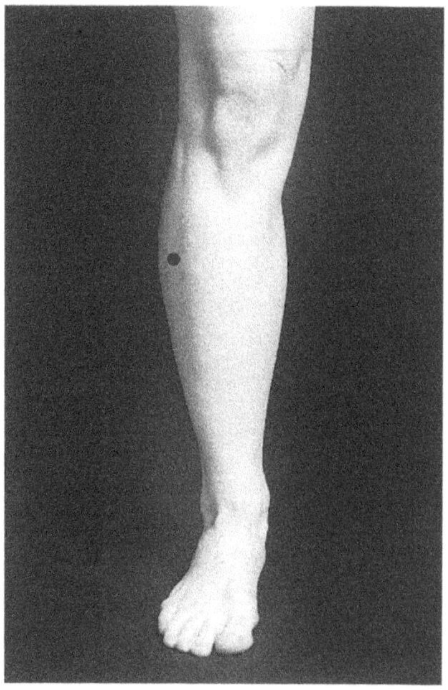

Innervation
Innervation is via the deep peroneal nerve, common peroneal nerve, peroneal division of the sciatic nerve, sacral plexus, and roots L_5, S_1.

Origin
The extensor digitorum longus originates from the lateral condyle of the tibia, the proximal three-fourths of the medial surface of the fibula, and the interosseous membrane.

Insertion
Insertion is into the dorsal digital expansion, which also receives contributions from the extensor digitorum brevis, lumbricals, and interosseous muscles. The expansion attaches to the bases of the middle phalanges with collateral slips that attach to the bases of the distal phalanges of the toes.

Activation Maneuver
Extension of the four lateral toes activates the muscles.

EMG Needle Insertion
Insert the needle 6–7 cm distal to the tibial tuberosity and 4–5 cm lateral to the shaft of the tibia. The muscle is superficial in this location, lying between the tibialis anterior and the peroneus longus (*Gray's Anatomy,* 1995).

Pitfalls
If the needle is inserted too laterally, it will be in the peroneus longus, which is innervated by the superficial peroneal nerve.

If the needle is inserted too anteriorly, it will be in the tibialis anterior, which is also innervated by the deep peroneal nerve.

Clinical Comments
Neurogenic changes on needle examination may be seen with lesions of the deep peroneal nerve, common peroneal nerve, peroneal division of the sciatic nerve, sacral plexus, or L_5, S_1 roots.

Extensor Hallucis Longus

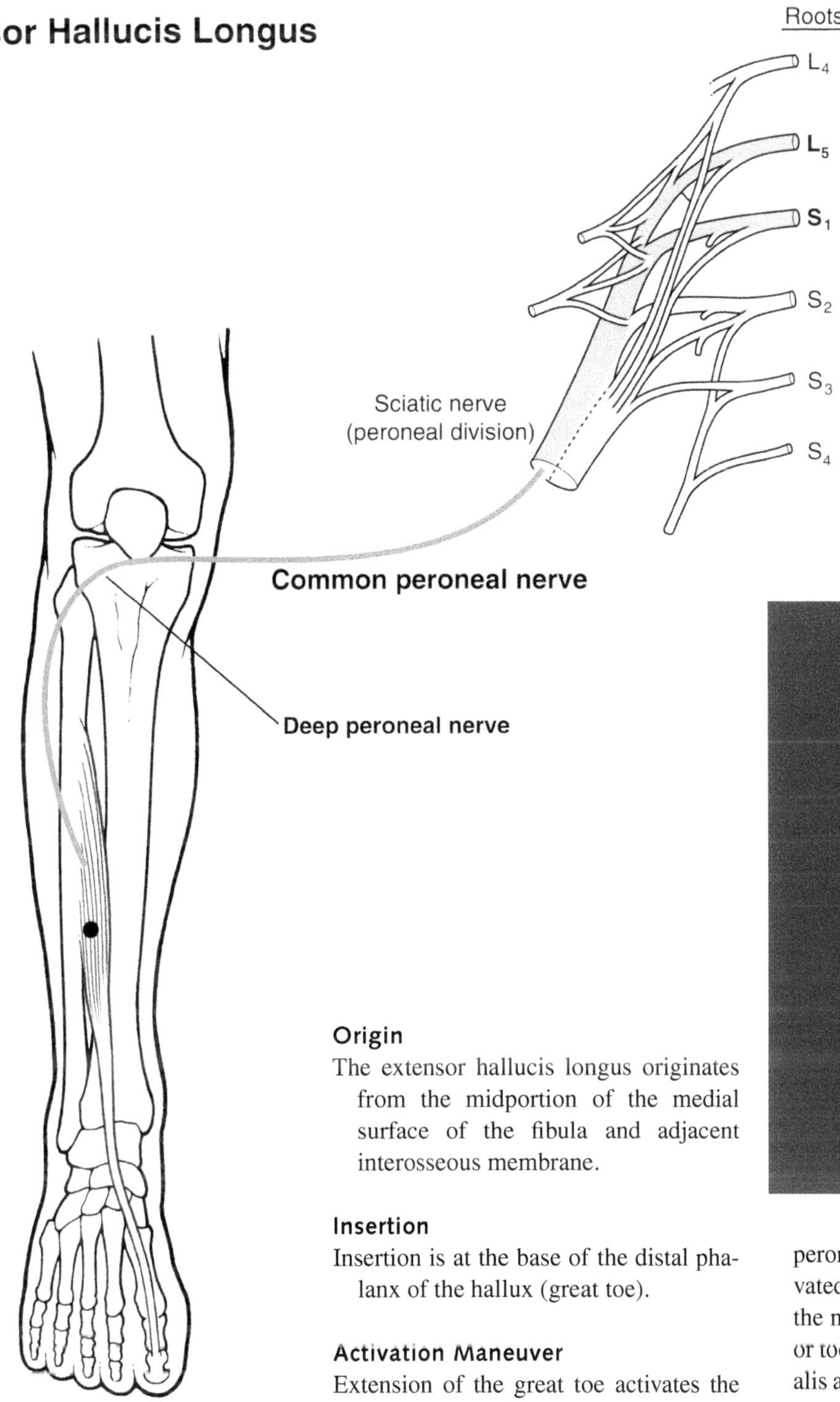

Innervation

Innervation is via the deep peroneal nerve, common peroneal nerve, peroneal division of the sciatic nerve, sacral plexus, and roots L_5, S_1.

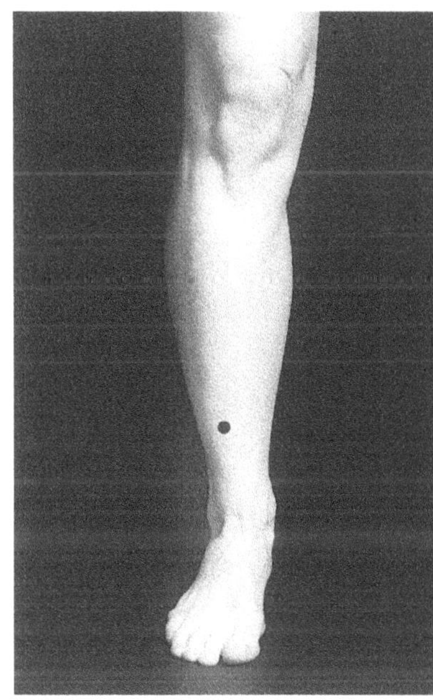

Origin

The extensor hallucis longus originates from the midportion of the medial surface of the fibula and adjacent interosseous membrane.

Insertion

Insertion is at the base of the distal phalanx of the hallux (great toe).

Activation Maneuver

Extension of the great toe activates the muscle.

EMG Needle Insertion

Insert the needle 7–9 cm proximal to the bimalleolar line of the ankle just lateral to the shaft of the tibia.

Pitfalls

There are no pitfalls. If the needle is inserted too laterally it will be in the peroneus tertius, which is also innervated by the deep peroneal nerve. If the needle is inserted too superficially or too proximally, it may be in the tibialis anterior or extensor digitorum longus, which are also innervated by the deep peroneal nerve.

Clinical Comments

Neurogenic changes on needle examination may be seen with lesions of the deep peroneal nerve, common peroneal nerve, peroneal division of the sciatic nerve, sacral plexus, or L_5, S_1 roots.

Peroneus Tertius

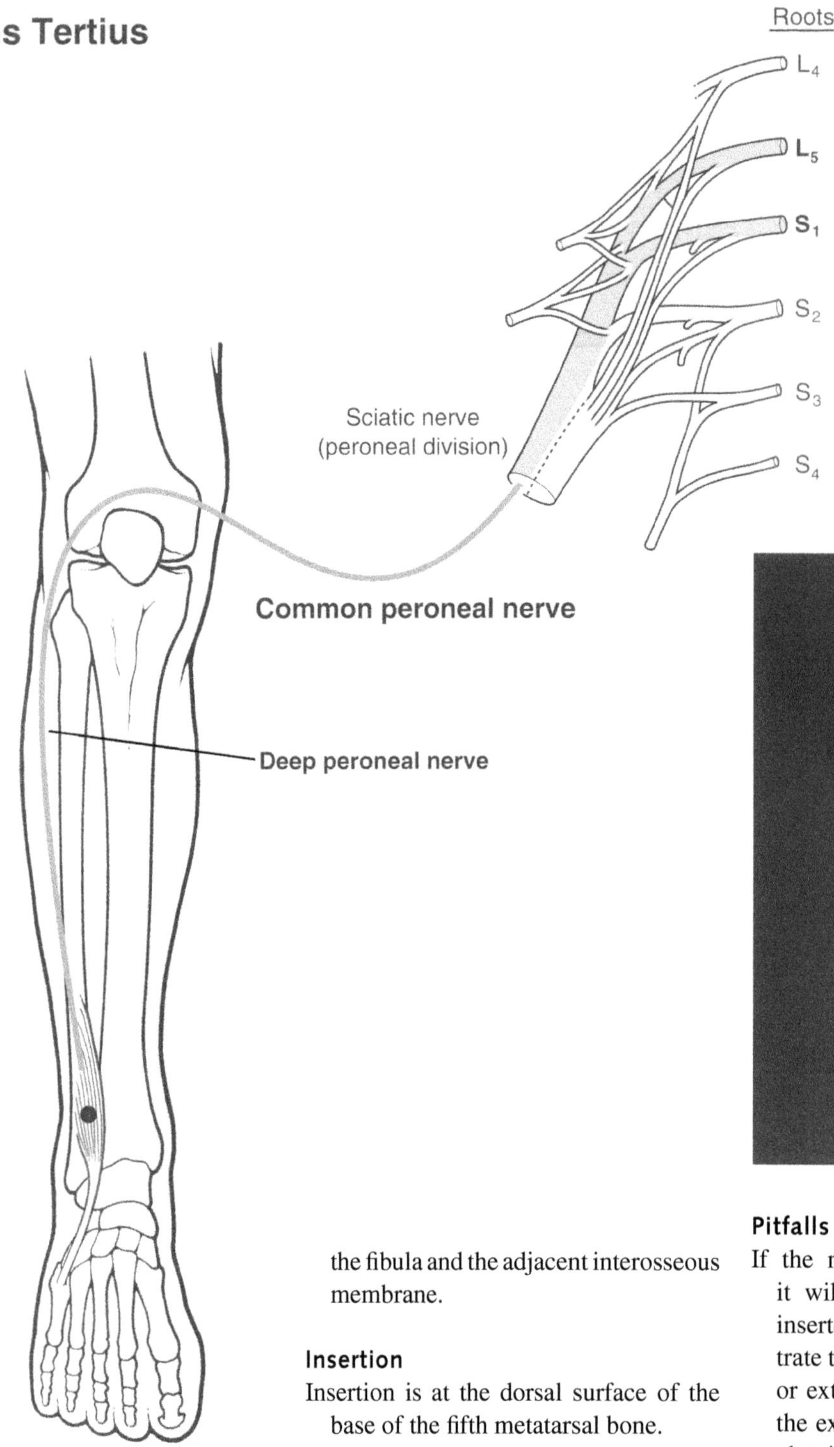

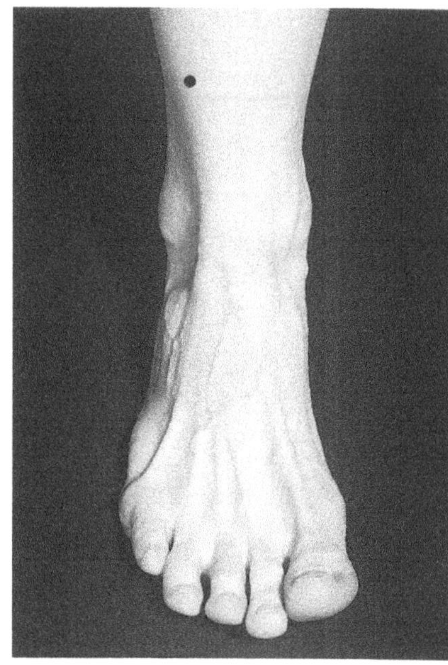

Innervation
Innervation is via the deep peroneal nerve, common peroneal nerve, peroneal division of the sciatic nerve, sacral plexus, and roots L_5, S_1.

Origin
The peroneus tertius originates from the distal fourth of the anterior surface of the fibula and the adjacent interosseous membrane.

Insertion
Insertion is at the dorsal surface of the base of the fifth metatarsal bone.

Activation Maneuver
Dorsiflexion and eversion of the foot activate the muscle.

EMG Needle Insertion
Insert the needle 6–8 cm proximal to the bimalleolar line of the ankle and 2–3 cm lateral to the shaft of the tibia.

Pitfalls
If the needle is inserted too laterally, it will encounter the fibula; if it is inserted too anteriorly, it may penetrate the tendons of the tibialis anterior or extensor digitorum longus or enter the extensor hallucis longus, which is also innervated by the deep peroneal nerve.

Clinical Comments
Neurogenic changes on needle examination may be seen with lesions of the deep peroneal nerve, common peroneal nerve, peroneal division of the sciatic nerve, sacral plexus, or L_5, S_1 roots.

Extensor Digitorum Brevis

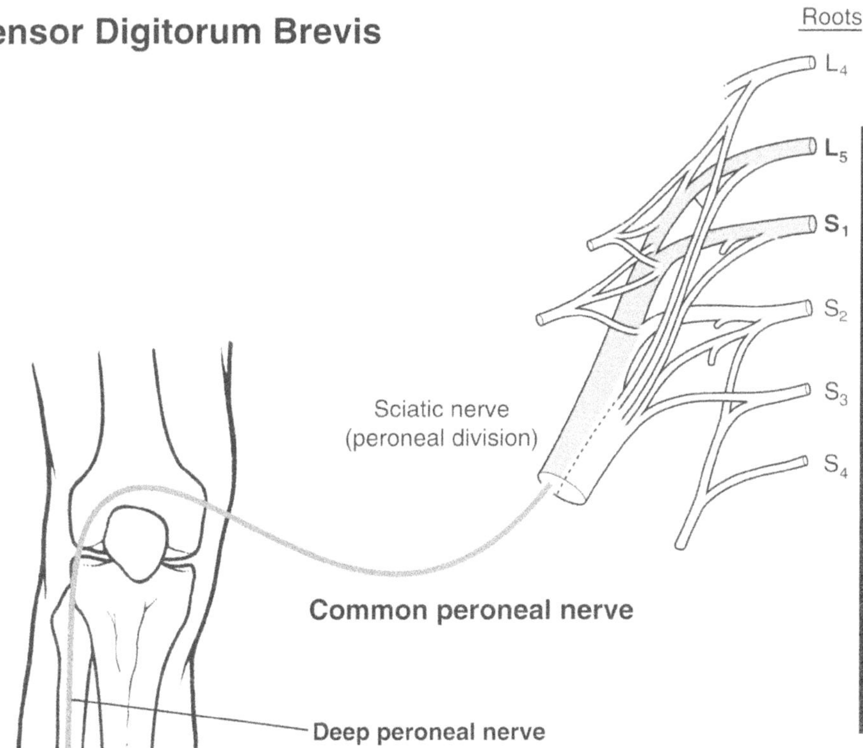

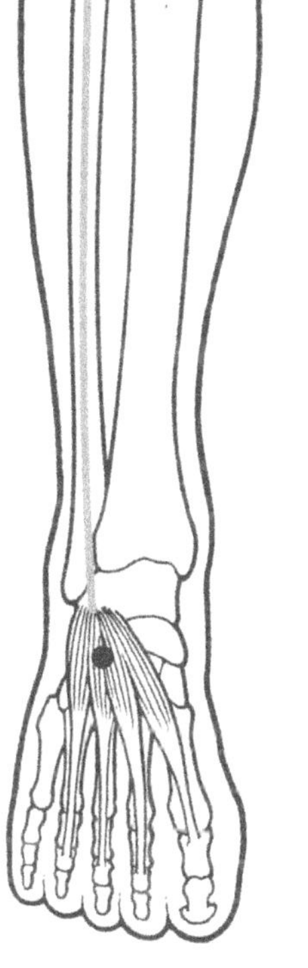

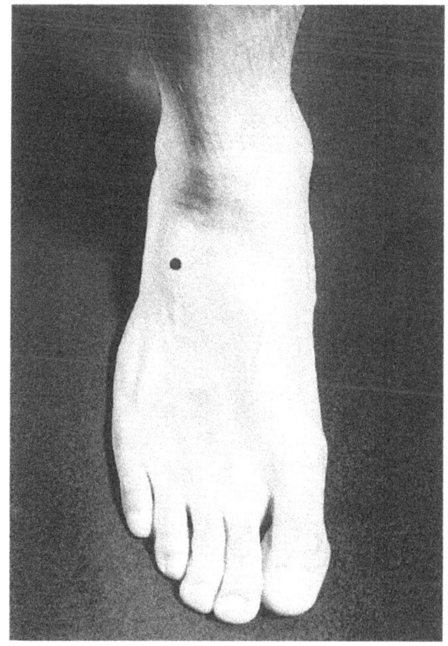

Innervation

Innervation is via the deep peroneal nerve, common peroneal nerve, peroneal division of the sciatic nerve, sacral plexus, and roots L_5, S_1.

In 20%–28% of subjects, an *accessory deep peroneal nerve* also supplies this muscle (Gutmann, 1993). The accessory deep peroneal nerve is an anomalous motor branch originating from the superficial peroneal nerve. It descends on the lateral aspect of the leg, passes posterior to the lateral malleolus, and proceeds anteriorly to supply the lateral portion of the extensor digitorum brevis.

Origin

The extensor digitorum brevis originates from the anterior and superolateral surfaces of the calcaneus.

Insertion

Insertion is into the dorsal digital expansion, which also receives contributions from the extensor digitorum longus, lumbricals, and interosseous muscles. The expansion attaches to the bases of the middle phalanges with collateral slips that attach to the bases of the distal phalanges of the toes. The extensor digitorum brevis contributes four tendons; three attach to the tendons of the extensor digitorum longus for the second through fourth toes, and one inserts into the base of the proximal phalanx of the hallux; this latter slip is sometimes termed the *extensor hallucis brevis*.

Activation Maneuver

Extension of the toes activates the muscle.

EMG Needle Insertion

Insert the needle into the small mound of muscle tissue located on the proximal lateral aspect of the dorsum of the foot.

Pitfalls

The muscle may be difficult to examine in patients with peripheral neuropathies or other conditions predisposing to atrophy (e.g., compression from chronically tight shoes).

Clinical Comments

Neurogenic changes on needle examination may be seen with lesions of the deep peroneal nerve, common peroneal nerve, peroneal division of the sciatic nerve, sacral plexus, or L_5, S_1 roots.

The extensor digitorum brevis is involved early in length-dependent peripheral neuropathies.

Neurogenic changes on needle examination may reflect chronic compression of the nerve or muscle from tight shoes or high-heeled shoes (Dawson et al., 1990).

This muscle is commonly used to record the compound muscle action potential during peroneal nerve conduction studies.

Peroneus Longus

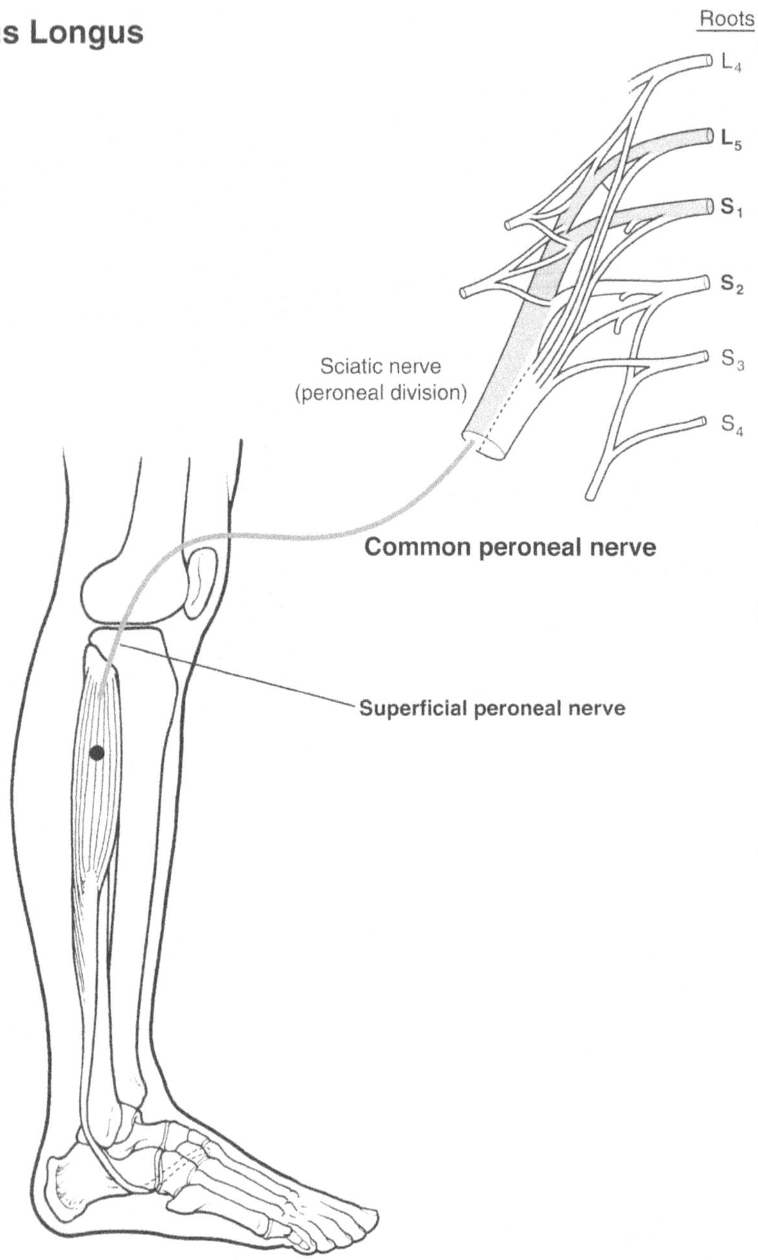

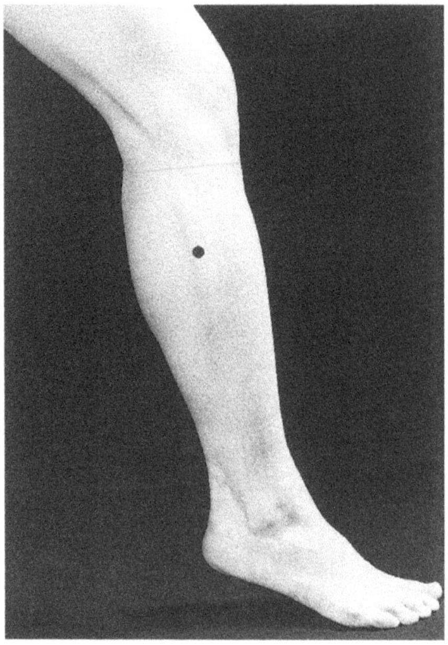

Innervation

Innervation is via the superficial peroneal nerve, common peroneal nerve, peroneal division of the sciatic nerve, sacral plexus, and roots L_5, S_1.

Origin

The peroneus longus originates from the head and proximal two-thirds of the lateral surface of the fibula.

Insertion

Insertion is at the lateral surface of the base of the first metatarsal bone and the medial cuneiform bone.

Activation Maneuver

Eversion of the foot activates the muscle. Note: This muscle can also *plantar flex* the foot because its tendon runs distally *behind* the lateral malleolus.

EMG Needle Insertion

Insert the needle 5–7 cm below the fibular head along the lateral aspect of the fibula.

Pitfalls

If the needle is inserted too posteriorly, it will be in the soleus or lateral gastrocnemius, which are supplied by the tibial nerve.

If the needle is inserted too anteriorly, it will be in the extensor digitorum longus, which is supplied by the deep peroneal nerve.

To minimize pitfalls, activation of the peroneus longus (i.e., eversion of the foot) should be performed while flexing the toes and slightly dorsiflexing the foot. This will avoid coactivation of the adjacent extensor digitorum longus and lateral gastrocnemius, respectively.

Clinical Comments

Neurogenic changes on needle examination may be seen with lesions of the superficial peroneal nerve, common peroneal nerve, peroneal division of the sciatic nerve, sacral plexus, or L_5, S_1 roots.

Peroneus Brevis

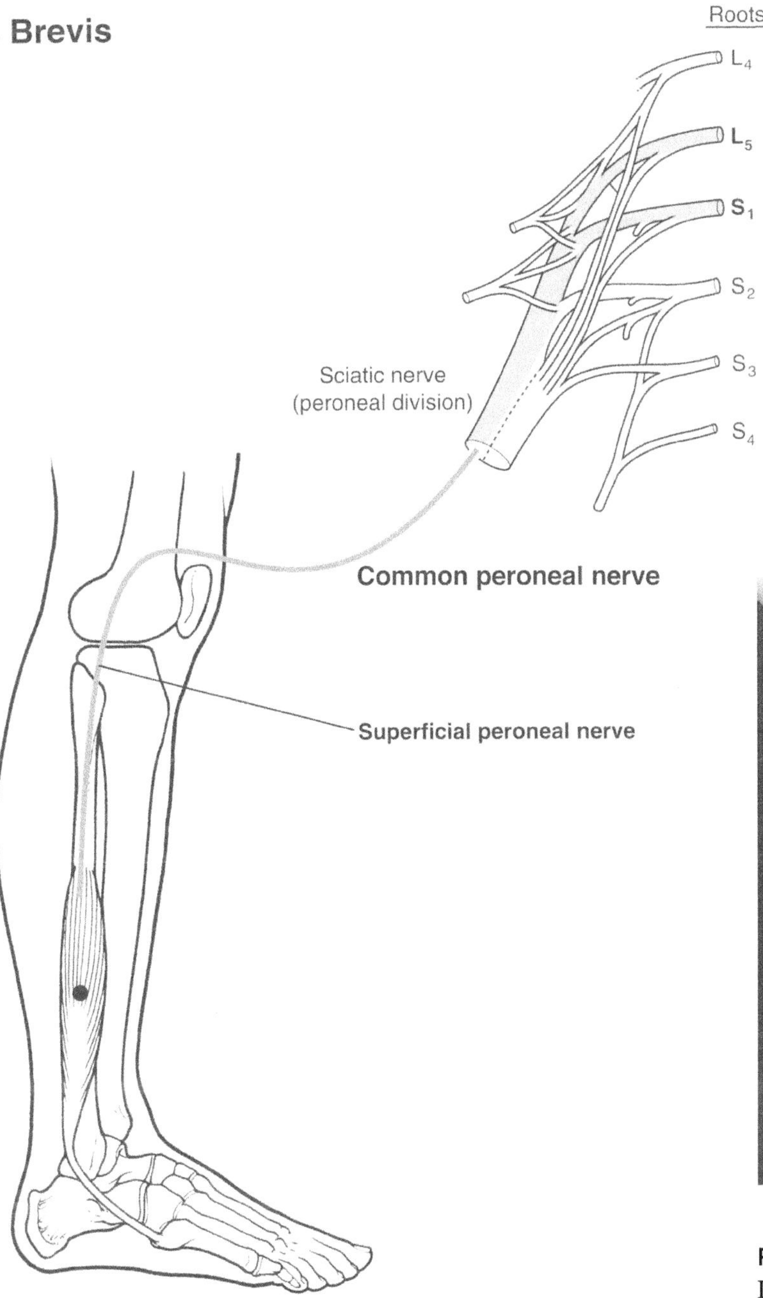

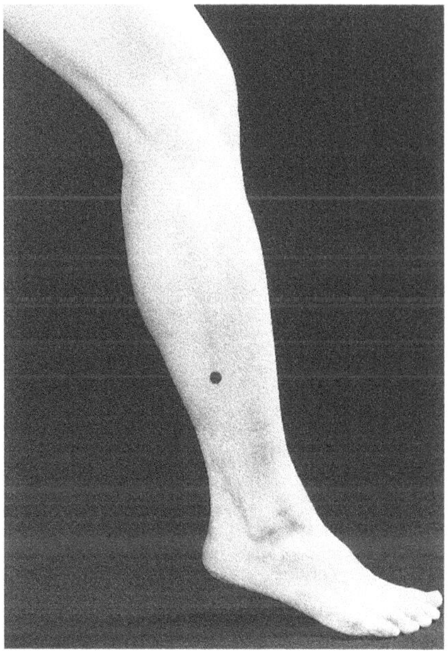

Innervation

Innervation is via the superficial peroneal nerve, common peroneal nerve, peroneal division of the sciatic nerve, sacral plexus, and roots L_5, S_1.

Origin

The peroneus brevis originates from the distal two-thirds of the lateral surface of the fibula.

Insertion

Insertion is at the lateral surface of the base of the fifth metatarsal bone.

Activation Maneuver

Eversion of the foot activates the muscle. Note: This muscle can also *plantar flex* the foot because its tendon, together with that of the peroneus longus, passes *behind* the lateral malleolus.

EMG Needle Insertion

Insert the needle 8–10 cm above the lateral malleolus just posterior to the lateral aspect of the fibula.

Pitfalls

If the needle is inserted anterior to the lateral aspect of the fibula, it will be in the peroneus tertius, supplied by the deep peroneal nerve.

If the needle is inserted too deeply, it will be in the flexor hallucis longus, which is supplied by the tibial nerve.

Clinical Comments

Neurogenic changes on needle examination may be seen with lesions of the superficial peroneal nerve, common peroneal nerve, peroneal division of the sciatic nerve, sacral plexus, or L_5, S_1 roots.

21 SUPERIOR GLUTEAL NERVE

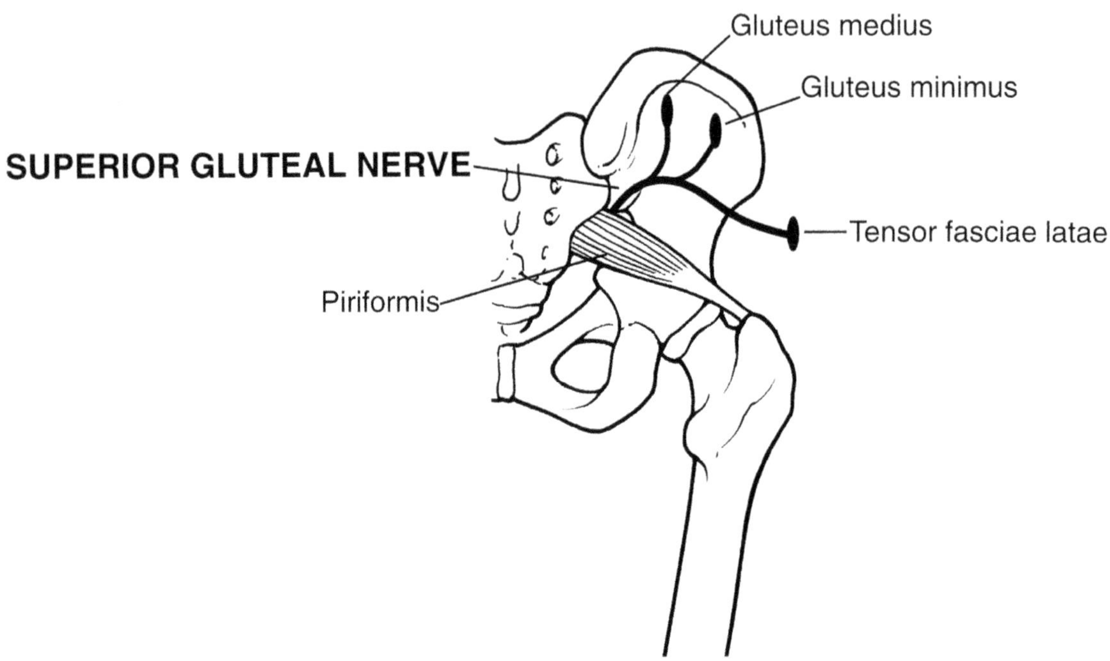

FIGURE 21-1 Diagram of the superior gluteal nerve (posterior view) and its branches.

THE SUPERIOR GLUTEAL NERVE arises from the posterior branches of the fourth and fifth lumbar and the first sacral ventral rami. It leaves the pelvis via the greater sciatic foramen above the piriformis muscle, with the superior gluteal vessels, and divides into superior and inferior branches. The superior branch follows the line of origin of the gluteus minimus to supply the gluteus medius. The inferior branch crosses obliquely between the gluteus minimus and gluteus medius, distributing filaments to both of these muscles before terminating in the tensor fasciae latae.

The gluteus medius and minimus play an essential role in maintaining the trunk upright when the opposite foot is in the swing phase of the gait cycle. In this phase, the weight of the elevated leg tends to make the pelvis sag downward. This is normally counteracted by the gluteus medius and minimus of the supporting side (i.e., on the standing leg side), which exert such a powerful traction on the hip bone that the pelvis on the unsupported side is actually raised slightly (*Gray's Anatomy,* 1995). This supportive effect of the glutei on the contralateral pelvis depends on preserved innervation to the two muscles and on the normal relationship between the components of the hip joint. When these conditions are not fulfilled, such as in lesions of the superior gluteal nerve, congenital dislocation of the hip, or nonunion fracture of the neck of the femur, the supportive effect of the glutei is abolished and the pelvis sinks on the contralateral foot during its swing phase. This results in a characteristic lurching gait (Trendelenburg's sign). Paralysis of the gluteus medius and minimus is the most serious muscular disability affecting the hip; paralysis of other muscles acting on the hip joint produces relatively little gait dysfunction.

The superior gluteal nerve, or its branches, may be involved by trauma and penetrating injuries, including pelvic fractures and misplaced intramuscular injections. The nerve is also prone to injury in the buttocks as it descends laterally between the gluteus medius and gluteus minimus. In this region, it is at risk during surgery on the hip (Kenny et al., 1999). However, in most cases of iatrogenic surgical injury, the damage tends to improve spontaneously and does not cause clinically significant long-term weakness of thigh abduction (Picado et al., 2007).

REFERENCES

Gray's Anatomy. 38th Edition. Churchill Livingstone, New York 1995, pp. 870–876, 1282–1288.

Kenny P, O'Brien CP, Synnott K, Walsh MG. Damage to the superior gluteal nerve after two different approaches to the hip. *J Bone Joint Surg* [Br] 1999;81-B:979–981.

Picado CH, Garcia FL, Marques W Jr. Damage to the superior gluteal nerve after direct lateral approach to the hip. *Clin Orthop Relat Res* 2007;455:209–211.

Preston DC, Shapiro BE. Electromyography and neuromuscular disorders. Clinical-electrophysiologic correlations. 2nd ed. Philadelphia, Elsevier Butterworth Heinemann, 2005.

Gluteus Medius

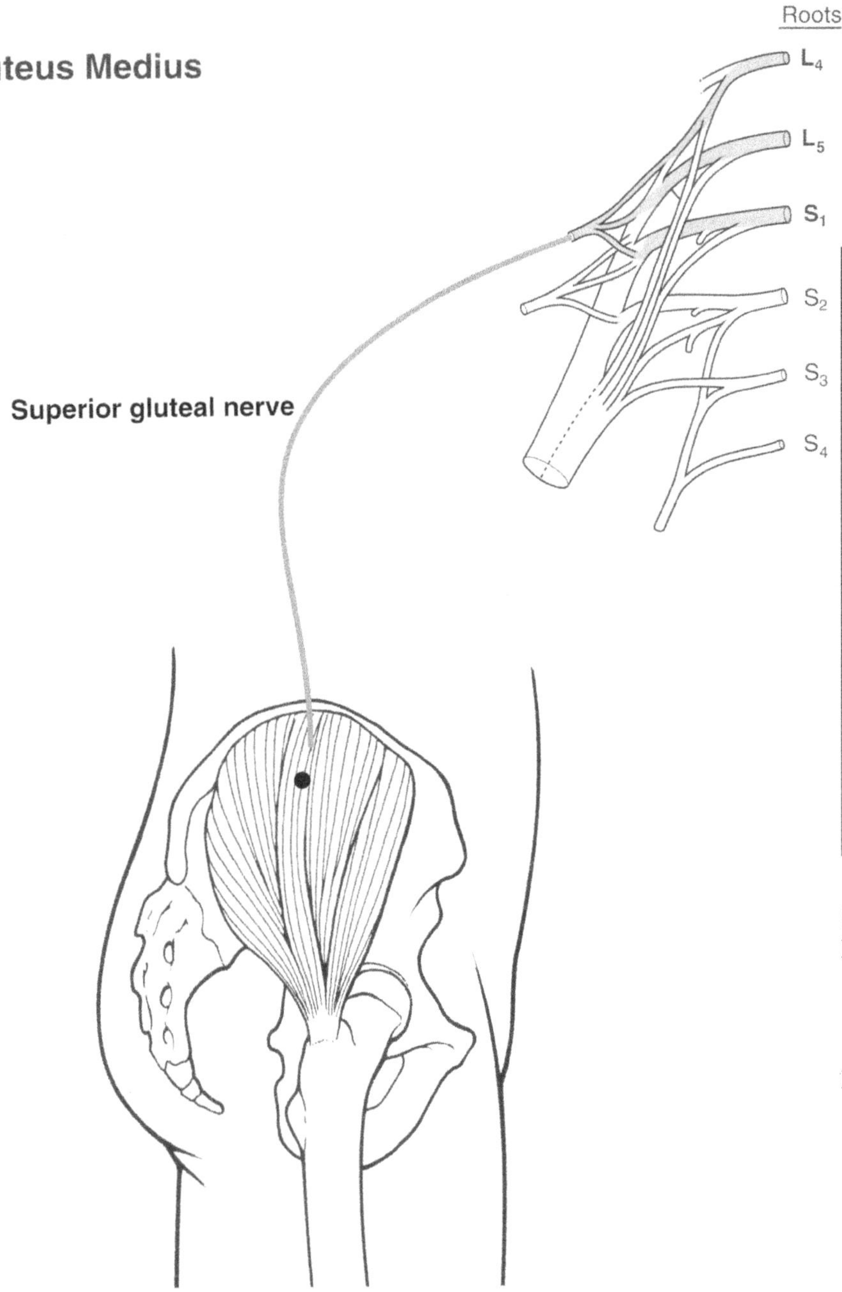

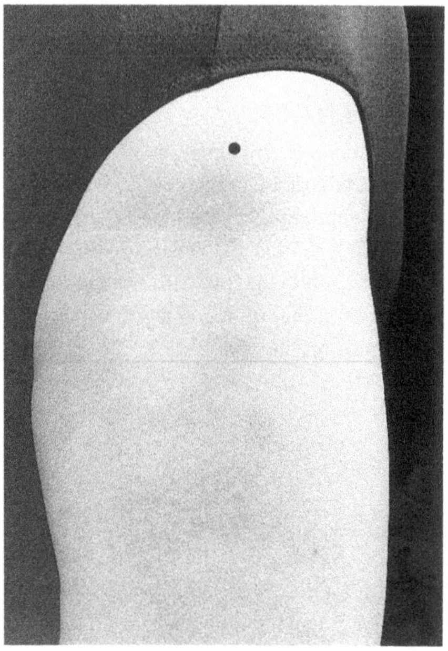

Innervation

Innervation is via the superior gluteal nerve, sacral plexus, and roots L_4, L_5, S_1.

Origin

The gluteus medius originates from the outer surface of the ilium between the iliac crest above and the anterior gluteal line below.

Insertion

Insertion is at the lateral surface of the greater trochanter of the femur.

Activation Maneuver

Abduction of the thigh activates the muscle. The anterior fibers may also contribute to medial rotation of the thigh.

EMG Needle Insertion

Insert the needle 2–3 cm distal to the midpoint of the iliac crest.

Pitfalls

If the needle is inserted too anteriorly, it may be in the tensor fasciae latae, which is also supplied by the superior gluteal nerve and L_4, L_5, and S_1 roots.

If the needle is inserted too posteriorly, it may be in the gluteus maximus, which is supplied by the inferior gluteal nerve and L_5, S_1, and S_2 roots. The posterior third of the gluteus medius is covered by the gluteus maximus.

Clinical Comments

Neurogenic changes on needle examination may be seen with lesions of the superior gluteal nerve, sacral plexus, or L_4, L_5, S_1 roots.

This is a good muscle to study for suspected L_4 or L_5 radiculopathy, because these roots primarily supply this muscle (*Gray's Anatomy,* 1995).

This is also a good muscle to study to differentiate a lumbosacral plexopathy from a sciatic nerve lesion (Preston and Shapiro, 2005).

Gluteus Minimus

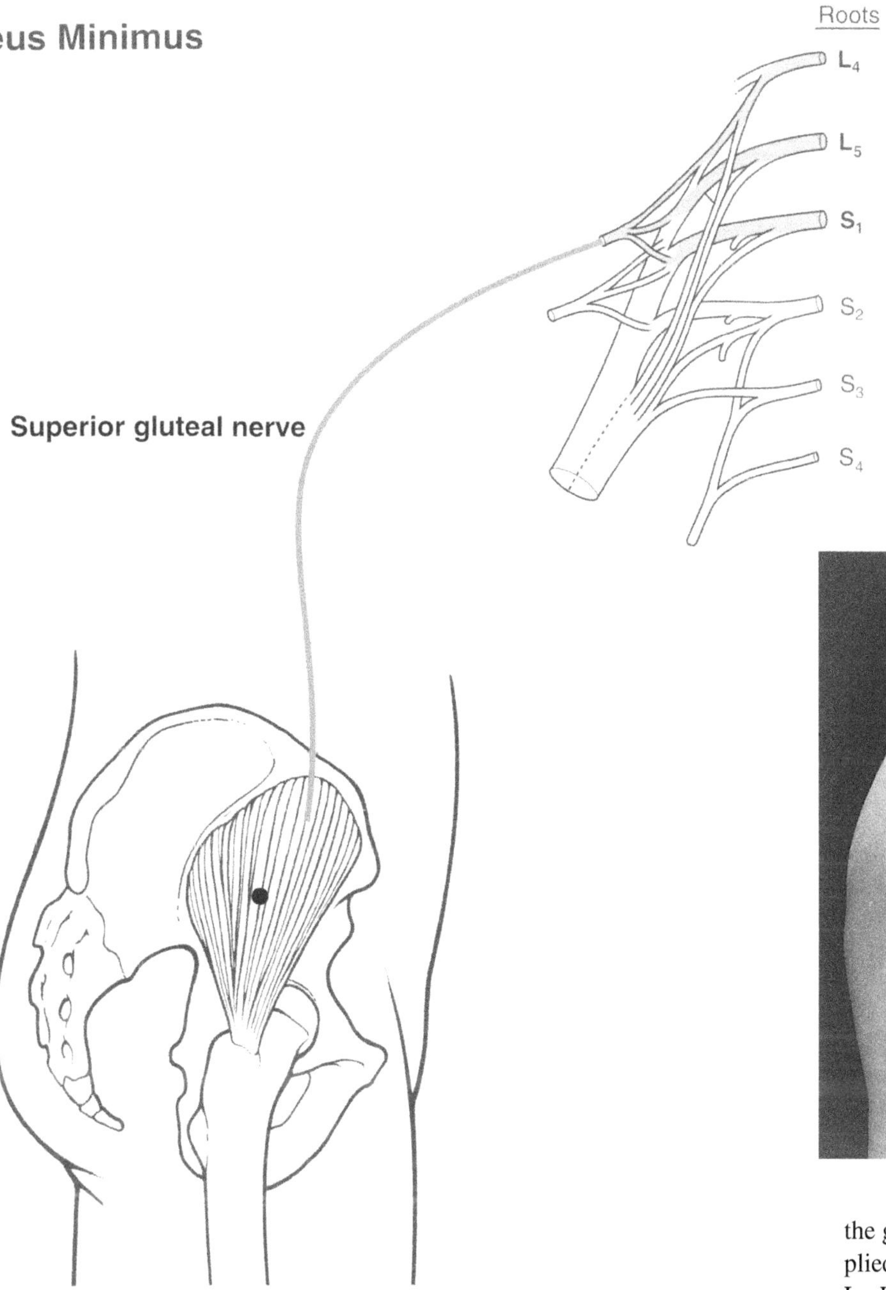

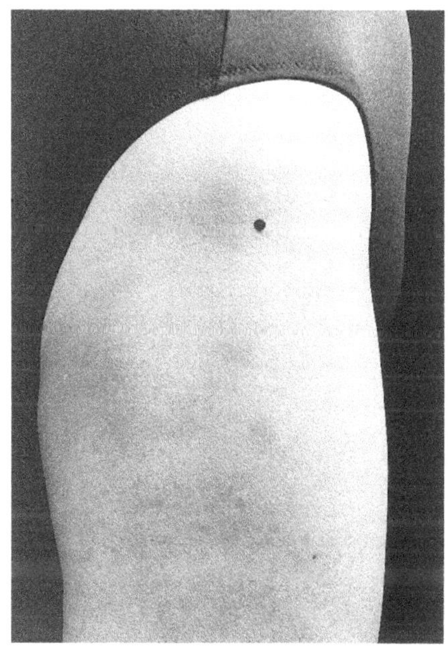

Innervation
Innervation is via the superior gluteal nerve, sacral plexus, and roots L_4, L_5, S_1.

Origin
The gluteus minimus originates from the outer surface of the ilium between the anterior and inferior gluteal lines.

Insertion
Insertion is at the anterolateral surface of the greater trochanter of the femur.

Activation Maneuver
Abduction of the thigh activates the muscle. The anterior fibers may also contribute to medial rotation of the thigh.

EMG Needle Insertion
Insert the needle midway between the iliac crest and the greater trochanter of the femur.

Insert to the bone and withdraw slightly.

Pitfalls
There are no pitfalls. If the needle is inserted too superficially, it may be in the gluteus medius, which is also supplied by the superior gluteal nerve and L_4, L_5, and S_1 roots.

Clinical Comments
Neurogenic changes on needle examination may be seen with lesions of the superior gluteal nerve, sacral plexus, or L_4, L_5, S_1 roots.

This is a good muscle to study for suspected L_4 or L_5 radiculopathy, because these roots primarily supply this muscle (*Gray's Anatomy, 1995*).

This is also a good muscle to study to differentiate a lumbosacral plexopathy from a sciatic nerve lesion (Preston and Shapiro, 2005).

Tensor Fasciae Latae

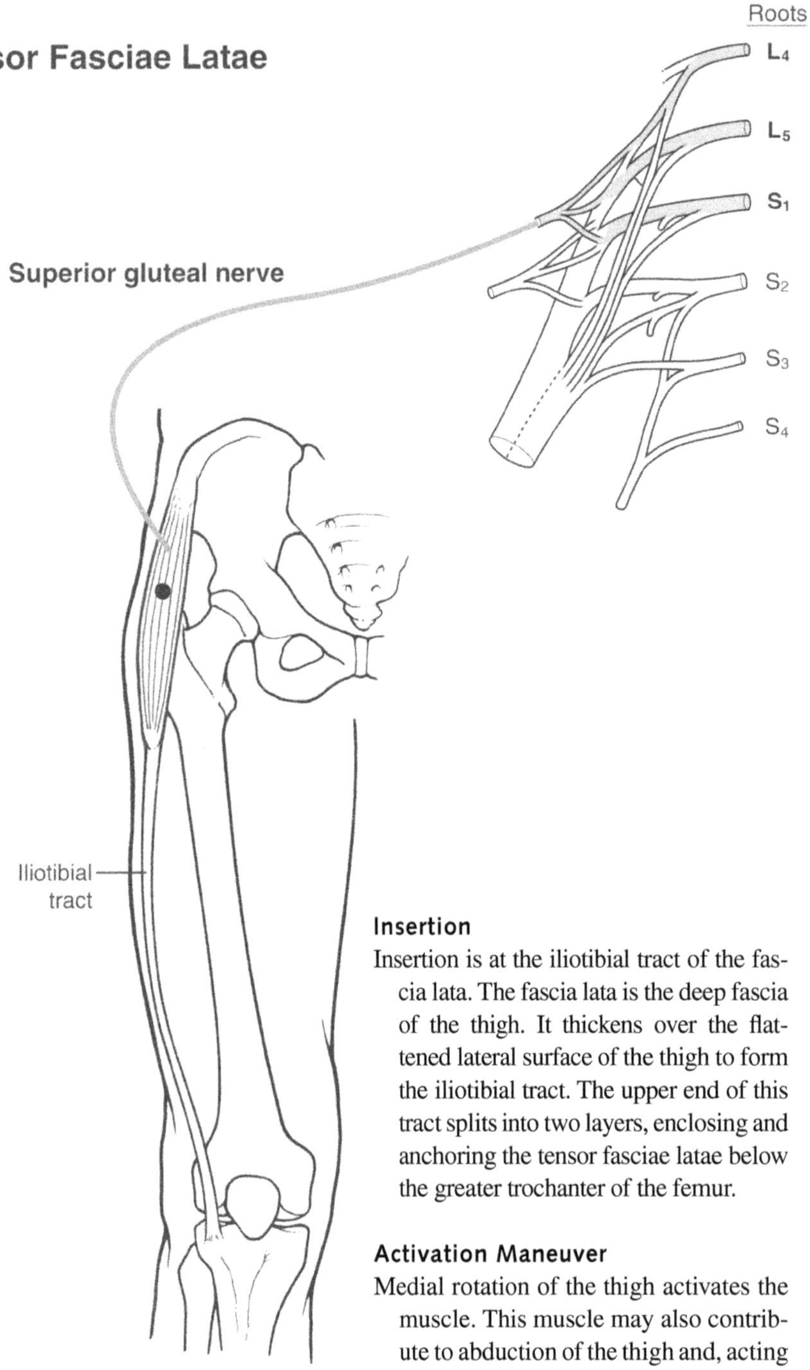

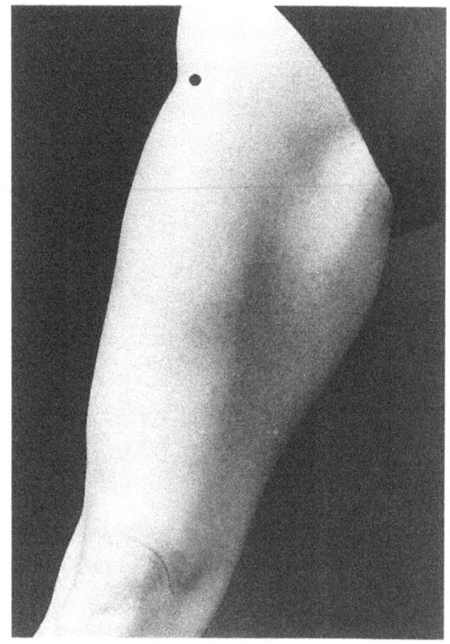

Innervation

Innervation is via the superior gluteal nerve, sacral plexus, and roots L_4, L_5, S_1.

Origin

The tensor fasciae latae originates from the anterior superior iliac spine and the outer lip of the iliac crest.

Insertion

Insertion is at the iliotibial tract of the fascia lata. The fascia lata is the deep fascia of the thigh. It thickens over the flattened lateral surface of the thigh to form the iliotibial tract. The upper end of this tract splits into two layers, enclosing and anchoring the tensor fasciae latae below the greater trochanter of the femur.

Activation Maneuver

Medial rotation of the thigh activates the muscle. This muscle may also contribute to abduction of the thigh and, acting through the iliotibial tract, it may also extend the knee with lateral rotation of the leg (*Gray's Anatomy,* 1995).

EMG Needle Insertion

Insert the needle midway between the anterior superior iliac spine and the greater trochanter of the femur.

Pitfalls

If the needle is inserted too medially, it may be in the rectus femoris or sartorius, both muscles innervated by the femoral nerve and L_2–L_4 roots.

If the needle is inserted too laterally, it may be in the gluteus medius, which is also supplied by the superior gluteal nerve and L_4, L_5, and S_1 roots.

Clinical Comments

Neurogenic changes on needle examination may be seen with lesions of the superior gluteal nerve, sacral plexus, or L_4, L_5, S_1 roots.

This is a good muscle to study for suspected L_4 or L_5 radiculopathy because these roots primarily supply this muscle (*Gray's Anatomy,* 1995).

This is also a good muscle to study to differentiate a lumbosacral plexopathy from a sciatic nerve lesion (Preston and Shapiro, 2005).

INFERIOR GLUTEAL NERVE

22

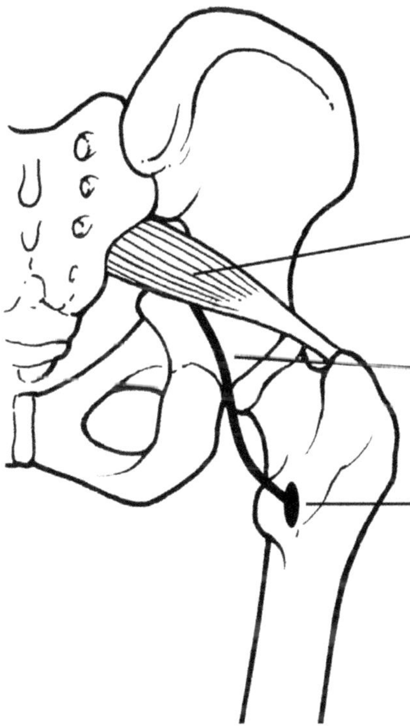

FIGURE 22-1 Diagram of the inferior gluteal nerve to the gluteus maximus (posterior view).

THE INFERIOR GLUTEAL NERVE arises from the posterior branches of the fifth lumbar and first and second sacral ventral rami (*Gray's Anatomy,* 1995). It leaves the pelvis via the greater sciatic foramen below the piriformis muscle and divides into a number of branches that enter the deep surface of the gluteus maximus. The gluteus maximus is the largest and most superficial muscle of the gluteal region. It forms the familiar prominence of the buttocks.

The inferior gluteal nerve, or its branches, may be involved by trauma and penetrating injuries, including pelvic fractures and misplaced intramuscular injections. The nerve is also prone to injury in the buttock as it descends laterally into the gluteus maximus. In this region, it is at risk during posterior and posterolateral surgical approaches to the hip (Goldberg and Goldstein, 1998; Apaydin et al., 2009). However, in most cases of iatrogenic surgical injury, the damage tends to improve spontaneously and does not cause clinically significant long-term weakness of thigh extension. Symptoms and signs of an inferior gluteal nerve lesion include difficulty climbing stairs or arising from a seated position, pain in the buttock region, weakness of hip extension, and atrophy of the buttock.

REFERENCES

Apaydin N, Bozkurt M, Loukas M, Tubbs RS, Esmer AF. The course of the inferior gluteal nerve and surgical landmarks for its localization during posterior approaches to hip. *Surg Radiol Anat* 2009;31:415–418.

Goldberg G, Goldstein H. AAEM case report 32: nerve injury associated with hip arthroplasty. *Muscle Nerve* 1998;21:519–527.

Gray's Anatomy. 38th Edition. Churchill Livingstone, New York, 1995, pp. 875–876, 1282–1288.

Sunderland S. *Nerves and Nerve Injuries.* Williams & Wilkins, Baltimore, 1968, p. 1076.

Villarejo FJ, Pascual AM. Injection injury of the sciatic nerve (370 cases). *Childs Nerv Syst* 1993;9:229–232.

Gluteus Maximus

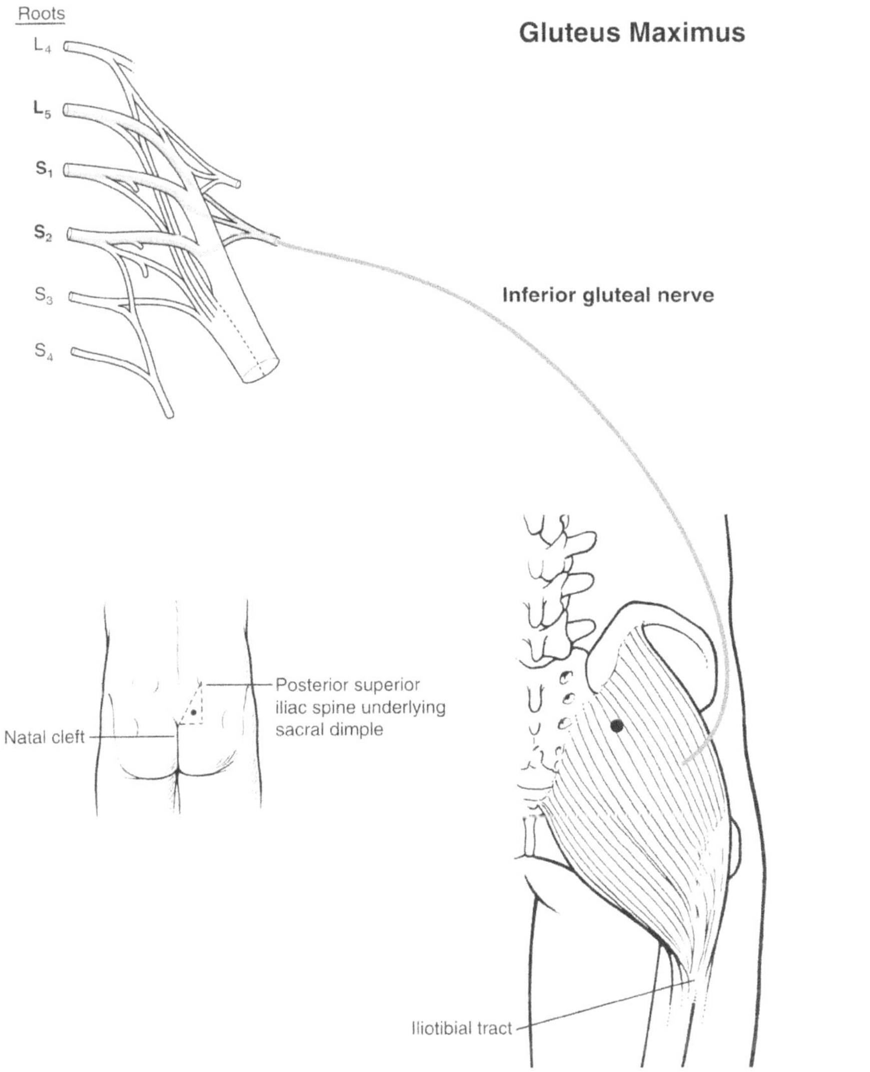

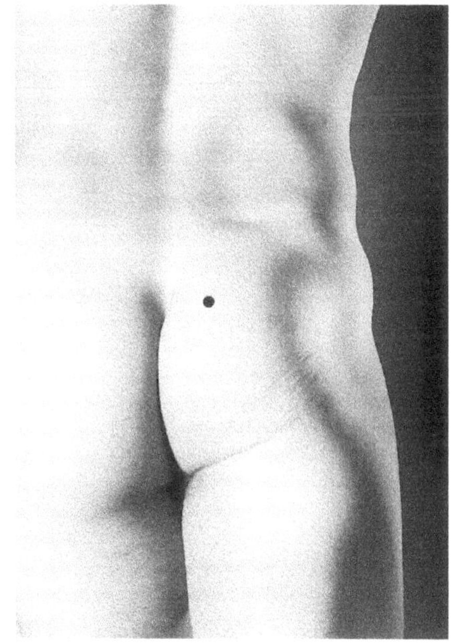

Innervation
Innervation is via the inferior gluteal nerve, sacral plexus, and roots L_5, S_1, S_2.

Origin
The gluteus maximus originates from the posterior gluteal line of the ilium and the posterior iliac crest above the line, from the aponeurosis of the erector spinae, from the lower part of the sacrum and the side of the coccyx, and from the sacrotuberous ligament and the gluteal fascia that covers the gluteus medius.

Insertion
Insertion is at the iliotibial tract of the fascia lata and the gluteal tuberosity of the femur. The fascia lata is the deep fascia of the thigh. It thickens over the flattened lateral surface of the thigh to form the iliotibial tract.

Activation Maneuver
Extension of the thigh with the knee flexed activates the muscle. The patient can also be asked to contract or tighten the buttock muscles. The gluteus maximus contributes to external rotation of the thigh and, acting through the iliotibial tract, stabilizes the femur on the tibia (*Gray's Anatomy,* 1995).

EMG Needle Insertion
Insert the needle inside an imaginary right triangle with the hypotenuse of the triangle formed by a line connecting the posterior superior iliac spine (underlying the sacral dimple) and the commencement of the natal cleft (corresponding to the third sacral spine). This will avoid the sciatic nerve, which exits the pelvis more laterally and inferiorly below the piriformis, and descends between the greater trochanter and ischial tuberosity.

Pitfalls
If the needle is inserted too laterally and inferiorly, it may encounter the sciatic nerve. Sciatic neuropathy from direct needle injury or associated hematoma is a potential complication (Sunderland, 1968; Villarejo and Pascual, 1993). It is therefore prudent to avoid needle examination of that portion of gluteus maximus that overlies the sciatic nerve (i.e., avoid the region below the piriformis and between the greater trochanter and ischial tuberosity. Muscles in this region intimately associated with the sciatic nerve include the gemellus superior and inferior, obturator internus, and quadratus femoris.)

Clinical Comments
Neurogenic changes on needle examination may be seen with lesions of the inferior gluteal nerve, sacral plexus, or L_5, S_1, S_2 roots.

This is a good muscle to study for suspected L_5 or S_1 radiculopathy because these roots primarily supply this muscle (*Gray's Anatomy,* 1995).

PUDENDAL NERVE

23

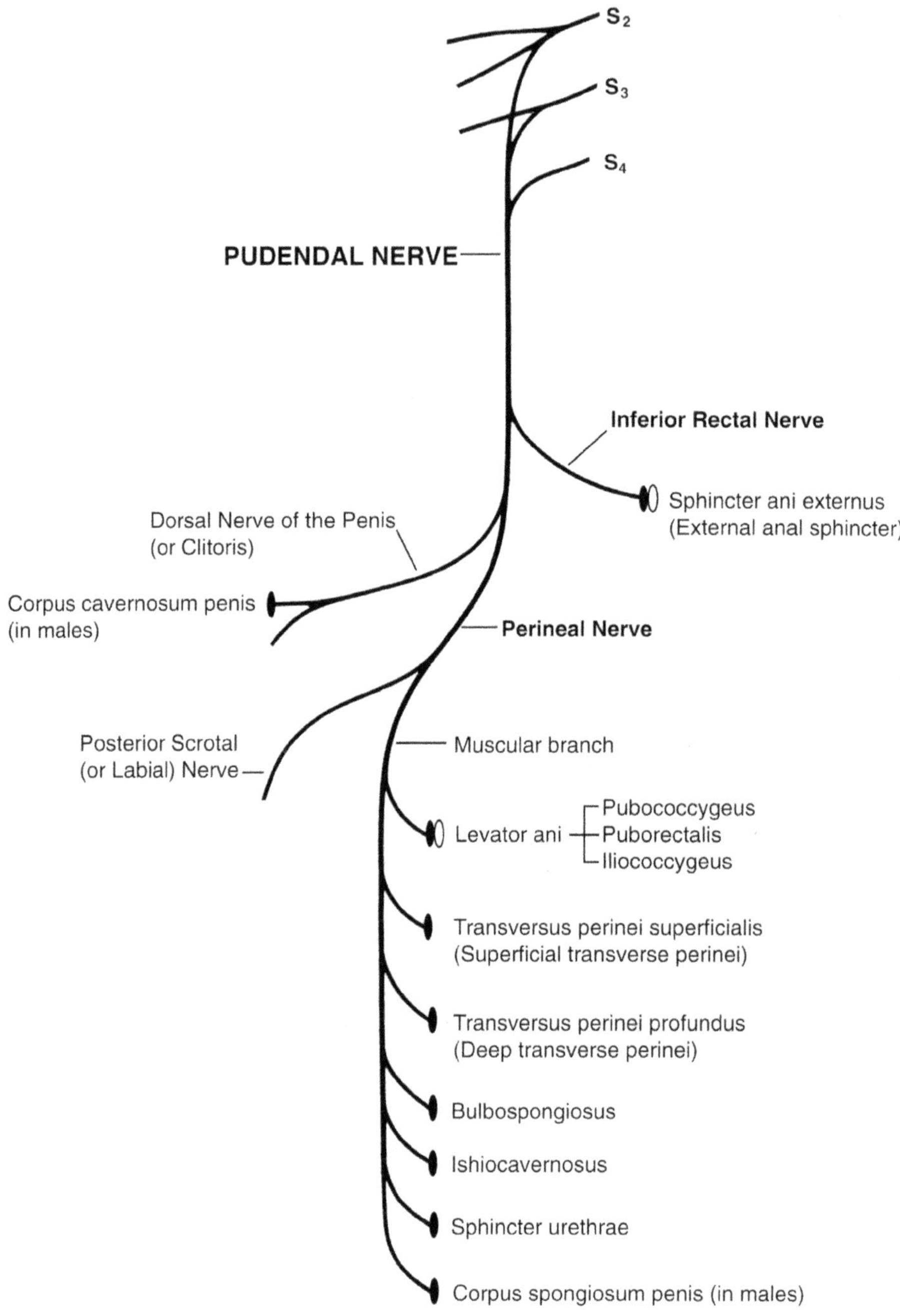

FIGURE 23-1 Diagram of the pudendal nerve and its branches. Note: The white ovals signify that a muscle receives part of its innervation via direct branches from the sacral plexus.

THE PUDENDAL NERVE is the direct continuation of the lower band of the sacral plexus, and is derived from the second, third, and fourth sacral ventral rami. It leaves the pelvis via the greater sciatic foramen below the piriformis to enter the gluteal region. It then crosses the spine of the ischium and reenters the pelvis through the lesser sciatic foramen. It accompanies the internal pudendal artery through the lesser sciatic foramen, passing into the pudendal canal (Alcock's canal) on the lateral wall of the ischiorectal fossa. In the posterior part of the canal it gives off the inferior rectal nerve. It then divides into two terminal branches, the perineal nerve and the dorsal nerve of the penis (or clitoris). In about 20% of subjects, the inferior rectal nerve arises directly from the sacral plexus (*Gray's Anatomy,* 1995).

The *inferior rectal nerve* pierces the medial wall of the pudendal canal, crosses the ischiorectal fossa with the inferior rectal vessels, and supplies the sphincter ani externus (external anal sphincter), the lining of the lower part of the anal canal, and the skin around the anus. The *perineal nerve*, the inferior and larger terminal branch of the pudendal nerve, runs forward with the perineal artery, dividing into posterior scrotal (or labial) nerve and muscular branches. The posterior scrotal or labial nerve connects with cutaneous branches of the inferior rectal nerve and posterior femoral cutaneous nerve to supply scrotal or labial skin. The muscular branches supply the anterior portions of the levator ani, transversus perinei superficialis (superficial transverse perinei), transversus perinei profundus (deep transverse perinei), bulbospongiosus, ischiocavernosus, and sphincter urethrae. In males, a branch also supplies the corpus spongiosum penis. The muscles of the pelvic floor, in particular the levator ani, also receive direct innervation from branches of the second, third, and fourth sacral nerves. This is an important concept because pudendal nervev injury does not necessarily cause dysfunction in the muscles of the pelvic floor (Retzky et al., 1996). The dorsal *nerve of the penis* is the deepest division of the pudendal nerve. It supplies the corpus cavernosum penis and passes forward to provide sensation to the dorsum of the penis. In females, the homologous *dorsal nerve of the clitoris* is very small.

Electrophysiologically, the muscles of the pelvic floor differ from most other skeletal muscles in that they exhibit constant EMG activity except during voiding and defecation (Retzky et al., 1996). The tonic activity in these muscles is necessary to continually support the viscera in the pelvic cavity.

Injury to the muscles or nerves of the pelvic floor often occurs during parturition. A tear involving the perineal body and perivaginal musculature may result in uterovaginal prolapse. This may often be prevented by incising the perineum (episiotomy) to provide a clean, easily reparable wound. Fecal incontinence due to anal sphincter damage or to a rectovaginal fistula may also occur following vaginal delivery or extension of a midline episiotomy (Fleshman, 1996).

PUDENDAL NERVE LESION

Etiology

Vaginal delivery (usually associated with third- or fourth-degree perineal tears) can cause a pudendal nerve lesion.

Pelvic tumors, including the delayed effects of pelvic radiation therapy, can be causative.

Other causes of pudendal nerve lesions are *(1)* iatrogenic (pelvic surgery), *(2)* blunt pelvic trauma or penetrating injures, *(3)* compression of the perineal branches during bicycle riding, and *(4)* chronic stretch injury, usually seen with repeated and excessive straining during defecation (Dominguez and Saclarides, 1996).

General Comments

The most common cause of injury to the pudendal nerve or to its branches is parturition. Damage occurs by mechanical disruption of muscle fibers or disruption of the innervation to skeletal muscle.

Conus medullaris or cauda equina injury may damage the anterior horn cells or sacral roots, which are the source of the pudendal nerve and sacral nerves that supply muscles of the pelvic floor.

Clinical Features

Fecal incontinence can occur due to anal sphincter disruption during delivery (often associated with extension of a midline episiotomy).

Passage of flatus or stool through the vagina (rectovaginal fistula) can occur due to obstetric injury.

Numbness or loss of sensation can occur in the perineal region.

Vaginal vault prolapse may be related to partial denervation of pelvic floor muscles during delivery (Timmons and Addison, 1996).

Impotence can occur. The bulbospongiosus assists in penile erection by compressing erectile tissue of the bulb and by compressing the deep dorsal vein of the penis. The ischiocavernosus maintains penile erection by compressing the crus penis.

Urinary incontinence can occur. The sphincter urethrae surrounds not only the lower urethra but also the bladder neck. It compresses the urethra, particularly when the bladder is full, to voluntarily delay voiding.

Weakness and atrophy of the muscles of the pelvic floor can occur, resulting in loss of support of the viscera in the pelvic cavity.

Note: Because fecal and urinary incontinence can occur, a useful mnemonic to remember is "S_2, S_3, S_4 keep it off the floor."

Electrodiagnostic Strategy

Use nerve conduction studies (pudendal nerve terminal motor latency) to evaluate a lesion of the pudendal nerve or its branches. Techniques have been developed for recording terminal motor latencies from both the inferior rectal branch and the perineal branch (Benson and Brubaker, 1996).

Pudendal somatosensory evoked potentials can evaluate pudendal sensory pathways (Haldeman et al., 1982).

Perform EMG needle examination in muscles innervated by the pudendal nerve or its branches. In pudendal nerve lesions associated with loss of motor fibers, EMG may show neurogenic changes (i.e., fibrillation potentials, polyphasic motor unit potentials, and neurogenic recruitment).

If EMG of the pelvic floor muscles is abnormal, and if the etiology is not clearly obstetric, study the muscles innervated by other sacral roots to exclude cauda equina or sacral root involvement (i.e., abductor hallucis, medial gastrocnemius, and paraspinal muscles).

Record the anocutaneous reflex ("anal wink") during the needle EMG examination of the anal sphincter. A tactile or noxious stimulus applied to the skin of the perineal region (e.g., stroking the skin around the anus) will elicit a reflex contraction of the anal sphincter muscle. The afferent limb of the reflex transmits orthodromic sensory impulses carried in the pudendal nerve to S_2–S_4 sacral segments in the spinal cord. The efferent limb of the reflex conveys orthodromic motor impulses to the anal sphincter. An intact anocutaneous reflex suggests preserved conduction in sensory and motor fibers of the pudendal nerve, sacral roots, and conus medullaris. The absence of this reflex indicates an interruption of the reflex arc, which may be in the sensory afferent limb, conus medullaris, or the motor efferent limb.

Record the bulbocavernosus (bulbospongiosus) reflex during the needle EMG examination of the anal sphincter (Blaivas et al., 1981). The test involves monitoring anal sphincter contraction in response to squeezing or electrically stimulating the glans penis or vulva. The reflex is spinally mediated and involves S_2–$S_{4,}$ with the afferent limb transmitting orthodromic sensory impulses carried in the pudendal nerve and the efferent limb conveying orthodromic motor impulses to the anal sphincter. The absence of this reflex indicates a lesion or injury to the conus medullaris or sacral nerve roots.

However, sacral reflexes are also absent after rostral spinal cord injury early during the spinal shock phase (Leis et al., 1996).

The anocutaneous and bulbocavernosus reflexes can also be performed during intraoperative neurophysiologic monitoring to verify function of sensory and motor sacral roots and conus medullaris (Vodusek and Deletis, 2002).

REFERENCES

Benson JT, Brubaker L. Electrodiagnostic assessment: A diagnostic adjunct. In Brubaker LT, Saclarides TJ (eds). *The Female Pelvic Floor: Disorders of Function and Support.* FA Davis, Philadelphia, 1996, pp. 100–108.

Blaivas JG, Zayed AA, Labib KB. The bulbocavernosus reflex in urology: a prospective study of 299 patients. *J Urol* 1981;126:197–199.

Dominguez JM, Saclarides TJ. Preprolapse syndromes. In Brubaker LT, Saclarides TJ (eds). *The Female Pelvic Floor: Disorders of Function and Support.* FA Davis, Philadelphia, 1996, pp. 283–288.

Fleshman JW. Fecal incontinence: Etiology and evaluation. In Brubaker LT, Saclarides TJ (eds). *The Female Pelvic Floor: Disorders of Function and Support.* FA Davis, Philadelphia, 1996, pp. 208–213.

Gray's Anatomy. 38th Edition. Churchill Livingstone, New York, 1995, pp. 830–835, 1780–1782.

Haldeman S, Bradley WE, Bhatia NN, Johnson BK. Pudendal evoked responses. *Arch Neurol* 1982;39:280–283.

Leis AA, Kronenberg MF, Stetkarova I, Paske WC, Stokic DS. Spinal motoneuron excitability following acute spinal cord injury in man. *Neurology* 1996;47:231–237.

Retzky SS, Rogers RM Jr., Richardson AC. Anatomy of female pelvic support. In: Brubaker LT, Saclarides TJ (eds). *The Female Pelvic Floor: Disorders of Function and Support.* FA Davis, Philadelphia, 1996, pp. 3–21.

Timmons MC, Addison WA. Vaginal vault prolapse. In Brubaker LT, Saclarides TJ (eds). *The Female Pelvic Floor Disorders of Function and Support.* FA Davis, Philadelphia, 1996, pp. 262–268.

Vodusek DB, Deletis V. Intraoperative neurophysiological monitoring of the sacral nervous system. In *Neurophysiology in neurosurgery: A modern intraoperative approach.* Deletis V, Shils JL, (eds.). Academic Press, 2002; pp. 153–165.[comp: set this section on a new page]

Sphincter Ani Externus (External Anal Sphincter)

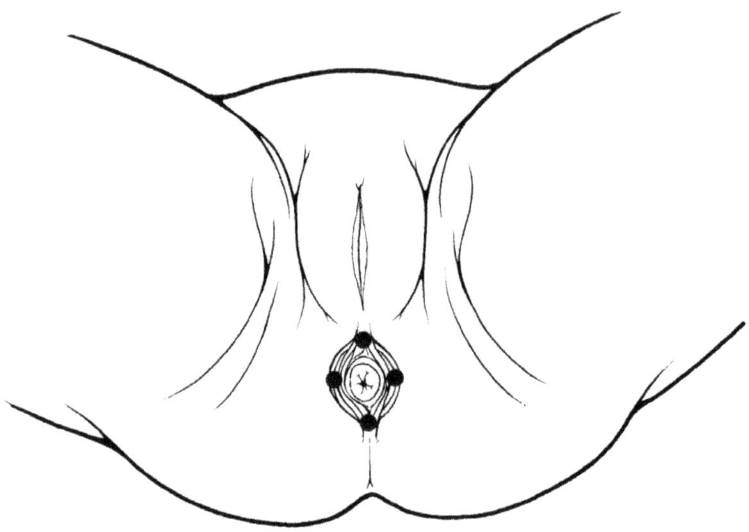

Innervation

Innervation is via the inferior rectal branch, pudendal nerve, sacral plexus, and roots S_2, S_3.

There is also a direct branch from the sacral plexus and root S_4.

Origin

The external anal sphincter is a tube of skeletal muscle with deep, superficial, and subcutaneous layers that surround the whole anal canal.

Insertion

Fibers from deep, superficial, and subcutaneous parts attach anteriorly to the perineal body and posteriorly to the coccyx.

Some fibers blend with the puborectalis or attach to the superficial transverse perineal muscles and to the anococcygeal raphe.

Activation Maneuver

This muscle exhibits constant EMG activity that keeps the anal canal closed except during defecation. To assess spontaneous activity such as fibrillation potentials, ask the subject to bear down as if having a bowel movement. To maximally activate the muscle, ask the subject to tighten or contract the anal sphincter.

EMG Needle Insertion

Insert the needle into the external anal sphincter at the 12:00, 3:00, 6:00 and 9:00 clock positions with the patient in the lithotomy position. This evaluation should ideally be performed with the gynecological surgeon present, particularly if surgery is planned to repair mechanical disruption of the muscle fibers or disruption of the innervation to the muscle.

The presence or absence of insertional activity in different segments of the muscle (reflecting the presence or absence of viable skeletal muscle) and the inability to voluntarily contract portions of the muscle are crucial information for the surgeon.

Pitfalls

The examiner should *not* insert his or her finger into the anus to guide the needle examination. This practice is unnecessary and poses a risk of needle injury to the examiner.

To lessen the risk of infection, cleanse the anal sphincter with alcohol to wipe away any fecal matter prior to needle insertion.

Clinical Comments

Neurogenic changes on needle examination may be seen with lesions of the inferior rectal nerve, pudendal nerve, sacral plexus, or S_2, S_3, S_4 roots.

Levator Ani

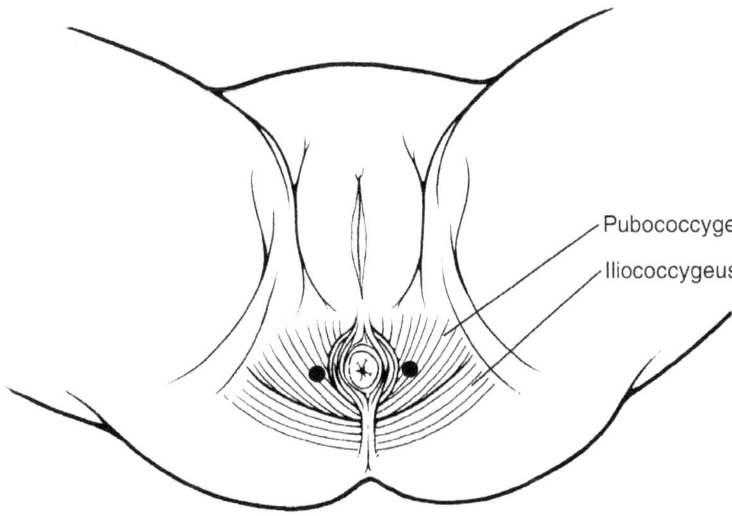

Innervation

Anteromedial portion: Innervation is via the perineal nerve, pudendal nerve, sacral plexus, and roots S_2, S_3, S_4.

Posterolateral portion: Innervation is via the direct branches from sacral plexus, and roots S_2, S_3, S_4.

Origin

The levator ani is a broad muscular sheet that forms the floor of the pelvic cavity. Right and left counterparts unite to support the viscera in this cavity and to surround the various structures that pass through it. The levator ani is separated into three muscular parts: pubococcygeal part (pubococcygeus), puborectal part (puborectalis), and iliococcygeal part (iliococcygeus).

The pubococcygeus arises from the back of the body of the pubis and passes back horizontally. The fibers form part of the periurethral, perivaginal, and perirectal musculature.

The puborectalis arises from the back of the body of the pubis (inseparable from the pubococcygeus at its origin) and joins its fellow muscle from the opposite side to form a sling around the anorectal junction.

The iliococcygeus arises from the obturator fascia between the obturator canal and the ischial spine.

Insertion

Most fibers of the pubococcygeus attach to the anterior surface of the coccyx. Some fibers insert into the walls of the vagina, perineal body, and rectum.

The puborectalis joins its fellow muscle from the opposite side to form a sling around the anorectal junction.

The iliococcygeus attaches to the sides of the last two segments of the coccyx.

Activation Maneuver

Muscles exhibit constant EMG activity and contribute to bowel and bladder continence; they must relax to permit voiding and defecation (Retzky et al., 1996). To assess spontaneous activity such as fibrillation potentials, ask the subject to bear down as if having a bowel movement. To maximally activate the muscle (particularly the puborectalis), ask the subject to tighten the anal sphincter.

EMG Needle Insertion

Puborectalis: Insert the needle into the posterior half of the external anal sphincter to a depth of 2–3 cm. The puborectalis lies deep to the external anal sphincter and is separated from it by a thin layer of fat and connective tissue that results in loss of insertional activity on needle examination.

Pubococcygeus: Insert the needle 1–2 cm on either side of the external anal sphincter. The pubococcygeus is the only muscle encountered.

Iliococcygeus: This muscle is thin, aponeurotic, and not easily accessible by routine needle examination.

Pitfalls

If the needle is inserted too deeply, it may penetrate the rectum and peritoneum.

Clinical Comments

Neurogenic changes on needle examination may be seen with lesions of the perineal nerve, pudendal nerve, sacral plexus, or S_2, S_3, S_4 roots.

24 LUMBAR PLEXUS

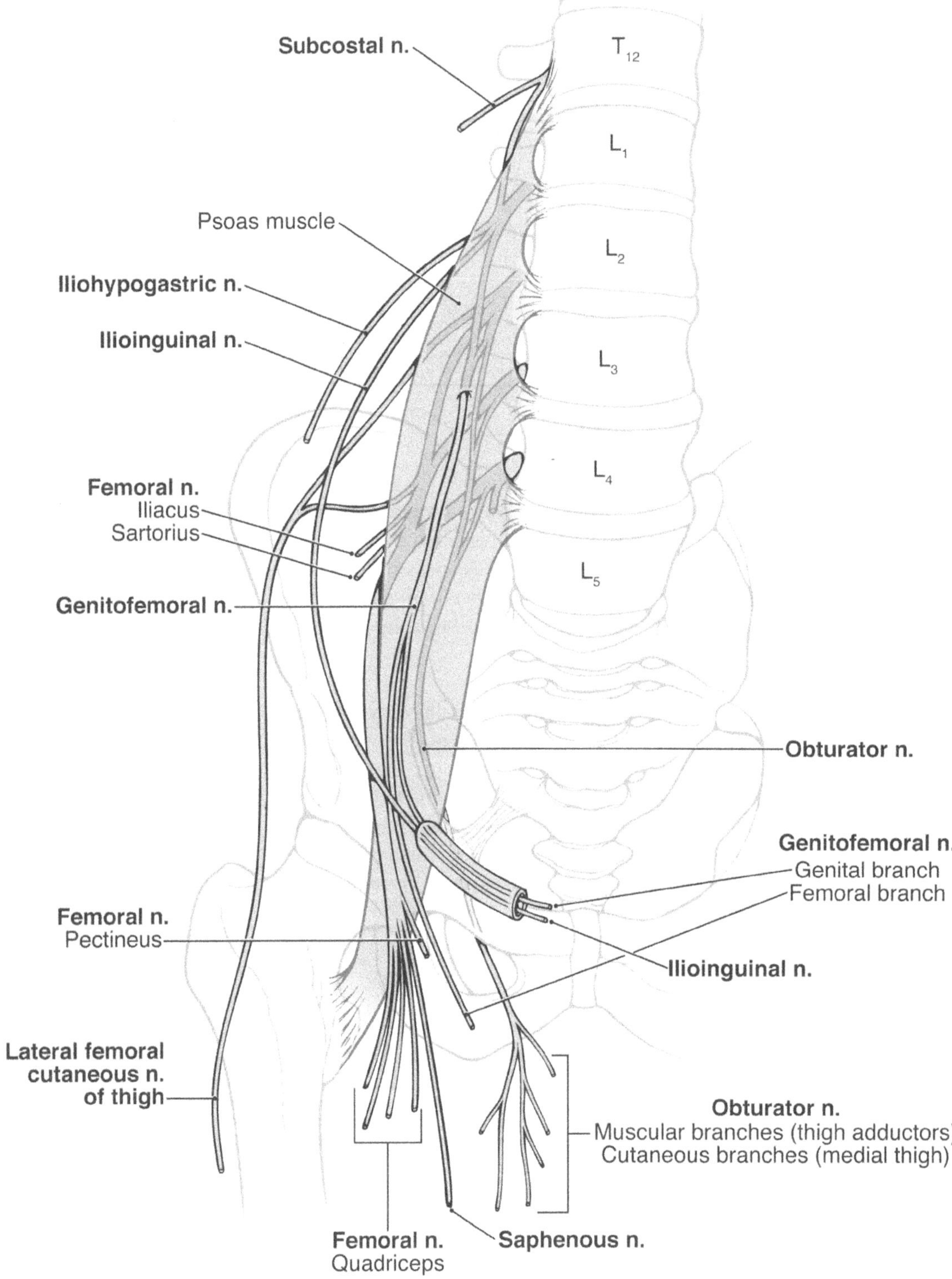

FIGURE 24-1 Diagram of the lumbar plexus (anterior view) and its branches. See color insert.

THE LUMBAR PLEXUS (Figure 24-1) is formed by the first three and most of the fourth lumbar ventral rami with a contributing branch from the twelfth thoracic ventral ramus (Hansen, 2010). The smaller branch of the fourth joins the fifth as the *lumbosacral trunk*, which joins the sacral plexus (see Chapter 17). Although the fourth lumbar ventral ramus is most often divided between the two plexuses, in a *prefixed* plexus the third may be the divided ramus whereas in a *postfixed* plexus the fifth ramus contributes to both plexuses. These variations modify the lumbar and sacral plexuses (*Gray's Anatomy,* 1995).

The lumbar ventral rami descend laterally into the psoas major muscle to form the lumbar plexus. In its usual arrangement, the first lumbar ventral ramus, joined by a branch from the twelfth thoracic, bifurcates into upper and lower parts. The upper part divides again into *iliohypogastric* and *ilioinguinal* nerves; the lower unites with a branch of the second lumbar ramus to form the *genitofemoral* nerve. The remainder of the second and third and part of the fourth lumbar ventral rami joining the plexus divide into ventral (anterior) and dorsal (posterior) divisions. The anterior division of the second to fourth ventral rami form the *obturator* nerve. The posterior division of the second to fourth ventral rami form the *femoral* nerve. Posterior branches of the second and third ventral rami also form the *lateral femoral cutaneous* nerve of the thigh. Muscular branches of the lumbar plexus directly supply the quadratus lumborum, psoas minor, psoas major, and iliacus (the latter also receives innervation from the femoral nerve). The *iliohypogastric* nerve contributes innervation to the transversus abdominis and to the internal and external oblique muscles. It then supplies cutaneous sensation to the posterolateral gluteal skin and the suprapubic skin. The *ilioinguinal* nerve also contributes innervation to the transversus abdominis and internal oblique muscles. It traverses the inguinal canal and emerges from the superficial inguinal ring to supply the proximomedial skin of the thigh and the skin covering the penile root and upper scrotum or that covering the moms pubis and the adjoining labium majus. The genital branch of the *genitofemoral* nerve supplies the cremaster muscle and provides cutaneous innervation to the scrotal skin in men or to the moms pubis and labium majus in women. The femoral branch supplies the skin over the upper part of the femoral triangle. Injury to the iliohypogastric, ilioinguinal, and genitofemoral nerves is almost always the result of direct trauma, usually related to surgery (inguinal herniorrhaphy, appendectomy, hysterectomy, caesarian section, and other gynecological operations, Kim et al., 2005; Loos et al., 2008).

The *lateral femoral cutaneous* nerve of the thigh descends behind the inguinal ligament about 1 cm medial to the anterior superior iliac spine. It divides into anterior and posterior branches, the former supplying skin over the anterior and lateral thigh as far as the knee and the latter supplying skin on the lateral surface of the thigh from the greater trochanter to about mid-thigh. A lesion of the lateral femoral cutaneous nerve, usually due to compression behind the inguinal ligament, produces impaired sensation with pain and paresthesias on the anterior and lateral aspects of the thigh. This condition is known clinically as *meralgia paresthetica*.

A lesion of the lumbar plexus produces a clinical picture similar to that seen with combined femoral and obturator nerve lesions, but with additional involvement of the above-mentioned branches. It is common for femoral nerve deficit to be accompanied by obturator nerve deficit (Dawson et al., 1990) because both arise within the substance of the psoas muscle. The femoral and obturator nerves are discussed individually in the Chapters 25 and 26, respectively.

LESION OF THE LATERAL FEMORAL CUTANEOUS NERVE (MERALGIA PARESTHETICA)

Etiology

Compression behind the inguinal ligament causes meralgia paresthetica.

Predisposing factors include obesity, recent weight gain, tight clothes (pants, girdles, belts, military body armor), pregnancy, and other conditions that cause direct pressure over the inguinal ligament (Deal and Canoso, 1982; Parmar, 2003; Fargo and Konitzer, 2007).

Conditions that result in acute angulation of the nerve across the inguinal ligament may also predispose to meralgia paresthetica (e.g., prolonged hyperflexion at the hip).

Iatrogenic meralgia paresthetica may occur after a number of orthopedic procedures, such as anterior iliac-crest bone-graft harvesting and anterior pelvic procedures. Prone positioning for spine surgery has also been implicated (Grossman et al., 2001).

Penetrating injuries, neuromas, or other mass lesions may involve the lateral femoral cutaneous nerve of the thigh.

General Comments

The lateral femoral cutaneous nerve of thigh is a pure cutaneous nerve derived from the L_2 and L_3 ventral rami (Figure 24-1).

Meralgia paresthetica is common.

Relief of pain and paresthesias after injection of a local anesthetic agent is helpful in establishing the diagnosis.

Meralgia paresthetica usually improves with nonoperative modalities, such as removal of compressive or aggravating agents (e.g., weight loss, avoid tight garments), nonsteroidal anti-inflammatory drugs, and local corticosteroid injections (Grossman et al., 2001).

Clinical Features

There is pain, numbness, or altered sensation (paresthesia, burning, tingling) localized to the anterior and lateral aspect of the thigh.

Patients can often identify exacerbating factors, such as certain body postures (walking, cycling, standing for long periods of time, sleeping in a fetal position), weight gain, or wearing tight clothes (hip-hugger or low-rise jeans, belts).

There is no muscle atrophy, weakness, or loss of the patellar reflex.

Electrodiagnostic Strategy

Perform lateral femoral cutaneous nerve conduction studies bilaterally. Unilateral absence or reduction suggests a lesion of the lateral femoral cutaneous nerve of the thigh.

Perform additional nerve conduction studies to exclude plexopathy, femoral neuropathy, or other mononeuropathies affecting the symptomatic lower limb.

Perform EMG needle examination in thigh and leg muscles to exclude plexus or root involvement.

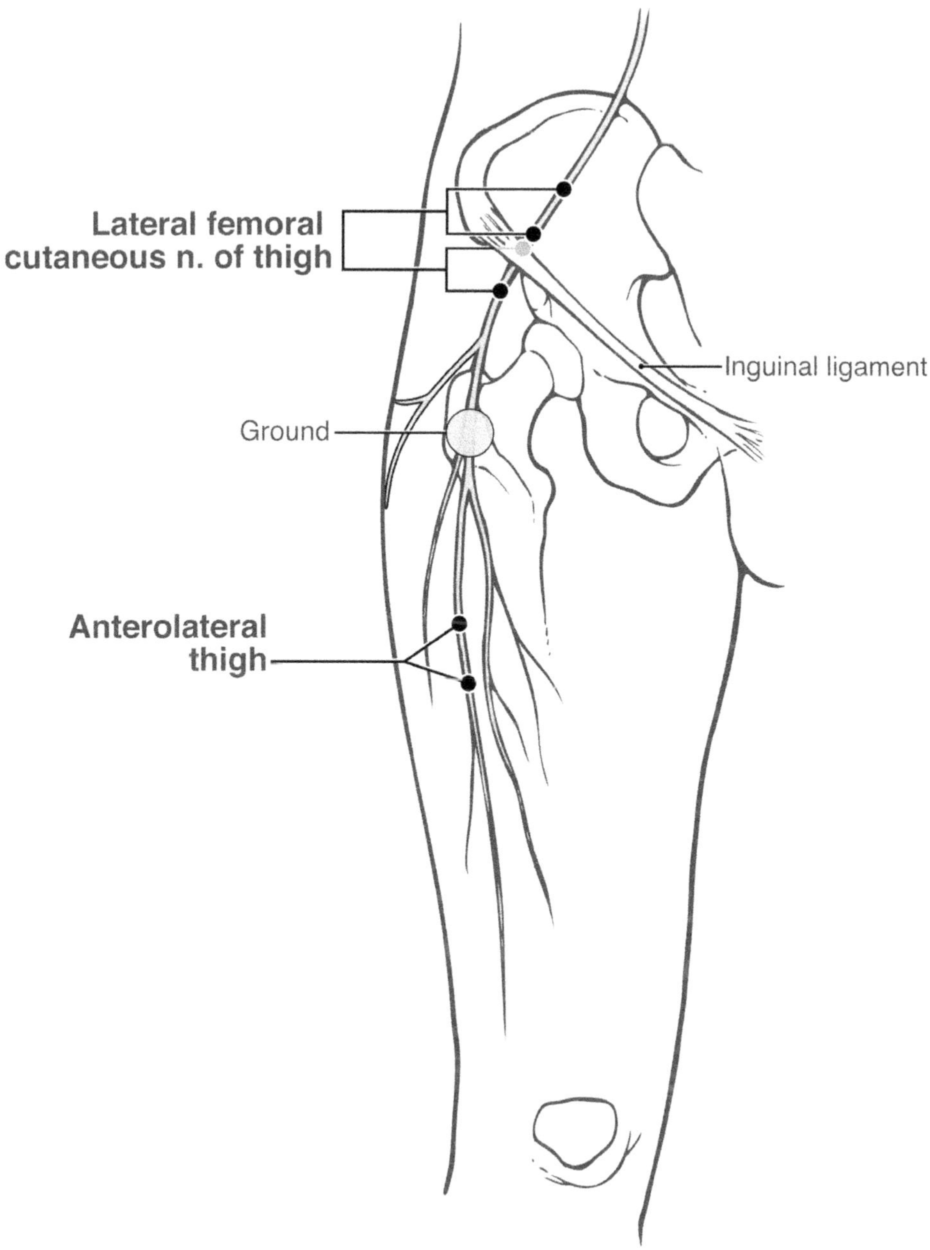

FIGURE 24-2 Lateral femoral cutaneous nerve conduction study (antidromic).

Recording

Active electrode: Place over the anterolateral thigh, 12 cm to 18 cm distal to the stimulating electrode.

Reference electrode: Place 3 cm distal to the active electrode.

Ground electrode: Place on the anterior thigh, between stimulating and recording electrodes.

Stimulation

Above or below the inguinal ligament: place cathode one fingerbreadth medial to the anterior superior iliac spine (above the inguinal ligament). Alternatively, place cathode one to two fingerbreadths below the anterior superior iliac spine (below the inguinal ligament). The stimulator may need to be moved slightly laterally or medially to elicit a maximal sensory response. The anode is 3 cm proximal to cathode.

Normal Values

Latency (ms) ≤ 3.0 (onset latency at distance 12 cm)
Amplitude (μV) ≥ 4.0
Conduction velocity (m/s) ≥ 40 m/s

Comments

This study is technically difficult to obtain even in some normal subjects because of obesity and anatomic variations of the nerve (Macnicol and Thompson, 1990). Accordingly, studies must always be performed bilaterally because side-to-side comparisons are more useful than normal value tables. An amplitude < 50 % of the unaffected side is evidence of abnormality (Seror and Seror, 2006).

If no sensory response can be obtained on the asymptomatic side, there is little value in testing the symptomatic side.

REFERENCES

Dawson DM, Hallett M, Millender LH. *Entrapment Neuropathies.* 2nd edition. Little, Brown, Boston, 1990, pp. 313–316.

Deal CL, Canoso JJ. Meralgia paresthetica and large abdomens. *Ann Intern Med* 1982;96:787–788.

Fargo MV, Konitzer LN. Meralgia paresthetica due to body armor wear in U.S. soldiers serving in Iraq: a case report and review of the literature. *Mil Med* 2007;172:663–665.

Gray's Anatomy. 38th edition, Churchill Livingstone, New York, 1995, pp. 1277–1282.

Grossman MG, Ducey SA, Nadler SS, Levy AS. Meralgia paresthetica: diagnosis and treatment. J Am Acad Orthop Surg 2001;9:336–344.

Kim DH, Murovic JA, Tiel RL, Kline DG. Surgical management of 33 ilioinguinal and iliohypogastric neuralgias at Louisiana State University Health Sciences Center. Neurosurgery 2005;56:1013–1020.

Knockaert DC, Boonen AL, Bruyninckx FL, Bobbaers HJ. Electromyographic findings in ilioinguinal-iliohypogastric nerve entrapment syndrome. *Acta Clin Belg* 1996;51:156–160.

Loos MJ, Scheltinga MR, Roumen RM. Surgical management of inguinal neuralgia after a low transverse Pfannenstiel incision. *Ann Surg* 2008;248:880–885.

Macnicol MF, Thompson WJ. Idiopathic meralgia paresthetica. *Clin Orthop Relat Res* 1990;254: 270–274.

Parmar MS. Hiphuggers' tingly thighs. CMAJ 2003;168:16.

Seror P, Seror R. Meralgia paresthetica: clinical and electrophysiological diagnosis in 120 cases. *Muscle Nerve* 2006;33:650–654.

Starling JR, Harms BA, Schroeder ME, Eichman PL. Diagnosis and treatment of genitofemoral and ilioinguinal entrapment neuralgia. *Surgery* 1987;102:581–586.

External Oblique, Internal Oblique, and Transversus Abdominis

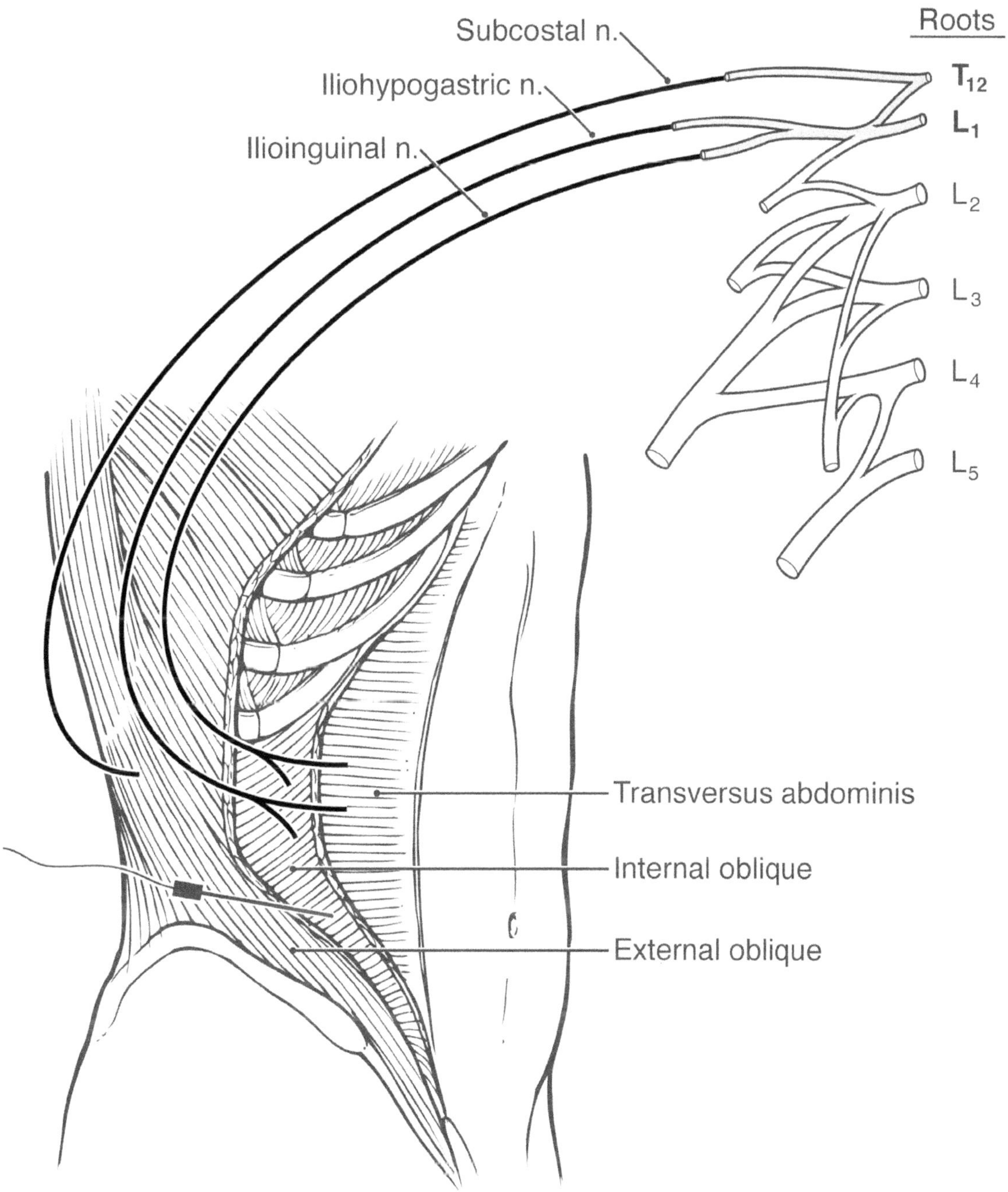

General Comments

The external oblique, internal oblique, and transversus abdominis are the three main muscles of the anterolateral abdominal wall. The external oblique is the largest and most superficial of the three flat abdominal muscles, with fibers that *descend* obliquely in a medial direction. The internal oblique is the intermediate muscle of the abdomen, lying just underneath the external oblique, with fibers that *ascend* obliquely in a medial direction. The transversus abdominis, named for the direction of its transverse fibers, is the innermost of the flat muscles of the abdomen, being placed immediately beneath the internal oblique (*Gray's Anatomy,* 1995).

Innervation

Innervation to the abdominal wall muscles is via the ventral rami of the lower six thoracic nerves, including the subcostal nerve (T_{12}). The iliohypogastric (T_{12}, L_1) and ilioinguinal nerves (T_{12}, L_1) also contribute innervation to the internal oblique and transversus abdominis muscles (and occasionally also to the external oblique).

Origin

The external oblique originates from the lower borders of the fifth to twelfth ribs before descending obliquely. The internal oblique originates from the anterior two-thirds of the iliac crest and inguinal ligament before ascending obliquely. The transversus abdominis originates from the internal surfaces of the lower costal cartilages, thoracolumbar fascia, inner lip of the iliac crest, and lateral inguinal ligament before coursing forward and medially.

Insertion

Insertion of external oblique is at the linea alba (a fibrous structure that runs down the midline of the abdomen formed by the fusion of the aponeuroses of the abdominal muscles), pubic tubercle, and anterior iliac crest. Insertion of internal oblique is at the inferior border of the tenth to twelfth ribs and linea alba. Insertion of transversus abdominis is at linea alba and pubic crest.

Activation Maneuver

These muscles compress and support the abdominal viscera, and flex and rotate the trunk. To assess the pattern of motor unit potential recruitment, ask the subject to tighten the abdomen or to initiate flexion of the trunk (i.e., to perform an abdominal crunch).

EMG Needle Insertion

Insert the needle obliquely, one-third of the distance between the iliac crest and the umbilicus.

Pitfalls

If the needle is inserted too deeply, it may enter the peritoneum. Entry of the needle into the peritoneum produces pain and loss of muscle insertional activity.

This is a technically difficult needle examination in obese individuals.

The close proximity of these flat muscles makes it difficult to isolate them individually by needle examination.

In subjects with a history of lower abdominal surgery, select a needle insertion site away from the surgical scar.

Clinical Comments

Iatrogenic injury to the iliohypogastric, ilioinguinal, and genitofemoral nerves is common, usually related to herniorrhaphy, appendectomy, or gynecological surgery. In cases of refractory neuralgia, significant pain relief may be achieved after neurectomy (Starling et al., 1987; Kim et al., 2005).

The iliohypogastric and ilioinguinal nerves may be damaged by T_{12} or L_1 radiculopathy, tumors, or trauma to the spine.

Sports injuries, such as trauma or lower abdominal muscle tears, may also result in injury to the iliohypogastric and ilioinguinal nerves.

Injury may also occur during pregnancy, attributed to the rapidly expanding abdomen in the third trimester.

Neurogenic changes on needle examination may be seen with lesions of the iliohypogastric or ilioinguinal nerves, upper lumbar plexus, or T_{12}, L_1 roots (Knockaert et al., 1996).

FEMORAL NERVE

25

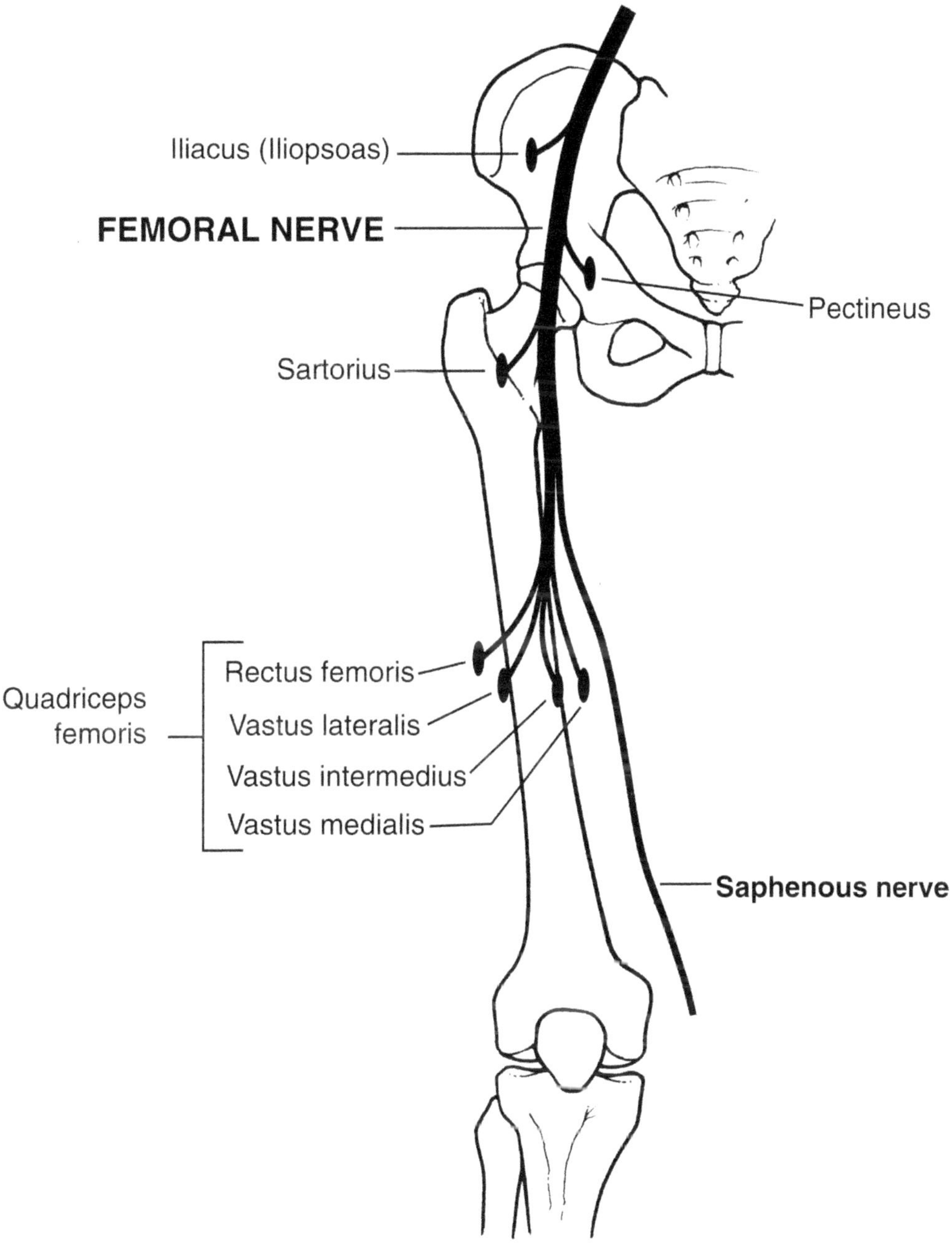

FIGURE 25-1 Diagram of the femoral nerve (anterior view) and the muscles that it supplies.

THE FEMORAL NERVE is the largest branch of the lumbar plexus. It arises from the posterior division of the second to fourth ventral rami, within the substance of the psoas major. It emerges from the psoas at its lower outer border in a groove between this muscle and the iliacus and descends along the groove to pass beneath the inguinal ligament to enter the thigh. In the iliac fossa, it supplies small branches to the iliacus muscle (the iliacus and psoas major act together, the combination being referred to as the *iliopsoas muscle*; *Gray's Anatomy,* 1995). While beneath the inguinal ligament, it gives off a branch that courses medially behind the femoral sheath to supply the pectineus muscle. On entering the femoral triangle, the femoral nerve lies on the iliacus muscle lateral to the femoral artery. About 4 cm distal to the inguinal ligament, it divides into anterior and posterior divisions that, in turn, subdivide to give out further branches. The anterior division divides almost immediately into a muscular branch to the sartorius and two cutaneous branches, the intermediate and medial cutaneous nerves of the thigh. The *intermediate cutaneous nerve of the thigh* provides sensation to the anterior surface of the thigh as far distally as the knee. The *medial cutaneous nerve of the thigh* innervates the medial and anteromedial aspects of the thigh and continues on to innervate the medial aspect of the leg just below the knee. The posterior division immediately divides into the saphenous branch and muscular branches. The *saphenous nerve* descends to the knee, where it becomes subcutaneous. It joins the saphenous vein, which it accompanies down the medial aspect of the leg. Branches of the saphenous nerve provide sensation to the skin on the medial aspect of the leg, and continue on to innervate the skin over the medial ankle and a portion of the medial foot. Muscular branches arise in spray fashion from the parent division and innervate the rectus femoris, vastus lateralis, vastus intermedius, and vastus medialis.

Anatomical features of clinical importance relate to the posterior abdominal wall, where a retroperitoneal hematoma or hemorrhage may compress the nerve (Sunderland, 1968). The appearance of signs or symptoms of a femoral nerve lesion in a patient with hemophilia, or who is receiving anticoagulant therapy, strongly suggests involvement of the nerve by a hematoma or hemorrhage. Compression of the nerve may also occur in this region from a benign or malignant tumor or an abscess. Beneath the inguinal ligament, the nerve may rarely be injured during inguinal or femoral hernia repair. Postsurgical femoral mononeuropathy has also been reported following positioning on the operating table in which the thigh is acutely flexed, as in the lithotomy position. In these cases, nerve involvement is likely related to acute angulation across the inguinal ligament (Sunderland, 1968). In the femoral triangle, gunshot wounds and other penetrating injuries are often fatal because the femoral artery and vein are also severed. Injuries distal to the site, where muscular branches arise in spray fashion, result in variable involvement of the branches; some will be spared while others will be involved depending on the precise site and nature of the injury.

Note: The short muscles around the hip joint—pectineus, obturator externus, quadratus femoris, gemellus superior, gemellus inferior, obturator internus, and piriformis—are largely inaccessible to direct observation. Because of the potential complications presented by their intimate relationship to important neurovascular structures, there is a relative lack of EMG data in humans.

FEMORAL NERVE LESION

Etiology

Retroperitoneal hematomas or hemorrhages that cause a femoral nerve lesion are usually seen in patients with hemophilia or who are receiving anticoagulant therapy.

Retroperitoneal tumors (benign or malignant) and abscesses are causative.

Femoral nerve lesions can be caused iatrogenically, during herniorrhaphy, appendectomy, hysterectomy, femoral angiography, or the postanesthesia state due to compression from acute angulation across the inguinal ligament (Garcimartin-Cerrón et al., 2002; Barner et al., 2002).

Other causes of femoral nerve lesions include *(1)* penetrating injuries, *(2)* aneurysm of the femoral artery, *(3)* neuralgic amyotrophy, and *(4)* diabetic amyotrophy (femoral nerve involvement is common).

Postpartum femoral neuropathy can be induced by prolonged lithotomy position (Hakim and Katirji, 1993).

General Comments

In diabetic amyotrophy, muscle weakness may first appear in the quadriceps muscles. Diabetic amyotrophy, however, is not simply a femoral mononeuropathy. Additional proximal muscles are involved, including gluteal, hamstring, adductor, and iliopsoas muscles (Chokroverty and Sander, 1996).

Clinical Features

The quadriceps muscles atrophy.

Paresis or paralysis of the quadriceps muscles produces weakness or an inability to extend the leg.

Paresis or paralysis of the iliopsoas, rectus femoris, and sartorius produces weakness during thigh flexion. If the iliopsoas is spared, as in a more distal lesion, loss of rectus femoris and sartorius is without noticeable effect (Sunderland, 1968).

Numbness or a loss of sensation can occur in the anterior and medial aspects of the thigh, and in the medial aspect of the leg in the saphenous nerve distribution.

The patellar tendon reflex is reduced or absent. This is a reliable objective sign of femoral neuropathy.

Electrodiagnostic Strategy

Use nerve conduction studies (saphenous sensory response and femoral motor response) to help determine a lesion of the femoral nerve or its branches.

Perform EMG needle examination in thigh muscles innervated by the femoral nerve or its branches. In lesions associated with loss of motor fibers, EMG may show neurogenic changes (i.e., fibrillation potentials, polyphasic motor unit potentials, and neurogenic recruitment).

If EMG of the quadriceps muscles is abnormal, study other proximal muscles (gluteal, hamstring, and adductors) and paraspinal muscles to exclude plexus or root involvement.

Femoral Motor Nerve Conduction Study

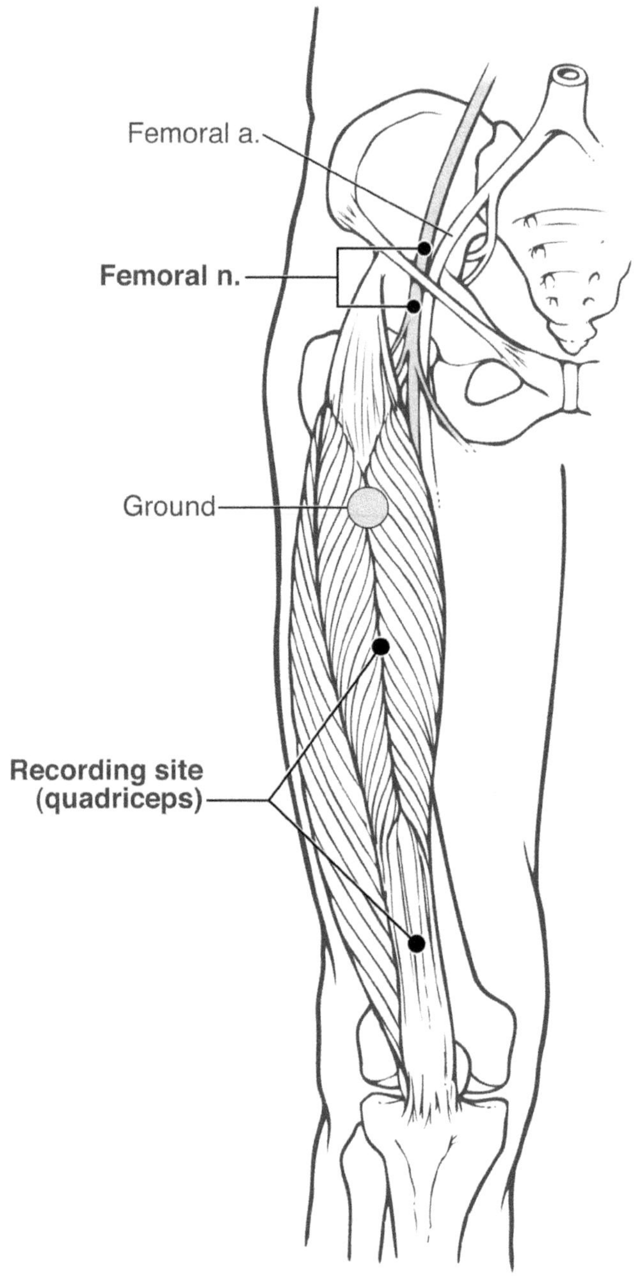

FIGURE 25-2 Femoral motor nerve conduction study.

Recording

Active electrode: Position over the rectus femoris or vastus lateralis muscles.

Reference electrode: Place distal to the active electrode over the quadriceps tendon.

Ground electrode: Place on the anterior thigh, between stimulating and recording electrodes.

Stimulation

Inguinal ligament: Place cathode just below the inguinal ligament, one fingerbreadth lateral to the femoral artery pulse. The anode is 3 cm proximal to the cathode.

Normal Values

Amplitude (mV) ≥ 3.5

Normal values differ depending on the distance used and the electrode placement. Femoral motor conduction studies should be performed bilaterally using identical technique. An amplitude ≤ 50 % of the unaffected side is evidence of abnormality and implies axonal loss injury (Preston and Shapiro, 2005).

Pitfalls

The femoral nerve lies just lateral to the femoral artery. Hence, palpation of the femoral pulse confirms proper placement of the cathode. This is particularly important in obese subjects, where greater pressure on the cathode, higher stimulus intensity, and increased duration may be required to evoke the motor response.

Saphenous Sensory Nerve Conduction Study

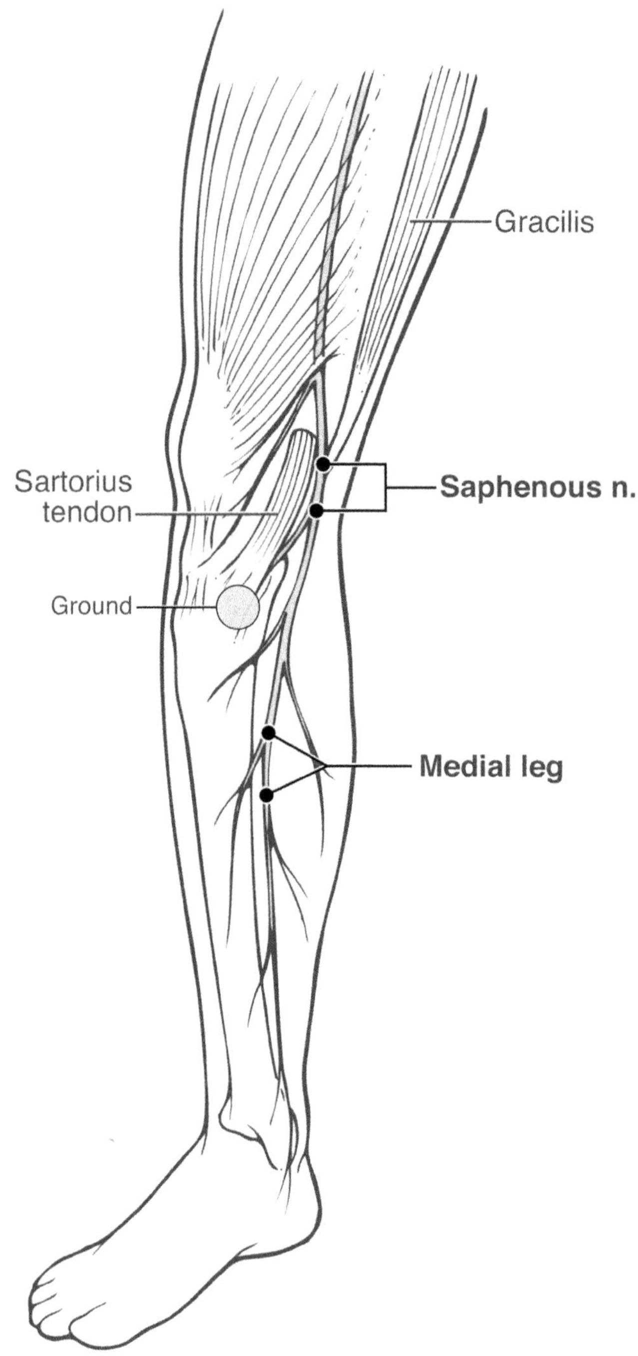

FIGURE 25-3 Saphenous sensory nerve conduction study (antidromic).

Recording

Active electrode: Place over the medial border of the tibia, 10 to 14 cm distal to the stimulating electrode.

Reference electrode: Place 3 cm distal to the active electrode.

Ground electrode: Place on the proximal leg, between stimulating and recording electrodes.

Stimulation

Knee: Place cathode over the medial aspect of the knee, just posterior to the tendon of the sartorius muscle, about 10 cm to 14 cm proximal to the recording electrodes. The stimulator may need to be moved slightly more posterior than anticipated to elicit a maximal sensory response. The anode is 3 cm proximal to cathode.

Normal Values

Latency (ms) ≤ 3.0 (onset latency)
Amplitude (μV) ≥ 4.0
Conduction velocity (m/s) ≥ 50 m/s

Comments

The normal amplitude of the saphenous SNAP has a large range and standard deviation. Even in some normal subjects, averaging of the saphenous sensory response may be necessary.

As with other sensory responses that are uncommonly studied, the saphenous sensory responses should be performed bilaterally because side-to-side comparisons are more useful than normal value tables that may not apply to your patient (Preston and Shapiro, 2005). An amplitude ≤ 50 % of the unaffected side is evidence of abnormality.

The saphenous response is useful in differentiating a postganglionic lesion associated with axonal loss, including femoral neuropathy or lumbar plexopathy, from a preganglionic lesion involving the L_4 root (the fibers underlying the saphenous nerve recording electrodes are derived primarily from the L_4 root).

REFERENCES

Barner KC, Landau ME, Campbell WW. A review of perioperative nerve injury to the lower extremities: part I. *J Clin Neuromuscul Dis* 2002;4:95–99.

Chokroverty S, Sander HW. AAEM case report #13: Diabetic amyotrophy. *Muscle Nerve* 1996;19:939–945.

Dawson DM, Hallett M, Millender LH. *Entrapment Neuropathies.* 2nd edition. Little, Brown, Boston, 1990, pp. 313–316.

Garcimartin-Cerron I, Tola-Arribas MA, Munoz-San Jose J. Neurological complications of cardiac catheterization. *Rev Neurol* 2002;35:470–474.

Gray's Anatomy. 38th Edition. Churchill Livingstone, New York, 1995, pp. 868–875, 1277–1282.

Hakim MA, Katirji MB. Femoral mononeuropathy induced by the lithotomy position: A report of 5 cases with a review of literature. *Muscle Nerve* 1993;16:891–895.

Preston DC, Shapiro BE. Electromyography and neuromuscular disorders. Clinical-electrophysiologic correlations. 2nd ed. Philadelphia, Elsevier Butterworth Heinemann, 2005.

Sunderland S. *Nerves and Nerve Injuries.* Williams & Wilkins, Baltimore, 1968, pp. 1105–1113.

Iliacus (Iliopsoas)

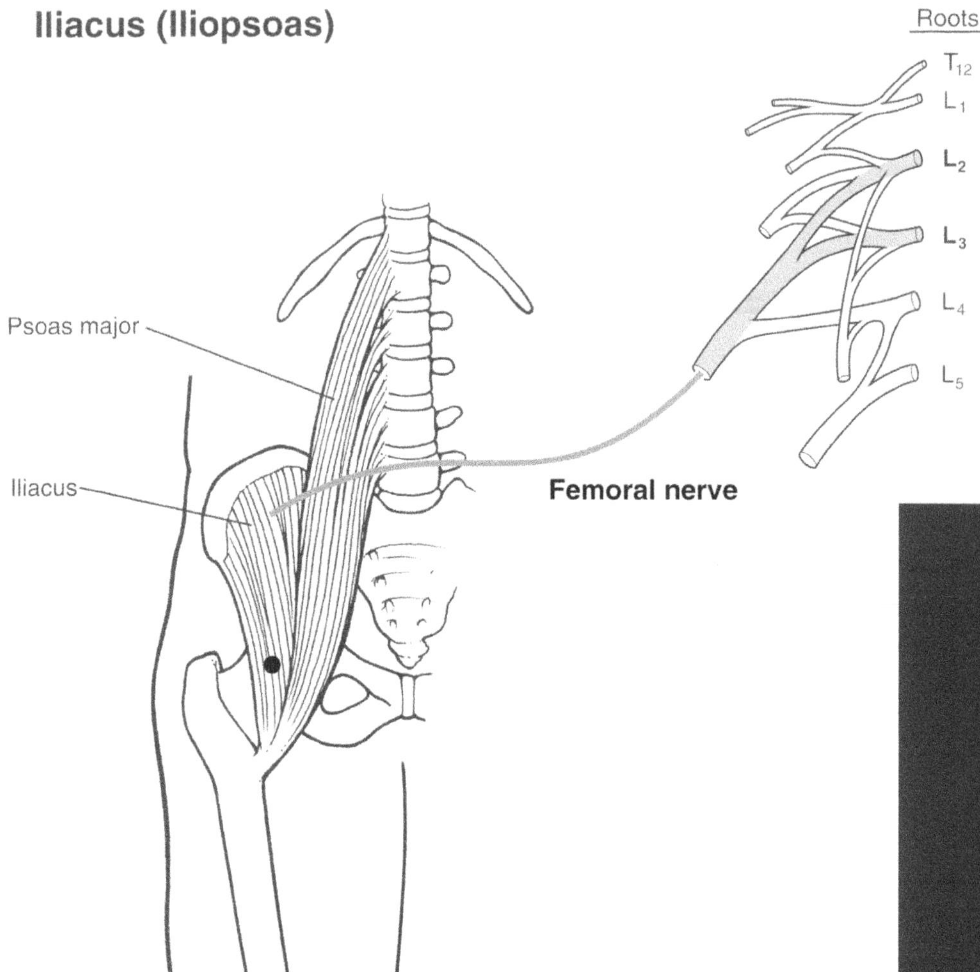

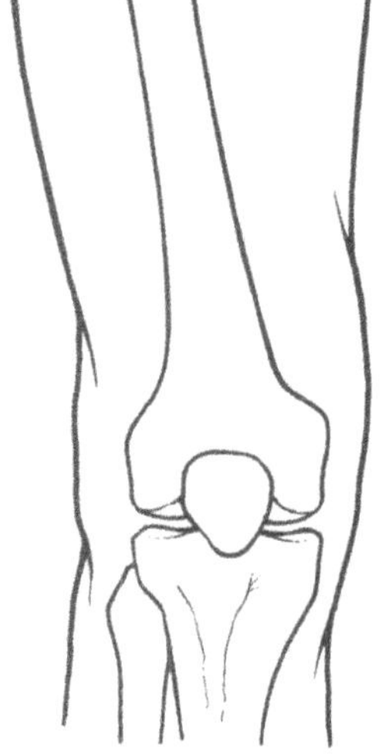

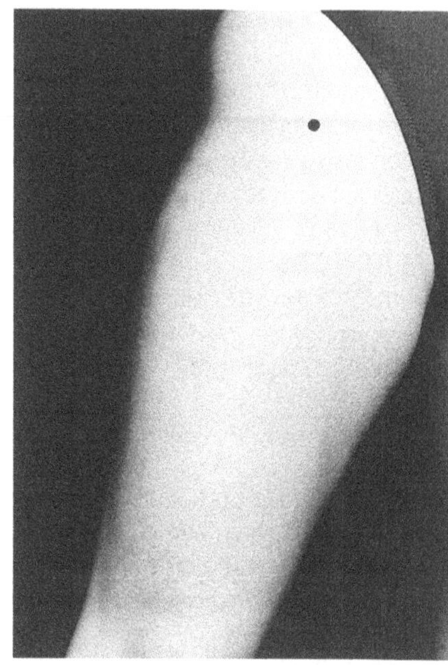

Innervation
Innervation is via the femoral nerve, posterior division of the lumbar plexus, and roots L_2, L_3. Note: Iliacus and psoas major act together, the combination being referred to as *iliopsoas*. However, direct branches from ventral rami of the lumbar spinal nerves L_1, L_2 and L_3 supply the psoas major.

Origin
The iliacus originates at the superior two-thirds of the iliac fossa, inner lip of the iliac crest, and upper surface of the lateral sacrum.

The psoas major originates at the transverse processes and bodies of all lumbar vertebrae and the body of the twelfth thoracic vertebra.

Insertion
The iliacus and psoas major insert together into the lesser trochanter of the femur (iliacus fibers are lateral; psoas fibers are medial).

Activation Maneuver
Flexion of the thigh upon the pelvis activates the muscle.

EMG Needle Insertion
Insert the needle 3–4 cm lateral to the femoral artery pulse just below the inguinal ligament.

Pitfalls
If the needle is inserted too medially, it may penetrate the femoral nerve or artery.

Clinical Comments
Neurogenic changes on needle examination may be seen with lesions of the femoral nerve within the abdomen (retroperitoneal hematoma or mass lesion), posterior division of lumbar plexus, or L_2, L_3 roots.

Pectineus

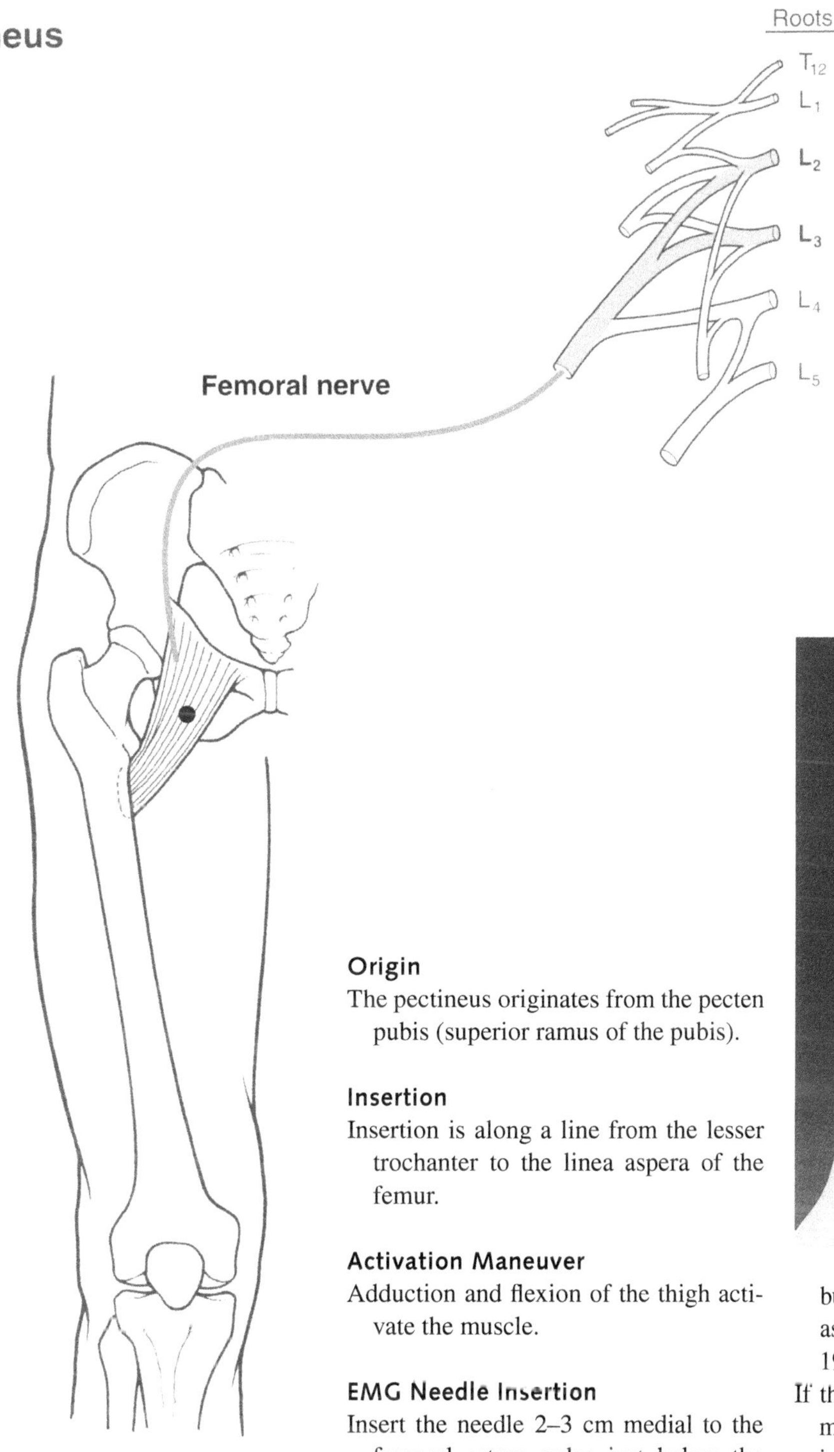

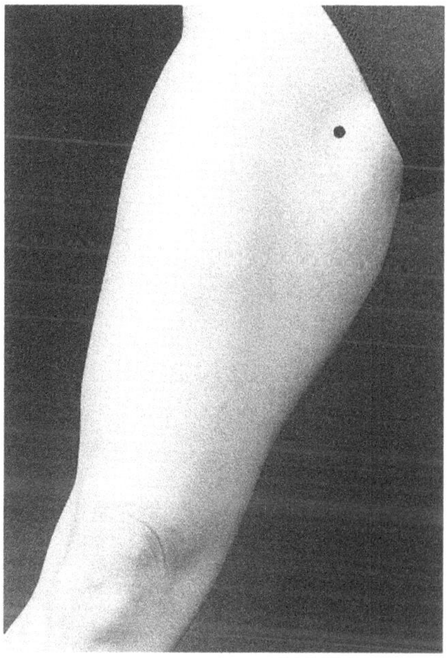

Origin

The pectineus originates from the pecten pubis (superior ramus of the pubis).

Insertion

Insertion is along a line from the lesser trochanter to the linea aspera of the femur.

Activation Maneuver

Adduction and flexion of the thigh activate the muscle.

EMG Needle Insertion

Insert the needle 2–3 cm medial to the femoral artery pulse just below the inguinal ligament.

Innervation

Innervation is via the femoral nerve, posterior division of the lumbar plexus, and roots L_2, L_3. This muscle may also receive a branch from the obturator nerve (*Gray's Anatomy,* 1995).

Pitfalls

If the needle is inserted too laterally, it may penetrate the femoral vein or artery; this muscle is often avoided in the EMG assessment, due to its relationship with the neurovascular bundle, which traverses the lateral aspect of the muscle (*Gray's Anatomy*, 1995).

If the needle is inserted too medially, it may be in the adductor longus, which is supplied by the obturator nerve.

Clinical Comments

Neurogenic changes on needle examination may be seen with lesions of the femoral nerve within the abdomen (retroperitoneal hematoma or mass lesion), posterior division of the lumbar plexus, or L_2, L_3 roots.

Sartorius

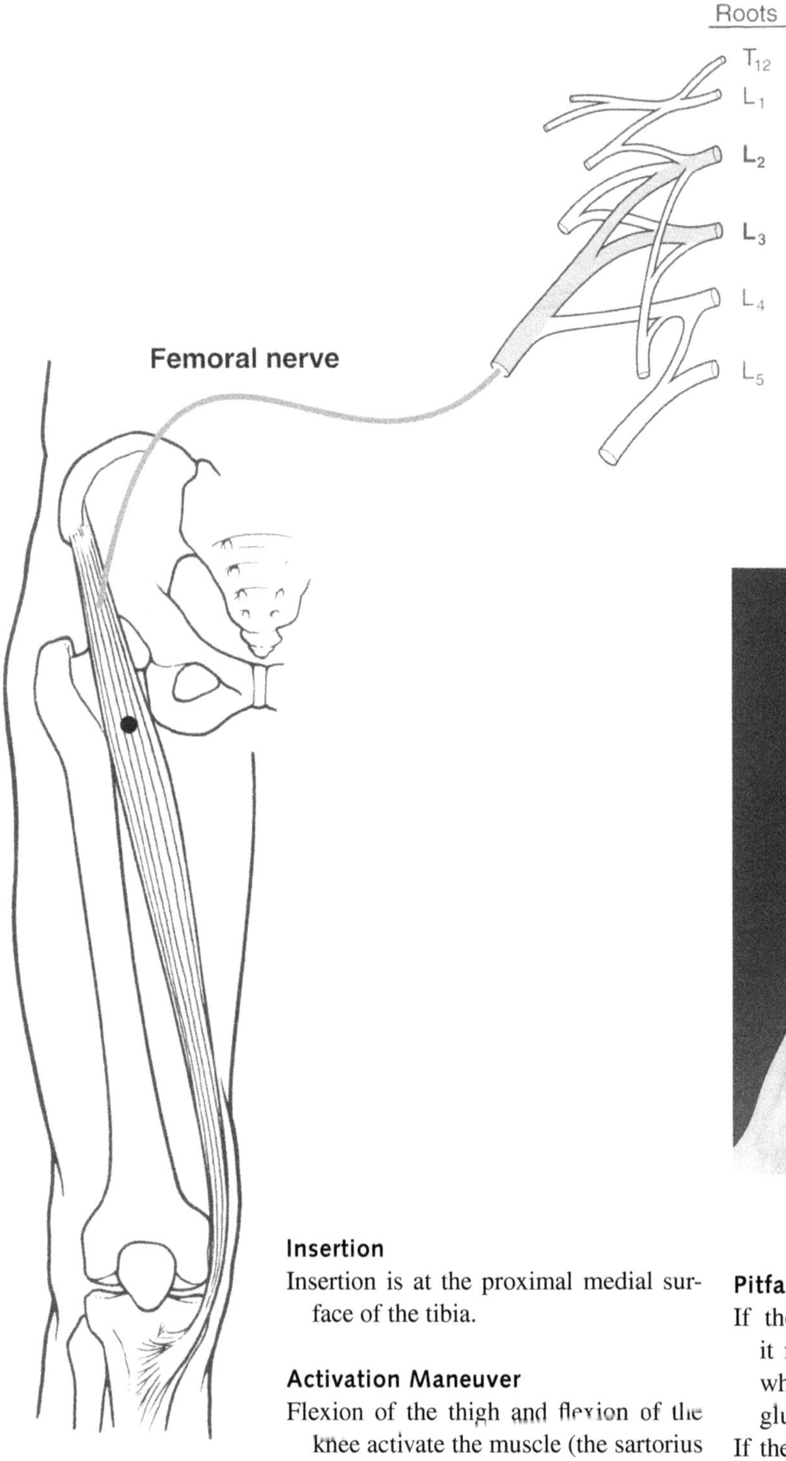

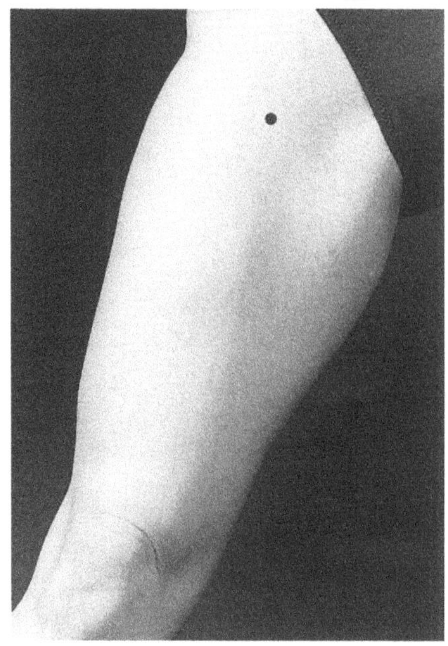

Innervation
Innervation is via the femoral nerve, posterior division of the lumbar plexus, and roots L_2, L_3.

Origin
The sartorius originates at the anterior superior iliac spine.

Insertion
Insertion is at the proximal medial surface of the tibia.

Activation Maneuver
Flexion of the thigh and flexion of the knee activate the muscle (the sartorius is a narrow strap muscle that crosses the hip and knee joints; it is the longest muscle of the body).

EMG Needle Insertion
Insert the needle 6–7 cm distal to the anterior superior iliac spine along a line to the medial epicondyle of the tibia.

Pitfalls
If the needle is inserted too laterally, it may be in the tensor fasciae latae, which is innervated by the superior gluteal nerve.

If the needle is inserted too medially or deeply, it may be in the iliopsoas or rectus femoris, respectively, which are also supplied by the femoral nerve.

Clinical Comments
Neurogenic changes on needle examination may be seen with lesions of the femoral nerve, posterior division of the lumbar plexus, or L_2, L_3 roots.

Rectus Femoris

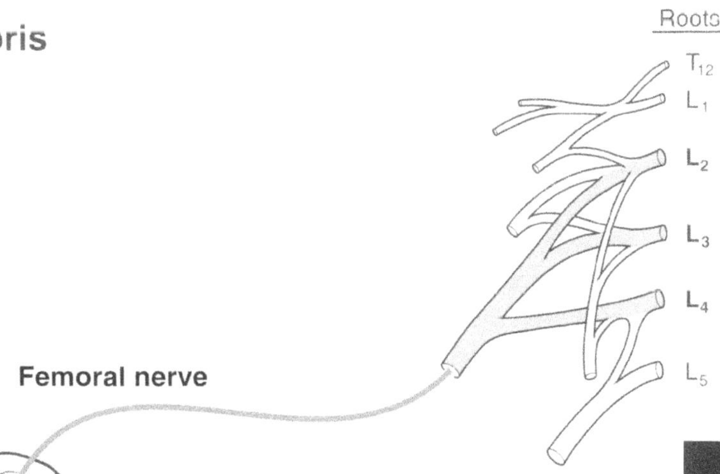

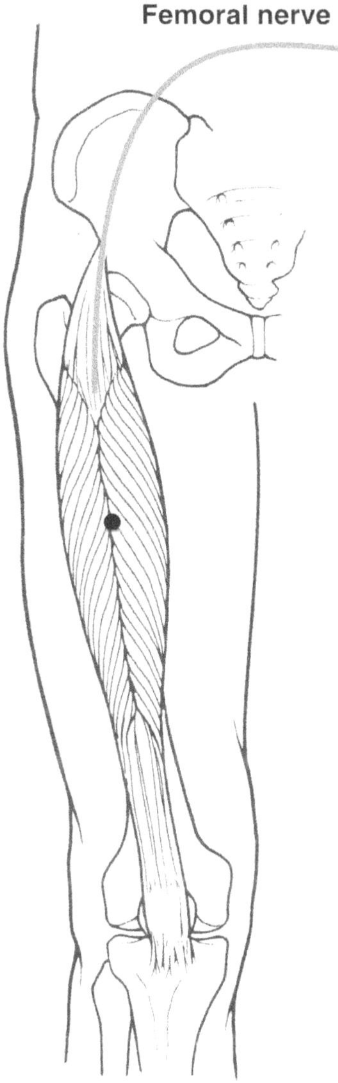

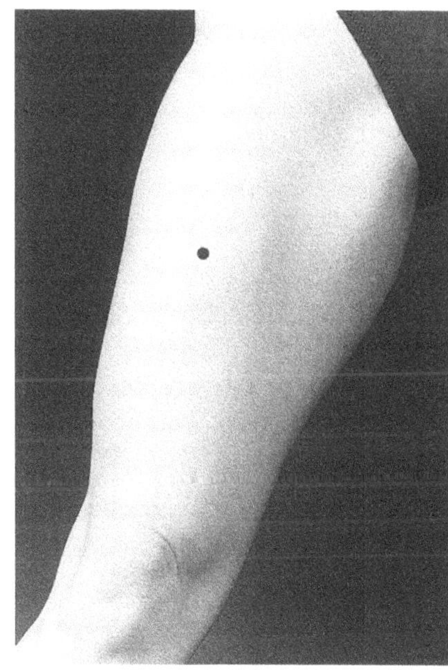

Innervation

Innervation is via the femoral nerve, posterior division of the lumbar plexus, and roots L_2, L_3, L_4.

Origin

The rectus femoris originates at the anterior inferior iliac spine and a groove above the acetabulum of the ilium. This is the only quadriceps muscle that arises from the ilium; the other three arise from the shaft of the femur. The muscle travels straight down the middle of the thigh; hence its name, *rectus femoris*.

Insertion

Insertion is at the base of the patella via the quadriceps tendon. Note: The tendons of the four quadriceps unite to form a single strong tendon attached to the base of the patella. The patella is, in fact, a sesamoid bone in the quadriceps tendon, and the ligamentum patellae, which extends to insert on the tubercle of the tibia, is the continuation of the tendon.

Activation Maneuver

Flexion of the thigh and extension of the knee activate the muscle (the rectus femoris crosses the hip and knee joints).

EMG Needle Insertion

Insert the needle into the anterior thigh midway between the anterior superior iliac spine and the patella.

Pitfalls

There are no pitfalls. If the needle is improperly inserted, it will still be in muscles supplied by the femoral nerve.

Clinical Comments

Neurogenic changes on needle examination may be seen with lesions of the femoral nerve, posterior division of the lumbar plexus, or L_2, L_3, L_4 roots.

Vastus Lateralis

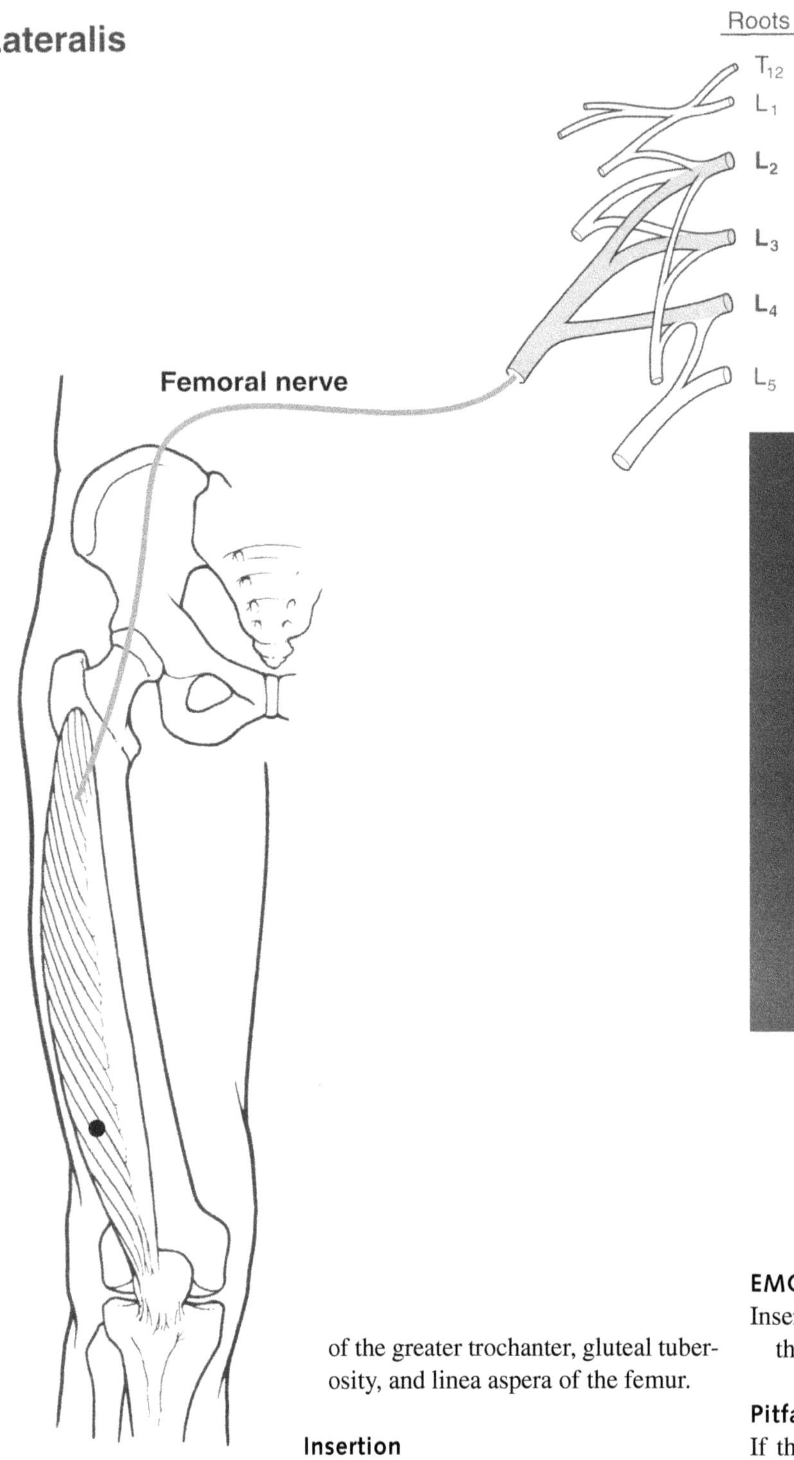

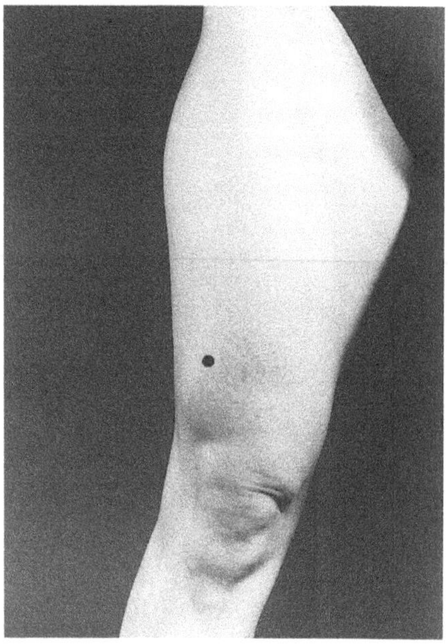

Innervation

Innervation is via the femoral nerve, posterior division of the lumbar plexus, and roots L_2, L_3, L_4.

Origin

The vastus lateralis originates from the intertrochanteric line, inferior border of the greater trochanter, gluteal tuberosity, and linea aspera of the femur.

Insertion

Insertion is at the tubercle of the tibia via the quadriceps tendon.

Activation Maneuver

Extension of the knee activates the muscle. Instruct the supine patient to press the knee down into the bed while lifting the heel of the foot off the bed.

EMG Needle Insertion

Insert the needle into the anterolateral thigh 8–10 cm above the patella.

Pitfalls

If the needle is inserted too posteriorly, it may be in the biceps femoris short head, which is supplied by the peroneal division of the sciatic nerve.

Clinical Comments

Neurogenic changes on needle examination may be seen with lesions of the femoral nerve, posterior division of the lumbar plexus, or L_2, L_3, L_4 roots.

Vastus Intermedius

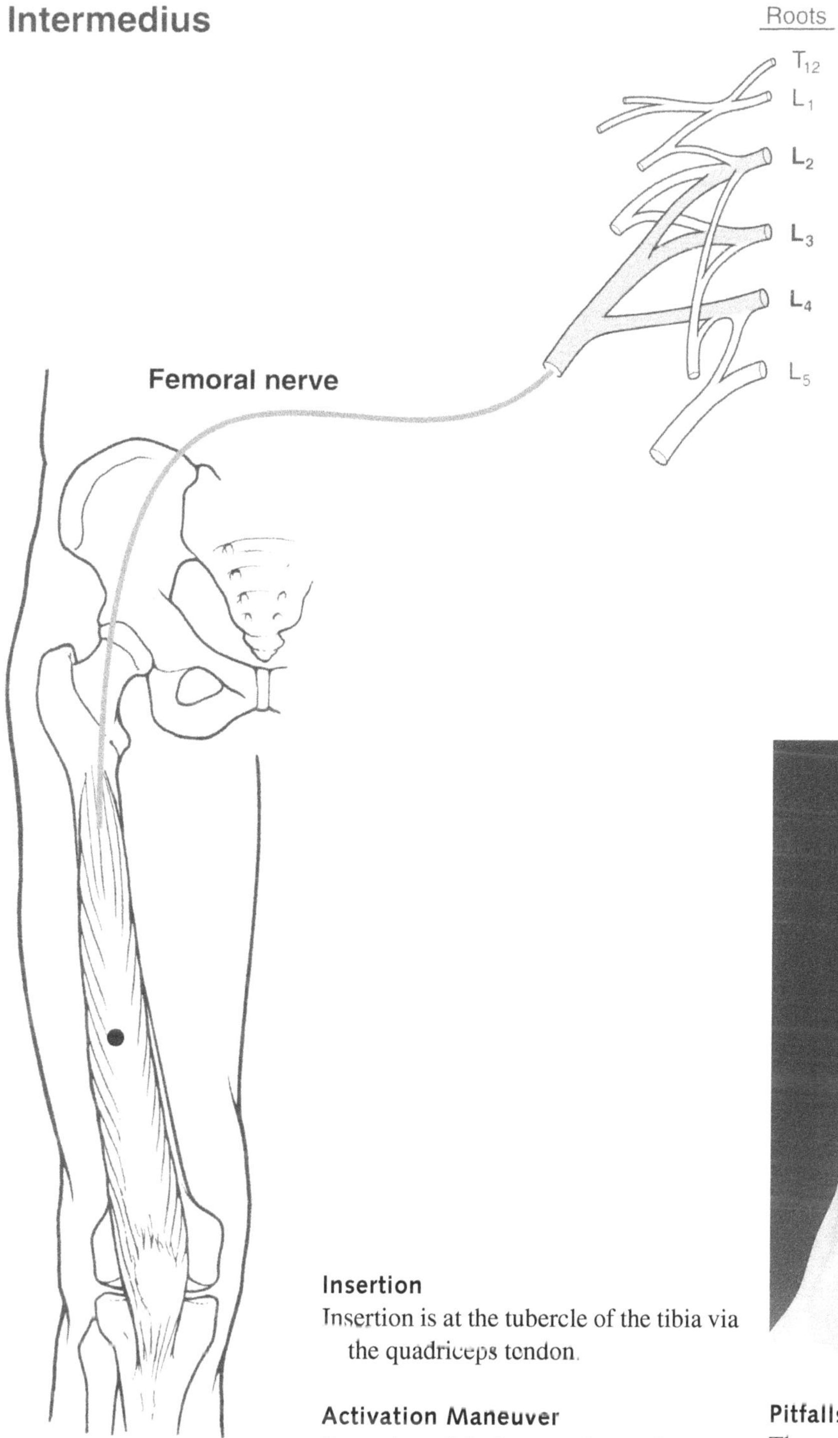

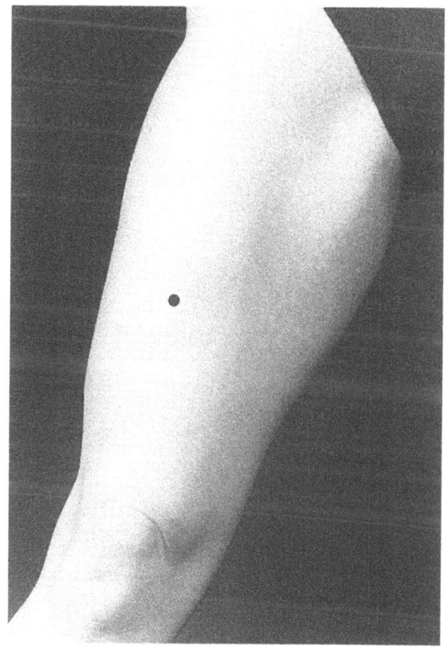

Innervation

Innervation is via the femoral nerve, posterior division of the lumbar plexus, and roots L_2, L_3, L_4.

Origin

The vastus intermedius originates at the anterior and lateral surfaces of the upper two-thirds of the femoral shaft.

Insertion

Insertion is at the tubercle of the tibia via the quadriceps tendon.

Activation Maneuver

Extension of the knee activates the muscle. Instruct the supine patient to press the knee down into the bed while lifting the heel of the foot off the bed.

EMG Needle Insertion

Insert the needle into the anterior thigh midway between the anterior superior iliac spine and the patella. This muscle lies deep to the rectus femoris.

Pitfalls

There are no pitfalls. If the needle is improperly inserted, it will still be in muscles supplied by the femoral nerve.

Clinical Comments

Neurogenic changes on needle examination may be seen with lesions of the femoral nerve, posterior division of the lumbar plexus, or L_2, L_3, L_4 roots.

Vastus Medialis

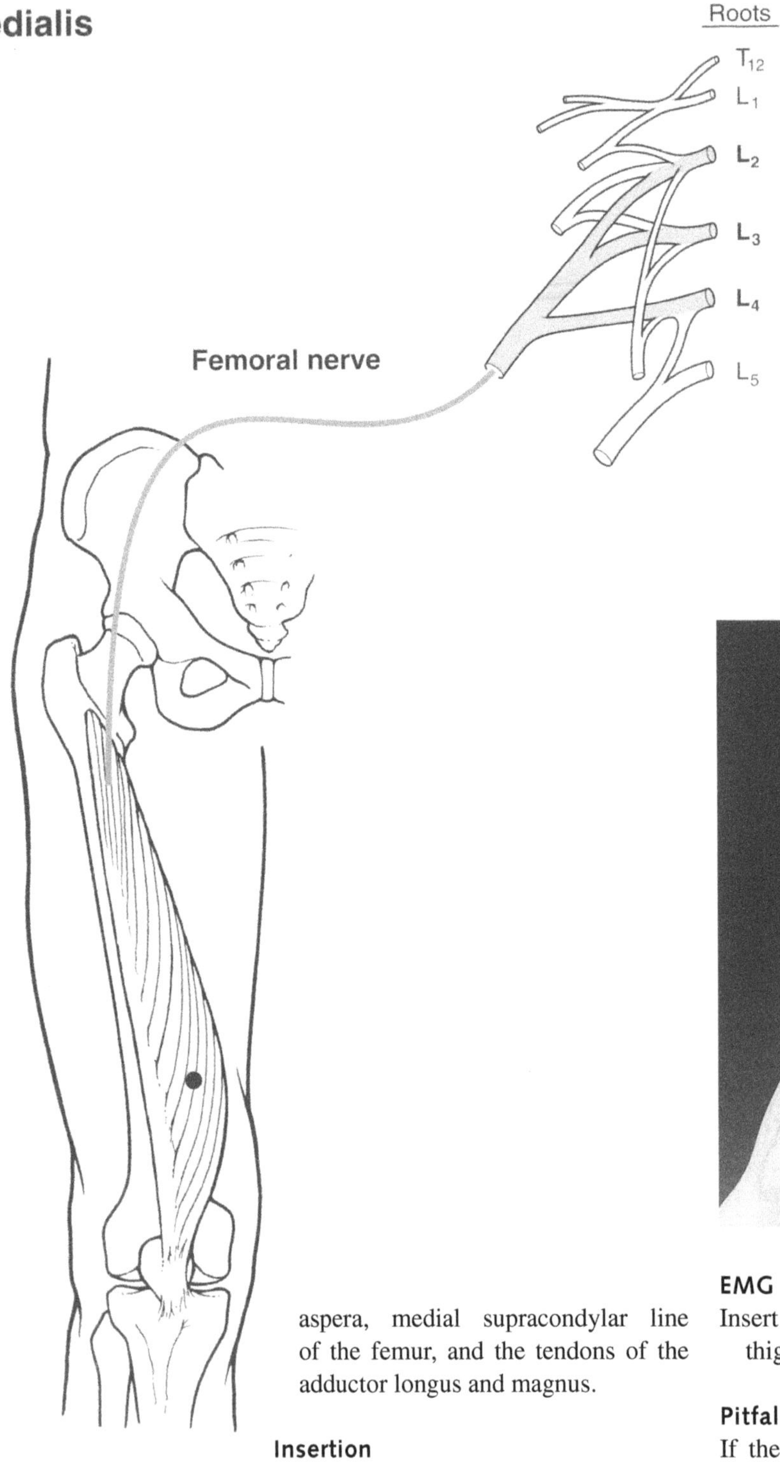

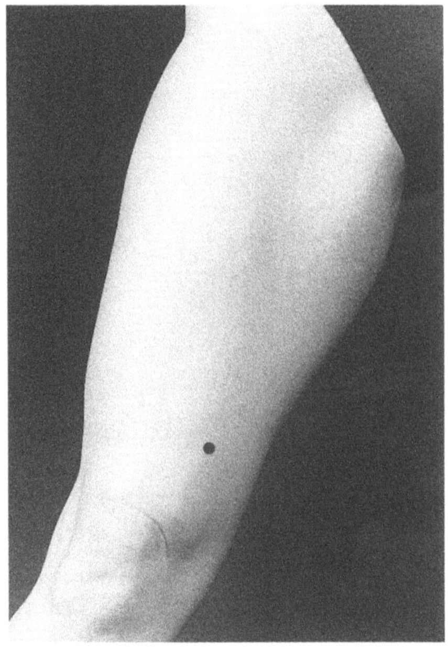

Innervation
Innervation is via the femoral nerve, posterior division of the lumbar plexus, and roots L_2, L_3, L_4.

Origin
The vastus medialis originates from the intertrochanteric line, spiral line, linea aspera, medial supracondylar line of the femur, and the tendons of the adductor longus and magnus.

Insertion
Insertion is at the tubercle of the tibia via the quadriceps tendon.

Activation Maneuver
Extension of the knee activates the muscle. Instruct the supine patient to press the knee down into the bed while lifting the heel of the foot off the bed.

EMG Needle Insertion
Insert the needle into the anteromedial thigh 5–7 cm above the patella.

Pitfalls
If the needle is inserted too superiorly and medially, it may be in the adductor magnus, which is supplied by the obturator and sciatic nerves.

Clinical Comments
Neurogenic changes on needle examination may be seen with lesions of the femoral nerve, posterior division of the lumbar plexus, or L_2, L_3, L_4 roots.

OBTURATOR NERVE

26

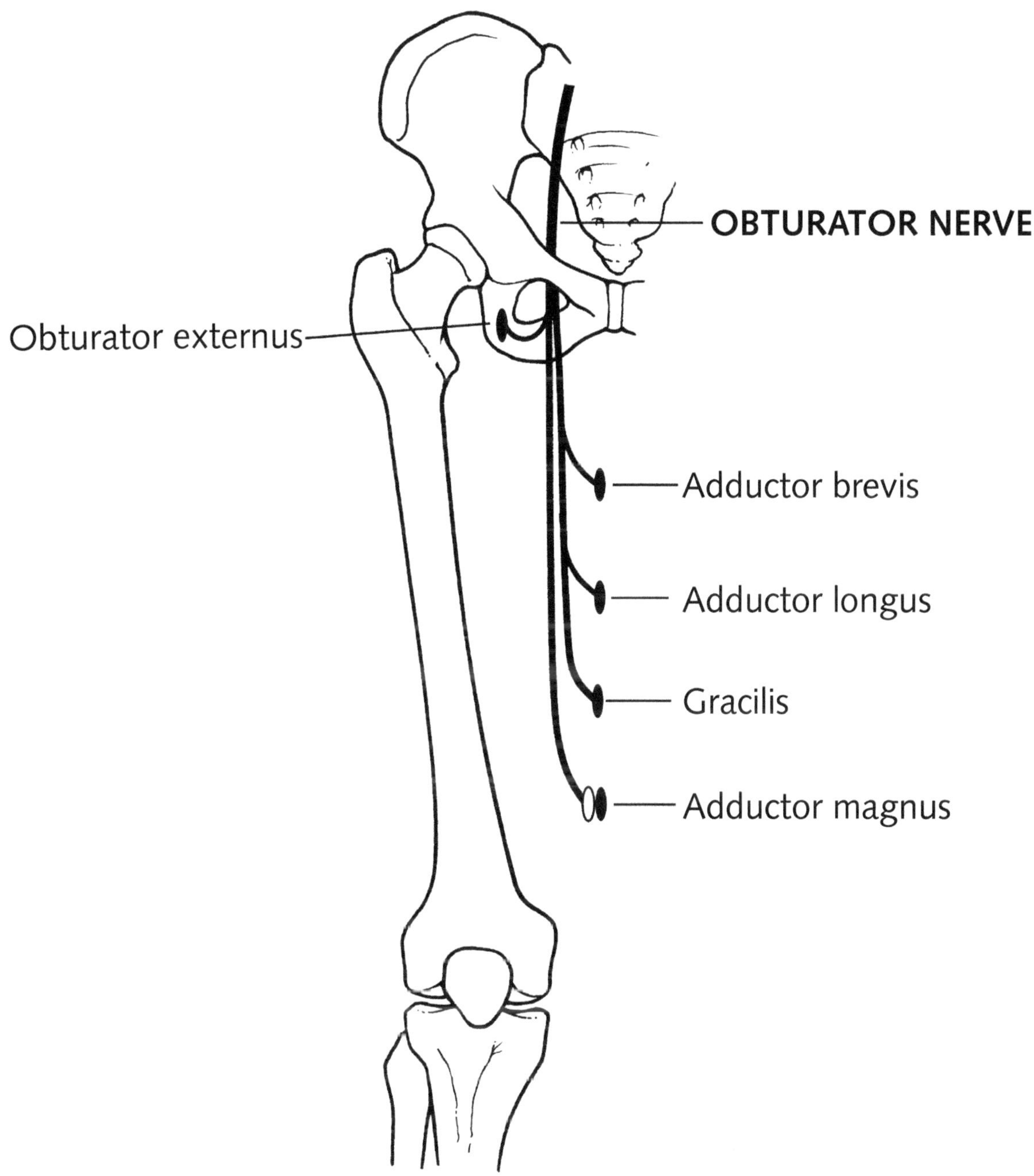

FIGURE 26-1 Diagram of the obturator nerve and the muscles that it supplies. Note: The white oval signifies that a muscle receives a part of its innervation from another peripheral nerve.

THE OBTURATOR NERVE arises from the anterior division of the second to fourth lumbar ventral rami. The contribution from the third or fourth ramus is the largest, and that from the second is often very small. The nerve descends within the substance of the psoas major, emerging from its medial border at the pelvic brim. It descends further along the ala of the sacrum to reach the lateral pelvic wall on the obturator internus muscle. It then sweeps forward within the pelvis to reach and pass through the obturator foramen to enter the thigh. Near the foramen it divides into anterior and posterior branches. The *anterior branch* supplies the adductor longus, adductor brevis, gracilis, and often the pectineus (*Gray's Anatomy,* 1995). At the lower border of the adductor longus, it communicates with the medial cutaneous and saphenous branches of the femoral nerve to supply the skin on the medial aspect of the thigh. The *posterior branch* supplies the obturator externus and adductor magnus muscles. It usually sends an articular branch to the knee joint. A small *accessory obturator nerve* may occasionally be present, arising from the anterior division of the third and fourth lumbar ventral rami to supply the pectineus and, rarely, the adductor longus muscles.

Anatomical features of clinical importance relate to the posterior abdominal wall, where the obturator nerve may be involved together with the femoral nerve in retroperitoneal lesions. In the pelvis, compression of the nerve may occur against the lateral pelvic wall. Here, the nerve may be in direct contact with the bone or separated from it by only a thin layer of muscle (Sunderland, 1968). It may be compressed by the fetal head during a difficult delivery or by a benign or malignant pelvic tumor or abscess. On the left side it may be involved by carcinoma of the sigmoid colon, and on the right by an inflamed appendix. At the obturator foramen it is intimately related to the superior ramus of the pubis, and fractures of the bone may damage the nerve. Postsurgical obturator neuropathy has also been reported following positioning on the operating table in which the thigh is acutely flexed, as in the lithotomy position. In these cases, nerve involvement is likely related to acute angulation where the nerve leaves the bony obturator foramen (Sunderland, 1968). Neurectomy has been performed to relieve adductor spasms in disorders associated with upper motor neuron dysfunction.

Note: The short muscles around the hip joint—pectineus, obturator externus, quadratus femoris, gemellus superior, gemellus inferior, obturator internus, and piriformis—are largely inaccessible to direct observation. Because of the potential complications presented by their intimate relationship to important neurovascular structures, there is a relative lack of EMG data in humans.

OBTURATOR NERVE LESION

Etiology

Retroperitoneal lesions can cause an obturator neuropathy. The obturator nerve may be involved together with the femoral nerve by hematoma, hemorrhage, tumor, or abscess.

There are iatrogenic causes, including pelvic or abdominal surgery (e.g., direct surgical trauma, stretch injury, suture entrapment, or retractor related; Cardosi et al., 2002) and intraoperative or postanesthesia traction injury due to sustained abduction or hyperflexion of the thigh (Litwiller et al., 2004).

Entrapment of the obturator nerve may occur by a thick fascia overlying the adductor brevis muscle. This should be considered as a potential cause of chronic groin pain in athletes (Bradshaw et al., 1997).

Trauma, including pelvic fractures and penetrating injuries, is a common cause of obturator nerve lesion.

Other causes of obturator neuropathy include *(1)* compression of the nerve against the lateral pelvic wall by the fetal head or pelvic masses, *(2)* obturator hernias, *(3)* obturator nerve ganglion, and *(4)* neuralgic amyotrophy (Sorenson et al., 2002; Tipton, 2008).

General Comments

It is common for an obturator nerve deficit to be accompanied by a femoral nerve deficit (Dawson et al., 1990). Lesions of the upper portion of the lumbar plexus usually affect both the obturator and femoral nerves, because both arise from within the psoas muscle.

Most lesions that involve the obturator nerve are traumatic in origin.

In diabetic amyotrophy, proximal muscles are involved, including those innervated by the obturator nerve (Chokroverty and Sander, 1996).

Clinical Features

Paresis or paralysis of adductor muscles produces weakness or inability to adduct the thigh and leg.

Numbness, loss of sensation, or altered sensation in the medial aspect of the thigh can occur.

Pain in the groin may radiate down the thigh.

Loss or asymmetry of the adductor tendon reflex may be observed.

Electrodiagnostic Strategy

Perform EMG needle examination in thigh muscles innervated by the obturator nerve or its branches. In lesions associated with loss of motor fibers, EMG may show neurogenic changes (i.e., fibrillation potentials, polyphasic motor unit potentials, and neurogenic recruitment).

Perform EMG of quadriceps muscles, other proximal muscles (gluteal, hamstring), and paraspinal muscles to exclude plexus or root involvement.

REFERENCES

Bradshaw C, McCrory P, Bell S, Brukner P. Obturator nerve entrapment. A cause of groin pain in athletes. *Am J Sports Med* 1997;25:402–408.

Cardosi, RJ, Cox CS, Hoffman MS. Postoperative neuropathies after major pelvic surgery. *Obstet Gynecol* 2002;100:240–244.

Chokroverty S, Sander HW. AAEM case report #13: Diabetic amyotrophy. *Muscle Nerve* 1996;19:939–945.

Dawson DM, Hallett M, Millender LH. *Entrapment Neuropathies*. 2nd edition. Little, Brown, Boston, 1990, pp. 313–316.

Gray's Anatomy. 38th Edition. Churchill Livingstone, New York 1995, pp. 868–875, 1277–1282.

Litwiller JP, Wells RE Jr, Halliwill JR, Carmichael SW, Warner MA. Effect of lithotomy positions on strain of the obturator and lateral femoral cutaneous nerves. *Clin Anat* 2004;17:45–49.

Sorenson EJ, Chen JJ, Daube JR. Obturator neuropathy: causes and outcome. *Muscle Nerve* 2002;25:605–607.

Sunderland S. *Nerves and Nerve Injuries*. Williams & Wilkins, Baltimore, 1968, pp. 1096–1104.

Tipton JS. Obturator neuropathy. *Curr Rev Musculoskelet Med* 2008;1:234–237.

Adductor Longus

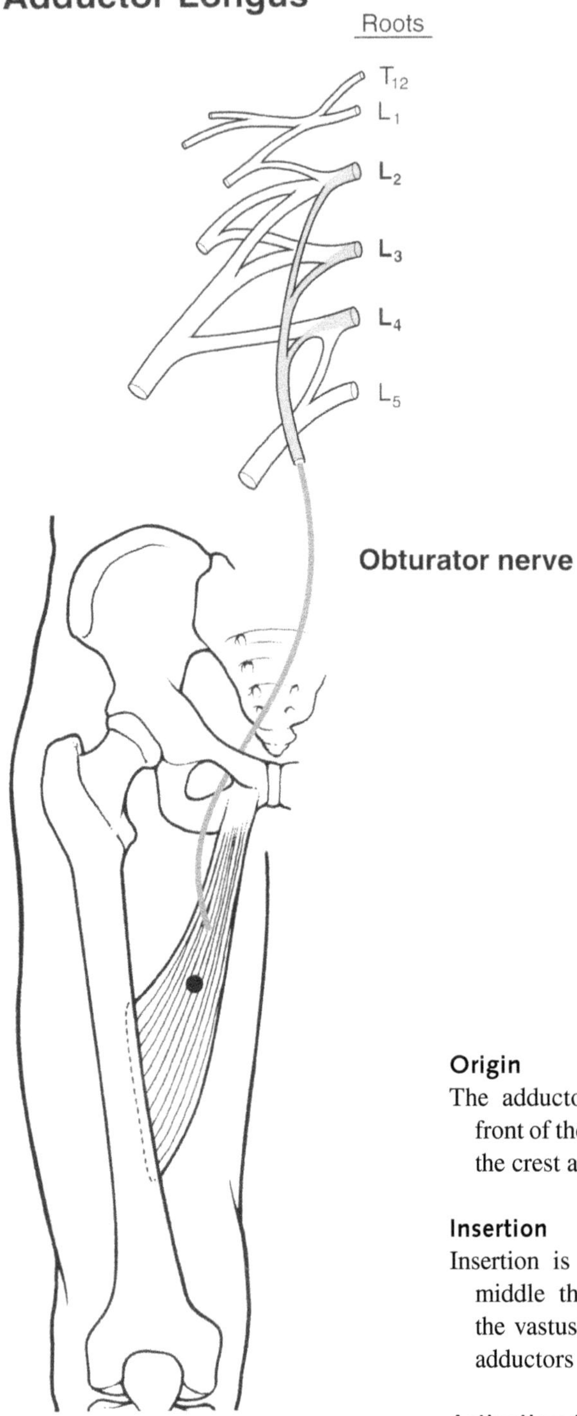

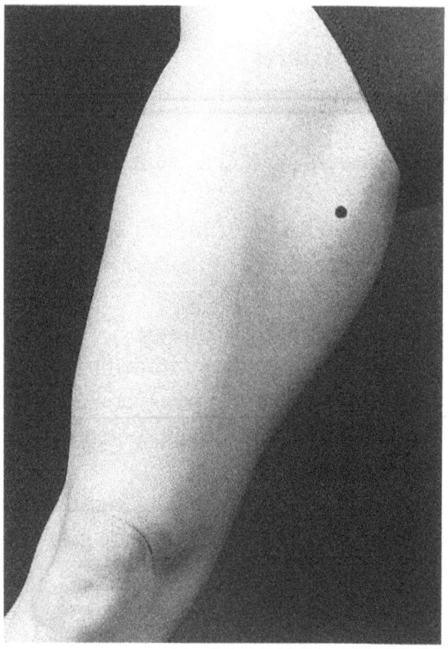

Innervation
Innervation is via the obturator nerve, anterior division of the lumbar plexus, and roots L_2, L_3, L_4.

Origin
The adductor longus originates at the front of the pubis, in the angle between the crest and the symphysis.

Insertion
Insertion is at the linea aspera in the middle third of the femur, between the vastus medialis and the other two adductors (magnus and brevis).

Activation Maneuver
Adduction of the thigh activates the muscle.

EMG Needle Insertion
Insert the needle into the medial thigh 6–8 cm distal to the origin of the tendon near the pubic tubercle. The tendon can be easily palpated.

Pitfalls
If the needle is inserted too medially and anteriorly, it may be in the sartorius, which is supplied by the femoral nerve.

If the needle is inserted too laterally, it may be in pectineus, which is supplied by the femoral nerve (the pectineus may also receive a branch from obturator nerve).

If the needle is inserted too medially or posteriorly, it may be in the gracilis or the other two adductors, which are also supplied by the obturator nerve (the adductor magnus also receives a branch from the sciatic nerve).

Clinical Comments
Neurogenic changes on needle examination may be seen with lesions of the obturator nerve, anterior division of the lumbar plexus, or L_2, L_3, L_4 roots.

Adductor Brevis

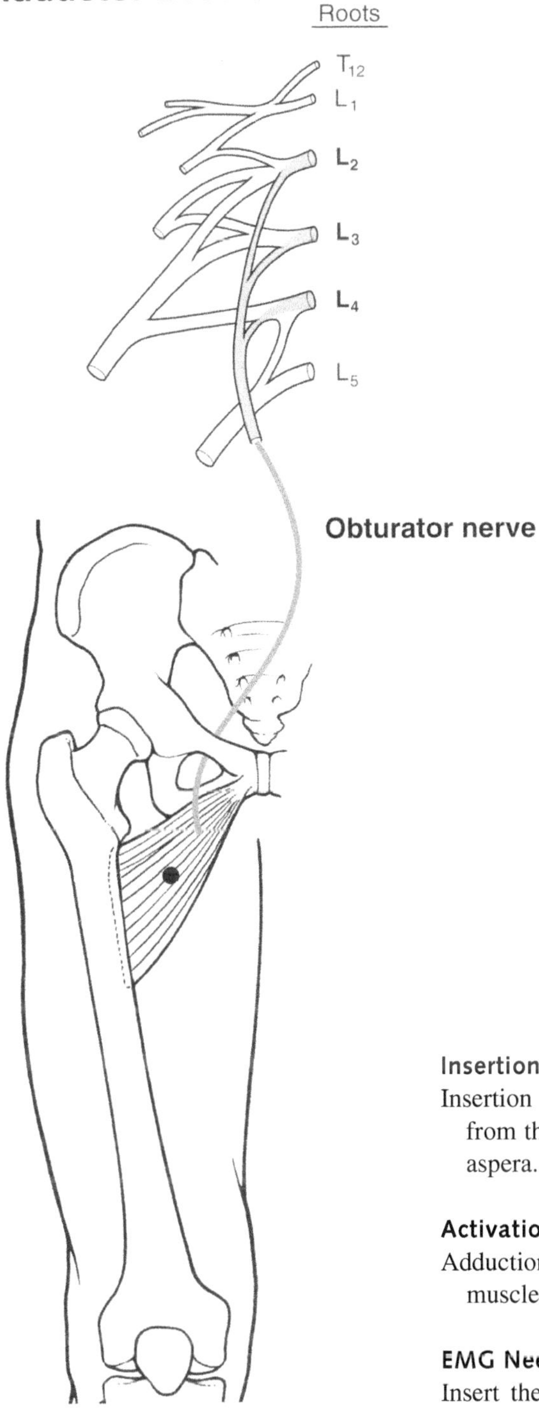

Innervation

Innervation is via the obturator nerve, anterior division of the lumbar plexus, and roots L_2, L_3, L_4.

Origin

The adductor brevis originates at the inferior ramus of the pubis.

Insertion

Insertion is into the femur, along a line from the lesser trochanter to the linea aspera.

Activation Maneuver

Adduction of the thigh activates the muscle.

EMG Needle Insertion

Insert the needle into the medial thigh 5–7 cm distal to the origin of the tendon of adductor longus, to a depth of about 4 cm. The adductor brevis lies deep to the pectineus and adductor longus.

Pitfalls

If the needle is inserted too superficially, it may be in the pectineus or adductor longus, which are supplied by the femoral and obturator nerves, respectively. The pectineus may also receive a branch from the obturator nerve.

If the needle is inserted too medially, it may be in the gracilis, which is also supplied by the obturator nerve.

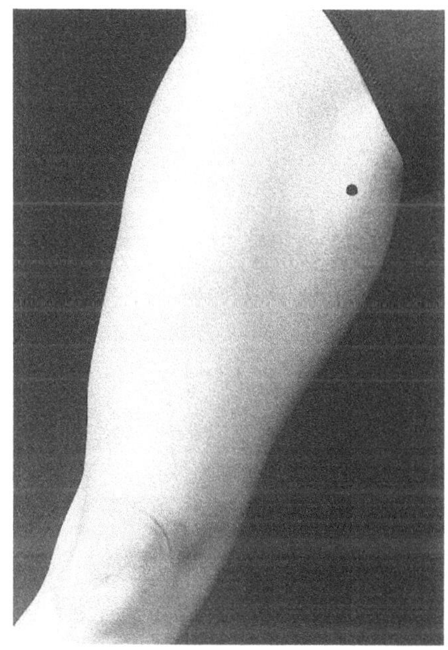

Clinical Comments

Neurogenic changes on needle examination may be seen with lesions of the obturator nerve, anterior division of the lumbar plexus, or L_2, L_3, L_4 roots.

Adductor Magnus

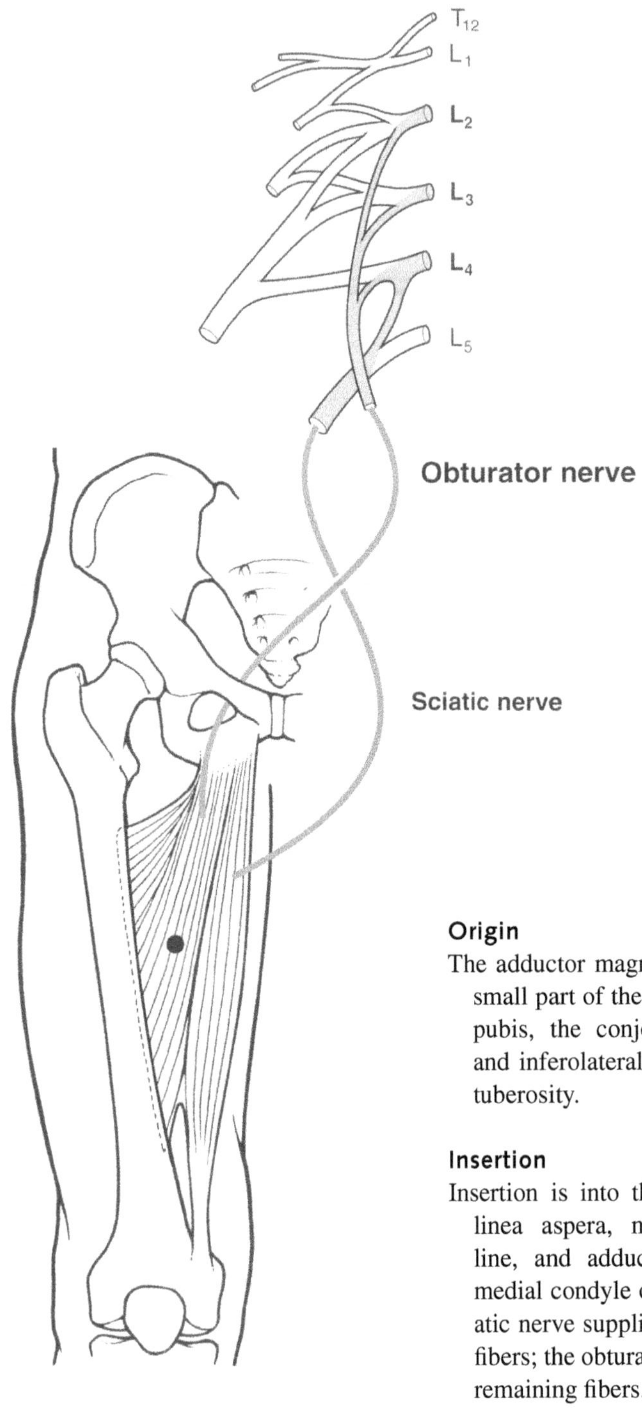

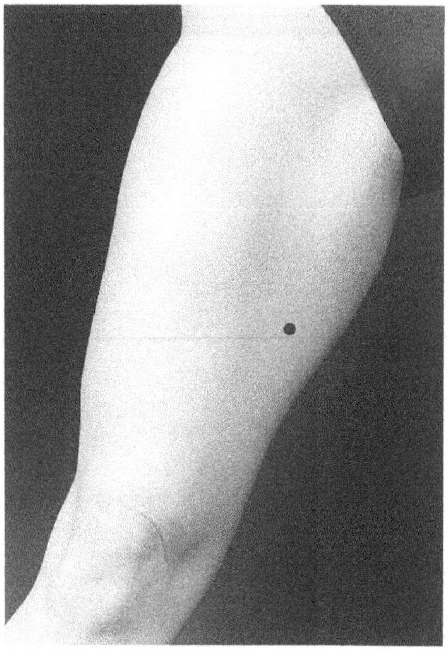

Innervation

Innervation is via the obturator nerve, anterior division of the lumbar plexus, and roots L_2, L_3, L_4.

Innervation is also via the sciatic nerve (tibial division), anterior division of the sacral plexus, and root L_4.

Origin

The adductor magnus originates from a small part of the inferior ramus of the pubis, the conjoined ischial ramus, and inferolateral aspect of the ischial tuberosity.

Insertion

Insertion is into the gluteal tuberosity, linea aspera, medial supracondylar line, and adductor tubercle on the medial condyle of the femur. The sciatic nerve supplies the ischiocondylar fibers; the obturator nerve supplies the remaining fibers.

Activation Maneuver

Adduction of the thigh activates the muscle.

EMG Needle Insertion

Insert the needle into the medial thigh midway between the pubic tubercle and medial condyle of the femur.

Pitfalls

If the needle is inserted too laterally and anteriorly, it may be in the sartorius, which is supplied by the femoral nerve.

If the needle is inserted too posteriorly, it may be in the semitendinosus or semimembranosus, which are supplied by the sciatic nerve.

Clinical Comments

Neurogenic changes on needle examination may be seen with lesions of the obturator nerve, anterior division of the lumbar plexus, or L_2, L_3, L_4 roots.

Neurogenic changes in ischiocondylar fibers may be seen with lesions of the sciatic nerve (tibial division), anterior division of the sacral plexus, or L_4 root. Morphologically, the ischiocondylar portion of the muscle may be considered to be a hamstring muscle, which explains its innervation from the sciatic nerve.

Gracilis

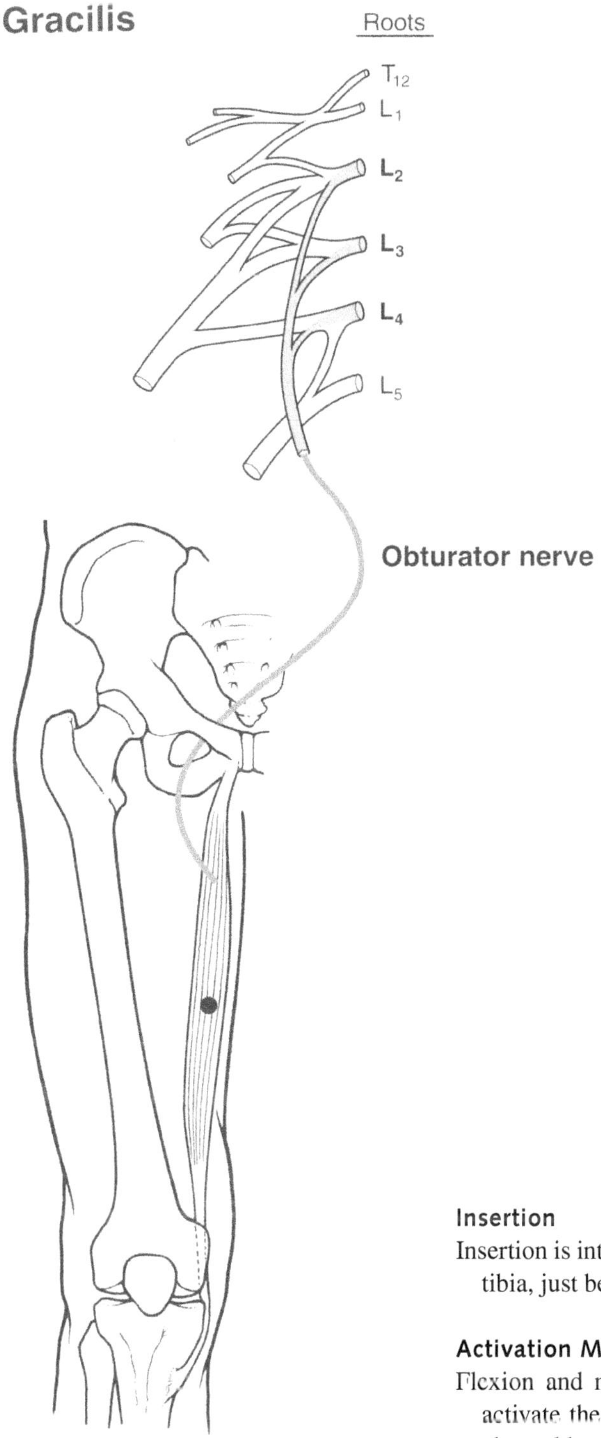

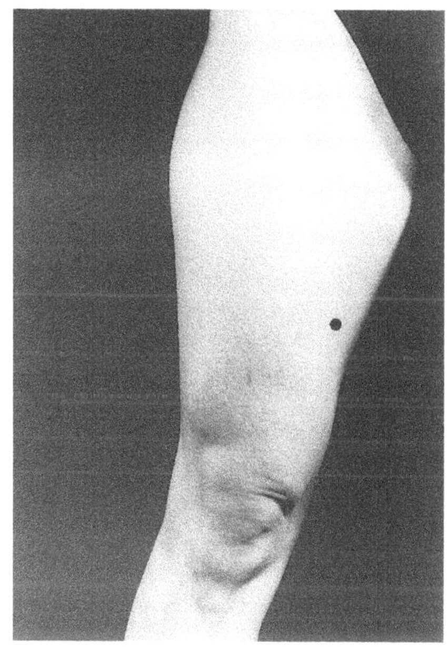

Innervation

Innervation is via the obturator nerve, anterior division of the lumbar plexus, and roots L_2, L_3, L_4.

Origin

The gracilis originates at the inferior ramus of the pubis and adjoining part of the ischial ramus.

Insertion

Insertion is into the medial surface of the tibia, just below the medial condyle.

Activation Maneuver

Flexion and medial rotation of the leg activate the muscle. The gracilis may also adduct the thigh (*Gray's Anatomy,* 1995).

EMG Needle Insertion

Insert the needle into the medial thigh midway between the pubic tubercle and medial condyle of the femur. The gracilis is the most superficial of the adductor group; it is thin and flat and may be missed by the needle.

Pitfalls

If the needle is inserted too anteriorly, it may be in the sartorius, which is supplied by the femoral nerve.

If the needle is inserted too posteriorly, it may be in the semimembranosus or semitendinosus, which are supplied by the sciatic nerve.

If the needle is inserted too deeply, it may be in the adductor magnus or the other two adductors, which are also supplied by the obturator nerve.

Clinical Comments

Neurogenic changes on needle examination may be seen with lesions of the obturator nerve, anterior division of the lumbar plexus, or L_2, L_3, L_4 roots.

27 PARASPINAL MUSCLES

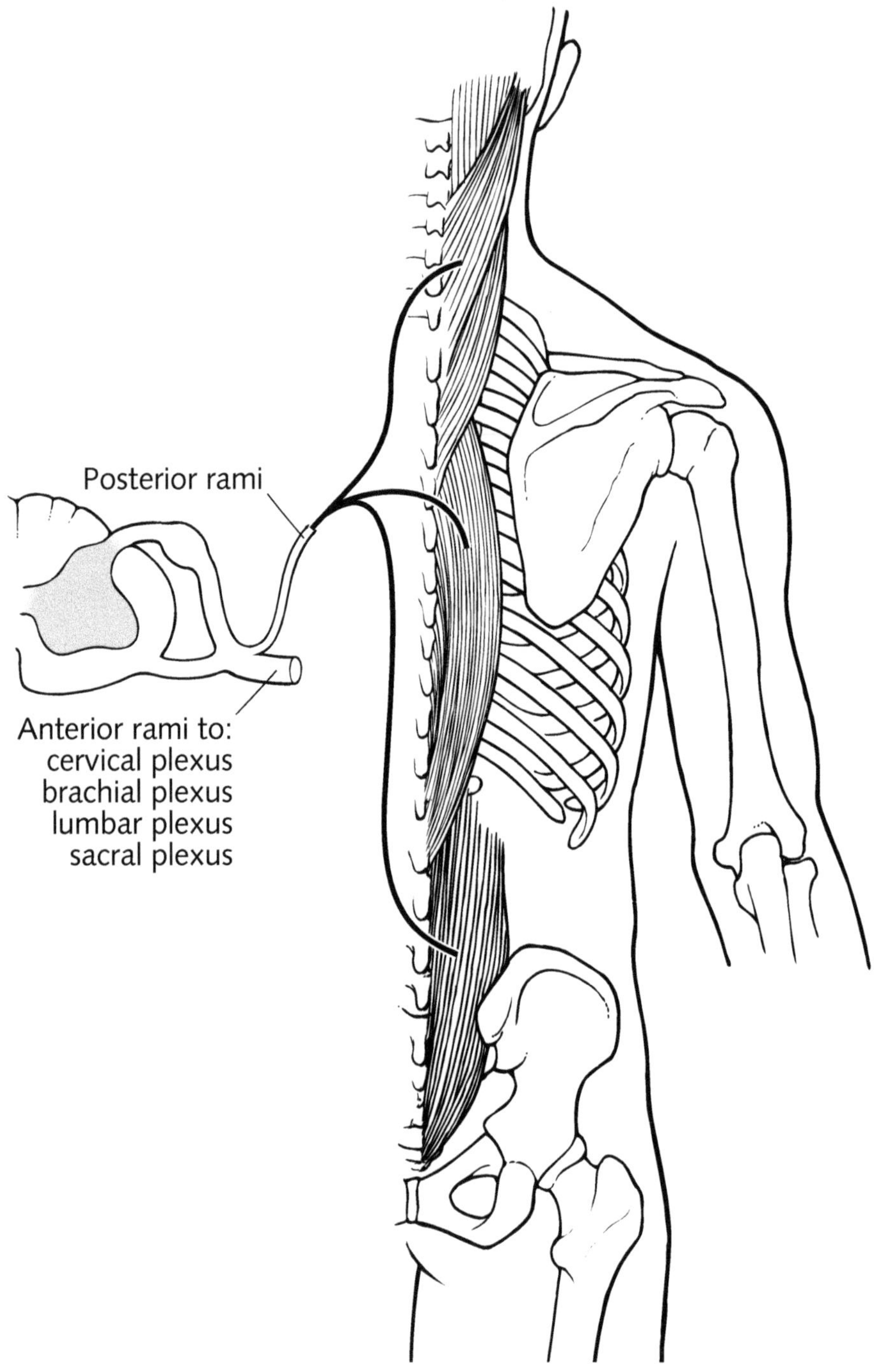

FIGURE 27-1 Diagram of the posterior rami supplying the paraspinal muscles in the cervical, thoracic, and lumbosacral regions.

VENTRAL AND DORSAL ROOTS form the spinal nerves that exit through the intervertebral foramina. There are 31 spinal nerves on each side: 8 cervical, 12 thoracic, 5 lumbar, 5 sacral, and 1 coccygeal nerve. Immediately after passing through the foramina, the spinal nerves branch into two divisions, the anterior and posterior rami.

The anterior rami form the cervical, brachial, lumbar, and sacral plexuses, which in turn give rise to the peripheral nerves in the neck and upper and lower limbs. The anterior rami of the thoracic spinal nerves become the 12 pairs of intercostal nerves that supply the intercostal and abdominal muscles. The posterior rami supply the paraspinal muscles in the cervical, thoracic, and lumbosacral regions. These muscles extend the head, neck, trunk, and pelvis. Because the posterior rami branch off the spinal nerve just distal to the intervertebral foramina, needle electromyogram (EMG) abnormalities in paraspinal muscles usually imply axonal loss at the root level (i.e., radiculopathy). However, radiculopathy causes EMG abnormalities in paraspinal muscles only after structural damage or axonal loss has occurred. Hence, the EMG may be normal when a compressing lesion irritates the root without causing axonal loss (Kimura, 1989). Moreover, the EMG in paraspinal muscles may be normal in the early stages of disease. Signs of denervation may not appear in paraspinal muscles for several days, and in limb muscles for several weeks, after severe root injury. Lesions limited to the plexuses or peripheral nerves do not produce EMG abnormalities in paraspinal muscles.

REFERENCES

Caress JB, Rutkove SB, Carlin M, Khoshbin S, Preston DC. Paraspinal muscle hematoma after electromyography. *Neurology* 1996;47:269–272.

Gray's Anatomy. 15th English Edition. Bounty Books/Crown Publishers, New York, 1977, pp. 336–350.

Haig AJ. Paraspinal denervation and the spinal degenerative cascade. *Spine J* 2002;2:372–380.

Honet JE, Honet JC, Cascade P. Pneumothorax after electromyographic electrode insertion in the paracervical muscles: Case report and radiographic analysis. *Arch Phys Med Rehabil* 1986;67:601–603.

Kimura J. *Electrodiagnosis in Diseases of Nerve and Muscle*. 2nd Edition. FA Davis, Philadelphia, 1989, p. 283.

Petrella JT, Giuliani MJ, Lacomis D. Vacuolar myopathies in adults with myalgias: value of paraspinal muscle investigation. *Muscle Nerve* 1997;20:1321–1323.

Streib EW, Wilbourn AJ, Mitsumoto H. Spontaneous electrical muscle fiber activity in polymyositis and dermatomyositis. *Muscle Nerve* 1979;2:14–18.

Tong HC, Haig AJ, Yamakawa KS, Miner JA. Paraspinal electromyography: Age-correlated normative values in asymptomatic subjects. *Spine* 2005;30:E499-E502.

Cervical Paraspinal

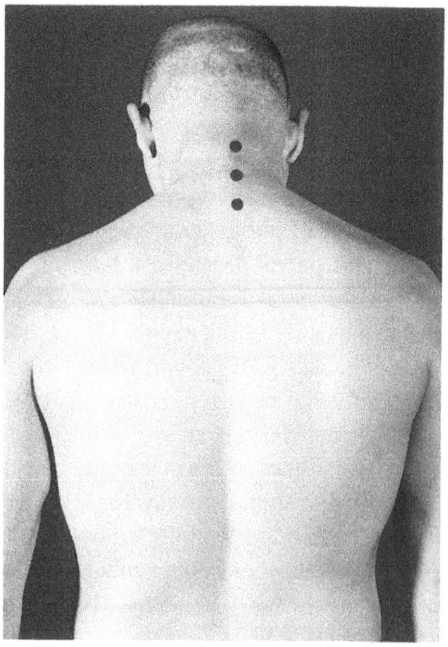

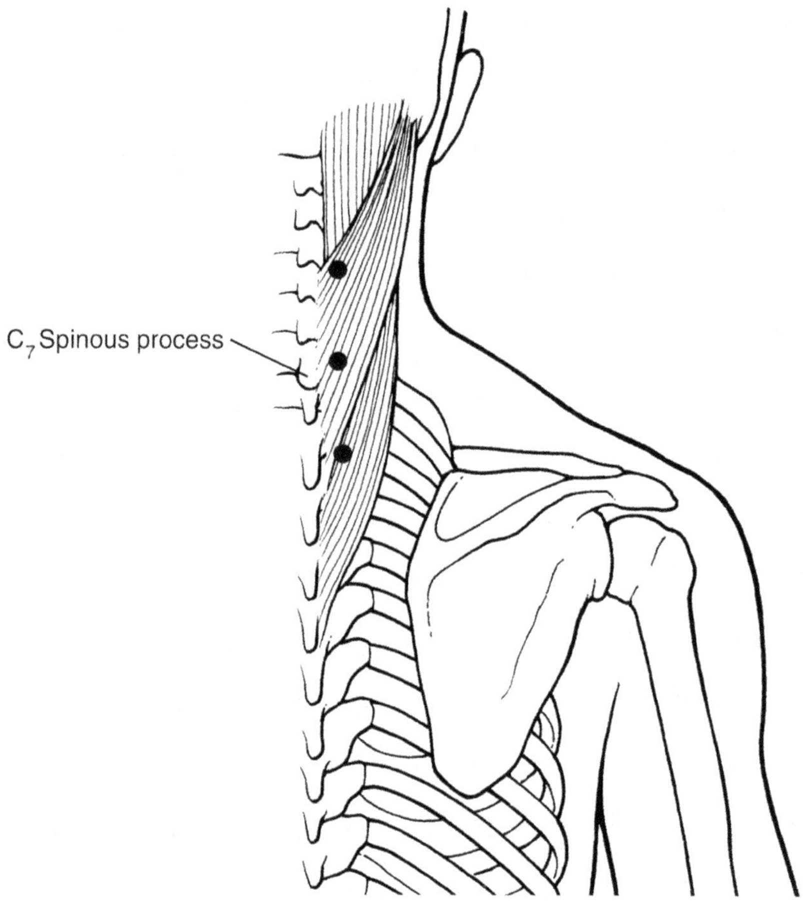

Innervation

Innervation is via the posterior primary rami of the cervical spinal nerves at the respective segmental levels.

Origin

The muscles of the paraspinal region are numerous and situated in superficial to deep layers (*Gray's Anatomy,* 1977). The most superficial muscles include the upper trapezius, levator scapulae, and rhomboids; the splenius capitis and erector spinae (longissimus dorsi, transversalis colli, spinalis colli) are intermediate in depth. The deeper muscles include the multifidus, supraspinales, interspinales, rectus capitis, and obliquus capitis, which lie deep against the vertebrae. The close proximity and overlap of the intermediate and deeper muscles makes it impossible to isolate them individually by needle examination. In general, however, the deeper muscles are shorter and receive a more discrete nerve supply from the corresponding posterior rami, whereas the more intermediate muscles are longer and receive a more overlapping nerve supply.

Insertion

It is not possible to describe all of the attachments of the muscles of the paraspinal region.

Patient Position

To achieve complete relaxation, the patient lies in the prone position with pillows underneath the chest and the forehead resting against the examining table. If full relaxation cannot be obtained, ask the patient to gently press the forehead against the table (this will cause reciprocal inhibition of the cervical paraspinal muscles). Alternatively, the patient may be in the side-lying fetal position. The examiner can apply gentle pressure against the patient's forehead to evoke reciprocal inhibition.

Activation Maneuver

Ask the patient to extend the head.

EMG Needle Insertion

Identify the C_7 spinous process (the most prominent process), and count the remaining spinous processes to determine the level of the spine to be examined. Insert the needle perpendicular to the skin, or slightly upward, about 2 cm lateral to the spinous process of the desired level. The needle should encounter the lamina of the vertebra to assess the deep muscles.

Pitfalls

If the needle is too superficial, it may be in the trapezius, levator scapulae, or rhomboids.

In about 20% of thin subjects, lung tissue extends above the clavicle with a distance from skin surface to lung tissue of about 3.3 cm (Honet et al., 1986). Rarely, pneumothorax can occur following needle examination of paraspinal muscles. One can minimize the risk of pneumothorax by inserting the needle close to the midline, particularly when studying the lower cervical or thoracic paraspinal muscles.

Rarely, paraspinal muscle hematoma may occur after needle examination. Caution is warranted when performing electromyography of paraspinal and other deeper muscles in anticoagulated patients (Caress et al., 1996).

The innervation to the cervical paraspinal muscles may extend one or two segments below a particular level. This anatomical variability makes it difficult to determine the precise localization in cases of radiculopathy.

Clinical Comments

Documentation of EMG abnormalities in paraspinal muscles suggests axonal loss affecting the spinal nerve proximal to its bifurcation into the posterior and anterior rami (i.e., at the root level).

In the early stages of radiculopathy, within 1–2 weeks of onset, EMG abnormalities may be limited to paraspinal muscles (Kimura, 1989). Hence, EMG of paraspinal muscles is crucial in the evaluation of cervical radiculopathy.

Some systemic conditions, most notably inflammatory myopathies (e.g., polymyositis), may affect the paraspinal muscles preferentially and sometimes exclusively (Streib et al., 1979; Petrella et al., 1997).

Thoracic Paraspinal

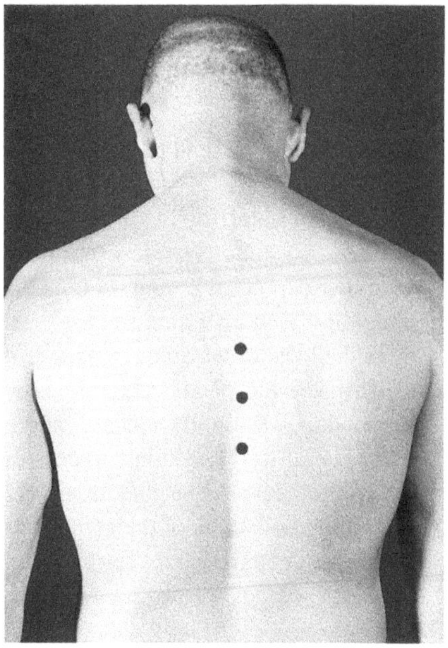

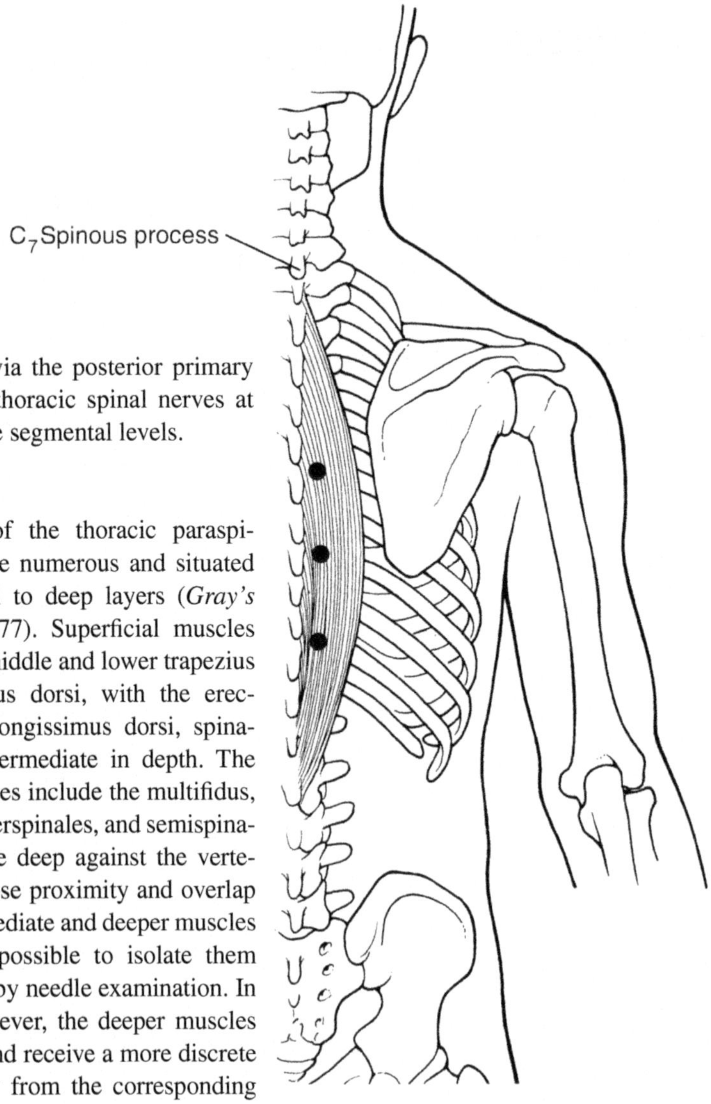

Innervation

Innervation is via the posterior primary rami of the thoracic spinal nerves at the respective segmental levels.

Origin

The muscles of the thoracic paraspinal region are numerous and situated in superficial to deep layers (*Gray's Anatomy,* 1977). Superficial muscles include the middle and lower trapezius and latissimus dorsi, with the erector spinae (longissimus dorsi, spinalis dorsi) intermediate in depth. The deeper muscles include the multifidus, rotatores, interspinales, and semispinales, which lie deep against the vertebrae. The close proximity and overlap of the intermediate and deeper muscles makes it impossible to isolate them individually by needle examination. In general, however, the deeper muscles are shorter and receive a more discrete nerve supply from the corresponding posterior rami, whereas the more intermediate muscles are longer and receive a more overlapping nerve supply.

Insertion

It is not possible to describe all of the attachments of the muscles of the paraspinal region.

Patient Position

The patient lies in the prone position with pillows underneath the chest, and the forehead resting against the examining table. Alternatively, the patient may be flat or in the side-lying fetal position.

Activation Maneuver

Ask the patient to gently arch the back.

EMG Needle Insertion

Identify the C_7 spinous process (the most prominent process), and count down the remaining spinous processes to determine the level of the spine to be examined. Insert the needle perpendicular to the skin, about 2 cm lateral to the spinous process of the desired level. The needle should encounter the lamina of the vertebra to assess the deep muscles.

Pitfalls

If the needle is too superficial, it may be in the trapezius or latissimus dorsi.

Rarely, pneumothorax can occur following needle examination of paraspinal muscles (Honet et al., 1986). One can minimize the risk of pneumothorax by inserting the needle close to the midline.

Clinical Comments

Documentation of EMG abnormalities in thoracic paraspinal muscles suggests axonal loss affecting the spinal nerve proximal to its bifurcation into posterior and anterior rami (i.e., at the root level).

Some systemic conditions, most notably inflammatory myopathies (e.g., polymyositis), may affect the paraspinal muscles preferentially and sometimes exclusively (Streib et al., 1979; Petrella et al., 1997).

Lumbosacral Paraspinal

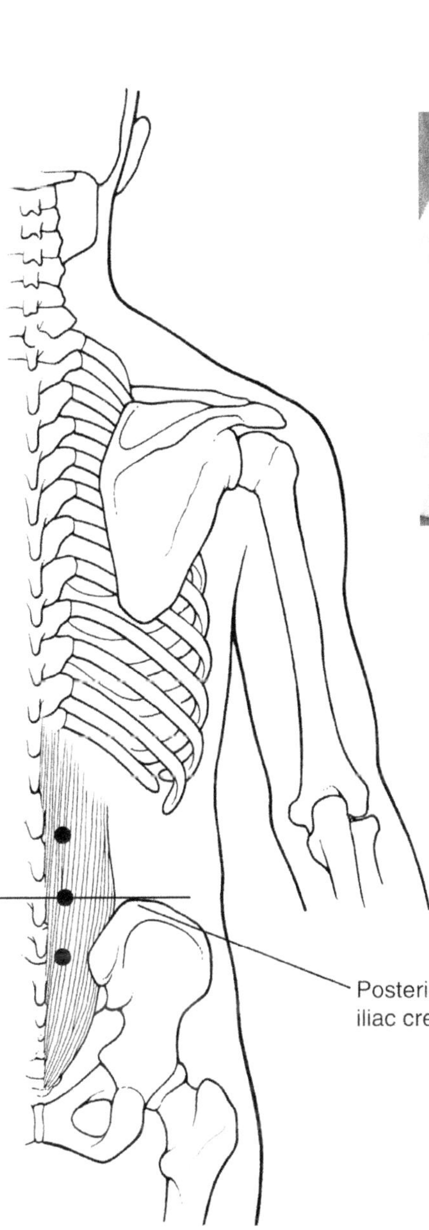

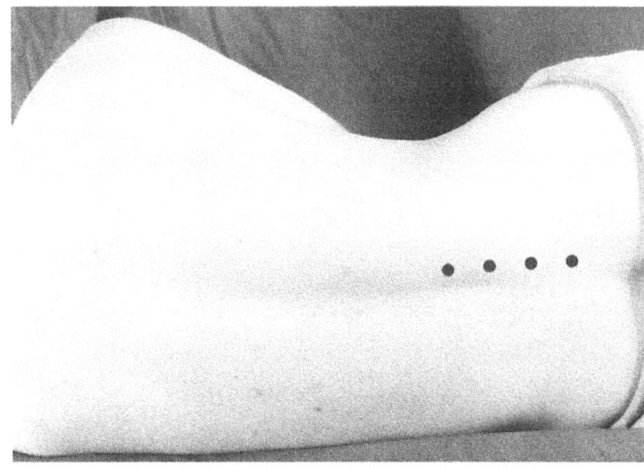

Innervation

Innervation is via the posterior primary rami of the lumbar and sacral spinal nerves at the respective levels.

Origin

The muscles of the paraspinal region are numerous and situated in superficial to deep layers (*Gray's Anatomy,* 1977). Superficial muscles include the latissimus dorsi; the erector spinae (longissimus dorsi, spinalis dorsi) are intermediate in depth. The deeper muscles include the multifidus and interspinales, which lie deep against the vertebrae. The close proximity and overlap of these muscles makes it impossible to isolate them individually by needle examination. In general, however, the deeper muscles are shorter and receive a more discrete nerve supply from the corresponding posterior rami, whereas the more superficial muscles are longer and receive a more overlapping nerve supply.

Insertion

It is not possible to describe all of the attachments of the muscles of the paraspinal region.

Patient Position

The patient lies in the prone position with pillows placed underneath the abdomen. Alternatively, the patient may be in the side-lying fetal position. In the latter position, the muscles on the side farthest from the table are generally relaxed.

Activation Maneuver

For the prone position, ask the patient to elevate the whole leg (perform hip extension). For the side-lying fetal position, ask the patient to perform hip extension against resistance by the examiner.

EMG Needle Insertion

Draw an imaginary line connecting the posterior superior iliac crests. This line intersects the lumbar spine at the L_3–L_4 intervertebral level. Count up or down the spinous processes to determine the paraspinal level to be examined. Insert the needle perpendicular to the skin, about 2 cm lateral to the spinous process of the desired level. The needle should encounter the lamina of the vertebra to assess the deep muscles.

Pitfalls

If the needle is too superficial, it may be in the latissimus dorsi.

To facilitate relaxation of these muscles, instruct the patient to push the small of the back against the examiner's hand.

The amount of lumbar paraspinal muscle denervation in asymptomatic older adults increases with age (Tong et al., 2005). However, the denervation seen in asymptomatic subjects is typically subtle and sparsely distributed (Haig, 2002). In contrast, paraspinal muscle denervation associated with radiculopathy, spondylosis, and other focal structural abnormalities of the spine is usually more localized and more pronounced (i.e., look for a "pocket" of focal denervation).

Clinical Comments

Documentation of focal EMG abnormalities in lumbosacral paraspinal muscles suggests axonal loss affecting the spinal nerve proximal to its bifurcation into the posterior and anterior rami (i.e., at the root level).

Some systemic conditions, most notably inflammatory myopathies (e.g., polymyositis), may affect the paraspinal muscles preferentially and sometimes exclusively (Streib et al., 1979; Petrella et al., 1997).

CRANIAL NERVES AND MUSCLES

28

CONDUCTION STUDIES OF CRANIAL NERVES XI (spinal accessory), VII (facial) and V (trigeminal) are routinely performed in an electrodiagnostic laboratory. Motor nuclei of cranial nerves XI, VII, V, and XII (hypoglossal) supply the muscles of the head and neck that are most commonly tested during needle electromyography (EMG).

Spinal accessory nerve. This nerve is composed of cranial and spinal portions. The smaller cranial portion arises from cells in the nucleus ambiguous and ultimately joins the vagus nerve to innervate laryngeal and pharyngeal muscles. The larger spinal portion originates from a long column of spinal motor neurons situated in the first five cervical segments. The spinal fibers ascend within the spinal canal to enter the cranial cavity through the foramen magnum, and then join with the cranial portion of XI and the vagus nerve to exit the skull through the jugular foramen. The spinal accessory nerve descends into the posterior triangle of the neck (an area bounded by the posterior border of the sternocleidomastoid muscle, the upper trapezius muscle, and the clavicle), passing deep to the upper portion of the sternocleidomastoid and innervating this muscle. At the midpoint of the sternocleidomastoid, the nerve is superficial and just posterior to the posterior border of the sternocleidomastoid. At this level, it is easily accessible to surface stimulation. The spinal accessory nerve continues distally to supply the trapezius muscle. Lesions of the spinal accessory nerve are often iatrogenic, due to surgical procedures in the posterior cervical triangle, most commonly lymph node biopsy or tumor excision. This type of injury affects the trapezius but spares the sternocleidomastoid. Neuralgic amyotrophy (Parsonage-Turner syndrome) may preferentially or selectively involve the spinal accessory nerve. Other causes of spinal accessory neuropathy include face lift surgery, carotid endarterectomy, penetrating wounds, traction injury, compression from shoulder straps, weight lifting, and tumors or aneurysms near the jugular foramen.

Facial nerve. In the caudal pons, the facial motor nucleus gives rise to the efferent fibers that form the facial nerve. This nerve supplies the muscles of facial expression, stapedius, platysma, posterior belly of the digastric, and the stylohyoid (*Gray's Anatomy,* 1977) The intrapontine portion of the facial nerve initially projects posteriorly to loop around the sixth nerve (abducens) nucleus. The long intrapontine course makes it vulnerable to various brainstem lesions, which cause a peripheral rather than central type of facial palsy. The facial nerve emerges from the brainstem near the caudal border of the pons, at the cerebellopontine angle. At this site, the nerve is prone to injury by acoustic neuromas or other cerebellopontine angle masses. After traversing the subarachnoid space, the facial nerve enters the internal auditory meatus. Here it begins the long and complex intraosseous course through the petrous portion of the temporal bone (facial canal). Within this segment lies the presumed site of the lesion in Bell's palsy. The facial nerve then exits the skull at the stylomastoid foramen and courses anteriorly to penetrate the superficial and deep lobes of the parotid gland. At this site, the nerve is vulnerable to injury by parotid tumors and blunt trauma. Other etiologies of facial nerve dysfunction include meningitis, borreliosis, tuberculosis, herpes zoster, AIDS, and sarcoidosis. A lesion involving facial motor neurons or fibers of the facial nerve within the brainstem or in their peripheral course produces paralysis of the muscles of facial expression. It may also produce hyperacusis due to paralysis of the stapedius muscle, which functions to dampen oscillations of the ear ossicles. Loss of taste sensation over the anterior two-thirds of the tongue occurs due to involvement of the chorda tympani branch of the facial nerve. Lacrimation and submandibular and sublingual salivary gland secretion are also impaired on the side of the lesion due to destruction of parasympathetic fibers. The particular deficit that results depends on the exact location of the lesion and its severity (for a review see Carpenter, 1976). In clinical practice, facial motor nerve conduction studies, blink reflex studies, and EMG of facial muscles are most commonly performed in patients with suspected Bell's palsy or in those with traumatic injury to the facial nerve.

Trigeminal nerve. In the mid-pons, the main sensory nucleus of the trigeminal nerve receives afferent impulses from the ophthalmic division of the trigeminal nerve that are relayed via an oligosynaptic arc to the facial motor nucleus. This reflex arc gives rise to the R1 component of the blink reflex. In the pons and medulla, afferent impulses are conducted through the descending spinal tract of the trigeminal nerve before they reach the caudal spinal trigeminal nucleus. Impulses are then relayed via medullary pathways that ascend bilaterally to reflexly activate the facial nuclei in the pons (Aramideh et al., 1997). This gives rise to the bilateral R2 components of the blink reflex. In practice, blink reflex studies are commonly performed in patients with suspected trigeminal nerve lesions, Bell's palsy, or in those with traumatic injury to the facial nerve. The motor nucleus of the trigeminal nerve, located in the mid-pons, gives rise to the efferent fibers that innervate the muscles of mastication (masseter, temporalis, and pterygoids), mylohyoid, anterior belly of the digastric, and the tensor tympani and tensor veli palatini. The motor fibers emerge from the brainstem near the lateral border of the pons and exit the skull through the foramen ovale. Together with the corresponding sensory fibers, they form the mandibular division of the trigeminal nerve, which is distributed to the above-mentioned muscles. Needle EMG of the muscles of mastication is most commonly performed in patients with suspected trigeminal nerve injury. Injury to the trigeminal nerve occurs with trauma (gun shot or stab wounds), surgery, infections (meningitis, borreliosis, tuberculosis, herpes zoster, and AIDS), sarcoidosis, acoustic neuromas, invasive tumors of the head and neck, and aneurysms. Clinical features of a trigeminal nerve lesion include numbness or loss of sensation over the face and weakness of closing the jaw.

Hypoglossal nerve. This motor nerve supplies the complex musculature of the tongue. The neuronal cell bodies that give rise to the nerve are found in the dorsal medulla in the hypoglossal nucleus. The nerve exits the cranium via the hypoglossal canal at the base of the skull. Injury to the hypoglossal nerve occurs with fractures of the base of the skull, tumors of the skull base, and aneurysms of the carotid artery. Hypoglossal nerve injury produces a lower motor neuron paralysis of the ipsilateral half of the tongue. Clinical signs include loss of movement, loss of tone, atrophy of muscle, and involuntary muscle twitches (i.e., fasciculations). Since the major muscle of the tongue, the genioglossus, controls protrusion of the tongue, a unilateral hypoglossal nerve injury will cause the protruded tongue to deviate to the side of the lesion. In practice, EMG of tongue muscles is often performed in patients with suspected motor neuron disease (amyotrophic lateral sclerosis).

Spinal Accessory Nerve Conduction Study

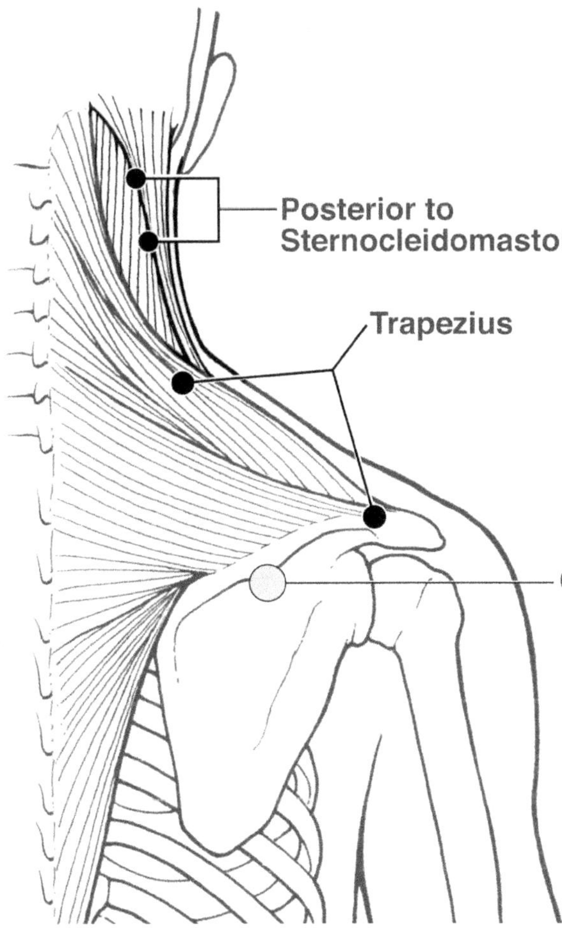

FIGURE 28-1 Spinal accessory nerve conduction study.

Recording

Active electrode: Position over the upper fibers of trapezius, just distal to the angle of the neck and shoulder.

Reference electrode: Place over the acromion process at the shoulder joint.

Ground electrode: Place over the upper scapular region.

Stimulation

Neck: Place the cathode just posterior to the posterior border of the sternocleidomastoid, midway between the mastoid process and the clavicle. At this level, the nerve is easily accessible to surface stimulation. The anode is 3 cm superior to the cathode.

Normal Values

Distal latency (ms): 2.0 to 3.0 ms (depending on distance between cathode and recording electrode).

Amplitude (mV): Spinal accessory motor conduction studies should always be performed bilaterally. An amplitude ≤ 50 % of the unaffected side is evidence of axonal degeneration (Kimura, 1989).

Comments

In a spinal accessory neuropathy, motor conduction studies of the spinal accessory nerve will be abnormal. On needle EMG examination, the trapezius may demonstrate denervation or neurogenic changes. The sternocleidomastoid may also demonstrate denervation or neurogenic changes, depending on the location of the lesion.

The spinal accessory nerve may be used as a proximal nerve in repetitive stimulation studies to look for a defect in neuromuscular transmission. Patients with myasthenia gravis may demonstrate a decrement on repetitive stimulation studies of the spinal accessory nerve, despite normal repetitive stimulation studies in distal nerves of the limbs (e.g., median or ulnar nerves in the hand). The setup for repetitive stimulation studies of the spinal accessory nerve is identical to the routine spinal accessory motor conduction study, although repetitive stimulation (5 stimuli at 3 Hz) is delivered instead of single shocks. Exercise is performed by instructing the patient to shrug or elevate the shoulder for 10-second, and the train of stimuli are repeated immediately after exercise to look for repair of the decrement (post-tetanic repair). Repetitive stimulation studies are then repeated at 1, 2, 3, and 4 minutes after one minute of sustained maximum voluntary contraction (e.g., sustained elevation of the shoulder), because some patients with myasthenia gravis may only demonstrate a significant decrement (greater than 10%) several minutes after sustained exercise.

Facial Motor Nerve Conduction Study

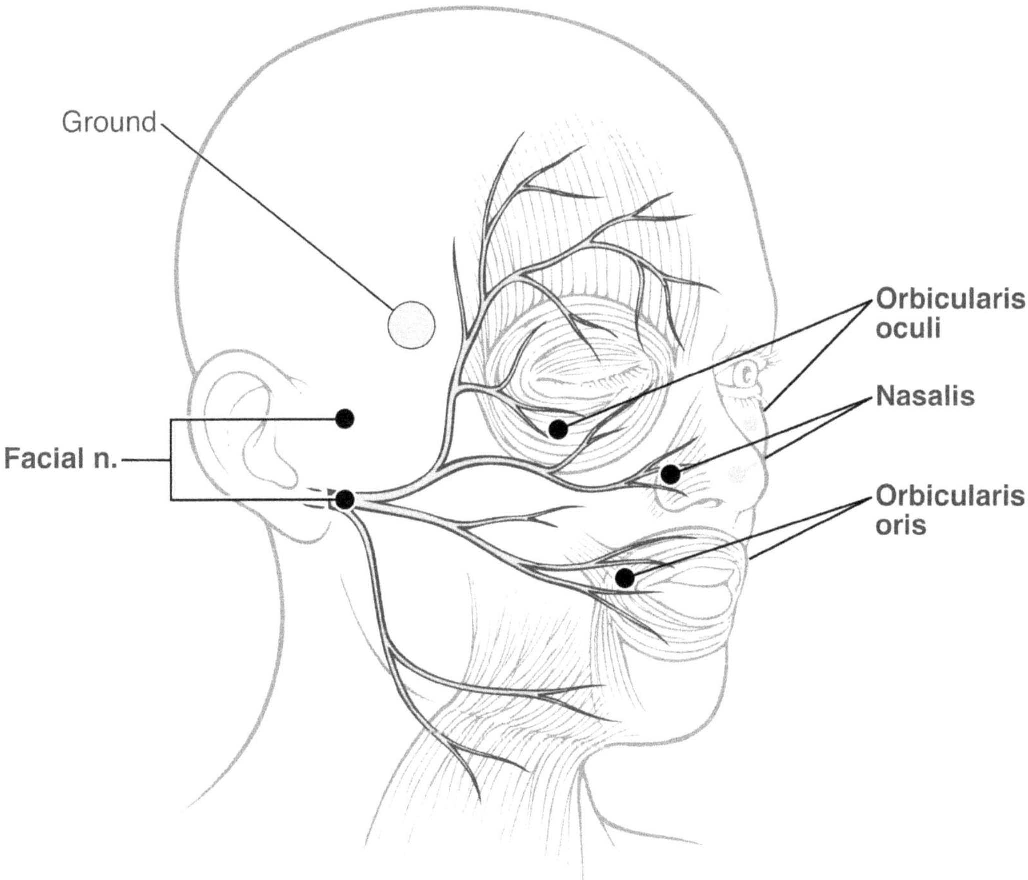

FIGURE 28-2 Facial motor nerve conduction study.

Recording

Active electrode: Position over the nasalis, orbicularis oculi, or orbicularis oris muscle. Reference electrode: Place over the same muscle on the opposite side.

Ground electrode: Place on the face, forehead, or chin.

Use a sweep speed of between 2 to 5 ms/division and a gain of 500 μV to 1 mV to maximally visualize the motor response.

Stimulation

Facial nerve: Place the cathode just below the ear in front of the ear lobe (this is anterior to where the facial nerve emerges from the stylomastoid foramen). The anode is 3 cm above the cathode.

Normal Values

Distal latency (ms): 3.4 ± 0.8 ms (mean ± 1 standard deviation, Kimura, 1989).
Amplitude (mV) ≥ 1.0 (usually 2 to 3 mV)

Facial motor conduction studies should be performed bilaterally. Once facial motor studies on one side are completed, change the stimulator to the other side while switching the active and reference electrodes. An amplitude ≤ 50 % of the unaffected side is evidence of axonal degeneration (Kimura, 1989).

Comments

The facial motor response is often designated as the *direct* response, to distinguish it from the reflex activation of facial muscles elicited by stimulation of the trigeminal nerve (blink reflex).

After complete section of the facial nerve at a proximal site, distal excitability may remain normal for up to 4 days before being lost due to Wallerian degeneration. Accordingly, a relatively preserved direct response one week after onset of symptoms suggests a favorable prognosis for recovery of function (Kimura, 1989).

The facial motor conduction study is most useful in assessing patients with Bell's palsy (seventh cranial neuropathy). Most patients referred to the EMG laboratory for facial palsy are sent to determine a prognosis for recovery of function (Gilchrist, 1993). The prognosis is directly related to the degree of axonal loss (axonopathy): the more severe the axonal loss, the worse the prognosis. The facial motor response is very useful in making this determination, provided that conduction studies are performed after Wallerian degeneration has occurred (seven or more days after onset of symptoms). One scheme for determining prognosis for recovery of function in Bell's palsy or other seventh cranial neuropathy is provided below:

- When the CMAP is absent or markedly reduced in amplitude (<10% of the unaffected side), prognosis for recovery of function will be *poor* with no recovery or delayed incomplete recovery (6 to 12 months), often characterized by visible synkinesis of facial muscles due to aberrant reinnervation (misdirected regrowth of nerve fibers).
- When CMAP amplitude is moderately reduced (20% to 40% of the unaffected side), prognosis for recovery of function will be *fair* or even favorable, although it will depend on reinnervation and regeneration, which may be slow (over several months) and incomplete, with possible residual synkinesis.
- When CMAP amplitude is mildly reduced (~50% of the unaffected side), prognosis for recovery of function will be *good*, with full recovery expected within a few months.
- When CMAP amplitude is preserved (comparable to the unaffected side), the facial palsy is caused by demyelination, and prognosis for recovery of function will be *excellent*, with complete recovery expected within 2 to 6 weeks (as with most neurapraxic injuries).

The facial nerve is commonly used as a proximal nerve in repetitive stimulation studies to look for a defect in neuromuscular transmission. Patients with myasthenia gravis may demonstrate a decrement on repetitive stimulation studies of the facial nerve, despite normal repetitive stimulation studies in distal nerves of the limbs (e.g., median or ulnar nerves in the hand). The setup for repetitive stimulation studies of the facial nerve is identical to the routine facial motor conduction study, although repetitive stimulation (5 stimuli at 3 Hz) is delivered instead of single shocks. Exercise is performed by instructing the patient to perform a brief (10-second) maximum contraction of facial muscle(s), and the train of stimuli are repeated immediately after exercise to look for repair of the decrement (post-tetanic repair). Repetitive stimulation studies are then repeated at 1, 2, 3, and 4 minutes after one minute of sustained maximum voluntary contraction (e.g., tightly closing eyes, wrinkling nose, or puckering lips), because some patients with myasthenia gravis may only demonstrate a significant decrement (greater than 10%) several minutes after sustained exercise.

Blink Reflex Study

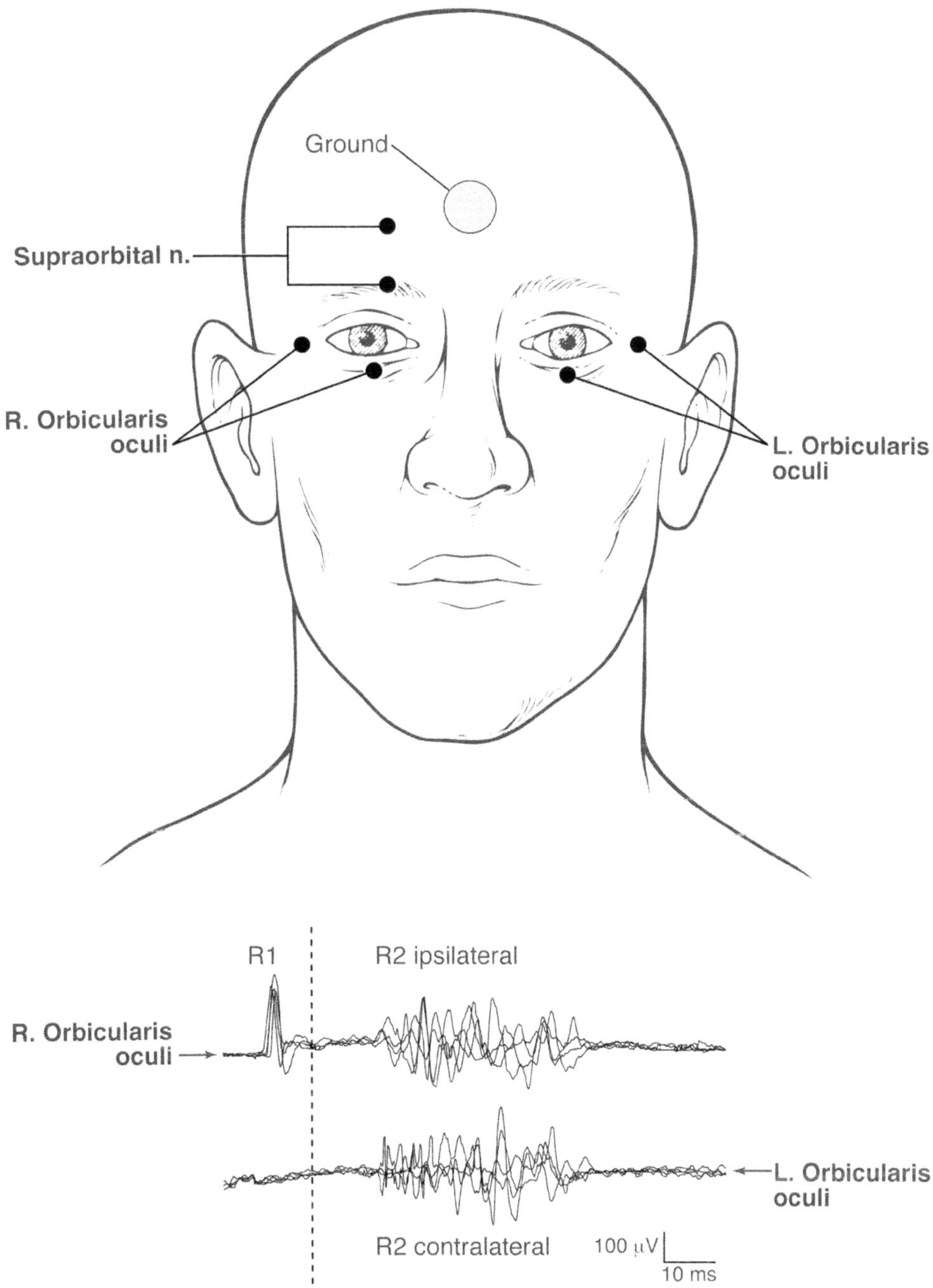

FIGURE 28-3 Blink reflex study.

Recording (2 channels)

Active electrodes: Place on the orbicularis oculi muscles bilaterally, just below the eyes. Reference electrodes: Place over the outer canthus of the eyes bilaterally. Ground electrode: Place on the forehead or the chin.

Use a sweep speed of between 10 ms/division and a gain of 100 to 500 μV to maximally visualize the desired responses.

Stimulation

Supraorbital notch: Place the cathode directly over the supraorbital branch of the trigeminal nerve. The supraorbital notch can be palpated along the medial eyebrow. The anode is on the forehead 3 cm above the cathode.

Stimulus intensities of 10 mA to 20 mA and 0.1 ms duration are usually sufficient to elicit stable blink reflex responses with repeated trials. Once the blink reflex study on one side is completed, the other supraorbital nerve should be stimulated, leaving the recording electrodes unchanged.

Normal Values (Kimura, 1989)

R1 latency (ms): 10.5 ± 0.8 ms (mean ± 1 standard deviation).
Ipsilateral R2 latency (ms): 30.5 ± 3.4 ms
Contralateral R2 latency (ms): 30.5 ± 4.4 ms

Amplitude (mV) is not usually measured, but decreased amplitude of all recordable responses is seen on the side of a seventh cranial nerve lesion.

Comments

The afferent arc of the blink reflex is mediated by sensory fibers in the trigeminal nerve, with the efferent arc mediated by motor fibers of the facial nerve.

A single stimulus to the supraorbital nerve elicits two distinct reflex components in the orbicularis oculi muscle, an R1 response that occurs at a latency of about 10 ms ipsilateral to the side of stimulation, and a second or late R2 response that is bilateral and appears after a latent period of about 30 ms.

The R1 response is a disynaptic reflex between the main sensory nucleus of the trigeminal nerve in the pons and the facial nucleus. Hence, the latency of R1 reflects the conduction time along the trigeminal and facial nerves and pontine relay. Although the R1 response is usually elicited only on the side of stimulation, occasionally a smaller contralateral R1 may be seen.

The R2 response is a polysynaptic reflex with afferent impulses conducted through the descending trigeminal spinal tract in the pons and medulla before reaching the caudal spinal trigeminal nucleus. Impulses are then relayed via medullary pathways that ascend bilaterally to activate facial nuclei in the pons (Aramideh et al,. 1997). Thus, the longer latency of the R2 response reflects the longer distance and polysynaptic connections of trigeminal fibers in the lower brainstem.

Clinically, there is no visible mechanical correlate to the R1 response. In contrast, the R2 responses are associated with eyelid closure.

Clinical Applications

The blink reflex is used to evaluate the function of both the trigeminal and facial nerves, and to provide an assessment of brainstem function, since the pons and medulla contain the central connections that generate the R1 and R2, respectively. Recognition of a particular pattern of blink reflex abnormalities can aid in the localization of a lesion and in establishing pathogenesis (Kimura, 1989; Aramideh et al., 1997).

Pattern of Blink Reflex Abnormalities

1. Efferent lesion: A lesion of the facial nerve (e.g., Bell's palsy) will result in delay or absence of all blink reflex responses (R1 and R2) on the paretic side, regardless of the side of stimulation. The abnormalities will be present during the first week of symptoms, at a time when the direct facial motor study is not useful because Wallerian degeneration is not complete (Kimura, 1989).
2. Afferent lesion: A lesion of the trigeminal nerve will result in delay or absence of the R1 response ipsilaterally and R2 bilaterally with stimulation of the affected side. Stimulation on the unaffected side elicits normal R1 ipsilaterally and R2 bilaterally.

3. Main sensory nucleus: A lesion at this site will result in delay or absence of the R1 response on the affected side, with normal R2 responses bilaterally.
4. Spinal trigeminal nucleus: A lesion at this site will result in a normal R1 response on the affected side, and delay or absence of R2 responses bilaterally with stimulation on the affected side.
5. Medullary uncrossed interneurons: A lesion at this site will result in a normal R1 response on the affected side with a delay or absence of the ipsilateral R2 response. The contralateral R2 response will remain normal if crossed interneurons are unaffected. On the side opposite the lesion, the R1 and R2 responses will be normal.
6. Medullary crossed interneurons: If only crossing fibers from one side are affected, the contralateral R2 response will be delayed or absent, while the ipsilateral R1 and R2 responses are normal.

The blink reflex is performed in a variety of neurological disorders including acoustic neuromas, multiple sclerosis, Guillian-Barré syndrome, other demyelinating neuropathies, and various brainstem lesions. In these disorders, the blink reflex shows various abnormalities (Kimura, 1989).

The blink reflex is often performed in conjunction with direct facial motor study, and is particularly helpful in evaluating facial palsy. However, the blink reflex as a prognostic study has not been particularly helpful (Gilchrist, 1993).

Pitfalls

In about 10% of normal subjects, single stimuli of appropriate intensity may fail to elicit an R1 response. In such cases, instructing the subject to perform minimal voluntary eye closure or to anticipate the next stimulus (e.g., count down to the next shock) will potentiate the R1 response (Leis et al., 1993). Paired stimuli with an interstimulus interval of 3 ms to 5 ms may also facilitate the R1 response (Kimura, 1989).

REFERENCES

Aramideh M, Ongerboer de Visser BW, Koelman JHTM, Majoie CBL, Holstege G. The late blink reflex response abnormality due to lesion of the lateral tegmental field. *Brain* 1997;120:1685–1692.

Gilchrist JM. AAEM case report #26: Seventh cranial neuropathy. *Muscle Nerve* 1993;16:447-452.

Gray's Anatomy. 15th English Edition. Bounty Books/Crown Publishers, New York, 1977, pp. 299–327, 720–756.

Carpenter MB. *Human Neuroanatomy.* 7th edition. Williams & Wilkins Co., Baltimore, 1976, pp. 346–349.

Kimura J. *Electrodiagnosis in Diseases of Nerve and Muscle.* 2nd ed., FA Davis Co., Philadelphia, 1989, pp. 307–331.

Leis AA, Kofler M, Stokic DS, Grubwieser GJ, Delapasse JS. Effect of the inhibitory phenomenon following magnetic stimulation of cortex on brainstem motor neuron excitability and on the cortical control of brainstem reflexes. *Muscle Nerve* 1993;16:1351–1358.

Sternocleidomastoid

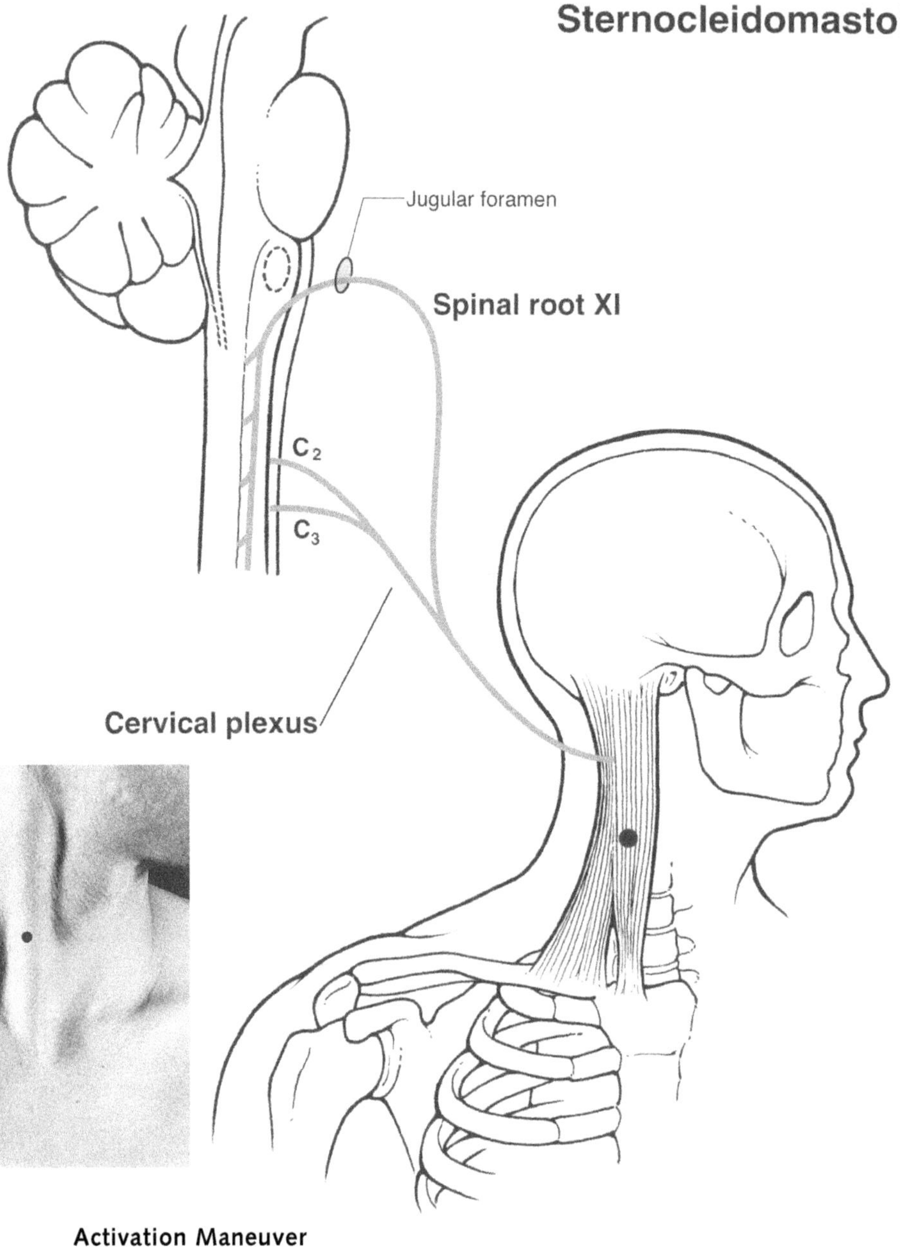

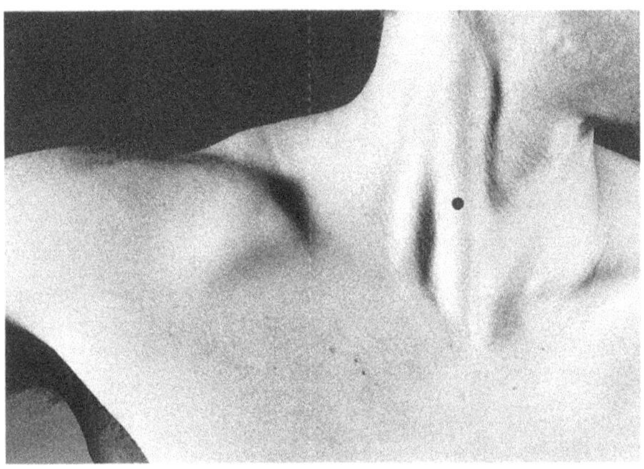

Innervation

Innervation is via the spinal accessory nerve and branches from the C_2, C_3, and sometimes the C_4 cervical spinal nerves (*Gray's Anatomy,* 1995).

Origin

The sternal head arises from the upper part of the manubrium sterni.

The clavicular head arises from the medial third of the clavicle.

Insertion

Insertion is at the lateral surface of the mastoid process.

Activation Maneuver

Rotation of the head (opposite to the muscle studied) activates the muscle.

EMG Needle Insertion

Insert the needle at the midpoint between the mastoid process and the sternal origin. Enter the muscle obliquely, and direct the needle parallel to the muscle fibers.

Pitfalls

If the needle is inserted too medially and anteriorly, it may penetrate the common, internal, or external carotid arteries.

Clinical Comments

Needle examination may show neurogenic changes when injury to the spinal accessory nerve or branches from C_2, C_3, and C_4 produces axonal loss. Note: The spinal accessory nerve may be damaged during lymph node dissection in the posterior triangle of the neck, sparing the sternocleidomastoid but affecting the trapezius (Donner and Kline, 1993).

Cervical dystonia (torticollis) often begins with tonic or clonic spasms of the sternocleidomastoid muscle.

Trapezius

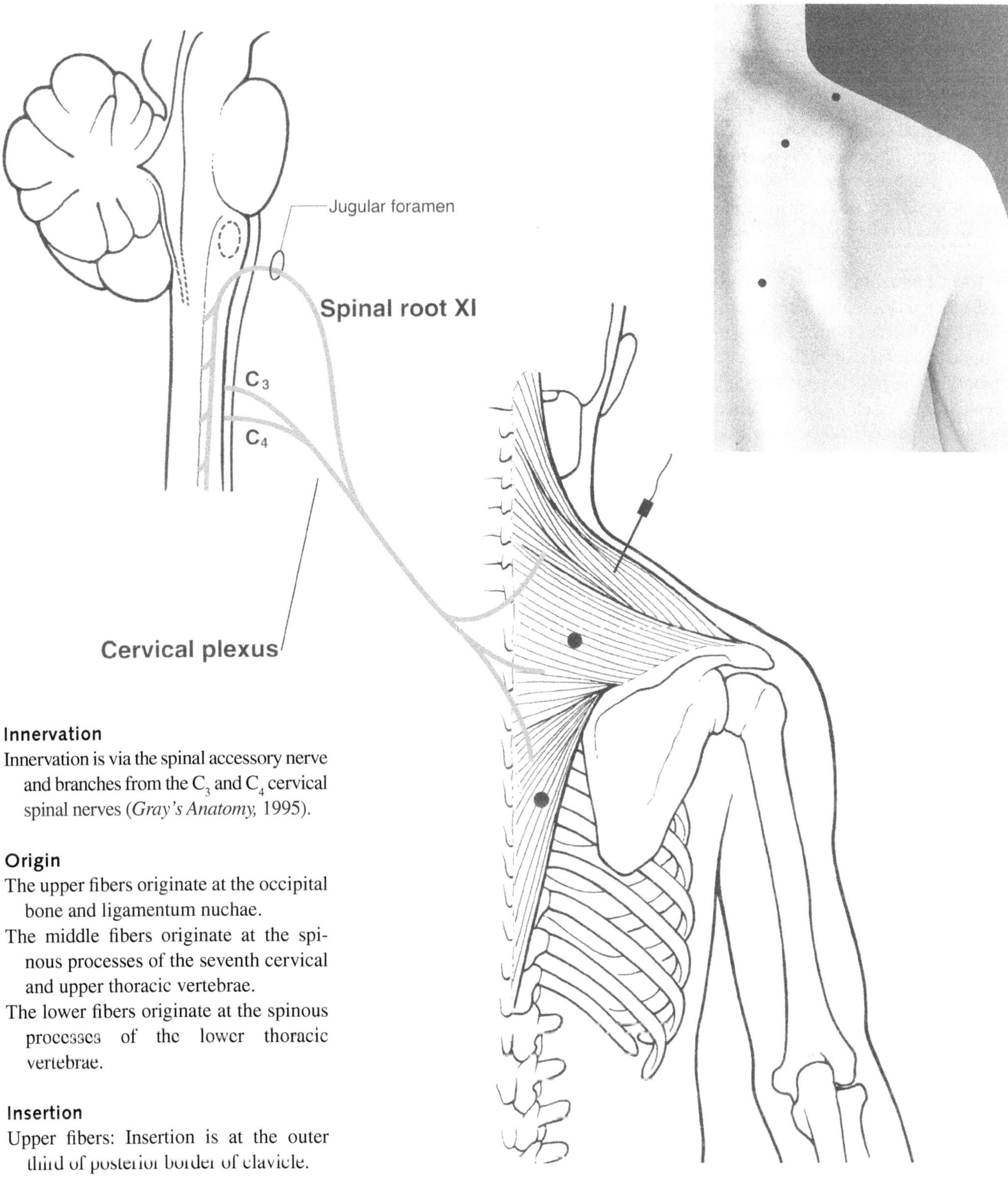

Innervation

Innervation is via the spinal accessory nerve and branches from the C_3 and C_4 cervical spinal nerves (*Gray's Anatomy,* 1995).

Origin

The upper fibers originate at the occipital bone and ligamentum nuchae.

The middle fibers originate at the spinous processes of the seventh cervical and upper thoracic vertebrae.

The lower fibers originate at the spinous processes of the lower thoracic vertebrae.

Insertion

Upper fibers: Insertion is at the outer third of posterior border of clavicle.

Middle fibers: Insertion is at the acromion process and the crest of the spine of the scapula.

Lower fibers: Insertion is at the medial surface of the spine of the scapula.

Activation Maneuver

Upper fibers: Shrug or elevate the shoulder.

Middle fibers: Retract the scapula.

Lower fibers: Rotate the scapula by elevating the arm.

EMG Needle Insertion

Upper fibers: Insert the needle at the angle of the neck and shoulder.

Middle fibers: Insert the needle midway between the spine of the scapula and the spinous processes at the same level.

Lower fibers: Insert the needle 3–4 cm lateral to the spinous processes of the lower thoracic vertebrae.

Pitfalls

Upper fibers: If the needle is inserted too deeply, it may be in the levator scapulae (supplied by the dorsal scapular nerve and C_3, C_4) or other neck muscles.

Middle fibers: If the needle is inserted too deeply, it may be in the rhomboideus major or minor, which are supplied by the dorsal scapular nerve.

Lower fibers: If the needle is inserted too deeply and caudally, it may be in the latissimus dorsi, which is supplied by the thoracodorsal nerve.

Clinical Comments

Needle examination may show neurogenic changes when injury to the spinal accessory nerve or branches from C_3 and C_4 produces axonal loss.

A common etiology of spinal accessory mononeuropathy is iatrogenic injury related to biopsy of cervical lymph nodes in the posterior triangle of the neck or benign tumor removal (Berry et al., 1991; Donner and Kline, 1993). This type of injury affects the trapezius but spares the sternocleidomastoid.

Neuralgic amyotrophy (Parsonage-Turner syndrome) may preferentially or selectively involve the spinal accessory nerve.

The nerve supply to trapezius is superficial in its course and is susceptible to closed traction injury or other direct trauma to the posterior cervical triangle.

Weakness of trapezius produces winging of the scapula (Martin and Fish, 2008), which manifests as lateral and upward displacement of the scapula (the superior angle is more lateral to the midline than the inferior angle). The winging is accentuated during lateral abduction of the arm.

Weakness of trapezius is also associated with drooping of the affected shoulder and an asymmetric shoulder shrug. Consistently, patients are limited in overhead activities on the affected side.

Frontalis

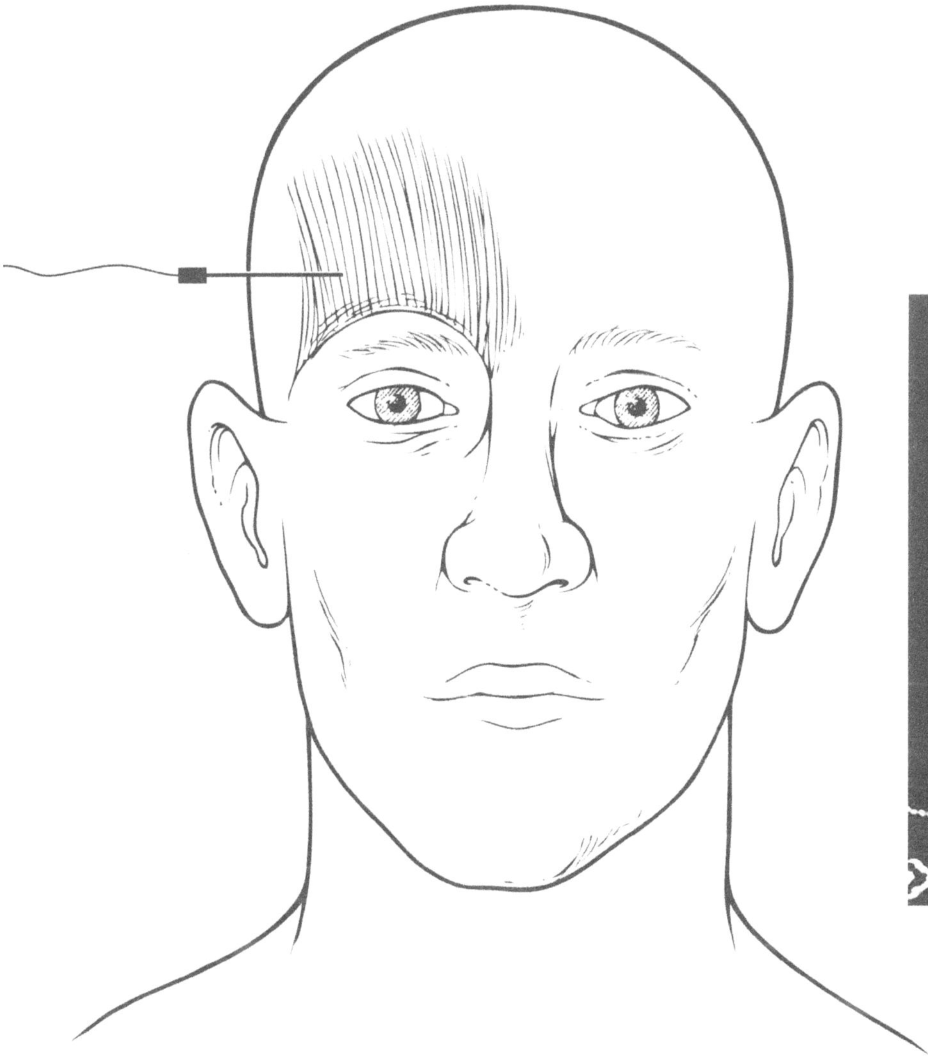

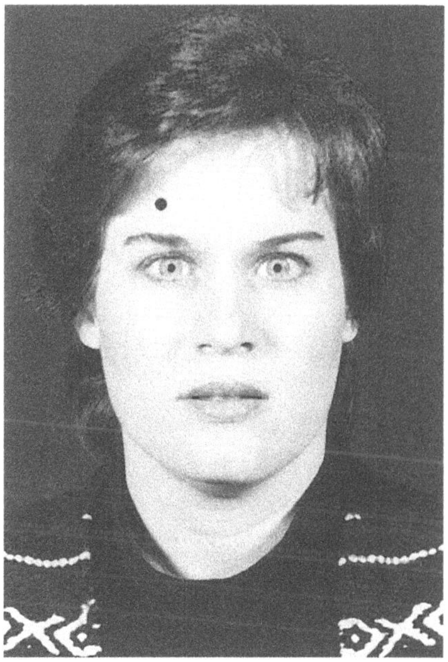

Innervation
Innervation is via cranial nerve VII (facial nerve).

Origin
The frontalis originates at the aponeurosis below the coronal suture.

Insertion
The fibers form a broad, thin, flat layer on the frontal scalp that merges with fibers from the orbicularis oculi and other facial muscles.

Activation Maneuver
Gentle raising of the eyebrows activates the muscle.

EMG Needle Insertion
Insert the needle at a 20- to 30-degree angle with the skin, 2 cm superior to the lateral half of the orbital margin.

Pitfalls
Do not insert the needle perpendicular to the skin. The muscle is very thin, and the needle must remain superficial.

Clinical Comments
Needle examination of facial muscles is usually performed in patients with suspected Bell's palsy or other injury to the facial nerve.

Neurogenic EMG changes (i.e., increased insertional activity, fibrillation potentials, excessive polyphasic motor unit potentials) occur when injury to the facial nerve or facial nucleus produces axonal loss.

In facial nerve disorders associated with profound axonal loss, including severe Bell's palsy, needle examination performed several months later is likely to show aberrant reinnervation (misdirected regrowth of nerve fibers).

Orbicularis Oculi

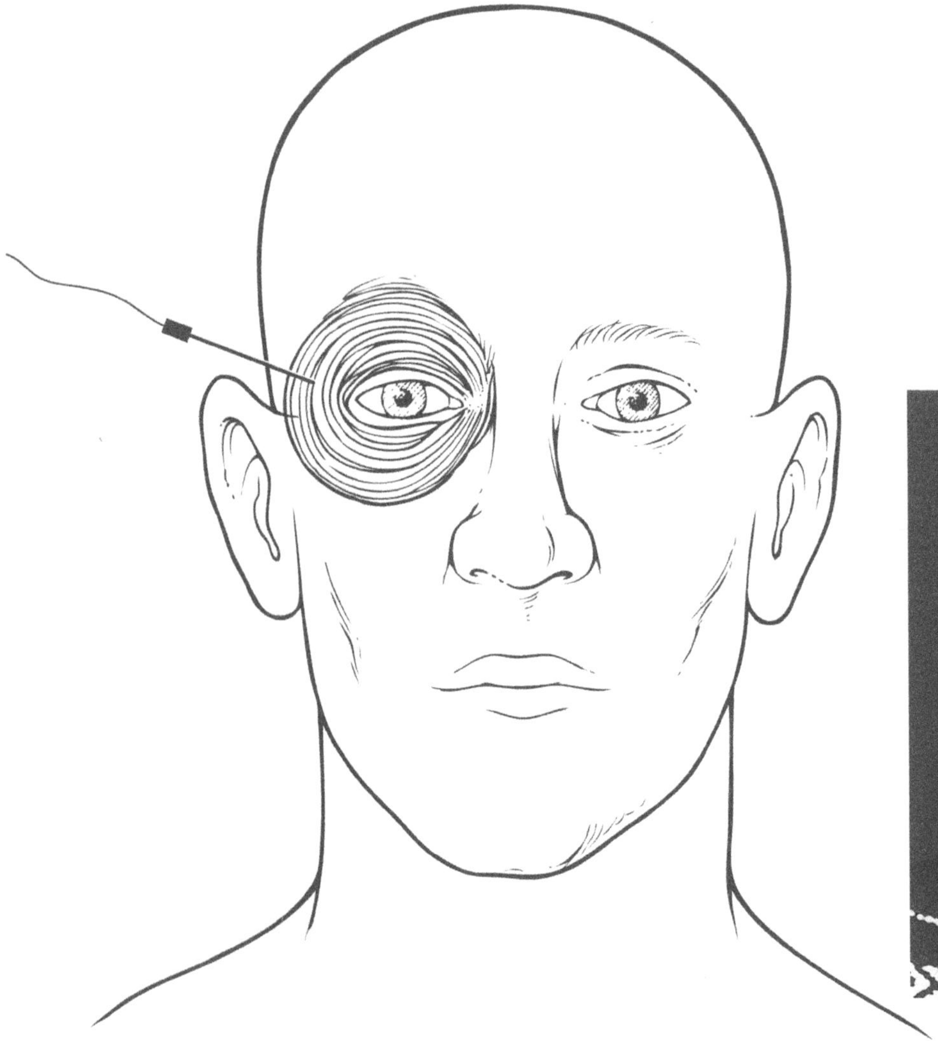

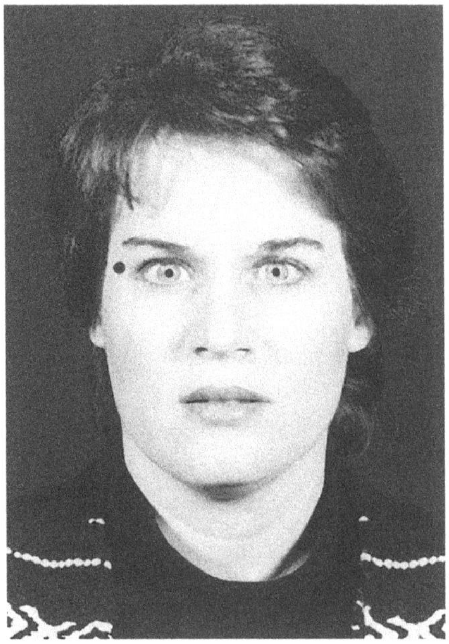

Innervation

Innervation is via cranial nerve VII (facial nerve).

Origin

The orbicularis oculi is a sphincter muscle that surrounds the orbit and eyelids (*Gray's Anatomy,* 1977). It arises from the frontal and maxillary bones.

Insertion

The fibers are directed outward, forming a broad, thin, flat layer that surrounds the orbit and eyelids.

Activation Maneuver

Gentle eye closure or blinking activates the muscle.

EMG Needle Insertion

Insert the needle at a 20- to 30-degree angle with the skin, lateral to the outer wall of the orbit, which is formed by the malar bone.

Pitfalls

Do not insert the needle perpendicular to the skin. The muscle is very thin, and the needle must remain superficial.

Excessive motion of the needle may result in hemorrhage ("black eye").

Clinical Comments

Needle examination of facial muscles is usually performed in patients with suspected Bell's palsy or other injury to the facial nerve.

Neurogenic EMG changes (i.e., increased insertional activity, fibrillation potentials, and excessive polyphasic motor unit potentials) occur when injury to the facial nerve or facial nucleus produces axonal loss.

In facial nerve disorders associated with profound axonal loss, including severe Bell's palsy, needle examination performed several months later is likely to show aberrant reinnervation (misdirected regrowth of nerve fibers).

Orbicularis Oris

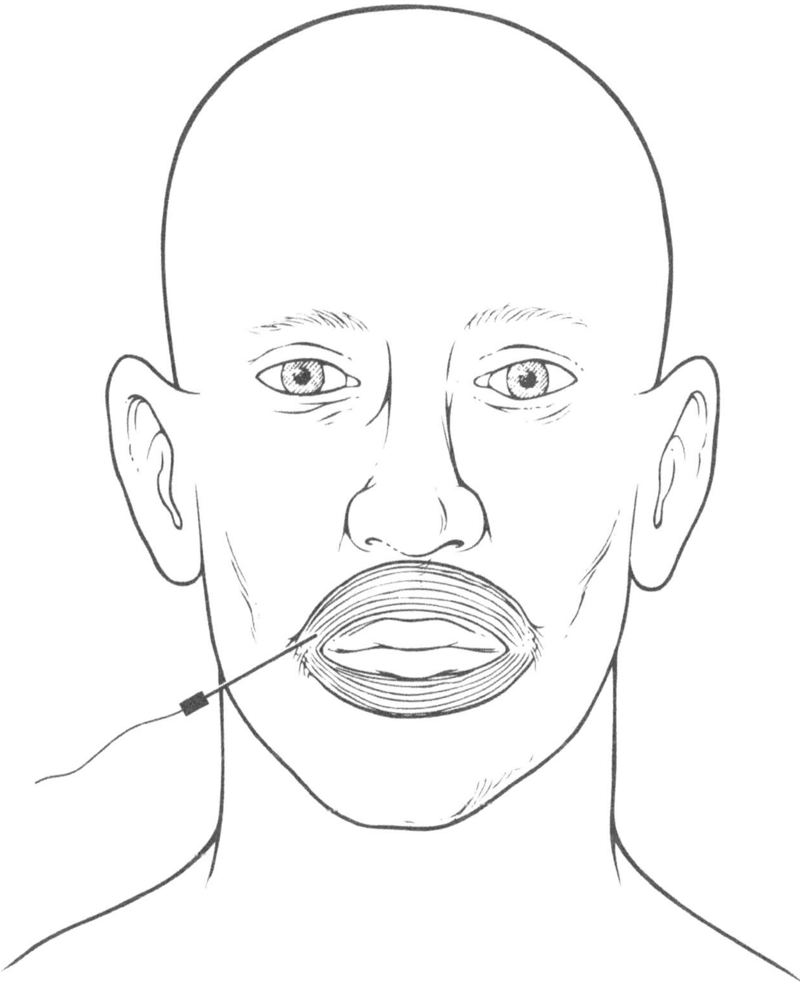

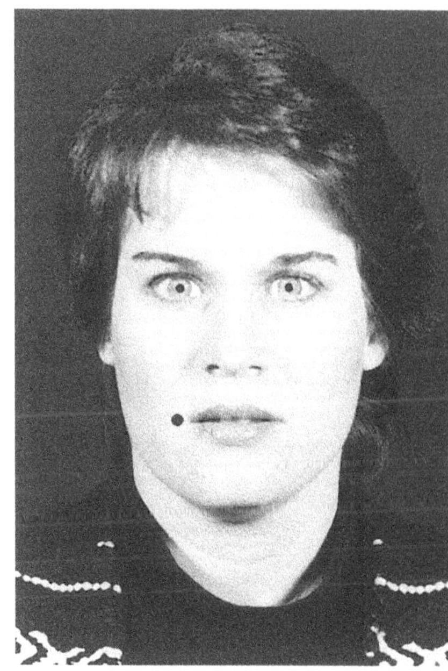

Innervation

Innervation is via cranial nerve VII (facial nerve).

Origin

The orbicularis oris consists of numerous strata of muscular fibers, having different directions, which surround the orifice of the mouth (*Gray's Anatomy*, 1977). These fibers are partially derived from other facial muscles that insert into the lips, and partly from fibers proper to the lips themselves.

Insertion

There is no single point of insertion.

Activation Maneuver

Gentle puckering of the lips activates the muscle.

EMG Needle Insertion

Insert the needle at a 20- to 30-degree angle with the skin, just lateral to the angle of the mouth.

Pitfalls

Do not insert the needle perpendicular to the skin. The muscle is thin, and the needle may penetrate the oral cavity.

Clinical Comments

Needle examination of facial muscles is usually performed in patients with suspected Bell's palsy or other injury to the facial nerve.

Neurogenic EMG changes (i.e., increased insertional activity, fibrillation potentials, and excessive polyphasic motor unit potentials) occur when injury to the facial nerve or nucleus produces axonal loss.

In facial nerve disorders associated with profound axonal loss, including severe Bell's palsy, needle examination performed several months later is likely to show aberrant reinnervation (misdirected regrowth of nerve fibers).

Masseter

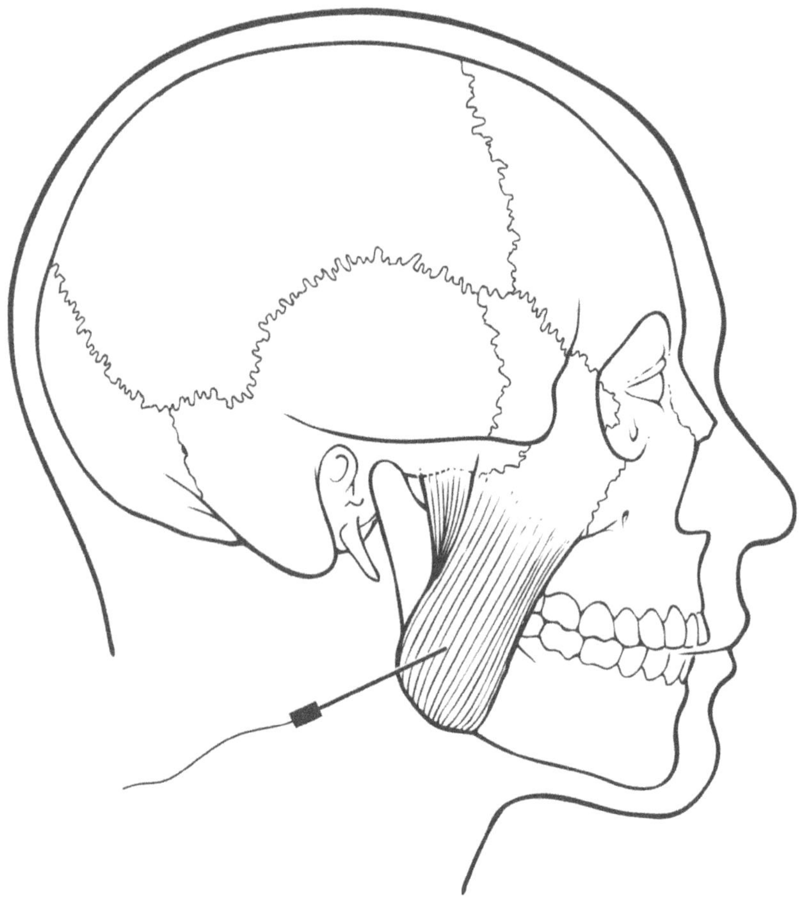

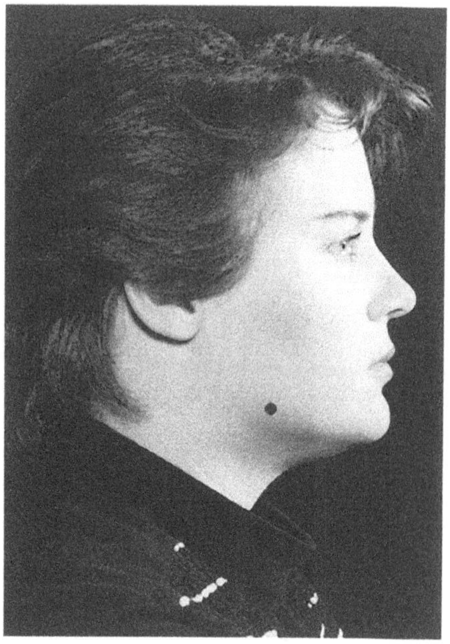

Innervation
Innervation is via the motor nucleus of cranial nerve V (trigeminal nerve).

Origin
The masseter originates from the malar process of the superior maxilla and the lower border of the zygomatic arch (*Gray's Anatomy*, 1977).

Insertion
Insertion is into the angle of the jaw, outer surface of the ramus, and coronoid process of the jaw.

Activation Maneuver
Jaw closure activates the muscle.

EMG Needle Insertion
Insert the needle 2–3 cm distal to the angle of the jaw and 2 cm cephalad to the lower edge of the mandible (the muscle belly is easily palpated when the patient clenches the teeth).

Pitfalls
If the needle is inserted too posteriorly, it may penetrate the parotid gland or duct that overlaps the posterior margin of the muscle.

If the needle is inserted too anteriorly, it may penetrate the buccinator muscle (supplied by the facial nerve) that lies beneath the anterior margin of the masseter muscle.

Clinical Comments
Needle examination of the masseter muscle is usually performed in patients with suspected injury to the trigeminal nerve.

Neurogenic EMG changes (increased insertional activity, fibrillation potentials, and excessive polyphasic motor unit potentials) occur when injury to the trigeminal nerve or motor nucleus produces axonal loss.

Tongue

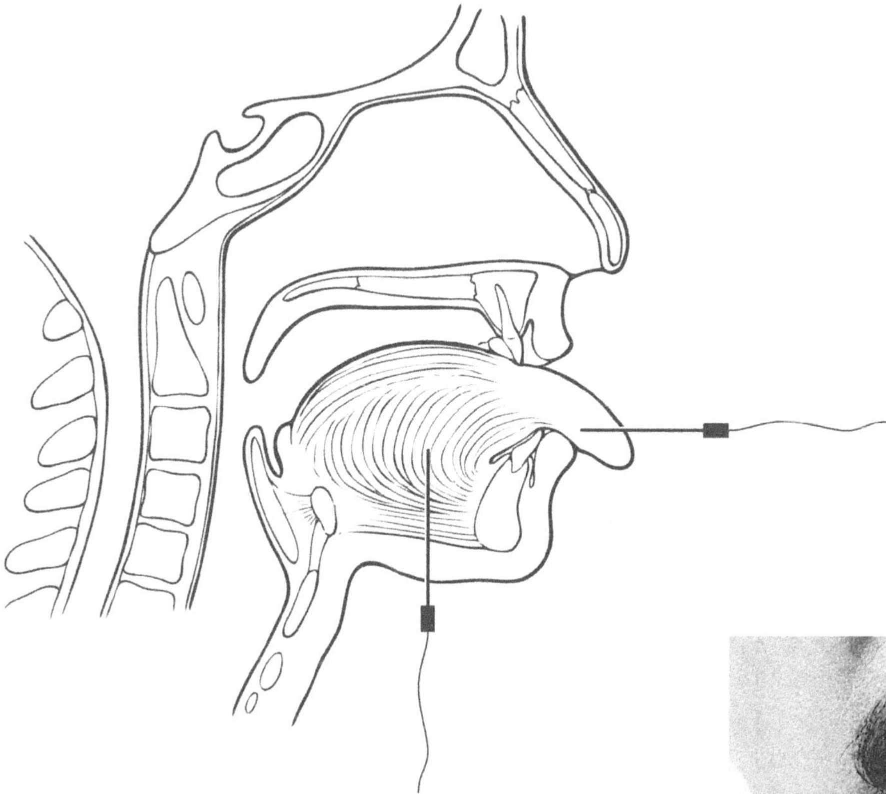

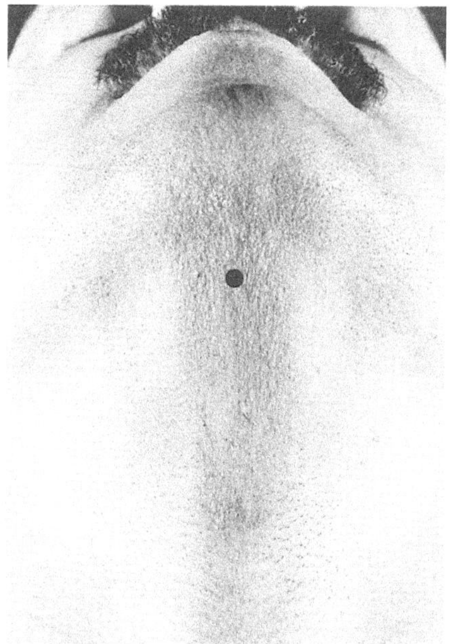

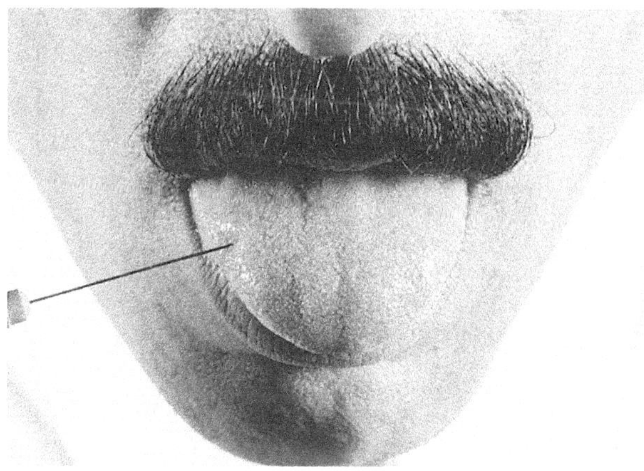

Innervation

Innervation is via cranial nerve XII (hypoglossal).

Origin

The tongue is composed of muscular fibers from multiple muscles arranged in various directions (*Gray's Anatomy*, 1977). This complex arrangement of the muscular fibers, and the various directions in which they run, give the tongue the ability to assume the various forms necessary for enunciating the different consonantal sounds.

The major muscle of the tongue, the *genioglossus*, arises from the superior genial tubercle on the inner side of the symphysis of the jaw.

Insertion

The genioglossus muscle spreads out in a fan-like form. The inferior fibers attach to the body of the hyoid bone, and the middle and superior fibers pass backward, upward, and then forward to enter the whole length of the undersurface of the tongue.

Activation Maneuver

Gentle protrusion of the tongue activates the muscle. Deviation away from the needle generates muscle activity.

EMG Needle Insertion

Insert the needle into the midline undersurface of the mandible 2–3 cm posterior to the tip of the chin. The needle may be angled to study the right or left genioglossus muscle.

Alternatively, the examiner can grasp the tongue with a gauze pad and insert the needle into the inferolateral portion of the tongue. To study spontaneous activity, ask the patient to gently retract the tongue so that it lies on the floor of the oral cavity.

Pitfalls

This study requires patient cooperation.

Clinical Comments

Needle examination of the tongue is often performed in patients with suspected amyotrophic lateral sclerosis.

Neurogenic changes (increased insertional activity, fibrillation potentials, and excessive polyphasic motor unit potentials) occur when injury to the hypoglossal nerve or nucleus produces axonal loss.

29 DERMATOMES AND PERIPHERAL NERVE CUTANEOUS DISTRIBUTIONS

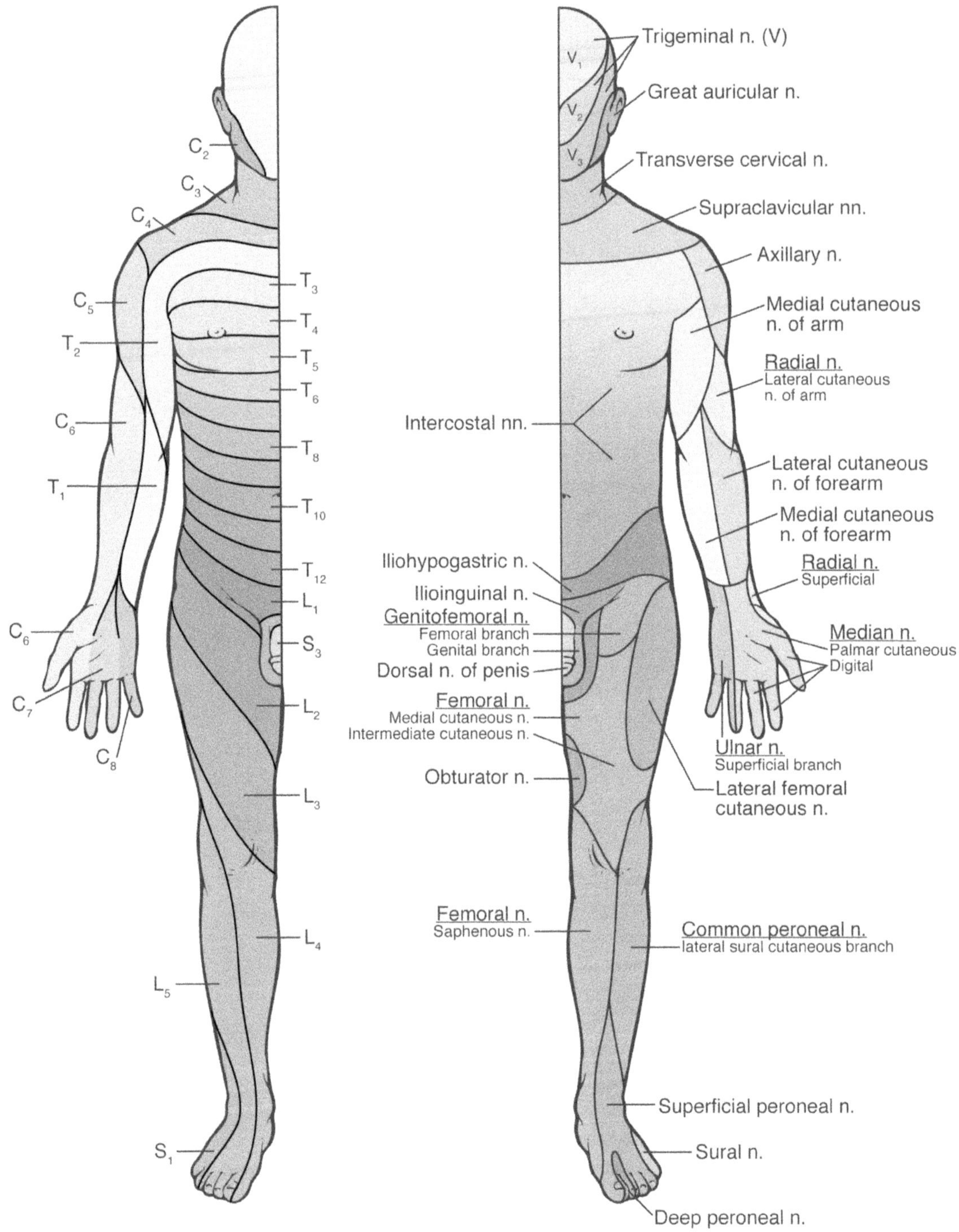

FIGURE 29-1 Approximate cutaneous distributions of dermatomes (left) and corresponding peripheral nerves (right, anterior views). There may be considerable variation or overlap between cutaneous distributions so that an isolated root or nerve lesion may result in a slightly different or smaller area of sensory deficits than indicated in these diagrams. See color insert.

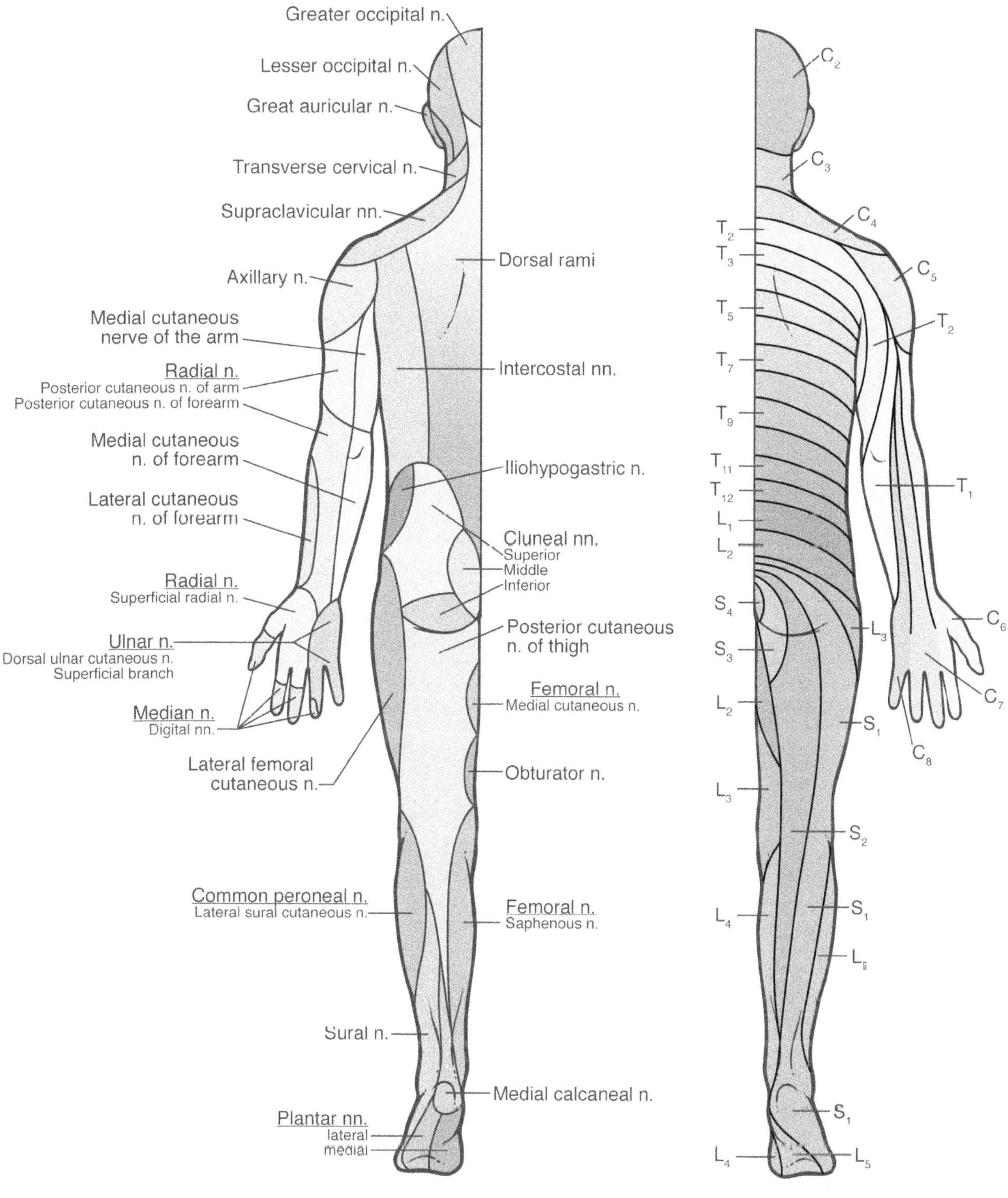

FIGURE 29-2 Approximate cutaneous distributions of peripheral nerves (left) and corresponding dermatomes (right, posterior views). There may be considerable variation or overlap between cutaneous distributions so that an isolated root or nerve lesion may result in a slightly different or smaller area of sensory deficits than indicated in these diagrams. See color insert.

INDEX

O

P

www.ingramcontent.com/pod-product-compliance
Ingram Content Group UK Ltd.
Pitfield, Milton Keynes, MK11 3LW, UK
UKHW051323180626
13230UKWH00006B/46

9 780199 754632